43.15

DS004-76

Property of US Army

Infection in Surgical Practice

Edited by

Professor J.D. Williams
Emeritus Professor of Medical Microbiology
University of London
UK

Mr E.W. Taylor
Consultant Surgeon
Inverclyde Royal Hospital
UK

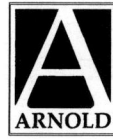

A member of the Hodder Headline Group
LONDON

First published in Great Britain in 2003 by
Arnold, a member of the Hodder Headline Group,
338 Euston Road, London NW1 3BH

http://www.arnoldpublishers.com

Distributed in the United States of America by
Oxford University Press Inc.,
198 Madison Avenue, New York, NY10016
Oxford is a registered trademark of Oxford University Press

Whilst the advice and information in this book are believed to be true and
accurate at the date of going to press, neither the authors nor the publisher can
accept any legal responsibility or liability for any errors or omissions that may be
made. In particular (but without limiting the generality of the preceding
disclaimer) every effort has been made to check drug dosages; however it is still
possible that errors have been missed. Furthermore, dosage schedules are
constantly being revised and new side-effects recognized. For these reasons the
reader is strongly urged to consult the drug companies' printed instructions before
administering any of the drugs recommended in this book.

British Library Cataloguing in Publication Data
A catalogue record for this book is available from the British Library

Library of Congress Cataloging-in-Publication Data
A catalog record for this book is available from the Library of Congress

ISBN 0 340 76305 1

1 2 3 4 5 6 7 8 9 10

Commissioning Editor: Serena Bureau
Project Editor: James Rabson
Production Controller: Bryan Eccleshall
Cover Design: Terry Griffiths

Typeset in 10/12 Minion by Integra Software Services Pvt. Ltd, Pondicherry, India
www.integra-india.com
Printed and bound in Italy

What do you think about this book? Or any other Arnold title?
Please send your comments to feedback.arnold@hodder.co.uk

Contents

Contributors

N.S. Ambrose
Department of Surgery, St James's University Hospital
Leeds, UK

G.A.J. Ayliffe
Hospital Infection Research Laboratory
City Hospital NHS Trust, Birmingham, UK

J.A.J. Barbara
National Blood Service North
London, UK

S.P. Barrett
Department of Medical Microbiology
Hammersmith Hospitals NHS Trust
London, UK

R. Bayston
Department of Medical Microbiology, Frenchay Hospital
Bristol, UK

E.M. Brown
Department of Medical Microbiology, Frenchay Hospital
Bristol, UK

J.P. Burnie
Infectious Diseases Research Group, University of Manchester
Manchester, UK

E.M. Cooke
Central Public Health Laboratory
Public Health Laboratory Service
London, UK

B.D. Cookson
Laboratory of Hospital Infection
Central Public Health Laboratory
London, UK

P.G. Davey
Department of Clinical Pharmacology and Pharmacy
Ninewells Hospital
Dundee, UK

L.A. Ficker
Department of Pathology, Institute of Ophthalmology
London, UK

R. Freeman
Public Health Laboratory, Newcastle General Hospital
Newcastle-on-Tyne, UK

J.D. Hansford
Hospital Infection Research Laboratory
City Hospital NHS Trust, Birmingham, UK

E. Houang
Department of Microbiology
Chinese University of Hong Kong
Shatin, Hong Kong

P.N. Hoffman
Laboratory of Hospital Infection
Central Public Health Laboratory
London, UK

A.D. Kitchen
National Blood Service North
London, UK

A.G. Lawrence
Chelsea and Westminster Hospital
London, UK

M.A.O. Lewis
Department of Oral Surgery
Medicine and Pathology Dental School
University of Wales College of Medicine
Cardiff, UK

R. Marwood
Chelsea and Westminster Hospital
London, UK

S. Mehtar
Microbiology Department
Pacalsdorp, South Africa

K.G. Naber
Department of Urology
Klinikum St. Elisabeth
Straubing, Germany

S.W.B. Newsom
Cambridge Regional Health Authority
Cambridge, UK

B.L. Oppenheim
Public Health Laboratory
Heartlands Hospital
Birmingham, UK

J. Philpott-Howard
Department of Medical Microbiology
Guy's, King's and St Thomas' School
of Medicine
London, UK

E.H. Price
Department of Medical Microbiology
Barts and the London NHS Trust
London, UK

R.J. Sage
Microbiology Department
Basildon and Thurrock General
Hospitals NHS Trust
Basildon, UK

P.J. Sanderson
Microbiology Department
Edgware Community Hospital
London, UK

D.V. Seal
Department of Pathology
Institute of Ophthalmology
London, UK

A.M. Sefton
Department of Medical Microbiology
Barts and the London Queen Mary's School of
Medicine and Dentistry
London, UK

G.R. Serjeant
Sickle Cell Unit
University of the West Indies
Kingston, Jamaica

G. Shone
Department of Otolaryngology
University Hospital of Wales
Cardiff, UK

E.W. Taylor
Department of Surgery
Inverclyde Royal Hospital
Greenock, UK

J.D. Williams
Federation of European Societies for
Chemotherapy and Infection
London, UK

M.E.R. Williamson
Directorate of Surgery
Royal United Hospitals
Bath, UK

A.P.R. Wilson
Department of Medical Microbiology
University College London Hospitals
London, UK

T.G. Wregheitt
Public Health Laboratory
Addenbrooke's Hospital
Cambridge, UK

General chapters

Infection control

J. PHILPOTT-HOWARD

1.1 INTRODUCTION

Infection control is the means whereby healthcare practitioners seek to minimize the risk to individuals of direct or indirect transmission of infection hazards from medical, surgical and biological **materials**, the **environment** and **other individuals** (patients or staff). In this context, 'hazard' and 'risk' need to be distinguished as the terms are not interchangeable. An organism such as HIV, or a disinfectant such as hypochlorite are, in themselves, hazardous but the risks of harm to healthcare workers from day-to-day contact with patients or disinfectants are almost negligible under normal working conditions. In contrast, varicella-zoster virus is less hazardous than HIV, but the risk of this viral infection for a non-immune staff member who is in close contact with a patient with chickenpox or shingles is very high. Under general legislation such as the Health and Safety at Work Act 1974, adequate protection against risk to health (in this case, from infectious agents) must be provided as far as is reasonably practicable. In hospital or in the community healthcare setting, this applies not only to the patient but also to healthcare workers and anyone else in the immediate vicinity.

Medical organizations have a 'duty of care' to ensure that the environment and any materials leaving the premises (e.g. clinical waste bags containing contaminated dressings, etc.) do not represent a significant risk to staff or to the public. In fact, it has been argued that most hospital waste is no more of a risk than domestic waste, since either could contain hazardous materials. The risk to anyone handling the bags is minimal because, apart from contaminated sharps or a disposable container

with a large volume of blood, it would be very difficult for blood-contaminated dressings to be a significant source of infection; moreover, domestic waste may contain blood-stained items. However, the regulations are strict and even items that only look as if they might be contaminated (e.g. a pair of surgical gloves that were opened but never used) must be placed in a yellow bag for incineration; if clinical waste appears in the hospital's domestic-type waste (which is often used for landfill) then the hospital, and responsible individuals, may be prosecuted and fined. The most important regulations are the Control of Substances Hazardous to Health (COSHH) Regulations, produced by the Health and Safety Commission; these apply to infectious material as well as chemical agents, which also includes disinfectants. The Department of Health also produces guidance on the handling of dangerous pathogens, and these also are important for healthcare organizations.

As far as hospital or clinic staff are concerned, their immediate source of guidance on what constitutes good infection control lies firstly in their basic professional training, and secondly in the provision of written policies and further education on what constitutes acceptable day-to-day practice. In practical terms, 'infection control procedures' can be distinguished from good clinical practice or technique, although there is some overlap. Good clinical practice will reduce the risk of infection for the individual patient on whom a procedure is performed, for example through adequate debridement of a wound or appropriate antibiotic prophylaxis. In contrast, the protection of the patient's wound through hand disinfection before and after wound examination, or the use of a 'no-touch' technique when applying dressings, are infection control procedures; it is these types of procedures that will be dealt with in this chapter. Even so, surgeons who wish to analyse their infection rates must recognize and distinguish between these two underlying causes of infection, since poor surgical technique (e.g. by a new and inexperienced surgeon) may increase the infection rate, even though staff rigidly adhere to all infection control procedures. Environment problems (such as failure of the operating theatre's air-conditioning), are rarely a cause of surgical infections except in sensitive specialities such as orthopaedic surgery.

Many hospital-acquired infections are a consequence of advances such as transplantation, chemotherapy and implanted devices, and are caused by organisms derived from the patient's resident microbial flora. Even so, it is estimated that one-third of all such infections are preventable.

1.2 GENERAL PRECAUTIONS FOR PREVENTING INFECTION IN SURGICAL PATIENTS

1.2.1 Background

All hospitals in the United Kingdom must have an Infection Control Doctor, and most have (or should have) at least one Infection Control Nurse. Together, they develop and manage important hospital policies such as the **Isolation Policy**, and ensure that all relevant staff have access to these policies, and to advice. The Infection Control Doctor advises the hospital's Chief Executive, and the Chief Executive is responsible to the Department of Health for making sure that adequate infection control arrangements are in place.

Within a hospital, those responsible for the provision of surgical services should liaise closely with infection control personnel, especially when drawing up infection control policies, and meet together when a specific cross-infection problem is suspected. Liaison can be done informally, or more formally by surgical representation on the Hospital Infection Control Committee. The Infection Control Doctor or Infection Control Nurse may also attend various committees when appropriate, for example the Operating Theatre, Medical Equipment and CSSD/TSSU User Groups. When new surgical facilities and new equipment are designed or purchased, infection control aspects must be discussed with the infection control team at an early stage. This is often forgotten, and it is not uncommon for a clinical or surgical suite to have inadequate handwashing facilities, or for new surgical and medical equipment, e.g. endoscopes to create unanticipated costly and potentially hazardous problems related to disinfection and sterilization. Attention to detail is essential, especially when writing maintenance and cleaning protocols for equipment; areas such as efficacy of disinfectant protocols are parti-cularly important. Factual errors may occur, for example distilled water is considered to be sterile by otherwise well-informed personnel.

Another area of key importance is the instruction of new healthcare staff in infection control procedures, particularly for individuals with limited surgical experience. Also, members of staff should benefit from refresher courses at appropriate intervals on infection control procedures. The key areas for training are listed below under Personnel Health.

1.2.2 Design and layout of wards

Any surgeon may be involved in the design of a new ward, and should have some idea of the key features of a surgical ward in relation to hospital-acquired infection. These include:

- provision of sufficient wash handbasins, with **one basin in easy reach of each bed**;
- an adequate number of siderooms, e.g. **at least six on a 25-bed ward**;
- avoidance of over-crowding, with an **inter-bed distance of at least 2 metres**; and
- **adequate ventilation**, especially in the siderooms where negative air pressure ducted to the exterior will be desirable for the isolation of certain patients (e.g. those colonized or infected with methicillin-resistant *Staphylococcus aureus* (MRSA), and essential for others (e.g. shingles or chickenpox).

Provision must be made for a sluice with a functioning bed-pan washer (which reaches 80°C for at least 1 minute), and enough space for storage and disposal of clinical waste and laundry bags. However, one of the key areas of infection control practice remains a constant difficulty in most hospitals, i.e. that of staffing levels; **understaffing** of the nursing establishment may lead to a **decline in standards of infection control** as staff take short-cuts to get through the workload; they will also have less time for training.

1.2.3 Infection control procedures on the ward

BASIC CLEANING AND WASTE DISPOSAL ON THE WARD

General: Floors should be damp-dusted to keep them free of dust. Hot water with detergent is suitable for most cleaning, except for body fluid spillages (see below). Alcohol spray can be used to clean surfaces being set up for procedures, e.g. clinical trolleys. Between patients, baths and showers are cleaned with hot water and a chlorine releasing powder. Handbasins and toilet fittings should be cleaned daily.

Waste and linen: The correct disposal procedures are as follows:

- *General clinical waste* Yellow plastic bags for incineration
- *Sharps* Sharps container
- *Glass and aerosol cans* Plastic bins that are clearly labelled 'Glass and aerosol cans: not to be incinerated'
- *Non-clinical waste* Black plastic bags
- *Confidential waste* Yellow plastic bags for incineration
- *Food waste* Return to kitchens
- *Radioactive waste* Advice to be sought from the Radiation Protection Officer
- *Labelling* All waste bags must be labelled with the ward name, and the date that the bag was left for collection.

ISOLATION OF PATIENTS IN SIDEROOMS

Isolation of patients in siderooms is indicated when a patient is known or strongly suspected to have certain infectious diseases which are identified in the isolation policy. The main indications for consultation of the policy are for the management of patients with diarrhoeal disease, uncontrolled bleeding, colonization or infection with multiply-resistant pathogens such as MRSA and *Klebsiella*, shingles, untreated tuberculosis, scabies, etc. The ward staff must inform the Infection Control Team of the details of such patients. Apart from these specific indications, it is also important to realize that isolation is required for a patient who has diarrhoea, uncontrolled bleeding or other dissemination of body fluids, whether or not the patient is known to be a carrier of an infectious agent. For example, the specific diagnosis of diarrhoea may take 3 or 4 days after a patient has been admitted, and such patients must be nursed in a sideroom. Even if the diagnosis is later shown to be unrelated to infection, for practical and aesthetic reasons these patients are better managed in a sideroom. Environmental contamination with faecal bacteria can also be a significant reservoir of infection, especially with organisms that resist drying, such as *Clostridium difficile*, enterococci and some coliforms such as *Klebsiella*.

Patients who are carriers of viruses such as HIV and hepatitis B do not need sideroom isolation unless there is uncontrolled dissemination of body fluids, or they have an additional specific infection that requires containment.

MRSA

New patients should be routinely screened for carriage of MRSA if they have been transferred from another hospital where MRSA occurs, or if the individual is known to have been MRSA-positive at any time in the past.

OTHER INFECTION SITUATIONS

Precautions are required for handling all needles, sharps, blood and body fluids, even from patients not known to be infected with an infectious agent. When a patient has been tested as hepatitis B- or HIV-positive, then in general the main safety procedure to be implemented is to ensure that hand disinfection and safe needle disposal are adhered to. Other measures may be required only in certain circumstances, for example additional protective equipment may need to be worn in the operating theatre since the dissemination of blood is so much greater than on the ward. Patients with other infections, such as chickenpox, are highly infectious and so it is unlikely that even 'good infection control practice' would be sufficient to prevent infection of susceptible staff. Patients are not being screened routinely for infectious agents such as hepatitis B or HIV unless this is indicated for clinical management of liver disease or an opportunist infection when data on the virus infection will significantly affect patient management.

DECEASED PATIENTS

Cadaver bags should be used for any dead bodies that are likely to leak body fluids.

1.2.4 'Cohort nursing' during an outbreak of infection on a ward

If several patients have the same infection, or are known to be carriers of an outbreak organism (e.g. MRSA), then **cohort nursing** may be appropriate. This will be arranged by the nurse manager in consultation with the Infection Control Team. Cohort nursing involves one nurse or group of nurses exclusively looking after the infected group of patients (usually in a four- or six-bedded bay), whilst separate nurses care for the uninfected; the two groups should avoid contact with each other in the ward environment.

1.2.5 Hand hygiene on the surgical ward

Good hand hygiene is the single most important measure for the control of infection in a hospital, and must be meticulously observed by all staff who come into contact with patients either directly or indirectly. Doctors are notoriously bad at observing good hand hygiene, and thus place their patients at tremendous risk of hospital-acquired infection, including life-threatening septicaemia.

Handwashing for at least 30 seconds with liquid soap and water is adequate for most types of patient contact, but when a procedure is performed in which hand contamination is likely, then disposable latex or vinyl gloves should be worn. If skin contamination with blood and body fluids occurs, a hand disinfectant such as aqueous or alcoholic chlorhexidine, or povidone-iodine, should also be used. Staff with broken skin on their hands such as eczema or a fresh cut (i.e. a wound that is less than 24 hours old) should keep the area covered with a waterproof plaster or with disposable gloves. Wearing of gloves protects the hands of the wearer, but it should be noted that **cross-infection** can occur if the individual moves between patients without changing gloves; also, gloves do not protect against needle and sharps injuries.

Very frequent hand-washing can be time-consuming and cause soreness of the hands. Many hospitals now promote hand disinfection with alcohol gels dispensed from bedside containers or personal dispensers. These gels contain emollients and may reduce skin irritation. The alcohol is also active against many bacteria and viruses.

SHARPS INJURIES

Sharps injuries are a major problem in hospitals and staff are at risk of infection with hepatitis viruses and HIV. Needles and sharps must be placed immediately in a sharps container by the individual who used them. The container should be brought to the bedside, and needles must not be left in trays. Needles must not be resheathed, but if resheathing is unavoidable then a safe, one-handed technique (or a special holding device) must be used. **Sharps containers must never be overfilled**, as this is a very common cause of accidents; they must be changed when three-quarters full.

BODY FLUIDS

Spillages of blood and body fluids must be disinfected with a chlorine-releasing product such as NDCC (sodium dichloroisocyanusate) granules. A 1 in 10 dilution in water of neat bleach is also effective. The spillage area is demarcated and a health worker, who has been trained to clear up spillages, wears disposable gloves and a plastic apron. If there is **broken glass** in the spillage, the glass **must** be picked up with a plastic scoop, and never with hands – even if gloves are worn. Small spillages that do not contain glass or sharps are treated with hypochlorite granules, left for 10 to 30 minutes depending on the size of the spillage, and then cleared up with paper towels. If there is a high volume of bleach (e.g. greater than 100 ml, and especially if it is urine), a significant amount of chlorine gas is released which is in itself a health hazard; large spillages should be soaked up with paper towels first. After removal of the spillage the surface should be cleaned with detergent. Used gloves, apron and paper towels should be placed in a yellow bag for incineration.

When body fluids are splashed onto intact skin they should be washed off with soap and water followed by a skin disinfectant. If a penetrating exposure occurs, e.g. needle injury or splashing onto open cuts, or onto mucous membranes, the individual must attend Occupational Health (or Accident & Emergency out of hours). Depending on the hepatitis status of the patient, and the degree of blood or body fluid exposure from the injury, the individual is given a booster dose of hepatitis B vaccine. If they are unvaccinated, a full accelerated course is given. In very infectious cases when the blood is from an e-antigen-positive carrier, especially in an unvaccinated individual, an intramuscular dose of anti-HBs immunoglobulin is also given. The medical microbiologist or virologist on call will advise on the most appropriate action to take. Anti-HBs immunoglobulin, if indicated, must be given within 24–48 hours of the exposure. Antiviral prophylaxis against HIV infection may also be required if the exposure involves blood from a patient known or strongly suspected to be HIV-positive. The risk of transmission is estimated to be 0.4%, but a large inoculation of blood from someone with a high viral load is of greater concern. At the time of writing, recommended prophylaxis for an HIV exposure includes zidovudine, a second nucleoside analogue and a protease inhibitor; however the most recent guidelines should be followed. The drugs must be given within an hour of the injury, so if the HIV status of the patient is unknown, the health worker may have to decide for themselves whether they want to take the drugs, with advice from the virologist or microbiologist. To date, there have been very few transmissions to healthcare workers, and the drugs available for prophylaxis are not without side effects. Each case must be considered individually with guidance from the most expert specialist available.

1.2.6 Disposal of body fluids

Gloves and a plastic apron must be worn when bed-pans, urine bottles and suction bottles are taken to the sluice room or bed-pan washer. Commodes are cleaned with hot water and detergent unless heavily contaminated, when detergent hypochlorite solution is used. Sealed drainage bottles should be discarded.

1.2.7 Dressing changes and invasive procedures

Sterile gloves should be worn by staff when they undertake invasive procedures, change dressings, clean wounds, and perform catheter and line care. Skin disinfection is not required prior to venepuncture or intramuscular injection, unless the skin is visibly dirty, or the procedure is performed on severely immunocompromised patients. Intravascular catheters must be inserted in a sterile field with proper skin disinfection, by a member of staff wearing a filtering mask and sterile gloves, with sterile paper or linen towels placed over a wide area (**at least the length of the catheter!**). The catheter must be adequately secured and a sterile dressing placed over the insertion site (dressings impregnated with chlorhexidine or iodine may be used).

1.2.8 Preparation for and transfer of the patient to theatre

Preoperative chlorhexidine showering is sometimes indicated for cardiovascular surgery, at the surgeon's discretion. The patient is sent to the anaesthetic room wearing a surgical gown, and covered by a clean sheet. The trolley, or bed in the case of some orthopaedic procedures, may be taken directly from the ward to the anaesthetic room. No special procedures are required for transfer to theatre of patients known to be infected with any organism, unless there is uncontrolled bleeding or dissemination of body fluids.

1.2.9 Prevention of infection in the operating theatre

See Chapters 2 and 5.

1.2.10 Personnel health; pre-employment health screening and immunization

Staff working in hospitals and clinics have always been at risk of certain infectious diseases. Outbreaks of hepatitis B in hospitals during the early 1970s lead healthcare workers to recognize the need for better practice when handling sharps, blood and body fluids. Awareness of the necessity of these precautions was a valuable preparation for health workers dealing with the onset of the AIDS epidemic a decade later, since measures for the control of hepatitis B were also appropriate for HIV. New pathogens will be identified in the future and might also be transmissible by a similar route. The introduction of hepatitis B vaccine in the 1980s prompted risk assessments of the work of hospital and other staff. Surveillance studies of the incidence of clinical hepatitis B infection indicated that the highest risk groups included surgeons, dentists and laboratory workers and others who regularly handle blood and body fluids, and these groups were given priority for vaccination.

Adequate occupational health screening at the time an individual starts work is essential, not only for that person but also for the protection of patients on whom 'exposure-prone procedures' (EPPs) are performed – especially with reference to hepatitis B and HIV. This is because infected surgical staff can transmit hepatitis B

viruses to patients during surgery and other EPPs. Occupational health screening must therefore take place on the first day of employment, or earlier if possible, since apart from hepatitis B it also includes an assessment of immunity to tuberculosis, polio virus and rubella; tests for some of these infections will be necessary in some individuals. In addition, the presence of skin disorders such as eczema, or a history of any underlying immunosuppressive disorder might require an assessment of the staff member's work, as they will be at increased risk of acquiring transmissible infections. For example, staff with eczema of the hands may need to wear disposable gloves more frequently than other staff since they are at a greater risk of acquiring blood-borne viruses through their damaged skin if blood or body fluids contaminate the eczematous lesions. Also, since the skin of such individuals is commonly colonized with *Staphylococcus aureus*, they may be responsible for nosocomial spread of this organism.

For the important inoculation-risk viruses, the risk of transmission from health worker to patient seems to be extremely small, and is certainly less than the risk of transmission in the reverse direction. In terms of the risk of **morbidity and mortality**, the transmission of '**conventional' pathogens** from staff to compromised patients is probably of much greater importance, particularly for **varicella-zoster virus**, **respiratory and enteric pathogens**, and **staphylococci**.

1.2.11 Procedure for screening new staff working in surgery

As noted above, all new staff must attend the Department of Occupational Health, whether medical, nursing or ancillary or clerical. It is the responsibility of the staff member's manager to ensure that the individual attends the Department. A health questionnaire will be completed by the employee, and this includes questions related to general health, past infections and immunization history. This information is completely confidential, and cannot be disclosed to a third party without the employee's consent.

STAFF ASSESSMENT

Clerical and administrative staff not in close contact with patients (e.g. secretaries): these staff should be questioned about their general health and past immunization record.
Staff in contact with patients or specimens: staff should be questioned on the following:

- General health, immunosuppressive treatment or disorders, pregnancy.
- Previous employment and training.
- Skin conditions, e.g. eczema of hands.

- History of infectious diseases and immunizations, especially: **tuberculosis**; **hepatitis B**; **varicella-zoster virus** (VZV), both chickenpox and shingles; rubella (if vaccine has never been given, the staff must be screened for antibodies and, if negative, then offered vaccine); **poliomyelitis** (the staff member should be offered vaccine if they have not received a primary course of vaccine or booster dose in the previous 10 years); **MRSA carriage** (if previously positive for carriage of MRSA, the Infection Control Team must be notified). Note that vaccine recommendations are liable to change.

Staff members must be told that they should not start work if they have acute or chronic diarrhoeal disease, or a febrile respiratory illness.

Staff who refuse immunizations: these staff may be prohibited from working in certain areas of the hospital, and their work should be reviewed by the Occupational Health Consultant.

Pregnancy: Pregnant staff must be advised by their manager of any particular risks encountered during their work, and the precautions that should be taken. In particular there is a remote but finite risk that a non-immune pregnant staff member may be exposed to patients or specimens with rubella, VZV and cytomegalovirus. Precautions that may be required are avoidance of direct contact (rubella, VZV) and attention to hand hygiene (cytomegalovirus).

Change in job description during employment: If an employee's job description changes significantly while they remain in employment in the hospital, they may need to be reassessed by the Occupational Health Department.

Agency staff: Agencies that provide temporary staff for the hospital should be informed of the staff screening policy, and only those agencies with an effective screening programme should be used, wherever possible. This is particularly important for hepatitis B immunization.

Training: The employee's manager is responsible for ensuring that the individual receives training in health and safety appropriate to the work to be undertaken. Basic training must include fire safety and manual handling. The following are of particular importance to infection control:

- Responsibilities of all employees under the Health & Safety at Work Act 1974: they are responsible for their own safety, and that of others.
- Control of Substances Hazardous to Health (COSHH) Regulations: especially handling of infectious material and hazardous chemicals (e.g. glutaraldehyde).
- The waste disposal policy: especially dealing with sharps, clinical waste, human tissues from surgery, and the procedure if there is a needlestick injury or

other high-risk exposure to blood and body fluids; they must report any accidents or illness to their manager and, if appropriate, to Occupational Health.
- Proper use of equipment and instruments.
- Hand disinfection and other infection control issues.
- General safety, e.g. fire, manual handling, etc.

Staff who know they are hepatitis B- or HIV-positive: This information must be declared and discussed in complete confidence with the Consultant in Occupational Health, either at the initial screening or later in their employment, when the staff member first becomes aware of their infection. The Department of Health has produced guidance on this issue. In general, such staff may require a work assessment and they must avoid exposure-prone procedures if they are hepatitis B- or HIV-positive. Retraining may be necessary, and the employer should provide this.

False declarations: Any employee who is found to have made a false declaration about their previous health record or who attempts to substitute blood samples (e.g. for hepatitis B screening) will be disciplined and may have to appear before their professional body.

1.3 SURVEILLANCE AND AUDIT IN SURGERY

1.3.1 Surveillance

Wenzel and others showed that even a **basic hospital infection control programme** is one of the most cost-effective clinical interventions in medicine, in terms of life-years saved. Every surgeon must place a high value on reducing infection in his or her patients, and an important part of this is the surveillance and audit of infection in the ward and hospital.

There have been numerous studies of rates of hospital-acquired (nosocomial) infection (HAI). National studies in both the USA and UK have estimated that 9–10% of inpatients developed an HAI during their stay. This may be an underestimate since shorter hospital admissions are now frequent; additional infections could be missed if they develop after discharge to the community or another hospital. Furthermore, since day surgery comprises up to 60–70% of all surgical procedures in many hospitals, patients with minor postoperative infectious complications would not be included. It is therefore difficult to obtain accurate data on postoperative infections, and the degree of difficulty of the task should not be underestimated. Comparison of data between surgical teams, departments or hospitals is even more complex since one has to allow for case mix and patient risk factors, which may be significantly different. Furthermore, even the definitions of 'wound infection' or 'catheter infection' are controversial, and require careful thought; adherence to definitions published in large studies is advisable. It should also be noted that a number of terms are used in relation to surveillance and audit; these include medical (or clinical) audit, clinical effectiveness, good practice guidelines, clinical guidelines and evidence-based medicine. For the sake of clarity only the terms surveillance and audit will be used, but all of the activities described below are intended to be seen as multi-disciplinary; in the context of surgical infection this includes both nursing, medical and laboratory-based staff, all of them working with audit assistants where available. Also, it applies to all types of departments, whether academic or not and regardless of size.

WHAT ARE SURVEILLANCE AND AUDIT?

Infection control surveillance can be defined as planned observation of the incidence or prevalence of infection in a defined at-risk patient population over a period of time. For example, surveillance may reveal that surgical team X has a wound infection rate of Y% over 6 months of observation and record-keeping. Alternatively, it may be noted that a ward has X cases of *Clostridium difficile* infection in a year. **Infection control audit** may include surveillance of laboratory results or a record of observations of surgical practice. **Audit** is the analysis of healthcare practice related to a standard, with an intervention and re-audit (the cycle of audit) to monitor the effects of any change of practice. For example, analysis of the pre-incisional skin disinfection methods may reveal a wide range of practices across a hospital or even a surgical team. If a standard practice can be agreed, or has been published, then guidelines can be implemented and re-audited at a later date. If there are no data on the subject in the literature so that evidence-based guidelines cannot be implemented, then a research programme may be needed, e.g. a randomized controlled study; it is highly unlikely that a basic question such as the ideal skin preparation method would be answered by a simple audit. Even so there may be grounds for recommending certain skin disinfectants based on cost if there is no good evidence that one agent (or combination of agents) is superior to another.

It should be noted that feedback to surgeons of infection rates acquired through surveillance is known to subsequently improve infection rates, probably through subtle changes in practice by those who perceive that they are experiencing 'high' rates of infection. Surveillance alone without intervention is almost certainly inadequate. This was clearly demonstrated in the SENIC studies in the United States in the late 1970s.

Surveillance or audit may also be prompted by the occurrence of a particular problem such as an outbreak of a certain type of clinical infection (e.g. diarrhoea). Alternatively, the laboratory may note the appearance of several infections with a multiply-resistant pathogen. In such cases all that is required is increased attention by the ward staff and infection control team to compliance with standard infection control procedures. Although surveillance and audit activities can be performed in these circumstances, there would be no need to prove that hand disinfection or environmental cleaning are inadequate, since for most organisms the source and route of transmission of infection are well recognized. However it is very important to incorporate a **degree of surveillance** into daily surgical practice, for example, as a regular component of surgical 'deaths and complications' meetings. Actual or suspected outbreaks of infection should be notified to the relevant infection control team for evaluation and investigation.

The ideal method of surveillance would at first sight seem to be centred on a constant ward- and laboratory-based recording of data so that all HAIs (i.e. those appearing postoperatively or 48–72 hours after admission) are documented and characterized. In practice this would be an enormous task in any hospital, and only limited surveillance is feasible. Studies have shown that laboratory-based surveillance for 'sentinel' pathogens and infections is probably the most cost-effective system for routine use, but it should be combined with specific ward surveillance for short periods of time as part of an audit. In most computerized laboratories is should not be difficult to find all *Staph. aureus* isolates for a particular ward or surgeon, but it is important that the surgical team recognizes the limitations of this data. For example, as discussed earlier, it may not include late infections presenting to other centres or GPs, and culture-negative (or unswabbed) wound infections would be missed. It should also be noted that for various reasons most laboratories do not keep all strains of *Staph. aureus* (except for MRSA), and there is no value in typing isolates unless a specific problem is being investigated by the Infection Control Team. All significant blood culture isolates, not including coagulase-negative staphylococci, are saved so if there is a high rate of septicaemias it facilitates the performance of typing. General laboratory data are limited to the organism identification and five or six sensitivities so that, although this can be helpful (e.g. the organism has an unusual antibiotic susceptibility profile), information on the precise nature of the transmission of staphylococcal infection on a particular ward is unlikely to be found. Also, many patients who become infected are themselves preoperative carriers of the infecting strain.

In addition to routine laboratory culture records, there is constant surveillance for 'sentinel organisms' such as Group A streptococci or gentamicin-resistant *Klebsiella*, which have the potential to a cause a serious cross-infection problem. Organisms that come in to this category are listed in Table 1.1.

Laboratory-based surveillance does not obviate the need for careful day-to-day ward-based observation for critical indicators of potential problems (Table 1.2).

In summary, specific surveillance and audit projects are carried out in addition to day-to-day surveillance

Table 1.1 *Typical 'sentinel organisms' included in laboratory surveillance*

Methicillin-resistant *Staphylococcus aureus*

Streptococcus pyogenes (Group A streptococci)

Penicillin-resistant **pneumococci**

Vancomycin-resistant **enterococci**

Clostridium difficile (toxin-positive faeces)

Aminoglycoside- (or totally beta-lactam-) resistant **aerobic Gram-negative rods**

Unusual **environmental Gram-negative rods**, especially when two or more occur in a short space of time

Any enteric pathogen, especially food-borne infections (*Salmonella, Campylobacter*) and those commonly spread from person to person (**rotavirus, small round structured virus (SRSV)**)

Legionella pneumophila

Mycobacterium tuberculosis

HIV, hepatitis B and C

Influenza

Varicella-zoster virus

Hospital-acquired **aspergillosis**

Table 1.2 *Criteria for ward-based observation and reporting infection problems*

A cluster of clinically diagnosed severe wound infections, especially in specialities such as cardiothoracic and orthopaedic surgery

Unexplained diarrhoea in a number of patients (e.g. more than 3)

Diarrhoea in staff members

Influenza-like illness in staff members

Postoperative synergistic gangrene

Postoperative tetanus (extremely rare)

activity. They are part of a total quality of care package and are an essential component of surgical team management. For the surgical team, the main tasks are to:

- Identify the most likely problem area with healthcare outcome and cost effects, and obtain the cooperation and agreement of colleagues at an early stage.
- Determine whether there are any written standards of relevance to the area of study.
- Ask simple important questions and define any terms used.
- List data to be collected (pilot the data collection form if the study is particularly large).
- Decide on the data analysis method – seek advice from a statistician if necessary.
- Prepare computer software, if used.
- Ensure that confidentiality of data is maintained, e.g. when calculating surgeon-specific infection rates.

- Collect, analyse and present data.
- Compare the results with published standards.
- Decide on the appropriate intervention and mode of implementation of change.
- Implement and plan to re-audit after a set time.

The correct analysis of epidemiological data is complex and should not be underestimated. The reader is referred to other texts on epidemiology and statistics for guidance. Staff who undertake such work should also be sensitive to any implied criticism of individuals, and information which may reflect badly on the hospital should be handled carefully. In the future it is likely that 'league tables' of hospital infection rates, mortality and other measures will become publicly available. For all of the reasons stated above, the **misuse of audit and surveillance data must be avoided**.

1.3.2 Audit

COLLECTION OF INFORMATION: BASIC DATA SETS

If there is a need to produce a set of data such as the extent of wound infection, then several methods are available by which this may be achieved:

- Point prevalence (cross-sectional) study: the proportion of patients infected at any particular time, e.g. on one day. This is not a rate since it is not time-dependent. It is particularly useful for identifying a point source for infection, such as surgical wound infection.
- Incidence: the rate of acquisition of infections over a time period per unit of population, e.g. per 1000 ward admissions per year; or, per 1000 patient-days.
- Cohort study: prospectively following a patient group based on a hypothesis derived from an incidence or prevalence study, e.g. looking at all admissions and comparing the infected and uninfected patients. Alternatively, the hospital acquisition rate could be determined, e.g. the number of MRSA-free patients who acquired MRSA during their stay in hospital.
- Case-control study: this is when affected and unaffected patients are matched by age, sex, underlying disorders, etc., to assess significant differences in procedural risk factors between the infected and uninfected patients. In general this is more suitable for determining the cause of a serious outbreak. For example, if there is a high incidence of unexpected septicaemias due to *Pseudomonas* spp., the case control study may reveal that all affected patients received a certain (contaminated) IV treatment whereas none of the case control patients did – in other words, a high **attack rate** was seen in the patients receiving the

IV treatment. Case control studies are commonly used in food-borne outbreaks when the contaminated food source is not immediately obvious. Significant association with a particular procedure can be revealed by logistic regression analysis.

This type of data is often combined with an analysis of the risk factors for infection which stratifies the patients according to some predetermined status, e.g. the APACHE score, Glasgow Coma scale. Smaller departmental audits are unlikely to yield sufficient patients for this kind of analysis, but the investigators should bear in mind the need to obtain and analyse data from comparable patients.

Common errors in audit and surveillance studies include:

- Use (or absence) of poor clinical and microbiological definitions of infection.
- Lack of distinction between infection and colonization, especially related to catheters and wounds.
- Comparison of dissimilar groups and lack of denominator data.
- Presence of confounding variables, e.g. a surgeon may have worse infection rates because he or she receives more difficult patients.
- Multiple counting of patients with separate episodes.
- Confusion of proportions of a population with rates of infection.
- Underestimation of the effect of direct feedback of infection rates on clinical practice.
- Data analysed too rigorously for the sample size.
- Over-extrapolation and generalization of specific surveillance data.
- Over-emphasis on environmental factors.
- Confusion between 'audit' and 'research'.

Most hospitals have audit departments with statistical back-up if required, and this can assist in the process of audit and surveillance, in order to avoid these pitfalls. It is of course important for surgical trainees to gain experience in audit methodology, and so it should be part of their training programme.

DESIGNING AUDIT QUESTIONNAIRES AND CHECKLISTS

This is not an easy task, as anyone who has sent out a questionnaire will testify. It is of course essential to use completely unambiguous statements or questions, and to provide alternatives for every possible response that a respondent might make. In general it is very useful to pilot the draft questionnaire with a few colleagues, so that contradictions and unsatisfactory phrasing can be removed; simplicity is essential, and the designer must have an idea of how the answers will be analysed. Free text comments are particularly difficult to analyse, but they can provide a very illuminating insight into the problem which is not revealed in the formal answers. Respondents must be assured that any comments are confidential. This may require security arrangements for the records. Statistically, it is better to have a smaller survey sample and attempt to obtain 100% compliance than to send out many questionnaires and have only a small percentage returned. An enticement to respond, such as a free prize draw, is particularly useful if you think the questionnaire will be of little interest! Also, a covering letter is useful, to explain why the study is being done and why it is important. Telephone surveys are also useful, for example for follow-up of discharged patients, but all the comments above still apply.

Once the data have been collected it is not always necessary to perform an analysis by anything other than a numerical summary using a paper and pencil. A computer database or spreadsheet program can be helpful in dealing with problems such as empty data fields. For the prospective collection of data, or a large audit, it is essential to have an audit clerk or secretary partly devoted to data entry.

1.4 FURTHER READING

Altman, D.G. (1991) *Practical Statistics for Medical Research*. Chapman & Hall, London.

Mayhall, G. (ed.) (1996) *Hospital Epidemiology and Infection Control*. Williams & Wilkins, Baltimore.

Philpott-Howard, J.N. and Casewell, M.W. (1994) *Hospital Infection Control: Policies and Practical* Procedures. Ballière-Tindall, London.

Wenzel, R.P. (ed.) (1993) *Prevention and Control of Nosocomial Infections*. 2nd edition. Williams & Wilkins, Baltimore.

In the UK, the NHS Executive has also published several pamphlets on Audit, Clinical Effectiveness and Clinical Guidelines.

Theatre design and measures to prevent infection in operating theatres

S.W.B. NEWSOM

2.1 INTRODUCTION

Up to 80% of infections following surgery occur from contamination in the operating theatre, although most of these are 'endogenous' and relate to microbes from the patient. Nonetheless, correct design (especially of ventilation) and accepted theatre procedures are important in the prevention of infection. In times gone by external light was regarded as essential, and theatres were often on the top of hospitals, with windows that could be opened for ventilation. In one hospital the windows overlooked a stables and allowed ingress of tetanus spores into the theatre air, while in more modern times top-floor theatres were found to contain air contaminated with staphylococci from the patients in the wards beneath (hot air rises). Today most – but not all – operating theatres are sealed and provided with plenum (positive-pressure) ventilation using filtered air. Thus, the most likely source of bacteria in the operating theatre comes from within it: the **personnel**, and occasionally the **equipment**.

Sometimes the cause of infection is obvious, as for example when a surgeon operated with a boil on his forearm caused by a strain of bacteriophage type-80 *Staphylococcus aureus* and infected all the patients on one operating list. However, it is often very difficult to prove that an infection has been acquired from theatre staff, and even harder to provide evidence-based data that a particular precaution has a statistically significant effect in reducing the infection rates. Lidwell (see Further reading) noted the following:

Number of observations required in each group in a randomized trial to demonstrate a significant difference with an even chance at the 5% level:

Reduction due to treatment	Incidence untreated	
	3%	10%
10%	25 000	6900
25%	3600	1100

Thus many of today's theatre designs and practises are based on data that needs further evaluation, or on 'rational' grounds. In addition some 'ritual' practises – time-honoured but with no value – may still be found, for example the storage of special instruments such as knives in cabinets containing paraformaldehyde tablets, or the use of 'tacky mats' at theatre doorways. Even when a major trial is performed correctly, the need for a multi-centre approach – often taking several years – may reduce the value of the data obtained. The only really comprehensive single-centre survey of a significant number of operations was published by Cruse and Foord in 1973, who studied the factors influencing the outcome of 23 649 surgical wounds.

The design and operation of a theatre suite can involve a wide range of personnel – architects, engineers, administrators, doctors and nurses – all of whom may be well motivated but not fully aware of the overall problems. A sudden rise in temperature of in-coming air, desirable perhaps in cardiac surgery after a patient has been cooled, can inactivate the airflow in a downflow theatre (hot air rises). Removal of plastic overshoes may result in the transfer of pathogenic bacteria from the floor (where they are probably harmless) onto staff hands, causing a potentially dangerous situation. The scrubbing brush of today is fortunately provided sterile and used only once; Figure 2.1 shows the effect of using a ward scrubbing brush kept in a bowl of disinfectant. Soap on the brush neutralized the disinfectant, and allowed a healthy growth of *Pseudomonas aeruginosa*, with the result that three patients required enucleation of infected eyes after surgery because the nurse had scrubbed with the brush before applying the first dressings.

Surgery continues to evolve. The insertion of prostheses continues to increase in both number and variety, 'keyhole' surgery is increasing, and in particular day surgery is encouraged. All of these stress the system. In particular the **intensive use of theatres** for day surgery means that the **microbial load** will be high, because the highest counts of bacteria in air are found when the patients are being moved in and out of the theatre, and during cleaning. Thus, it is wrong to expect that a lower standard of theatre for day surgery will suffice. Similarly, the highest count ever recorded in theatre air by the author was in a small room provided with ventilation designed as a labour ward, but used for Caesarian sections. During the operation the room housed up to ten staff (the usual theatre team and students, plus paediatricians who resuscitated the baby in the corner of the room). The increase in prosthetic surgery has been accompanied by a rise in infections caused by the coagulase-negative staphylococci.

This chapter will consider provision of a safe theatre environment for the patient. The first section deals with the provision of a suitable facility; this will then be followed by preparation of the patient; the role of the

staff; and finally the actual operation. Subsequent chapters will deal with some of these topics in more detail.

The whole topic of operating theatres has been considered by a working party convened by the Hospital Infection Society in the UK. The working party (2001) has completed a draft report, which hopefully will be published in the *Journal of Hospital Infection*. The report will be of a very practical nature – for example the importance of doing negative controls when testing air in an operating theatre is stressed, as it is clearly vital to ensure that the bacteria found come from the theatre environment and NOT from the tester. It should provide an excellent source for further reading.

2.2 OPERATING THEATRE DESIGN

2.2.1 General principles

In the 1960s the Medical Research Council proposed six basic requirements for an operating theatre suite, namely:

1. Independence from general hospital traffic and air movement.
2. Continuous progression from the entrance through zones of increasing sterility to the operating table and instrument 'laying-up' area.
3. Ability for 'clean' personnel to move from one clean area to another within the suite (clean corridor).
4. Removal of 'dirty' materials without passing through the clean area ('dirty corridor').
5. Air movement from cleaner to dirtier areas.
6. Heating/ventilation systems which ensure safe and comfortable conditions for both patients and staff.

These principles form the basis of modern theatre design. However, a slightly simpler approach can be taken where pre-set instrument trays are provided, and much of the material is disposable. In such cases a 'bagged disposal' system may obviate the need for a dirty corridor, and 'laying-up' may be performed actually in the theatre rather than in a 'preparation room'. Figure 2.2 shows details of the airflow through a conventional theatre, and through a simplified lay-out.

2.2.2 Ventilation: conventional versus ultraclean

Ventilation is one of the key properties of the operating theatre with respect to control of air-borne infection. The air outside the hospital (except beside an exhaust duct) is likely to contain very few bacteria, which are carried on particles of dust, skin scales, etc. A depth filter in the theatre air supply duct able to remove particles

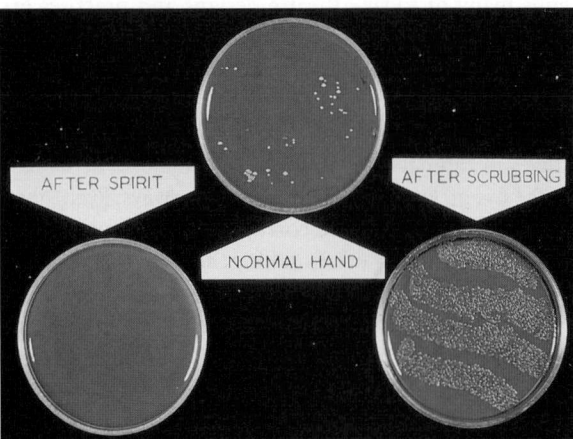

Figure 2.1 *The effect of scrubbing with a contaminated brush obtained from a surgical ward washbasin.*

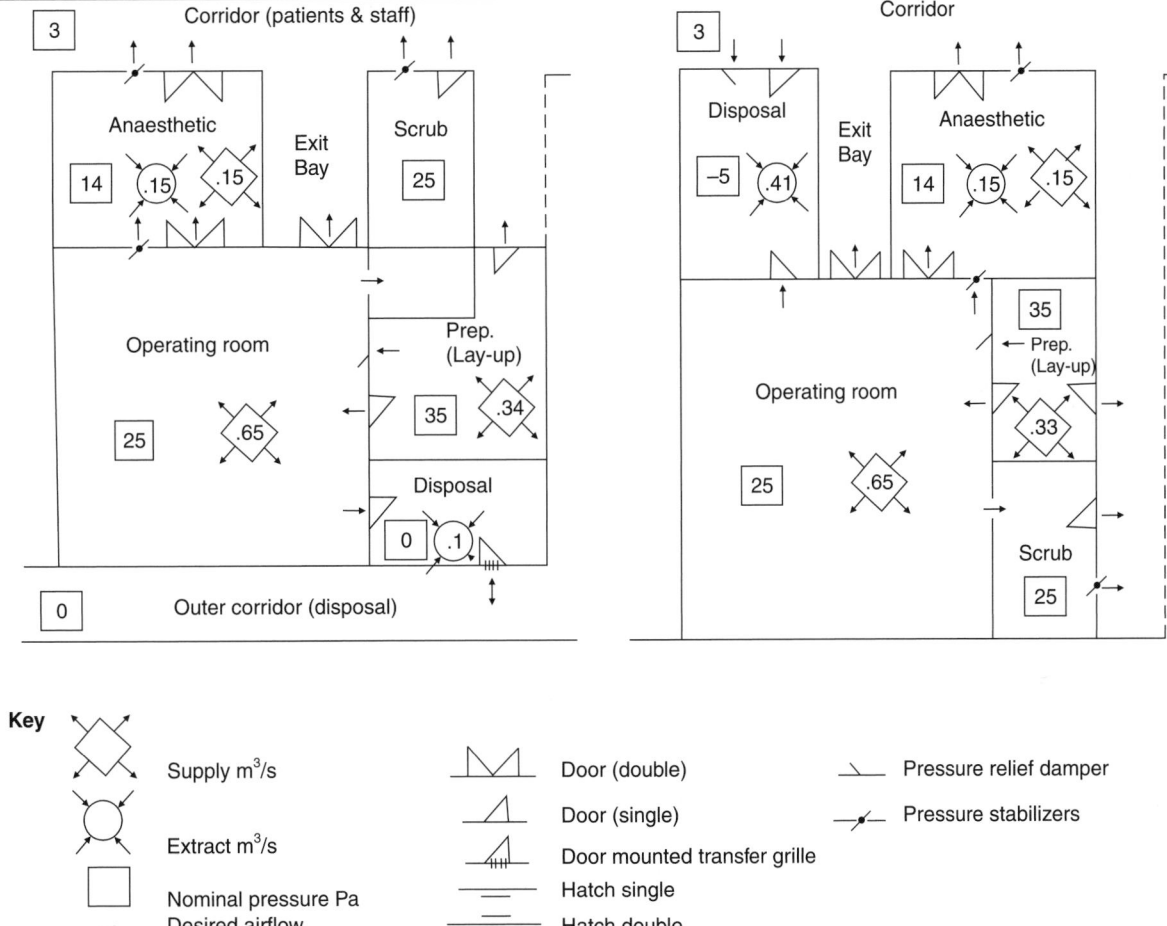

Key

Supply m³/s	
Extract m³/s	
Nominal pressure Pa	
→ Desired airflow	
Door (double)	
Door (single)	
Door mounted transfer grille	
Hatch single	
Hatch double	
Pressure relief damper	
Pressure stabilizers	

Figure 2.2 *Two possible theatre airflow patterns. Left: Conventional two-corridor, Right: Single corridor.*

of 5 μm in diameter will allow provision of air free of bacteria, although not necessarily of fungal spores. Assuming the theatres are at a positive pressure to the rest of the hospital, the loading of air-borne bacteria must come from theatre staff. Thus, the prime aim of the theatre ventilation is to flush out these mainly staff-originating bacteria, so preventing them falling into the wound. A secondary aim is to provide a positive pressure across openings, so that when doors are opened ingress of bacteria in hospital air is prevented. Originally, theatre airflow was described in air changes, with 20 per hour being specified; more recently however, the volumes of air to provide pressure differences over open doors have been specified (15 air changes per hour is still required to purge anaesthetic gases). The aim in a conventional theatre is to reduce bacterial counts to <180 cfu m⁻³ in the air during normal working. This is done by using a **turbulent flow** of air – usually supplied from four evenly spaced diffusers in the ceiling to flush any particles in the air out through floor-level balanced exhaust flaps leading to ancillary rooms. The **ultraclean operating theatre** is much more complex and like an industrial 'clean room', with a design specification to reduce bacterial load to <10 cfu m⁻³.

To achieve, this a **laminar flow** of air at high speed is passed over the wound. The volume of air required would swamp the normal theatre heating/cooling mechanisms, and so the air must be recirculated. As this air has passed through the theatre it has become contaminated from the theatre personnel, so it must be passed through a high-efficiency filter (0.5 μm) before being returned to the theatre. The filters remove the bacteria and also provide a back-pressure that ensures that the airflow is even and laminar. Such theatres are necessarily complex. Different enclosure configurations have been used, including a tent over just the surgical team, or including the whole theatre, having a horizontal or vertical flow of air; and sometimes including several operating bays in a single large room.

THE ULTRACLEAN THEATRE

The ultraclean operating theatre was first introduced as part of the development of a successful hip-replacement programme by Charnley, and has been used particularly for orthopaedic operations since then. The Medical Research Council performed a major controlled trial on theatre type and other parameters in relation to deep infection after hip replacement surgery in the 1970s using centres in the UK and Sweden. A simplified view of the trial results is shown in Figure 2.3. The overall reduction in deep wound infection was very impressive, and the investigators concluded that the ultraclean theatre was of significant value. Many new ultraclean suites have been commissioned for orthopaedic surgery following these results. However, the study remains controversial because the use and type of antibiotic prophylaxis was left to individual surgeons. Addition of the effect of an ultraclean operating theatre to that of antibiotics did not show as much of a decrease in wound infection as might have been expected. Furthermore, the antibiotic prophylaxis schedules used were uncontrolled in that they varied between units and were not necessarily the best available. The reports of the trial and subsequent studies are well worth reading.

HYBRID THEATRES

Some conventional theatres have been provided with a so-called 'laminar flow' air supply. This is done by having a panel above the operating table with a perforated supply port through which an even downflow of air is provided. The air is not recirculated, and the flow rate equates with that of a normal theatre. Some designs (for example the 'Allander' theatre from Sweden) do perform better than the conventional turbulent-flow theatre. However, there is a great danger in believing that the words 'laminar flow' equate with 'ultraclean'. This is not so, and the increased complexity of this type of design may be counter-productive. The author had to commission one such suite of operating theatres, which even after 13 adjustments to the ventilation plant did not function as well as a conventional turbulent-flow theatre. As originally provided, the ventilation produced fierce columns of air aimed behind the surgeon's head, while the air over the table was stagnant, thus offering the possibility of washing bacteria off the surgeon and onto the patient (Figure 2.4).

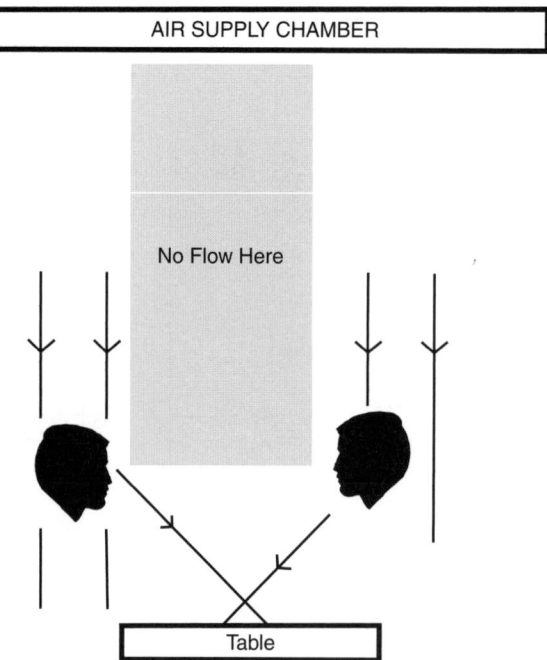

Figure 2.4 *Badly designed airflows from so-called 'laminar flow' supply over surgeon's head.*

ULTRAVIOLET IRRADIATION

Irradiation by ultraviolet rays can sterilize air, and provision of UV-irradiated air might be used to replace or supplement filtration, and the flushing out of theatre air. However, there are some significant problems with this approach. The UV generators have a limited life, but continue to emit visible rays after the germicidal rays have waned; also the radiation is only effective on microbes on clean surfaces, as the rays will not penetrate dirt. Finally, the rays may be toxic to humans and the protective clothing required for the theatre staff is cumbersome. A recent report suggests that wound bacterial counts at the end of an operation were reduced by using ultraviolet irradiation. This type of theatre is not much used at present, although the concept should be monitored for developments.

2.3 COMMISSIONING OF NEW OPERATING THEATRES

2.3.1 Design

The Department of Health has issued guidance on the General Design of operating theatres in Health Building Note No. 16 – Operating Department, and more detailed advice on ventilation as Part of Health Technical Memorandum 2025, on 'Ventilation in Healthcare Premises'. As health service planning in the UK has been devolved downwards and dedicated regional planning teams disbanded, the value of such documents has become greater, and anyone involved in theatre planning

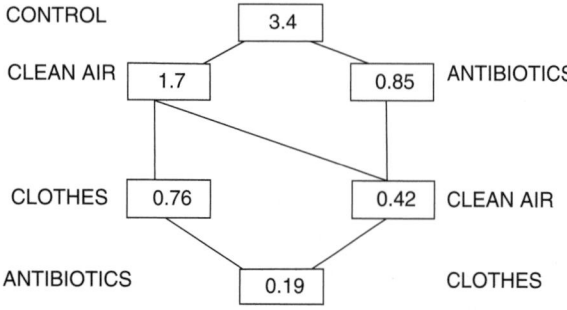

Figure 2.3 *MRC Trial on infection in orthopaedic surgery. Figures = % of deep infections prevented by interventions.*

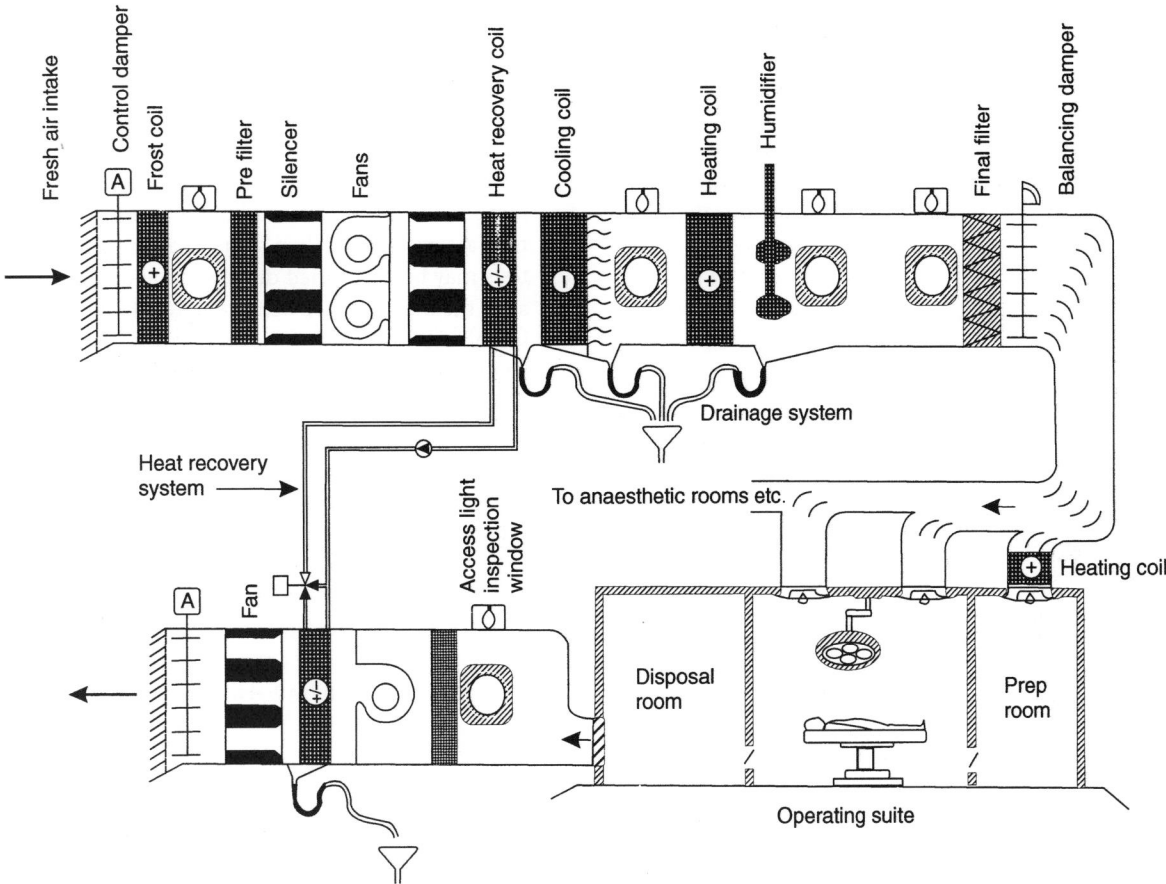

Figure 2.5 *Plan of a theatre ventilation plant.*

should be aware of their existence. The microbiologist should be aware of the sections on basic design, and on ventilation; together with recommendations for testing on commissioning and thereafter. The most important aspect, viz: the design of the ventilation plant, is properly an engineering problem. The plan of such a plant (Figure 2.5) is necessarily complex. Some simple points however require emphasis, especially as the design may imply a maintenance schedule beyond the competence of a hospital's engineering facilities.

The **air intake** should be protected from rain, and preferably should not be immediately downwind of the hospital incinerator or other source of particulates. The pre-filter, which is meant to exclude leaves, birds, etc. and prolong the life of the main filter, should be readily accessible. A blocked pre-filter can inactivate the whole ventilation plant, and eventually be subjected to such

suction from the fans that it buckles and no longer acts as a filter. **Humidification** of the air is important; however, problems have arisen when contaminated water is used for this purpose. The best means of humidification is injection of steam, but modern hospitals often have no steam supply. Where no steam is available a 'spinning disk' humidifier is required, which in turn, may require a demineralizing plant to provide adequate quality water, but with the added hazard of a potential for contamination. Contamination can also arise from water condensing on the cooling coils in summer, and so plant drainage is important. A final safeguard is to ensure that the main filter is at the theatre end of the system in the positive-pressure airstream so that contaminated air cannot leak into the ducting. The filter is specified to remove particles >5 μm from the air; there is no need in this system for the 0.5 μm 'high-efficiency' filter, which would require more powerful fans and would block up more quickly, and so be counter-productive. Such filters are purely for the ultraclean theatre.

Controls for **temperature** and humidity are required, together with monitors of the **pressure** across the filters. A popular energy-saving measure is to have a 'set-back' position to run the fans at half-speed when theatres are not in use. As there will be no bacterial challenge in an empty theatre, an airflow just enough to maintain a positive pressure across the doors is quite adequate to maintain very low particle counts throughout the night.

2.3.2 Commissioning

Although much of the commissioning involves monitoring air movements, and is an engineering function, microbiological commissioning of new or refurbished theatres is important. Time should be allowed after completion of the building works and before the theatre staff move in, for a thorough microbiological check. The phone call to say – 'please can you get your tests over by lunch time doctor, as we have to remove a scratched door for repair and are handing over tomorrow' – must be resisted at all costs. A week is not an unreasonable time to request. The plant should have been operational for at least 24 hours, and all cleaning completed before testing.

Four types of test are required:

1. *Cleanliness/cleanability.* All surfaces should be examined for cleanability, and all horizontal surfaces for dust. A wet swab is almost as good as a bacterial culture. The sealing of ledges around X-ray display stands, etc. should be checked.
2. *Air distribution.* Portable smoke generators (e.g. Drager . . .) help to define patterns of airflow. Balanced-flap exhaust valves should be checked (to ensure that they swing freely), together with the flow round doors, starting with those between the theatre suite and hospital corridor (to ensure that the theatres are at a positive pressure). Look for opening windows in ancillary rooms in the theatre suite such as the recovery area, which could unbalance the airflows. Air distribution in the theatre itself can be checked using smoke, and rates of flow through exhaust flaps measured with an anemometer to ensure that the flow is balanced. In one operating theatre tested by the author, 90% of the air was exhausted from one end of the room, leaving a large 'dead space' within the theatre that had little air movement.
3. *Air quality.* This can be measured simply and directly using a particle counter. A more relevant measurement is of the number of bacterial colony-forming units (particles) in the air, which is best measured by a 'slit sampler' (Cassella) in which the air is accelerated over an agar plate at such a speed as to deposit any bacteria-containing particles

on the surface. The plate is next incubated for 48 hours and any colonies present counted. The new and empty theatre suite (apart from the testers) should contain virtually no bacteria in the air. A more relevant test is to see if the theatres can deal with a bacterial challenge similar to that released during an operation. The simplest challenge is to ask four members of the theatre staff to don theatre clothing then spend time in the theatre, first standing around and then walking around while air samples are taken. Provided that the results of these tests are acceptable, then some final confirmatory tests may be performed during actual operations after the theatres have been accepted. However, if the initial tests give cause for concern, it is possible to enlarge on these by performing a mock operation.

4. *General construction.* A careful inspection may reveal constructional defects not apparent to others. For example, doors that do not shut properly or where the automatic closing devices have not been properly fitted. Another more subtle observation was of the electric fittings seen in Figure 2.6. The covers had all been fitted upside down, so that instead of protecting the sockets from any water used for washing walls down, the water would actually collect under the cover and be held in by it – a Health and Safety risk.

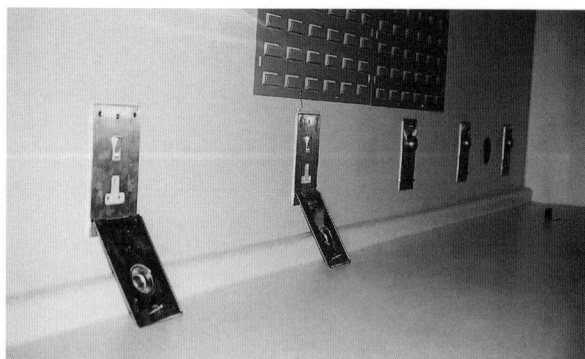

Figure 2.6 *How not to install shielded electric fittings in theatre – the shields are upside down!*

A more detailed account of commissioning operating theatres is provided by Holton and Ridgway (1993).

2.4 USE AND MAINTENANCE OF OPERATING THEATRES

All too often, the careful planning of theatre ventilation is completely neutralized by the users. The basic premise is that bacteria in theatre air emanate from movement of staff, and hence the value of ventilation is forgotten.

Thoughtless and **excessive movement** may provide an increased bacterial challenge. For example, siting the nurse 'runner' in the farthest corner of the theatre so that picking up a swab from the floor beside the surgeon and hanging it on a rack behind the scrub nurse entails walking twice round the whole theatre. Another common sight is the temporarily free surgeon or anaesthetist who walks around the other theatres to check progress or to have a chat. **Interference by staff** with the proper function of the ventilation is also common, and happens through ignorance. The simplest example is **leaving doors open**, though this is now rarer with better-designed theatres (but the 'balanced flaps' employed to allow air out of the theatre are frequently out of order). A common sight is a flap that has been cleaned and then either replaced the wrong way round, or not fitted properly onto its swivel, so that it will not open. A more subtle problem encountered by the author was the deliberate blocking off of a flap which opened from the theatre into a dirty corridor where the air was discharged under a table and over the feet of an Operating Department Assistant who sat at the table to make records.

Maintenance of theatre **ventilation** is the province of the engineers, but occasionally requires some **microbiological input**. The main problems are likely to relate to filters. The simplest is blockage of a pre-filter. The life of such a filter will vary very considerably with the local conditions, being shortest in a city-centre environment. The pre-filter should either be readily accessible or monitored by a pressure gauge. A blocked filter will mean that airflow is markedly reduced; if unchecked the air pressure will build up enough to destroy the filter, and allow unfiltered air into the system. Blockage of the main filter is less likely; such filters are monitored and are often provided with a roll of filter material that moves on automatically when the pressure-drop across the currently used part increases. Excess moisture is another occasional problem, as it can cause rusting in ducts, and if the main filter is wrongly sited would allow the ingress of contaminated air to the theatre.

Opinions differ on the value of routine **microbiological monitoring** of operating theatres. Regular testing of an ultraclean theatre is often at three-monthly intervals. For a standard theatre regular testing is not required, but can be useful in checking the ventilation, and for reassuring the theatre staff. Any monitoring performed should be as non-invasive as possible. Thus, a noisy slit sampler would be unacceptable. Exposure of blood agar 'settle plates' on suitable horizontal surfaces has been used, but this is an unsatisfactory indicator of microbial contamination as only large particles will settle out. Moreover, it is a slow and insensitive method. Exposure of a standard (9 cm-diameter) culture plate will only sample the equivalent of 0.0018 m³ of air per hour. Thus, an electromechanical sampler is preferable, and although the RCS sampler (Biotest Folex, Birmingham, UK) is not as accurate as a slit sampler for sampling small particles, it is quite adequate for use in the theatre and has the advantages of being non-invasive (almost soundless) and small (the size of a large torch).

Theatres should be checked after major maintenance or alterations, although if the ventilation plant is not involved, the most important aspect is a check on the cleaning, particularly of horizontal surfaces. There is some value in an occasional visit by the Infection Control Team to observe theatre practises as 'fly-on-the-wall' outsiders. Physical examination of the theatre environment may reveal problems that have been unsuspected by the theatre team, such as damaged door seals, or accumulations of dust in out-of-the-way places.

2.5 THEATRE MANAGEMENT

The use of operating theatres requires staff to adhere to rigorous codes of practise, in which ritual has had a significant role. While operations on infected patients are usually put last on the list, and in any event theatres must be tidied between operations, it is not often realized that the bacteria on the floor are unlikely causes of wound infection, unless stirred up by the cleaning process; most of the bacteria in the theatre air come from movements of the staff. The provision of **set-back controls** to run the ventilation at reduced speed when the theatre is out of use requires a staff member to be available to turn the speed up before the theatre is used.

2.6 SURGICAL TECHNIQUE

Cruse and Foord noted that the **length of an operation** was a risk factor. After clean operations, wound infection rates were 1.3%, 2.7% and 3.6% for those lasting 1, 2 and 3 hours, respectively. Others have noted the increased risk of longer (>2 hours) operations. Cruse and Foord cited the following time-associated risk factors: increased exposure to potential contaminants; tissue damage from exposed wound tissues becoming desiccated; increased suturing and electrocoagulation; and finally a diminution of host defences mediated by blood loss or shock. In cardiac surgery an increase in leakage of endotoxin from the gut into the blood due to splanchnic ischaemia has also been involved.

Surgical technique is probably the most important of all risk factors. Reoperation to control postoperative haemorrhage is always associated with a higher degree of infection. Cruse and Foord noted that the length of time spent on a particular operation by different surgeons was important – too fast was almost as dangerous as too slow. Some surgeons puncture their gloves significantly more often that others. Familiarity of the operating team with the relevant procedures is also important; Farber *et al.* found a highly significant relationship between wound infections and the number of procedures performed for straightforward operations such as appendectomy or herniorrhaphy.

A piece of equipment or fixtures can be a source of bacterial contamination, but this should now rarely be the case. However, occasional anecdotal reports have pinpointed theatre equipment as sources of outbreaks of infection.

In the past, some ventilators were virtually unsterilizable, and even today some of the materials used in new equipment may be difficult to sterilize. The dangers from anaesthetic equipment have been reduced by using vapour condenser humidifiers in the ventilation circuitry, because these also act as antimicrobial filters. The provision of sterile services (see Chapter 3) has ensured that most equipment used is now properly sterilized. However, some problems – old and new – remain, such as keeping certain valuable items within the theatre environs. Until recently, exposure of some carbon steel theatre knives and other equipment to 'paraform' or paraformaldehyde tablets in a sealed box in the theatre was used for 'sterilization', but this has been shown to be a valueless procedure. A recent equipment-associated problem is the use of highly expensive/sophisticated equipment which is leased for a single use, delivered to the theatre during the operation by the agent, and then removed for use elsewhere immediately afterwards. The surgeon may not be able to specify a 'sterilizing' process, and those used by the hirer may not in fact be acceptable.

2.7   CONCLUSIONS

Surgery is a costly business requiring a high-technology environment, and skilled workers. Nonetheless, the best that can be said about exogenous wound infections is that there is an 'irreducible minimum'. The main risk factor for surgical wound infection is human, a simple but important example being excess movement by staff during an operation. If an 'outbreak' of infection should occur, then the first step in investigation is to note, What has changed? The answer lies usually in the staff, less so in the procedures, or least in the matrices of the theatre itself. As hospital stays become increasingly shorter, the danger of missing a problem becomes greater, as does the need for audit.

2.8   FURTHER READING

Cruse, P.J.E. and Foord, R. (1980) The epidemiology of wound infection. A ten-year prospective study of 62 939 wounds. *Surg. Clin. North Am.*, **60**, 27–40.

Health Technical Memorandum 2025, Ventilation in Healthcare Premises. NHS Estates, UK Health Departments (1994), HMSO, London.

Holton, J. and Ridgway, G.L. (1993) Commissioning operating theatres. *J. Hosp. Infect.*, **23**, 153–160.

Lidwell, O.M. (1963) Methods of investigation and analysis of results. In *Infection in Hospitals*, ed. R.E.O. Williams and R.A. Shooter, Blackwell Publications, Oxford, 43.

Lidwell, O.M., Lowbury, E.J.L., Whyte, W., Blowers, R., Stanley, S.J. and Lowe, D. (1982) The effect of ultraclean air in operating rooms on deep sepsis of the joint after total hip or knee replacement: a randomised study. *Br. Med. J.*, **285**, 10–14.

Medical Research Council Operating-Theatre Hygiene Sub-committee (1962) Design and ventilation of operating suites for control of infection and for comfort. *Lancet*, **2**, 945–948.

Rotter M.L. (1981) Povidone-iodine and chlorhexidine gluconate containing detergents for disinfection of hands. *J. Hosp. Infect.*, **1**, 273–276.

Taylor, G.J.S., Leeming, J.P. and Bannister, G.C. (1992) Assessment of airborne bacterial contamination of clean wounds. Results in a tissue model. *J. Hosp. Infect.*, **22**, 241–249.

3

Sterilization, disinfection and sterile supplies

G.A.J. AYLIFFE AND J.D. HANSFORD

Medical equipment has become increasingly complex, expensive and difficult to clean. Many items are heat-labile and delicate, and cannot be steam sterilized rapidly for immediate reuse. This applies particularly to endoscopes and accessories used for minimally invasive surgery and for diagnostic purposes. Difficulty in cleaning and heat lability have been responsible for a considerable increase in the use of expensive single-use items.

In addition, patients have become more susceptible to infection due to an increase in invasive procedures, immunosuppression and major surgery which is often carried out on elderly and less-fit patients. The emergence of HIV, often associated with tuberculosis or other mycobacterial infections, the greater awareness of the transmissibility of hepatitis B and C viruses, and the potential hazards of legal claims for negligence (see Chapter 7) have all increased the need to ensure that medical devices are rendered safe for use on patients and for handling by staff.

Safety of medical devices can be assured by tightly controlled and validated cleaning, disinfection, packaging and sterilization carried out by well-trained staff in sterile services departments, operating theatres, endoscopy departments and in industry. However, the final responsibility for patient safety rests with the clinicians and nursing staff using the equipment. Unsatisfactory aseptic techniques can rapidly eliminate any benefits gained from the safe and efficient processing of instruments.

SECTION I: STERILIZATION AND DISINFECTION

3.1 INFECTION RISKS FROM MEDICAL EQUIPMENT AND THE ENVIRONMENT

These risks are categorized in Table 3.1 as **high, intermediate, low** and **minimal**. Although surgical instruments and other invasive devices are classified as high risk, infections due to inadequately sterilized items are very rare. Steam sterilization (Table 3.2), if well controlled, virtually eliminates any infection risk from the treated item. Infections following inadequate autoclaving have mainly been associated with 'sterile fluids' in which some Gram-negative bacilli have survived the faulty process and subsequently grown to large numbers. Outbreaks of infection, such as septicaemia, have been reported from contaminated intravenous fluids, and infections have been associated with contaminated eye drops and disinfectant solutions. Infection is more likely to follow low-temperature processes than autoclaving as the margin of safety is reduced. An inadequate autoclaving process in which a temperature of only 100°C is reached will still kill most non-sporing bacteria and viruses, whereas a failure of ethylene oxide at 37°C may allow bacteria and viruses to survive at this lower temperature. Nevertheless, a well-controlled ethylene

Table 3.1 *Classification of infection risk of medical devices and surfaces*

Risk category	Application	Some examples
High risk	Items in contact with a break in the skin or mucous membrane or introduced into sterile cavities or vascular systems	Surgical instruments, laparoscopes, arthroscopes, implants, infusions, injections, needles and syringes, catheters, swabs, surgical dressings, sutures
Intermediate risk	Items in contact with mucous membranes, body fluids or items contaminated with particularly virulent or readily transmissible organisms	Respiratory and anaesthetic equipment, used surgical instruments (prior to handling), gastrointestinal endoscopes, bronchoscopes, thermometers, vaginal speculae
Low risk	Items in contact with intact, healthy skin	Stethoscopes, sphygmomanometer cuffs, operating tables, wash bowls, baths
Minimal risk	Items not in close contact with patient or their immediate surroundings	Floors, walls, furniture, ceilings, sinks and drains

Table 3.2 *Process options for decontamination of medical devices in high-risk category*

Sterilization is preferred			
Heat-tolerant items			
Autoclaving	121–124°C	for	15 minutes (sterilization time)
	134–137°C	for	$3\frac{1}{2}$ minutes (sterilization time)
Hot-air oven	160°C	for	2 hours (sterilization time)
	170°C	for	1 hour (sterilization time)
	180°C	for	30 minutes (sterilization time)
Heat-sensitive items			
Ethylene oxide	37–55°C	up to 6 hours ⎫	plus degassing and
Low-temperature steam and formaldehyde	73–80°C	up to 3 hours ⎬	quarantine time
Gas plasma (new process)	45°C	50–90 minutes	
Sporicidal disinfectants			
2% glutaraldehyde		10 hours ⎫	
0.2–0.35% peracetic acid		10 minutes ⎬	holding time
1000–10 000 p.p.m. av chlorine dioxide		10 minutes ⎭	
Superoxidized water (Sterilox)		5–10 minutes	

oxide process is unlikely to be associated with infection from a well-cleaned item. Immersion in a chemical disinfectant is less satisfactory, since items are not packaged, and recontamination can occur on rinsing; also the processes are usually less well-controlled than with gaseous or heating methods.

3.1.1 Infection from high-risk items

Hospital-acquired infection due to spore-bearing organisms, e.g. *Clostridium perfringens* and *Cl. tetani*, are surprisingly rare even after exposure of instruments to inadequate sterilization methods. This is probably because few spores are present on well-cleaned instruments before sterilization or immersion in a chemical agent. Postoperative clostridial infections that have been reported are mainly endogenous in origin, although anaerobic spores are frequently isolated in the environment of the operating theatre.

Recent studies on the incidence of infection following invasive endoscopy, e.g. cholecystectomy, are few and there is little evidence in these studies that infections were due to inadequate decontamination of the endoscopes. Most of the available information is not recent and is from large retrospective questionnaire surveys. In one of these surveys of over 12 000 arthroscopies, there were five infections, four of which were caused by *Staphylococcus aureus*, probably of endogenous origin. Another survey of over 100 000 laparoscopies showed a complication rate of 3–4 per 1000 operations, but only 7/320 of the infections reported were considered to be due to unsterile instruments. Similar results have been obtained in other surveys, and in most of them endoscopes have been disinfected by immersion in 2% glutaraldehyde for 10–15 minutes and not subjected to a sterilization process. Although the infection risk is low, sterilization by heat is preferred, and whenever possible manufacturers should be encouraged to produce autoclavable endoscopes and accessories. Cystoscopes are inserted into a normally sterile body cavity and are considered to be high risk, although until recently they have not usually been sterilized. Infection acquired from inadequately decontaminated cystoscopes were often reported in the 1950s. These were usually immersed in mercuric oxycyanide or aqueous quaternary ammonium compounds which have a poor spectrum of antimicrobial activity. Thorough cleaning and immersion in 70% alcohol for 5 minutes, or more recently 2% glutaraldehyde for 10 minutes has almost eliminated the risks of instrument-associated infection. Unfortunately, glutaraldehyde is an irritant and is sensitizing to the skin, eyes and respiratory tract, and precautions must be taken to protect both patients and staff. Autoclavable rigid fibre-optic laparoscopes, arthroscopes and cystoscopes are now available and should be purchased whenever possible. Flexible fibre-optic endoscopes do not withstand thermal disinfection or sterilization and have to be processed by chemical methods.

3.1.2 Infection from intermediate-risk items

Most infections from medical equipment are included in this group, the main reasons for infection being inadequate cleaning, the use of an inappropriate disinfectant, or storage in moist conditions.

ENDOSCOPES

The narrow channels of flexible endoscopes are particularly difficult to clean and dry. Infections arising from items in this category have been considerably reduced in recent years by use of improved cleaning methods in automated machines, and more effective disinfectants.

Infections following gastroscopy and bronchoscopy have mainly been due to opportunist Gram-negative bacilli, e.g. *Pseudomonas aeruginosa*, *Serratia marcescens* and *Klebsiella* spp. These have usually multiplied during storage overnight or longer in moist endoscope channels, or water bottles and their channels. Infection commonly occurs in immunocompromised patients or following endoscopic retrograde cholangio pancreatography (ERCP). *Salmonella* infections, including one instance of *Salmonella typhi*, have also followed the use of inadequate disinfectants, e.g. hexachlorophane, quaternary ammonium compounds, aqueous chlorhexidine and povidone-iodine. Infection has sometimes occurred after apparently an adequate immersion time in an effective disinfectant, but with inadequate pre-cleaning.

Evidence of transfer of *Mycobacterium tuberculosis* during bronchoscopy is scanty, and only two instances of infection have been reported due to inadequate disinfection or cleaning. Other mycobacteria have been isolated from bronchial washings causing pseudo-outbreaks. These usually arise from contaminated rinse water in a washer disinfector. The organisms are often present in biofilms on the inner surface of the washing container or associated pipework. *Mycobacterium chelonae* isolated from the rinse water of washer disinfectors have shown an increased resistance to glutaraldehyde. However, reports of clinical infections from these atypical mycobacteria are rare.

Transmission of other organisms have rarely been reported. Patients with gastric haemorrhage frequently undergo gastroscopy, but transmission of HIV has not been reported. Hepatitis B transmission has been reported in one well-documented case but not hepatitis C, although infections may not have been associated with a previous endoscopy because of the long incubation periods, and prospective studies have not been carried out. Other organisms isolated after endoscopy, but not necessarily associated with clinical infection, include *Bacillus* spp., fungi, e.g. *Trichosporon beigelii* and *Rhodotorula rubra*, *Helicobacter pylori*, cryptococci and strongyloides. Infection has been rarely reported after colonoscopy or sigmoidoscopy, but there is a potential risk of transmission of *Salmonella* spp., *Campylobacter* and *C. difficile*.

INFECTIONS ASSOCIATED WITH RESPIRATORY TRACT INFECTION

Hospital-acquired pneumonia is commonly associated with endotracheal intubation, tracheostomy, mechanical ventilation, and treatment in an intensive care unit. Infection is usually caused by endogenous Gram-negative bacilli, such as *Escherichia coli* or *Klebsiella*, colonizing the throat and often the stomach. The organisms acquired from respiratory equipment are usually opportunistic pathogenic Gram-negative bacilli, e.g. *Ps. aeruginosa*, *S. marcescens* or *Acinetobacter* spp. that have grown overnight or for longer periods in tubing, rebreathing bags, Ambu bags, humidifiers, or within the ventilator or an anaesthetic machine. Contaminated aerosols generated from nebulizers containing stagnant fluids have caused lower respiratory tract infections, but with improved equipment design this is now infrequent.

3.2 PREVENTION OF INFECTION BY DECONTAMINATION OF EQUIPMENT

Decontamination is a process which removes or destroys microorganisms or other contaminants to render equipment safe to use or handle. It consists of cleaning, disinfection or sterilization.

Cleaning is a physical process which removes contaminants, including microorganisms, dust, soil and organic material, e.g. blood and sputum, that protects microorganisms. It is an **essential prerequisite to disinfection or sterilization** and should be **meticulous.** Microorganisms survive poorly and do not proliferate on clean, dry surfaces.

Disinfection is a process used to reduce the number of microorganisms, but not usually spores; it does not necessarily eliminate all microorganisms, but reduces their number to a level which is not harmful to health. Mycobacteria often show an inceased resistance to disinfectants and the term **high-level chemical disinfection** is sometimes used to include a process which is effective against *M.tuberculosis* and the more resistant enteroviruses.

Sterilization is a process used to render an object free from all living organisms, but it usually excludes the inactivation of prions which are highly resistant to most sterilization processes.

Of these processes, sterilization is the most effective method of destroying organisms, whilst cleaning is the least, although effective cleaning will usually remove most microorganisms.

The decontamination processes are shown in Tables 3.2 and 3.3. The choice of method depends on many factors in addition to the infection risk, and includes the tolerance of the item to moisture, heat, pressure and chemicals and the time available for processing. Toxicity and allergenicity must be considered when chemical methods are used. The process must be effective against the relevant pathogens and opportunist organisms present in the environment.

Heat sterilization is preferred, but if the item is heat-sensitive then chemical agents must be used.

Validated, well-controlled automated processes are the safest and most reliable options.

Autoclaves and other machines used for processing equipment should be well maintained.

Sterilization is usually considered to be a process which will kill 10^6 spores of a type highly resistant to the process, e.g. *Bacillus stearothermophilus* for heat sterilization and

Bacillus subtilis var. *niger* for ethylene oxide. This obviously represents a considerable overkill, since thorough washing of surgical instruments will remove most organisms, including spores.

In practice, it may be preferable to decide on a rapid and safe process at the point of use, rather than returning equipment to the Sterile Services Department for processing strictly in accordance with the risk categories. However, processing in the Sterile Services Department is preferable if possible, especially as one may also be limited by legal constraints.

3.2.1 Decontamination of high-risk devices

HEAT STERILIZATION

Heat sterilization at 134°C is the most widely used method for sterilizing surgical instruments, operating theatre clothing and linen. A porous load autoclave (i.e. a machine which draws a vacuum) is required to remove air from packaged equipment, clothing or fine tubing. A downward displacement autoclave, which does not draw a vacuum, may be useful in a theatre suite for dropped instruments, bowls and other utensils, operating at 121°C for 15 minutes. In clinics, small bench-top autoclaves *in-situ* are suitable for the sterilization of unwrapped instruments.

All parts of the Health Technical Memorandum 2010, which incorporates harmonized European Standards, BS EN 554, are now published and implemented. The design brief requires that time/temperature recorders (or computer printers) be fitted to autoclaves.

The time/temperature recorder will indicate that all stages of a cycle have been completed, and prescribed tests at intervals (e.g. use of thermocouples) will validate the process. Autoclave tape reacting with moist heat will indicate that an item has been through the autoclaving process, although it does not confirm sterilization. Chemical indicators are available which respond to time and temperature, and may be useful in clinics for daily use with bench-top autoclaves, but they will not detect

Table 3.3 *Process options for decontamination of medical devices in intermediate-risk category*

Disinfection is usually adequate		
Physical methods		
Boiling water		5–10 minutes
Low-temperature steam	73–80°C	10 minutes
Washer/disinfectors	70–100°C	up to 3 minutes (depending on temperature)
Chemical methods		
2% glutaraldehyde		4–20 minutes
0.2–0.35% peracetic acid		5 minutes
1000–10 000 p.p.m. av chlorine dioxide		5 minutes
70% alcohol		5–10 minutes

air removal. The Bowie Dick (or similar) test is carried out daily to demonstrate air removal in porous load autoclaves. In this test, a sheet with a chemical indicator is part of a pack conforming to BS EN 867 4 2001 or a pack of white cotton sheets of a size and depth specified in BS 5815 may be used by engineers using thermocouples to record the temperature profile in the pack. Similar information may be obtained from electronic test devices. This pack is placed in an empty chamber and put through a specific 'Bowie Dick test cycle' or, if this is not an option, the full sterilization cycle and then examined for any non-uniformity of colour change in the chemical indicator. In the UK, spores are not usually used for testing heat sterilization, and physical methods of measuring the process are preferred. However, spore strips are used in many countries, often in addition to other tests.

Fluids are sterilized at 115°C for 30 minutes, and temperatures are monitored with thermocouples placed in a bottle of fluid in an appropriate site in the autoclave. Dry-heat sterilizers are less efficient sterilizers than autoclaves and have longer cycles at higher temperatures, e.g. 160°C for 2 hours, 170°C for 1 hour and 180°C for 30 minutes (Table 3.2). They are mainly used when the presence of moisture is undesirable or likely to be ineffective, e.g. for delicate sharp instruments or in pharmacies for sterilizing ointments and powders.

ETHYLENE OXIDE

Ethylene oxide is the main process used for low-temperature sterilization. This is a toxic and potentially explosive gas, requiring special facilities to ensure safety of the operator and adequate removal of gas from the sterilized equipment. Post-sterilization aeration is usually necessary for one or more days to elute residual ethylene oxide. The aeration time depends on the turnover of air in the aerating chamber, the temperature, and on the material of the item sterilized. Spores and difficult test pieces are required to test for effectiveness of the sterilization process, and these require incubation for 2–5 days to ensure the safety of the sterilized material.

Ethylene oxide is suitable for sterilizing packaged items, but is not appropriate if rapid use is required. Loads are usually processed at 37–55°C, with a total time of 4–6 hours. The special facilities and expertise for using ethylene oxide are usually only present in large Sterile Service Departments (SSDs).

LOW-TEMPERATURE STEAM AND FORMALDEHYDE (LTSF)

The process is not frequently used in the UK, but is more common in some other European countries. It is a relatively low-temperature process operating at 73–80°C. Instruments can be wrapped and used soon after processing. Spore tests are necessary to ensure sterilization, and

these require incubation for 2–5 days. Formaldehyde is an irritant and is toxic, and special arrangements are required for its removal. LTSF was originally used for sterilizing rigid endoscopes, but most of these are now autoclavable and this is the preferred option.

LOW-TEMPERATURE STEAM (LTS)

LTS without formaldehyde at the same temperature (73–80°C) for 10 minutes may be used for high-level disinfection, and would be suitable for disinfecting rigid endoscopes and precleaned respiratory equipment.

GAS PLASMA STERILIZATION

Since ethylene oxide and formaldehyde are toxic, an alternative non-toxic gaseous agent is being sought for low-temperature sterilization. Gas plasma sterilization is a new method in which hydrogen peroxide or peracetic acid vapour is used as a substrate gas, and then radiofrequency emissions or microwaves are used to change it into plasma. Plasma consists of charged molecules, which include free radicals capable of destroying microorganisms. It requires a relatively short sterilization time and the end products are non-toxic. However, there are problems of penetration of narrow tubing, particularly if closed at one end, and the effects on materials need further study. It may be a suitable replacement for ethylene oxide, but it is expensive.

OTHER GASEOUS METHODS

Machines using vaporized hydrogen peroxide alone or ozone are also being tested, but also have problems in completely penetrating narrow tubing and with material incompatibility.

SPORICIDAL LIQUID AGENTS

These have the disadvantage that instruments cannot be wrapped for processing, and recontamination may occur particularly from the environment on rinsing to remove irritant residues (unless it takes place in a closed machine). Glutaraldehyde (2%) has been the agent of choice although other effective agents are now available and may be preferred. Glutaraldehyde produces toxic vapours, and can cause allergic reactions of skin and respiratory tract, but it does not damage materials and has been used for many years. Glutaraldehyde should be handled with gloves which are resistant to penetration, and should be used in an atmosphere which removes toxic vapours, e.g. an enclosed machine or a ventilated cabinet. It has a relatively slow sporicidal action, and at least 3 hours immersion is required. The manufacturers often recommend 10 hours, which is too long for practical use. However, as already discussed, spores do not usually represent a clinical problem and invasive endoscopes are usually immersed for 10–20 minutes. Immersion for 20 minutes or longer provides high-level disinfection. The spores of *C. difficile* are effectively killed in less than 10 minutes.

If an alternative to glutaraldehyde is considered, it should be checked with the manufacturer that it is effective, safe and compatible with the endoscope and processing equipment.

Peracetic acid has been used for many years, but only recently have preparations become available commercially that are suitable for clinical use. Its main advantages over glutaraldehyde is a rapid sporicidal action and lack of toxicity of end products. Peracetic acid (0.2–0.35%) is sporicidal in 10 minutes and disinfects in 5 minutes. The smell is rather unpleasant, but there is no evidence of toxicity at the concentrations used. It can damage certain materials, although endoscopes appear not to be functionally damaged by the commercial preparations available. Damage to some washing machines has been reported. An enclosed automated disinfection/sterilization machine (Steris) is available and appears to be microbiologically effective. It does not have a washing cycle, is expensive, but reduces any hazards to processing staff. Commercial preparations of peracetic acid are expensive, and in-use solutions are stable for only a few days.

Chlorine dioxide is a chlorine-releasing agent that has recently been introduced for sterilizing medical equipment. It is rapidly active against spores, e.g. 1000–10 000 p.p.m. (or possibly lower concentrations of av chlorine dioxide) is sporicidal in 10 minutes. It is potentially corrosive, but commercial preparations contain anticorrosive agents. Further experience is required to ensure that instruments and processing equipment will not be damaged.

Superoxidized water e.g. Sterilox is a novel system which is highly effective against bacterial spores, mycobacteria and viruses. It is relatively non-stable and should not be stored for more than 24 hours.

Orthophthalaldehyde (OPA) is a similar compound to glutaraldehyde but is more active against mycobacteria and less active against spores. It is stable and does not require activation.

3.2.2 Decontamination of intermediate-risk items

Autoclaving is still the method of choice, but heat at lower temperatures or chemical disinfection is usually adequate. Water at 70–100°C, preferably in an automated machine, or low-temperature steam at 73–80°C is preferable to chemical disinfection. Boiling water for 5–10 minutes is an effective method of disinfection and avoids the necessity for rinsing. The process should be well controlled using a timer, and instruments should be completely immersed. However, prewashing at low temperature is required to remove protein which will be coagulated at temperatures below that required for disinfection. Washer/heat disinfectors are commonly used for decontamination of soiled instruments, respiratory circuits, crockery and cutlery, bed-pans, other human waste receptacles and soiled linen (Table 3.3). Temperatures of 70°C for 3 minutes or 80°C for 1 minute or other appropriate time/temperature combinations should be adequate to disinfect items in a washing machine.

ENDOSCOPES

Heat-labile endoscopes are usually disinfected by a chemical method, although combined heating (below 60°C) and a lower concentration of the chemical agent is sometimes used. Gastrointestinal endoscopes are usually cleaned and disinfected in an automated machine, but even if a machine is used thorough brushing is still required. Exposure to 2% glutaraldehyde for 10 minutes is recommended by the British Society of Gastroenterology. This exposure time should be effective against non-spore-forming bacteria, fungi and viruses, including HIV and probably hepatitis B, particularly as most of the microorganisms will be removed by pre-cleaning. This protocol has been in use for many years and there have been no reports of infection due to failures in disinfection. However, an exposure time of 10–20 minutes is recommended in many countries. An exposure time of at least 20 minutes is recommended to achieve an adequate effect against *M. tuberculosis,* and is used routinely for bronchoscopes. Other mycobacteria may be more resistant to glutaraldehyde, and 60 or more minutes of exposure may be required after an endoscopy on a patient with an *M. avium-intracellulare* infection. The processing of endoscopes with glutaraldehyde should be carried out in a ventilated room or cabinet which reduces environmental levels to that required by health and safety authorities.

Rinse water in automated machines should be bacteria-free, and it is usually heat-sterilized or filtered. Machines should preferably have a self-disinfecting cycle to prevent biofilm formation and to ensure that they do not become a source of recontamination. Rinsing a bronchoscope at the end of the cleaning and disinfection cycle with alcohol followed by forced air-drying should eliminate surviving Gram-negative bacilli or mycobacteria.

Although glutaraldehyde remains the disinfectant of choice, other agents (e.g. peracetic acid and chlorine dioxide) are being used (Table 3.3). Their use needs careful monitoring (as already discussed) to detect damage to endoscopes and machines, as well as harm to staff.

Alcohol (70% ethyl, 60% isopropyl) is a useful agent for the rapid decontamination of instruments, but endoscopes should not be immersed for longer than 5 minutes to avoid possible damage to lens cement. It is effective against non-spore-forming bacteria, including mycobacteria, and most viruses (apart from some enteroviruses). It is unlikely to harm staff, and rinsing after use is not

Table 3.4 *Properties of disinfectants*

	Corrosion of metals	Irritant/ sensitizing	Inactivated by organic matter	Stability
Glutaraldehyde (2%)	No	Yes*	No (fixative)	Moderate 14–28 days
Peracetic acid (0.2–0.35%)	Slight	Slight	No	No (1–3 days)
Alcohol** (70%)	No**	No	Yes (fixative)	Yes (enclosed container)
Chlorine-releasing agents (100–1000 av Cl)	Yes	Yes	Yes	No (1 day)
Clear soluble phenolics (1–2%)	Slight	Yes	No	Yes
Quaternary ammonium compounds	No	No	Yes	Yes

*Skin, eyes and respiratory tract.
**May damage lens cement of endoscopes; flammable.

necessary. The main disadvantage is flammability; burns have occurred during diathermy if alcohol pools or collects in drapes and is accidentally ignited.

RESPIRATORY AND OTHER ITEMS

Whenever possible autoclaving or heat disinfection should be used for disinfecting respiratory equipment or instruments, such as vaginal speculae, whenever possible to avoid problems of irritation if rinsing is inadequate following chemical disinfection, especially glutaraldehyde. Heat disinfection in a washer disinfector renders items safe to handle and free from infection risk. The use of filters to protect ventilators from contamination reduces the necessity to decontaminate them after each patient use.

Single-use respiratory equipment, speculae and other items are available, but consideration should be given to costs, risk management and manufacturers' advice (see below).

3.2.3 Decontamination of low-risk items

Thorough cleaning and drying should be adequate, although occasionally disinfection may be required if the item is contaminated with potentially virulent or readily transmissible organisms or is used on immuno-compromised patients. Thermometers, stethoscope chest pieces, trolley tops and electrical equipment can be disinfected with 70% alcohol. Immersion for 5 minutes is preferred to wiping if this is practicable. Chlorine-releasing compounds (500–1000 p.p.m. av Cl) for 10 minutes can be used following pre-cleaning on items not corroded by them, e.g. tonometers and catering equipment. They can also be used for disinfecting baths, mattress covers washbasins and toilets, if disinfection is required.

Chlorine-releasing compounds are cheap and effective against most bacteria, fungi and viruses, including HIV, hepatitis viruses and enteroviruses, but are readily inactivated by organic matter. Corrosion of metals and some other materials reduces their value in the decontamination of medical equipment.

3.2.4 Decontamination of minimal-risk items

The dry environment such as floors, walls, furniture, ceilings and other environmental sites, e.g. sinks and drains, not in close contact with the patient are not important sources of infection, and routine cleaning should be adequate. Spillage of body fluids should be rapidly removed by cleaning by an operator wearing gloves. Disinfection of contaminated surfaces may sometimes be required. A solution or powder containing a chlorine-releasing agent (5000–10 000 p.p.m. av Cl) added to the spillage is usually recommended, but disinfection after cleaning with 1000 p.p.m. av Cl may be preferred. Phenolic solutions (1–2%) are sometimes used, particularly for bacterial contamination. However, they tend to be less active against viruses, especially enteroviruses, but are not readily inactivated by organic materials.

Fogging or **fumigating** with formaldehyde or other agents is of doubtful value, and should be avoided. Other agents with a narrow spectrum of activity or slow inaction such as chlorhexidine, triclosan, quaternary ammonium compounds and povidone-iodine should not be used for environmental disinfection, but may be used for skin disinfection or for clinical purposes if indicated.

3.3 PROBLEMS OF PRIONS

Device-associated infections caused by prions, e.g. Creutzfeld–Jakob disease, are rare, but a few have been reported following neurosurgical procedures. Prions are resistant to glutaraldehyde, ethylene oxide and routine autoclaving processes. They may be inactivated by high concentrations of oxidizing agents, e.g. chlorine-releasing agents (20 000 p.p.m. av Cl for 1 hour), but these are corrosive to most instruments. Immersion in 2 M sodium hydroxide for 1 hour has also been suggested. Thorough washing of instruments several times followed by autoclaving at 134°C for at least 18 minutes should render them safe, although survival of the more resistant prions has been reported even after this process. Autoclaving at 134°C in 2 M sodium hydroxide has also been suggested, but could damage the autoclave. Destruction of the instruments is recommended in specific circumstances. Variation in resistance to heat and chemicals depends on the type of prion, the amount of brain tissue used in the test, and the method of testing so that interpretation of laboratory tests is difficult.

3.4   SINGLE-USE ITEMS AND RE-PROCESSING

The number of disposable items of medical equipment used in hospitals continues to increase. Although these have often improved the safety of devices, costs can be very high and some hospitals re-process certain items labelled 'single-use'. If an item is labelled single-use by the manufacturer, they are no longer responsible for any deficiencies if the item is re-processed. It is therefore important that the responsibility for re-processing is taken by the hospital and not only by the user or processor. A **Device Assessment Group**, consisting of the Infection Control Doctor and Nurse, the Supplies (Procurement) Officer, the Sterile Services Manager, Risk Manager and other processors, e.g. Endoscopy Nurse, if relevant, a clinician representing the directorate concerned and a risk assessment officer, is suggested. The group reports to the Hospital Manager or Chief Executive, who may take legal advice if necessary.

The item is assessed by the group for risks of infection or toxicity to the patient associated with reprocessing and the possibility of damage to the item causing physical harm to the patient. Risks of infection or from a damaged item are obviously much higher from a device used intravascularly than those in contact with intact mucous membranes. Contact with intact skin is a lower risk, although toxicity could still be relevant in all items.

The device is assessed for cleanability and suitability for sterilization or disinfection. The main difficulty is assessing the effect of repeated processing on structure, function or release of toxic substances. The manufacturer has to provide this information if the item is sold as reusable, and this might persuade him/her to label it single-use. However, manufacturers should be encouraged to produce re-processible items and to provide these data. Careful costing should be

undertaken, taking into account all possible costs, including transport, packaging, training and safety of staff, testing and validation, and waste disposal before a decision is made. In the UK and in some other countries the re-processing of single-use items for re-use is now banned.

SECTION II: STERILE SUPPLIES

The first requirement of sterile supplies is the provision of equipment for performing aseptic procedures to the practitioner in containers and packets labelled by the supplier or manufacturer with details of the contents, production date, lot number and sterilization process indicator. This common approach is an element of quality systems adopted by commercial suppliers of intended single-use items and facilitates re-processing of surgical instruments and equipment after patient use. The choice of packaging, containers, trays, plastic and paper bags is determined by the need to protect contents whilst allowing effective access to sterilization agents.

3.5   COMMERCIAL PRODUCTS

The range of sterile products available from commercial manufacturers continues to increase.

Sterile dressings, catheters and cannulas, as well as single-use instruments may be added to procedure packs during the course of a ward or clinic procedure. Specifications for the contents are decided by the purchaser. The supplier, or an agent, may be the contractor for a local, regional or national contract. Manufacturers and suppliers are chosen where possible from those whose production methods and facilities comply with the European Medical Devices Directive EEC 93/42, or comply with the 'essential requirements' of European Standards, and may claim CE mark registration for their products. The associated quality assurance system specifies that a traceability record from raw material supplier to purchaser is maintained by the manufacturer for the expected lifetime of the product. The quality and materials used in the product can, at any stage, be compared to the accepted specification, National or International standards.

Manufacturers whose products are heat- and moisture- resistant will use steam under pressure to sterilize. The majority of commercially available packs contain items intended for single use of heat-labile and moisturesensitive materials requiring sterilization by low-temperature methods, ionizing irradiation, electron beam or ethylene oxide gas. The choice is indicated by the lowest denominator of material tolerance and the availability and capacity of processing plant.

In addition, a wide range of sterile medical devices are marketed for diagnostic, protective or therapeutic use. Most have a specific application including protective clothing for practitioners, diagnostic aids, implants and prostheses. Packaging materials are selected to ensure compatibility between the needs of the product and the chosen method of sterilization.

At each user point established policies and procedural techniques for opening packs and the aseptic use of sterile medical devices will guide the practitioner. In selected cases the product traceability link ends with entries to patients' records.

3.6 RE-PROCESSED INSTRUMENTS AND EQUIPMENT (MEDICAL DEVICES)

The second major requirement for sterile or disinfected supplies are operating theatres or 'in-house' units (e.g. Endoscopy) which provide a specialist service. A wide range of items are produced by the Sterile Services Department often located close to its major users, the operating theatres, intensive and special baby care units, but it may also supply other hospitals and clinics. The staff, management and technicians, may either be hospital personnel or be employed by a contractor managing the facility. A department supplying purchasers beyond its own Employing Authority must, since June 1998, comply with the same European Directive (EEC 93/42) or 'essential requirements' of relevant European Standards as commercial manufacturers. Differences between manufacturing practices in commercial and 'in-house' facilities will diminish although 'in-house' units will continue to be responsible for handling contaminated used items. Progressive departments will operate a recognized quality system in a controlled environment with regulated procurement and work practices; approved documentation with formal liaison and communication with users, monitoring and modifying practice to meet agreed criteria and requirements, are all subject to internal and external audit.

The prime functions of the Sterile Services Department are:

to re-process surgical instruments, holloware and equipment after patient use; to supply other sterile and disinfected items, single-use and re-usable items for the conduct of 'high' and 'intermediate' risk procedures in approved locations (e.g. hospitals), the community and occupational health facilities.

3.7 ORGANIZATION AND WORKFLOW

Each production process will follow a logical sequence of documented work practices known as 'standard operating procedures' that are followed by all staff. These are essential components of any quality system, and a basis for staff training programmes.

Re-processing items after patient use carries potential or actual risks. Receptacles used during the procedure must be emptied of surplus fluid and all single-use items disposed of at user level. Users are responsible for checking that all returned items are complete, wrapped and secured in colour-coded bags, containers or trolleys according to local practice before transport and the start of the re-processing cycle. Returned items are identified with the last user by document or a computerized tracking system. Staff responsible for transporting and sorting equipment will be trained in handling techniques, and safeguarded against infection risk by prophylactic vaccinations and the wearing of specified protective clothing to protect against the infection risk of items being transported or handled.

Immunization should include tetanus, hepatitis B and BCG (if the subject is not immune to tuberculosis). The occupational health service will provide advice where necessary.

Staff entering the '**decontamination area**' will wear hair covers, full-length protective gowns, gloves and washable footwear. Headwear and some gowns may be 'single-use'; other items are washable and re-usable. The gown will have a high collar line and give all-round cover with full-length tapered sleeves. Preferred materials are lightweight fine woven poly cotton fibre with good resistance to fluid penetration. Face visors are usually mounted on a head band and can be worn over spectacles. Washable and fibre-free household gloves and shoes with a protective toe cap complete the protection to be worn whilst sorting and preparing items returned for processing. Punctured or leaking gloves should be replaced without delay. If other items become torn or soiled by splashing or spillage they too should be replaced. All re-usable items will be discarded, cleaned and disinfected at the end of the work session.

Devices for re-processing are received into the department's 'decontamination area' and physically segregated from other work areas. All surfaces should be washable and frequently cleaned.

Returned goods are checked in (any missing items being reported) and sorted and the majority loaded into baskets exposing the maximum surface area to the action of thermal washer/disinfectors. Tubular items are mounted on manifolds. Thermal disinfection is the preferred option for decontamination, or making items 'safe to handle', as discussed previously. The operating cycle removes all loose soil before cleaning in detergent or enzyme detergent solution; some types incorporate ultrasonic action to enhance cleaning. The first rinse stage follows removing traces of detergent solution and increasing the surface temperature of the load before the final rinse at one of the three recognized time/temperature values, 71°C for 3 minutes, 80°C for 1 minute, or 93°C for 12 seconds. All temperatures are recorded from the surface of the load.

Large-capacity machines are not suitable for some endoscopes, delicate and micro-surgery instruments, long or cannulated instruments, and large items of equipment. These may be cleaned manually using warm detergent solution, followed by rinsing in hot water in double sinks. Non-linting cloths and soft brushes are used to remove soil. Mains connected jet spray guns may be used to force-rinse cannulated instruments, the distal end being below the fluid level in the rinse tank.

Bench-top ultrasonic tanks, some fitted with dedicated manifolds to hold tubing and endoscopes, are effective in loosening stubborn soils. Ultrasonic cavitation is the product of high-frequency waves generated within the tank, that rise to the surface where circular ripple patterns show that pressure variations have caused implosions with sufficient force to release soil from hard and inaccessible surfaces.

Both manual and ultrasonic cleaning systems remove soil. This is a pre-condition for effective disinfection. They do not themselves disinfect. Some items may be further processed through a thermal washer/disinfector, while others may require chemical disinfection by methods described in the previous section.

It is important for the protection of staff, and the working environment, that all items entering the next processing stage – the 'clean production' or 'packing area', should be 'disinfected', that is, 'safe to handle'.

The **clean production** or **packing area** has the cleanest environmental conditions in the department, and will usually be provided with pressurized filtered air. It is linked to the raw material store and the staff changing and gowning area. The supply of raw materials, stripped of transit packaging, is limited by demand and is delivered through transfer hatches. Work stations are equipped for processing instrument sets, supplementary items, ward and clinic supplies. The number and movement of gowned personnel in the area is restricted to reduce the dissemination of particles. Staff are not permitted to wear cosmetics or jewellery other than plain wedding rings in this 'clean area'. The approach will be routed through a changing area with washhand basins and possibly showers. Full-length fibre-free gowns or overalls with sleeves and no pockets, full hair cover and shoes of leather or non-shedding composite material are worn.

Staff should work to a programme that responds to the availability of items for re-processing and give priority to urgent demands on the service.

The functions performed continue the logical workflow, as follows:

1. Cleaned trays, holloware and instruments are received, the latter visually checked for soiling before arrival.
2. Checks are carried out that each instrument or set is complete, clean on visual examination and dry.

Illuminated magnification is available on selected benches to confirm cleanliness or function in critical areas.

3. Function tests are performed on critical instruments; for example, the sharpness of scissors and osteotomes, freedom but security of movement of joints, correct apposition of serrated surfaces, the conductivity and insulation integrity of diathermy instruments and lubrication of selected moving parts are carried out according to manufactures' instructions and local practice. More sophisticated tests will be conducted by medical engineers.
4. Assembly and packaging of re-usable and single-use items is carried out which follows the agreed configuration and range. Vented protective covers may be fitted to pointed and sharp-edged instruments.
5. Instrument sets are prepared from a comprehensive range of instruments, the selection and number determined by agreement with practitioners performing the procedure. The instruments are arranged on a lined stainless steel or alloy tray, with (or supplied separately) absorbent dressings, tubing, sundries and drapes for the patient and equipment in the immediate vicinity of the sterile field.

The original design of modular trays was developed for the Edinburgh Royal Hospitals in the early 1960s. The design has been subject to modification. Some prefer instruments to be packed separately from drapes and dressings, giving greater flexibility and choice.

Small collections and single instruments, required by individual practitioners or those stored in readiness for use in emergencies, may also be assembled on trays.

Sets of instruments are accompanied by a 'contents list' checked and signed by at least one technician. A process indicator is included as evidence to the 'scrub nurse' of processing. The check list is used to confirm that all items are present before the set is prepared for re-processing.

Instrument sets and packs for aseptic procedures have traditionally been double wrapped in non-linting, non-reflective material or fabric. One layer should conform to a recognized specification as a microbiological barrier.

Alternatively, and particularly designed for those preferring separation of instruments from drapes and dressings, a comprehensive instrument and holloware set may be fitted into the inner basket of a two-part instrument container. Each or one part of the container incorporates a short-life or single-use microbial filter. The two parts, lid and base, fit together with a gasket between parts and are locked by a tamper-proof seal prior to sterilization.

Endoscopes with a dedicated range of instruments and connections may be packed as a set in sterilizable pre-formed moulded cases.

The custom of arranging instruments in sequence of usage, including a range of size options where appropriate, is extended to supplies for wards, clinics and community services, the configuration of all composite packs being agreed with end-users or representatives. The agreed design must facilitate the easy removal of residual air and the circulation of the sterilant.

A further design consideration is the weight of the finished product which should be within the European limits for lifting and handling.

The technique for wrapping open trays and composite packs based on a sterile field recognizes two alternatives known as the 'envelope fold' and the 'parcel fold'. Packaging must protect and prevent movement of the contents and be secured firmly to maintain microbial protection of the contents after sterilization.

Every service will include a range of specialized items such as micro-surgery instruments for ENT, ophthalmic, minimal access surgery procedures; orthopaedic surgery, radiological investigations, procedures using radioactive materials, and equipment for laser surgery. Such instruments may be owned by or loaned to the hospital. Manufacturers are obliged to provide information on recommended methods for cleaning, disinfecting and the sterilization of their products, and these recommendations must be followed to ensure functional efficiency. Inspection and function tests will precede assembly and packaging. All points and sharp edges must be protected against possible damage. The order or configuration of the items may be indicated by a pre-formed tray or container supplied with the goods. Whatever the packaging method, sufficient space must be allowed for the free circulation of the sterilant. When the assembled items have been checked, documented, the packaging secured and labelling completed, the pack or tray may be sterilized.

Heat-sensitive items may be packed in trays or packs for processing by ethylene oxide or low-temperature steam and formaldehyde. Individual items may be packed in sheet sterilization paper, bags or 'see-through' sterilization packaging. Dedicated sterilization process indicators should be included with the contents and also applied to the outer packaging.

Other low-temperature processes such as gas plasma require specific packaging materials which will be indicated by the sterilizer manufacturer.

The hospital-based department is able to obtain and supply in sterile form the specialized dressings and medical sundries needed in small quantities required by specialized users, e.g. organ transplant units and researchers. Such items are outside the scope of commercial suppliers of procedure packs and supplementary items. Multiples of the same item may be placed, for convenience during further processing and transport, in transit bags or boxes.

Many supplies for wards and clinics can be packed in gussetted bags made from sterilization paper; these are closed by turning down the top of the bag three times and securing with process indicator tape. The same range of bag sizes is available with an adhesive band crossing the top of the bag. This, when passed between the heated jaws of a sealing machine will be crimped to form a durable seal. The specification for these bags includes a chemical process indicator. For items requiring easy recognition, reels and pouches are available with a sterilization paper backing with printed process indicator and a clear-front film enabling the contents to be seen. This packaging can be closed by turning over the top edge and closing with tape, or alternatively it can be heat-sealed.

3.8 THE TERMINAL PROCESS

Packed items are loaded for sterilization – the majority by steam under pressure. To be fully effective and economical, loads must make the best use of available space without overcrowding or compression. Both the design configuration of individual items and their loading pattern must permit the unhindered movement of air and steam. Crowding will compromise effective processing, including the flashing off of water vapour at the end of the cycle.

Heat- or pressure-sensitive items should be processed using either low-temperature steam and formaldehyde gas or ethylene oxide. Both processes are monitored by biological indicators included with the load and subsequently cultured, which delays the return of items to users. Both processes are subject to Health and Safety at Work limits to environmental pollution which must be monitored. Other low-temperature processes, e.g. gas plasma, are being evaluated as possible useful alternatives.

3.9 ACCEPTANCE OF THE LOAD

The processed load when removed from the steam sterilizer will be hot. Flexible wrappings will be vulnerable to damage until cool. All stock will be subject to 'acceptance of load' procedures including examination of the print-out, or trace for the specific sterilizer cycle to ensure compliance with expected norms of time, temperature and pressure. Checks should be made to ensure that all packaging is secure, undamaged and dry; that labels and indicators correctly identify the item's content, sterilization cycle and process; and that the user destination is clearly marked.

When these checks are complete, items are placed on racks to cool before despatch to users in closed trolleys or containers. Additional protection can be added to goods travelling by an outside route by adding (when cold) paper or plastic transit (or dust) covers.

3.10   SHELF LIFE

Packaging materials conforming to EN 868, together with packaging techniques correctly executed, will ensure that undamaged goods stored away from direct sunlight in well-ventilated conditions on shelving above ground level will maintain the microbial integrity of the contents.

3.11   SUMMARY

The range of commercially manufactured packs and single items is expanding and changing to meet consumer demand and accommodate new technologies. Hospital-based departments can concentrate their productive effort on the re-processing of re-usable instruments and equipment returned after patient use. The Sterile Services Department has the capability of effectively decontaminating items and other device-related risks sent to it thereby preventing potential infection risks affecting others.

The user should discuss with the Sterile Services Manager and Infection Control Team the methods for processing medical devices before purchase.

3.12   FURTHER READING

Ayliffe, G.A.J., Coates, D. and Hoffman, P.N. (1993) *Chemical Disinfection in Hospitals.* Public Health Laboratory Service, London.

Ayliffe, G.A.J., Babb, J.R. and Taylor, L.J. (1999) *Hospital-acquired Infection. Principles and Prevention.* 3rd edition, Butterworth, Oxford.

Ayliffe, G.A., Fraise, A.P., Geddes, A.M. and Mitchell, K. (2000) *Control of Hospital Infection. A Practical Handbook,* 4th edition. Chapman & Hall, London.

Babb, J.R. and Bradley, C.R. (2001) Choosing instrument disinfectants and processors. *Brit. J. Infect. Control.* **2**, 10–13.

British Society of Gastroenterology (1998) Working Party Report. Cleaning and disinfection of equipment for gastrointestinal endoscopy, Gut, **42**, 585–593.

BS. EN. 868, Parts 4–11. *Packaging materials for sterilization.* British Standards Institute, London.

BS EN 46002. *Application of EN 29002 (BS 5750) to the manufacture of medical devices.* British Standards Institute, London.

Department of Health (1994) *Hospital Technical Memorandum (HTM) 2010. Sterilization, 4 parts.* HMSO, London.

Department of Health, Medical Devices Agency (1996) *Sterilization, Disinfection and Cleaning of Medical Equipment.* Guidance on decontamination from the Microbiological Advisory Committee, Department of Health, London.

Department of Health, Medical Devices Agency (1996) *Decontamination of endoscopes.* Department of Health, London.

Department of Health, Medical Devices Agency SN (1999) 32, Sept 1999. *Storage of Medical Devices.*

Department of Health, Medical Devices Agency (2000) 04. *Implications and Consequences of Reuse.*

Institute of Sterile Services Management Standards and Practices for Sterile Services Personnel. MAT Working Party Report (2000) Decontamination of minimally invasive surgical endoscopes and accessories. *J. Hosp. Infect,* **45**, 263–277.

NHS Executive (1999) Variant Creutzfeld-Jacob disease (VCJD). Minimising the use of transmission. NHS Executive London.

Russell, A.D., Hugo, W.B. and Ayliffe, G.A.J. (eds) (1999) *Principles and Practice of Disinfection, Preservation and Sterilization,* 3rd edition, Blackwell Scientific Publications, Oxford.

Isolation strategies for containment of infection and protective isolation

P.N. HOFFMAN AND B.D. COOKSON

4.1 INTRODUCTION

Isolation of patients can be divided functionally into two broad headings: **source** isolation; and **protective** isolation. The objective of source isolation is to prevent the transmission of an infection, proven or suspected, from a particular patient to other patients. The objective of protective isolation is to prevent infectious disease developing in an unusually susceptible patient.

Source isolation is the more common of the two types. The segregation of people with infections to prevent their spread has a long history – the stigma associated with the isolation of lepers and plague sufferers is apparent throughout the ages. However, it was not until the 1940s that the 'barrier' precautions established in the infectious fever hospitals were applied to the general hospital setting. The past 50 years has seen several revisions to the approaches used, these having been informed by improvements in the understanding of the epidemiology of the spread of pathogens in the hospital environment.

4.2 SOURCE ISOLATION

Guidelines for infection containment have been published by the Centers for Disease Control and Prevention

(CDC) in Atlanta, USA. These guidelines have, as far as possible, used an evidence-based approach, but the amount of evidence for much of what is advocated is surprisingly slim. More recently there has been an increased emphasis on the local adaptation of guidelines based on risk assessment, resources, infection occurrence and healthcare workers' views.

The prevention of transmission of a particular infectious agent depends on blocking the specific routes by which its transmission is effected (an example of this is given in Table 4.1). Taken to a logical conclusion, this results in each infectious agent having its own isolation requirements – referred to as *disease-specific isolation precautions*. The logic of this approach results in a multiplicity of sets of requirements which in practice are complex for wards to adhere to. In addition, there is the complication that – for a significant time period – isolation precautions have to be established on the basis of symptoms and suspicion rather than diagnosis. However, the various modes of spread can be persuaded to fall into a small series of categories, such as the 1983 CDC classification in which there are seven *category-specific isolation precautions*. These are listed in Table 4.2 and comprise: *strict, contact, respiratory, tuberculosis, enteric, drainage/secretion* and *blood/body fluids* isolation categories. These have some pragmatic advantages: isolation is effected on the basis of symptoms before a confirmed diagnosis, and there is also the likelihood of increased compliance as

Table 4.1 *Disease Transmission Modes. The probable modes of spread of some infections relevant in hospitals*

Infection	Transmission routes			
	Hands/instruments	Air	Faecal–oral	Blood (percutaneous)
*Aspergillus**		X		
Campylobacter	X		X	
Candida	X			
Clostridium difficile	X		X	
Cryptosporidium	X		X	
Diphtheria	X	X		
E. coli (enteropathogenic)	X		X	
Hepatitis A	X		X	
Hepatitis B/C	X			X
Herpes simplex	X			
HIV				X
Influenza	X	X		
*Legionella**		X		
Listeria (neonatal)	X			
Measles	X	X		
Meningitis (meningococcal)	X	X		
Meningitis (viral)	X	(?)	X	
Mumps	X	X		
Pertussis	X	X		
Q fever	X	X	X	
Respiratory syncitial virus	X	X		
Rubella	X	X		
Salmonella	X		X	
Shigella	X		X	
Scabies (crusted)	X	X		
Staphylococci	X	X		
Streptococci	X	X		
Tuberculosis (open)		X		
Varicella-zoster virus	X	X		

*From environment, not patient-to-patient.
(Based on the approach used by Ayliffe, G.A.J., Lowbury, E.J.L., Geddes, A.M. and Williams, J.D. (1992) *Infection Control; A Practical Handbook*, 3rd edition. Chapman & Hall, London. ISBN 0412284405)

ward staff have to familiarize themselves with fewer isolation categories than the disease-specific approach.

Whatever the approach adopted, the principles remain the same. The processes comprising isolation of infectious diseases can be classified under several subheadings: **administrative controls, isolation strategies, handwashing, personal protective equipment** and **isolation procedures**. All of these have to be considered in the decision-making process for appropriate isolation of particular diseases in particular patients or categories of patient (see Table 4.2).

4.2.1 Administrative Controls

Having an ideal set of isolation policies will be of no use if they are not put into effect when required. The term **administrative controls** covers when and how patients should be isolated, including local isolation policies and procedures. These will cover the forms of isolation that symptoms or diagnoses should elicit, and when that isolation need no longer apply to a particular patient. There must be systems in place which ensure that all the relevant healthcare workers are involved in the design,

Table 4.2 *Isolation categories*

Requirement	Isolation category						
	A	B	C	D	E	F	G
Own room	Yes	Yes	Yes	Under negative pressure	+/−	No	No
Handwashing	Yes	Yes	Yes	Yes	Yes	Yes	Yes
Gloves	Yes	+/−	+/−	+/−	Yes	+/−	Yes
Gowns	Yes	+/−	No	+/−	+/−	+/−	+/−
Masks	Yes	+/−	+/−	+/−	No	No	No
Waste/equipment*	Yes	Yes	Yes	Yes	Yes	Yes	Yes

Yes: necessary; No: not required; +/−: optional or if direct patient contact.
*Special decontamination for reusable equipment.

Isolation categories and important examples of organisms:

A Strict isolation: disseminated varicella-zoster, pneumonic plague, haemorrhagic fevers (these also need negative-pressure isolation).

B Contact isolation: rubella, disseminated herpes, cutaneous diphtheria, antibiotic-resistant organisms such as MRSA and *Klebsiella* spp.

C Respiratory isolation: measles, mumps, pertussis, meningococcal meningitis and invasive disease, pneumococcal meningitis.

D Tuberculosis: Negative-pressure isolation, particularly if known or suspected to be multiply drug-resistant, also for haemorrhagic fevers.

E Enteric precautions: *Salmonella*, O157, hepatitis A and other infectious gastrointestinal diseases.

F Drainage and secretion precautions: any other infections producing such fluid not included in the other categories.

G Blood or body fluid, e.g. hepatitis B, C and HIV, leptospirosis, malaria.

(Based on the approach used in Meers, P., MacPherson, M. and Sedgewick, J. (1997) *Infection Control in Healthcare*. Stanley Thornes, Cheltenham. ISBN 0 7487 3318 3)

review and audit of these policies and procedures. This will determine compliance and the success (or otherwise) of outbreak prevention.

4.2.2 Isolation Strategies

ISOLATION ON A WARD

In this category of isolation, procedures and personal protective equipment (gloves, aprons, etc.) can be used to prevent disease transmission from one (source) patient to other (susceptible) patients. This is often referred to as 'barrier nursing' and is usually reserved for the less transmissible infectious diseases – diseases where either excretion of organisms is not great, can be controlled, or a large microbial inoculum is required to produce an infection. For example, if a patient develops mild, controlled diarrhoea, they would not normally be moved to a sideroom. Infection control precautions will centre around the use of *gloves* and *aprons*, along with hygienic procedures such as *handwashing*. These precautions form a useful, universal level of basic infection control precautions for routine use. Such isolation on the ward requires both trained and competent ward staff and a compliant, controlled patient. If the patient has a tendency to wander, is confused, uncooperative or can disperse bacteria or viruses whilst remaining stationary (for example, has uncontrolled diarrhoea or projectile vomiting), then isolation on the ward may not be appropriate.

ISOLATION IN A WARD SIDEROOM

Isolation of patients with transmissible infections in a ward sideroom is desirable from several management aspects, mainly: (i) in encouraging staff to adhere to the same infection control precautions used on an open ward; (ii) in helping to restrict mobile patients; and (iii) in physically restricting gross dispersion via faecal incontinence, uncontrollable vomiting or dispersion of contaminated skin scales.

Space tends to be at less of a premium in a sideroom than on an open ward, so there is more likely to be a point for provision and disposal of gloves and aprons by the room entrance, and a convenient handwash basin, than in an open ward. The presence of an anteroom, although not essential, is generally thought to help staff compliance with isolation procedures.

COHORTING ON A WARD

In outbreak situations, when the number of patients requiring isolation exceeds available siderooms, one can consider the cohorting of affected patients in a section of open ward (preferably a defined area such as a bay). The term implies that the nursing staff are 'dedicated' to treat solely these patients. In another form of this strategy, certain nursing staff perform close contact procedures on affected patients (e.g. wound dressings, tracheal suction) and are only allowed to perform procedures not requiring direct contact on unaffected patients, e.g. administrative procedures. This approach is sometimes referred to as *targeted nursing*. Staff adherence to isolation precautions is vital. Elderly-care patients become confused in siderooms and may do better cohorted in four- or six-bedded bays. The use of a sliding door to the bay area is sometimes successful for controlling their wandering to other ward areas.

ISOLATION WARDS

The other option in outbreak situations is physically to separate those with and without infection in different wards. This option offers superior separation, but at the costs of higher staffing and rendering the ward used unavailable for other purposes until the number of patients remaining who still require isolation is sufficiently low that they can be moved to conventional siderooms. It is conventional to move patients with the infection from their resident ward to the isolation ward, rather than to move non-infected patients, but both approaches are feasible.

NEGATIVE-PRESSURE ISOLATION

Accommodating a patient with untreated open tuberculosis in an isolation room under negative pressure is advisable. The consequences of failing to do so may be catastrophic if the organism is multiply antibiotic-resistant, especially if other patients on the ward are immunocompromized (e.g. with HIV) and thus highly susceptible to infection. In such accommodation, air is discharged from the room to the outside causing the air in adjacent ward areas to flow into the room. Thus, air with entrained infectious particles is kept away from susceptible patients. An anteroom or lobby, although not essential, is a convenient area to don and dispose of gloves and other personal protective equipment, and to wash hands. A bathroom and toilet integral to the room is essential. An indicator of the pressure differential between the room and the anteroom or ward should be in place to show continuously that the room is under negative pressure and staff must be properly instructed in reading and recording the results. The experience of the authors and others has shown that, whilst some rooms may be labelled 'negative pressure' and may indeed once have been so, it is not unusual for them to be at positive pressure, totally defeating their intended purpose. Air in these areas does not normally have to undergo filtration either as it is supplied or extracted. Such rooms will normally have around 15 air changes per hour. Whether this provides sufficient dilution of air-borne respiratory pathogens to ensure the safety of staff and visitors inside the room is probable, but unproven. Some centres advocate the use of filtering facemasks by staff and visitors (particularly if immuno-compromized) when inside the room.

PATIENT PSYCHOLOGY

A much neglected area has been the involvement of patients in the containment process. Patients can play a role in reminding hard-pressed staff that they should wash their hands before and after patient contact. Patients, and indeed their friends and relatives, should be given appropriate literature, explanations and opportunities to discuss their questions, feelings and fears. There should be a culture within the hospital which encourages patients to question and to be confident that their quality of care will not suffer as a result of carrying a particular pathogen or as a result of asking questions or reminding staff to comply with infection control policies.

4.2.3 Hand hygiene

The microorganisms found on skin can be divided into two categories: *resident* and *transient* organisms. Resident organisms are those which have skin as their habitat – they are present superficially but also more deeply in the sebaceous and other glands and hair follicles of the skin, and cannot be removed completely by any skin disinfection process.

Transient organisms do not have skin as their natural habitat, can be acquired by touch, are superficially located, and can be removed readily by simple handwashing.

The function of **handwashing** in isolation is to remove the 'transient' contaminants acquired directly or indirectly from the patient. It does not require disinfectant soap (as used in surgical scrubs), which acts against the 'resident' microbial microflora of the hands and can be poorly accepted by some users. A soap or detergent that is cosmetically acceptable to staff is preferable, as are good quality single-use hand-drying paper towels. Convenient and frequent positioning of handwashing sinks greatly enhances compliance. Alcohol, usually around 70% isopropanol or ethanol (with or without additional microbicides) used as a handrub can be a convenient substitute for handwashing, but is poor at penetration of organic matter, so where there is obvious soiling of hands, handwashing is essential. Such handrubs can be accomplished more rapidly than a water-based wash and the alcohol containers can be placed around a ward, for instance on bedside lockers or on infant incubators, more frequently than handwash basins would be found.

4.2.4 Personal Protective Equipment (PPE)

The use of PPE should never be the sole strategy for isolation, but can be useful in addition to other measures. PPE includes the use of gloves, aprons and masks. Their sheer visibility has perhaps resulted in a higher position in the safety hierarchies of the strategies brought into play to prevent transmission of infectious disease in hospitals. However, PPE can be amongst the most fallible of these strategies: gloves are prone to develop holes, are easily penetrated by sharps, and they may not be changed or removed when appropriate – increasing rather than decreasing transmission. Aprons are readily pushed aside or torn during close-contact procedures such as lifting a patient; filter masks will allow air to leak in around the edge and can become dislodged during use.

GLOVES

Staff hands have long been acknowledged (since Oliver Wendell Holmes and Ignaz Semmelweiss in the mid-19th century) as potent vectors of infection. Gloves should be made of a good quality latex with a long cuff to protect the wrist and lower forearm, and must be used correctly or they will be ineffective. Thus, they should be donned for contact with contaminated items such as a used bed-pan or soiled bedclothing, and removed as soon as possible thereafter. They should not be used to touch any other items such as handles or telephones. The use of gloves does not remove the need for handwashing, as hands can become covertly contaminated though the pinholes which gloves frequently develop, or by inadvertent contact between the hand and outer surface of gloves after their removal.

Allergies to latex proteins carried on starch particles amongst healthcare staff are increasing, coincidental with increased glove usage. Symptoms are often respiratory, and sufferers can be affected by other peoples' glove-use as much as their own. In view of this problem non-starched gloves, or **hypoallergenic gloves** that have been washed thoroughly during manufacture before starch application, are recommended. Alternatives to latex are being sought.

APRONS AND GOWNS

Single-use plastic aprons will protect staff clothes from contamination by contact during activities such as lifting a patient or changing bedclothes. Obviously they can only protect the areas covered and usually exclude the shoulders, forearms and back, and can be pushed aside easily or torn. Fabric gowns offer greater all-round protection, but are more cumbersome and expensive and hotter.

FILTER MASKS

Traditional surgical masks do not provide an adequate degree of filter protection. Filter masks have a possible role for the protection of staff from some of the infectious diseases more highly transmissible by the respiratory route. They may have a use for staff and visitors when in the negative-pressure rooms of patients dispersing respiratory pathogens such as multiply drug-resistant tuberculosis (MDRTB). However, there will always be some leakage of unfiltered air through gaps between the mask and face.

Their use is not necessary for procedures on patients affected by methicillin-resistant *Staphylococcus aureus* (MRSA) and other antibiotic-resistant organisms for procedures likely to generate aerosols, such as tracheal suction and wound irrigation.

FACE PROTECTION

Protective eyewear (glasses or visor) is necessary only if there is a possibility of splashing of body fluid to the eyes or face. Half-masks of the surgical type can be used to provide protection of mouth and nose against splashing in conjunction with eye-protective glasses. This combination accomplishes as protective an effect as the less comfortable full-face visors which are often perceived as having too 'industrial' an image in the hospital ward setting.

4.3   ISOLATION PROCEDURES

CLINICAL WASTE

A patient in isolation will generate clinical waste in three categories: (i) **used dressings** and **blood-stained articles**; (ii) **used sharps**; and (iii) **urine, faeces** and **their containers**. The first category of waste should be placed in yellow clinical waste sacks destined for incineration. The second category, used sharps, offers the highest infection potential of clinical waste. They must be placed into sharps containers by the user immediately after use and will also be disposed of by incineration. Urine and faeces can be disposed of to the public sewer system, as can their containers if single use, via a macerator. The macerator must be checked regularly for leaks in the lidseal that may allow emission of aerosols from the maceration chamber. If reusable, bed-pans and urinals, together with their contents, must be placed into a bedpan/urinal washer-pasteurizer. This will flush the contents to the sewer and clean adherent soil from the item. They must include – usually as the final rinse – a stage where the minimum surface temperature of all items is either 80°C for at least 1 minute or 90°C momentarily. For both macerators and washer-pasteurizers, it is important that bed-pans and urinals are not left lying around but are processed promptly.

LAUNDRY

Treatment of laundry generated by patients in isolation need only differ from other laundry if it presents a particular risk to either the hospital staff who transport it or the laundry staff who may come into contact with it during linen sorting or washing machine maintenance. This category of linen is called, somewhat misleadingly, 'infected' linen. It comes from patients with proven or suspected enteric fever, other *Salmonella* infections, *Shigella*, hepatitis A, B or C, HIV, open tuberculosis and other readily transmitted infectious diseases. A local policy can formulate a list of organisms considered relevant, but this should be done using the same rationale as in the list above. 'Infected' linen must be placed in red bags that are either water-soluble or have water-soluble stitching and so can be loaded into washing machines without further handling. Linen containing liquid that may escape from normal laundry bags should be placed in normal linen bags (usually coloured white) with an impervious inner lining. Linen from known or suspected viral haemorrhagic fever patients must be steam-sterilized within the isolation unit before being sent for laundering.

EQUIPMENT DECONTAMINATION

Wherever possible, a patient in isolation should have dedicated equipment not shared with those outside isolation. Where this is not possible, thorough washing of items that come into contact with intact skin should be adequate. If an item has contact with mucous membranes, such as thermometers or laryngoscopes, some form of heat or chemical disinfection is appropriate; steam sterilization is ideal, but cannot be used for some items, e.g. thermometers.

4.4 PROTECTIVE ISOLATION

This is the opposite of source isolation and comprises the protection of patients unusually vulnerable to infection, such as the neutropaenic, or bone marrow and liver transplant patients. These patients are at risk of infection both by pathogens commonly causing infection in hospitals and, more problematically, by common organisms not noted for their pathogenicity. The sources of these organisms can be within the patient (see Chapter 10) or acquired from their environment, principally by inhalation and ingestion. Uncooked foods such as salads or most cheeses should be avoided; freshly and completely cooked food being safest. Present-day infection risks are far lower than in the early days of transplantation and cytotoxic therapy, as levels and duration of immunosuppression are less profound and of shorter duration. However, infection of the lungs with *Aspergillus fumigatus* derived from the air is often a problem. Inhalation of fungal spores normally present in the air can only be prevented from transmission through high-efficiency particulate air (HEPA) filters and ensuring that the only air present in patient rooms has been thus treated. This is achieved by supplying filtered air to the room under positive pressure, i.e. the isolation room is at a higher pressure to its surroundings so that air flows outwards, excluding ingress of contaminated air. As with negative-pressure rooms (see above), a pressure differential indicator should be in place to show that the room is under positive pressure, and staff instructed in its reading and recording the results. Other normal infection control precautions to block transmission must be strictly enforced to protect the susceptible patient. No special precautions for laundry or clinical waste are necessary.

4.5 INFECTIOUS CASES IN THE OPERATING THEATRE

Surgical procedures breach the skin and mucous membranes – the most effective barriers against infection – and may further compromise host defences with the implantation of foreign materials (cardiac pacemakers, orthopaedic prostheses and even stitches can reduce the bacterial inoculum required to initiate infection). It is thus essential that precautions are taken to prevent infection acquired in the theatre. The two most relevant sources are from the patient's own microflora (e.g. skin and gut) and from dispersed contaminated microscopic skin fragments ('skin scales') from staff in the theatre. Concerns also exist about air-borne transmission from infected or contaminated patients to those operated on subsequently. However, the rate of air changes normally found in operating theatres are such that air-borne contamination will be reduced to less than 1% of that originally present in about 15 minutes. So, in a properly ventilated theatre, the risk of infection transmission from patient to patient is more likely to occur via improperly decontaminated instruments than via the air.

4.6 DISPOSAL OF THE DEAD

In general, any risk of infectious disease transmission from the dead is less than that from the living. Imposition of unnecessary and intrusive barriers can interfere with the grieving processes of those close to the deceased. Nevertheless, in death, as in life, precautions to prevent transmission of disease can be relevant; these have been reviewed comprehensively elsewhere.

4.7 FURTHER READING

Garner, J.S. (1996) Hospital Infection Control Practices Advisory Committee. Guideline for isolation precautions in hospitals. *Infection Control and Hospital Epidemiology*, **17**, 53–80, and *American Journal of Infection Control*, **24**, 24–52.

Garner, J.S. and Simmons, B.P. (1983) CDC guidelines for isolation precautions in hospitals. *Infection Control*, **4**, 245–325.

Hannan, M.M., Azadian, B.A., Gazzard, B.G., Hawkins, D.A. and Hoffman, P.N. (2000) Hospital infection control in an era of HIV infection and multi-drug resistant tuberculosis. *Journal of Hospital Infection*, **44**, 5–11.

Healing, T.D., Hoffman, P.N. and Young, S.E.J. (1995) *CDR Review*, **5**, R61–R68.

Teare, E.L., Stone, S. and Cookson, B. (2001) On behalf of the Hand Hygiene Liaison Group. Hand Hygiene. *British Medical Journal*, **323**, 411–412.

5

Risk factors for infection and sepsis

E.W. TAYLOR

5.1 INTRODUCTION

Infection remains the most common postoperative complication after almost all forms of surgery. Many patients admitted to hospital as emergencies have infective pathology such as acute appendicitis, peritonitis and empyema. These patients already have infection, and the surgical intervention and antibiotic therapy are aimed at curing that pathology. However, many patients come into hospital for elective surgical treatment of non-infective pathology and are at risk of surgical wound and other nosocomial infections. These include pneumonia and urinary tract infections, as well as intra-abdominal infections, septicaemia and, ultimately, the risk of systemic inflammatory response syndrome and multiple organ dysfunction leading to death. It has been estimated that 10% of patients entering hospital develop one or more nosocomial infection. Infection costs hospitals a great deal of money, principally because of the additional bed days but also because of further surgical intervention, antibiotic and other pharmacy costs and laboratory and X-ray costs to investigate the infection.

Patients now stay in hospital a considerably shorter length of time after elective surgery than they did in the past. Many procedures are now undertaken as day cases, and it is easy for the surgeon to be unaware that these patients develop infections which present later in the community. From 40–60% of postoperative surgical wound infections present in, and are treated in, the community. It is only by careful continued surveillance once the patient has gone home that such infections are accurately audited. The problems of determining the true inci-

dence of infection are compounded in patients in whom prosthetic implants are inserted and in whom surveillance might need to continue for a year before the true incidence of infection can be determined.

This chapter will review the risk factors for infection postoperatively, and also examine the factors that determine which patients go on to develop systemic sepsis, multiple organ failure.

5.2 DEFINITIONS

5.2.1 Infection

Infection is the invasion and multiplication of micro-organisms in body tissues which may be clinically inapparent, or result in local cellular injury because of competitive metabolism, toxins, intracellular replication or antigen – antibody response.

The ancients described infection as having the characteristics of *dolor, rubor, color, tumor et functio laessa* – that is pain, redness, heat, swelling and loss of function. These characteristics remain applicable to soft tissue and joint infection but may no longer be adequate to define infection of the parietes such as meningitis, pneumonia, peritonitis, etc., or postoperative periprosthetic infection.

A **wound infection** should have a **purulent discharge** or **spreading erythema** indicative of cellulitis, but it is important to realize that this may be **primary**, or **secondary** to some other underlying complication. A wound infection should be diagnosed principally on clinical grounds, and microbiology should support the diagnosis but not define it. It is important to realize that infection is only one form of complication that can occur to a wound. Dehiscence may occur because of infection, but may equally occur because of breakage of the suture used to close the wound, or of the sutures or skin clips being taken out too soon, or of sutures cutting out of tissues, etc. Similarly, patients who have an underlying anastomotic dehiscence with leak of gastric, pancreatic, intestinal or faecal material, and patients who have urinary or biliary leaks underlying their wounds, will develop a wound infection though this is really secondary to the underlying complication.

Many patients come into hospital with infective pathology, and this **community-acquired infection** must be distinguished from **hospital-acquired** or **nosocomial infection**. Infection appearing 72 hours after admission or in a patient readmitted with active infection that results from an earlier hospital admission should be classified as primary nosocomial infection.

5.2.2 Bacteraemia

Bacteraemia is a transient condition in which bacteria are released into the bloodstream from an infected or contaminated focus. This may occur transiently following insertion of a urethral catheter, drainage of an abscess, or even during the cleaning of teeth. It is usually of no great significance as the bacteria are rapidly removed by the recticuloendothelial system, ingested by macrophages and destroyed. However, bacteraemia may become significant if the bacteria lodge on a damaged heart valve or recently implanted prosthesis, cardiac pacemaker, etc., in which case the bacteria may seed at this site and create infection.

5.2.3 Septicaemia

This is a more significant and serious condition to which the term **sepsis** may more accurately be applied. Septicaemia is diagnosed if rigors occur together with one or more of the following signs: **fever** >38°C on more than one occasion within a 24-hour period, **hypotension** and **oliguria**. Rigor may not be detected if the patient is under sedation or paralysed and receiving artificial ventilation, or it simply may not be noticed by the nursing attendants. Laboratory confirmation of viable microorganisms (bacteraemia) or their products such as endo- and exotoxins, antigens or antibodies in the blood is desirable, but should not be essential to make the diagnosis.

5.2.4 Systemic Inflammatory Response Syndrome (SIRS)

This term has been used to describe the generic inflammatory response triggered by a variety of infective and non-infective events. SIRS is defined by the presence of two or more of the following signs:

- body temperature >38°C or <36°C;
- pulse >90 beats/minute;
- a respiratory rate >20 breaths/minute;
- Pa_{CO_2} <32 mmHg; and
- a white cell count >12 000 or <4000 per mm³.

This condition may lead to adult respiratory distress syndrome (ARDS), renal, hepatic, cardiac, gastrointestinal or cerebral failure summated in the condition known as **multiple organ failure** (MOF).

Shock is associated with ARDS and MOF. Shock is defined as an oxygen consumption (V_{O_2}) inadequate to meet peripheral tissue oxygen demands and a low V_{O_2} early after injury predicts both MOF and death. A low V_{O_2} is the result of not being able to achieve an early hyperdynamic state (cardiac index > $4.5\, l\, min^{-1}\, m^{-2}$). This is most consistently shown by a low gastric intermucosal pH reflecting splanchnic hypoperfusion, whereas other measurements of haemodynamics are less reliable.

Four stages of increasing severity have been identified: (i) SIRS; (ii) sepsis; (iii) severe sepsis; and (iv) septic shock. SIRS, as defined above, may not have an infective origin but is described as **sepsis** when there is. Severe sepsis is SIRS with developing organ failure, and septic shock when this is further complicated by hypotension.

5.3 RISK FACTORS FOR INFECTION

There are three major sources of risk factors related to the development of a postoperative wound infection: (i) bacterial contamination; (ii) the surgical wound; and (iii) the host resistance or immunocompetence of the patient.

5.3.1 Bacterial contamination

The body's tissues can normally cope with bacterial contamination up to 10^5 organisms per gram of tissue before infection occurs. Bacterial contamination may be either **exogenous**, that is, the organisms gain access to the tissues from the environment, healthcare workers, contaminated equipment or other sources outwith the patient's body: or it is **endogenous**, that is, the organisms which contaminate the wound are already present in or on the patient's body.

5.3.2 Exogenous risk factors: preparation of theatre staff

THEATRE ENVIRONMENT

The ventilation in the operating theatre should provide a near-sterile environment for the operation to be undertaken, and one in which it is comfortable for the surgical team to work. In addition, anaesthetic gases should be removed. Most operating theatres now have a filtered air system in which the air is passed through high-efficiency particulate air (HEPA) filters; these ensure that less than one *Staphylococcus aureus* or *Clostridium* organism is present per cubic metre of air. In addition, the rapid turnover of air (30 changes per hour) ensures that there are less than 35 bacteria-carrying particles (BCPs) per cubic meter of air circulating in the operating theatre. These data can be checked using a Casella filter, and this quality standard should be checked on initial commissioning of the operating theatre and whenever any major structural work is carried out in the theatre complex. The bacterial filters should be changed at standard intervals.

Bacteria-carrying particles are shed by the operating theatre team, and **movement within the operating theatre should be kept to a minimum**. The **number of staff** in the theatre should also be minimized.

STERILITY OF INSTRUMENTS

The **instruments** used to perform an operation, the linen, drapes, etc., should be autoclaved and sterile. Quality standards have been set and frequent checks should be made to ensure that the autoclave process meets these standards. All implants and disposable equipment used during the course of operations are now provided sterile in double-wrapped containers. The Trust purchasing these services and this equipment should ensure that the Providers meet the required standards.

Equipment used for **minimal access surgery**, such as laparoscopes, arthroscopes, etc., are now manufactured such that they can be autoclaved, and these pieces of equipment should be cleaned and then autoclaved before reuse.

DISINFECTION OF HANDS

In the 1860s Semmelweis operated using the 'chlorine covers' that he had developed for hygienic hand disinfection to prepare his hands for safer gynaecology, and hand disinfection has been in use ever since. Today, a 'belt and braces' approach is provided by covering the disinfected hands with gloves. However, as glove punctures can occur in up to 38% of operations (depending on the type of operation and type of glove), and up to 1000 bacterial cells may escape through a puncture, it seems reasonable to ensure optimal surgical hand disinfection before donning gloves (see also Chapter 2). Cruse and Foord showed that this mattered in real life when they found a clean wound infection rate of 1.7% to be increased to 5.7% when a glove puncture had been noted at operation.

The **skin flora** on the hands can be divided into two: (i) the more superficial 'transient' bacteria (often those recently picked up from the environment); and (ii) the permanent resident flora established in micro-colonies and spreading into hair follicles and pores. The transient flora is readily removed by washing with soap and water. However, the resident flora, which includes coagulase-negative staphylococci and some Gram-negative bacteria (especially *Acinetobacter* spp.) are less readily dislodged. Although *Staph. aureus* can be grown from the hands of ≥40% of healthcare workers on most occasions, this seems to be more the result of repeated contamination in the hospital environment, than a true 'residence' on the skin. As the main causes of postoperative infections in clean surgery are staphylococci, it seems reasonable to select hand-degerming agents with a predominantly anti-Gram-positive activity. The agents currently in use in the UK include chlorhexidine and povidone-iodine.

When choosing a suitable agent as an antibacterial, three properties might be considered: **immediate action**; **persistent action** (3 hours covers most operations); and **cumulative action**. Clearly, a good agent will have both rapid and persistent actions. The value of accumulation of the agent on the hands is less sure as it means that the effect would be variable, being least for example on a Monday morning. It might also result in destruction of the 'colonization resistance' provided by resident skin flora, allowing the possibility that more pathogenic microbes might become established. A fourth property is also very important, namely **user acceptability**. A combination of fair skin and prolonged exposure to UV radiation in summer means that Scandinavians are particularly prone to skin problems. Indeed, in a Nordic individual one chlorhexidine preparation actually caused an *increase* in skin flora due to the damage caused to the skin by its prolonged use. As a general comment it is almost impossible to find a single product that is acceptable to all theatre staff, and a choice should be available.

A double-blind controlled clinical trial comparing different surgical scrub preparations with wound infection as the marker is not practicable. Hands lend themselves to laboratory tests, and three approaches to testing hands after disinfection and wearing of gloves have been made. First, measurement of the bacteria found inside a glove juice after use by resuspending them in a recovery fluid (containing neutralizers for the antibacterial activity) which is also put into the glove and massaged around the fingers in a standard way (the glove juice method). Second, removal of the glove and sampling of the fingertips by kneading them in a recovery fluid. Third, by making impressions of the hand after the glove has been removed to test for bacteria and for residual antiseptic. In all cases both immediate and 3-hour testing is required so that the persistent effect is included in the test.

Figure 5.1 shows the relative effectiveness of different agents when tested by the fingertip kneading method. (The figure is reproduced by permission of

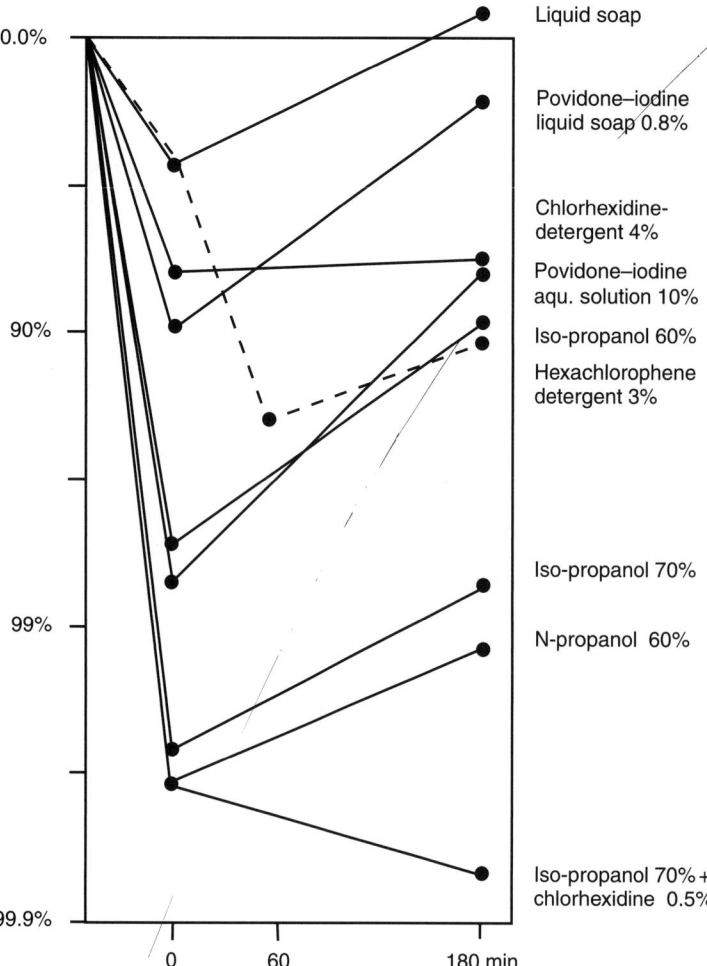

Figure 5.1 *The effect of different agents in reducing normal hand flora (expressed as percentage reduction) when tested using the method of Rotter, measured immediately after surgical hand disinfection, and after wearing gloves for three hours.*

Prof. M. Rotter, who first described this approach.) The relative strength of the different agents is well portrayed. Povidone-iodine/detergent scrub has good immediate activity, but by 3 hours most of this has worn off, and sampling at the end of longer operations may reveal bacterial multiplication on the hands. Interestingly, 10% aqueous povidone-iodine had a much better effect, possibly due to the increased concentration, and also absence of interference from the detergent. Chlorhexidine (4%) in detergent is slightly worse at immediate killing, but has a much more persistent effect (and a cumulative effect). Iso-propanol, an alcohol, if used at 70% concentration as a scrub is very effective, and iso-propanol containing 0.5% chlorhexidine is the best of all in that it has a good immediate effect followed by prolonged persistence. The other advantage of alcohol preparations is speed, in that a 1-minute 'scrub' time is all that is required compared to 3 (or even 5) minutes with detergent scrubs. However, problems may occur with flammability when alcoholic preparations are stored, and because of this *n*-propanol (which is slightly less flammable) is preferred in some countries. Furthermore, it is much easier to miss out part of the hands with an alcoholic preparation, which is usually colourless.

A practical approach to surgical hand disinfection would be to start the day by using a detergent scrub together with an orange stick to clean behind the nails, and then to use an alcoholic rub between operations. Keeping the fingers pointing upwards during the procedure is important, as it prevents re-contamination of the hands by water dripping down from the forearms.

A simple way to test the efficiency of any surgical scrub is to make an impression plate from the hands after an operation. Figure 5.2 shows an impression from a hand made on a 25 cm² square plate filled with a nutrient agar after using a chlorhexidine scrub for 3 minutes, then wearing a surgeon's glove for 1 hour. Subsequently, a similar impression is made on a plate which is then layered with a strain of *Staph. epidermidis* in agar to reveal any persistent antibacterial activity on the hands. In this way the effectiveness of the scrub is clearly portrayed.

GLOVES

Rubber gloves were first used earlier this century by Halstead to protect patients from the operator. Since

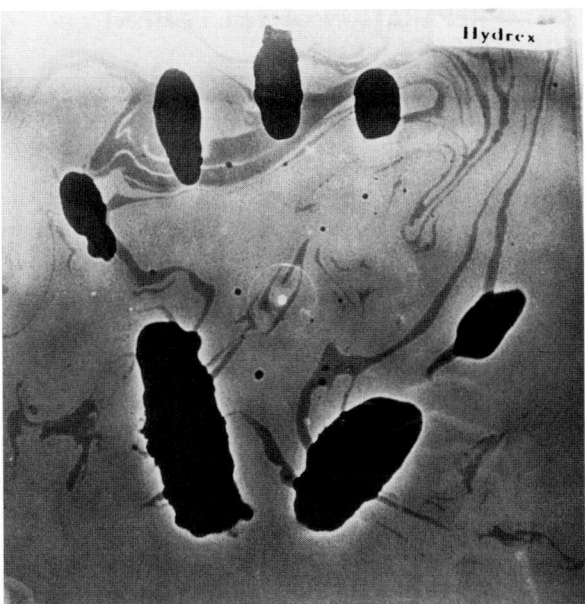

Figure 5.2 *Simple method of detecting antimicrobial activity on the hands. Hand print on 25 cm² agar plate seeded with a culture of* Staphylococcus aureus *after washing with chlorhexidine surgical scrub.*

then, advances in manufacture have led to thin latex gloves, which at first were donned with the aid of a talc or starch powder. However, worries about the formation of starch granulomas, and adhesions in abdominal surgery led many surgeons to use 'starch-free' gloves. In addition to this the widespread use of latex gloves throughout healthcare premises as part of 'Universal precautions' highlighted the problem of **latex allergy**. The allergens are the latex proteins, and in Finland 8% of theatre staff reacted to a latex skin test, compared with 0.8% of matched controls. The latex proteins can be adsorbed on to starch particles, and further studies have shown that inhalation of such particles can cause occupational asthma. Thus, the case for powder-free gloves is supported from several aspects.

Several alternative gloves are now available. **Powder-free gloves** require a 'slippery' coating to facilitate donning. Indeed, one such glove has a coating that includes cetylpyridinium chloride, a quaternary ammonium compound, which itself has antibacterial properties. Increased washing of the latex during manufacture results in gloves with a reduced load of latex proteins and accelerators, and several **'hypoallergenic' gloves** are now available. Washing itself has been associated with problems from contamination of gloves with endotoxin in the rinse water, so 'pure' water is required. Recent developments include gloves which are 'supersensitive', and gloves made from non-latex materials such as a synthetic elastomer designed for the allergic surgeon.

Double-gloving has also become common. This was originally used by orthopaedic surgeons for hip joint replacements, to reduce any danger to the patient from punctures, and to allow for easy removal of gloves coated with cement powder. However, a significant increased usage factor is now to protect the surgeon from contracting viral infection from the patients. Paradoxically, wearing a slightly smaller glove as the outer layer makes for more comfort. A recent development of double gloving is the use of a coloured 'marker' glove as an inner glove. Such 'Reveal' gloves outline in colour any ingress of fluid, so making punctures easy to discover.

THEATRE TEXTILES

This section includes comments on staff dress, patients drapes and instrument wraps (see also Chapter 3). The standard cotton surgeon's gown, although cheap, has many disadvantages in that it is not moisture-proof (allowing strike-through of blood) and has a wide weave which allows the wearer's skin bacteria to leak out. Indeed, a 'wick' effect may actually draw bacteria through the cloth. The bacteria are largely carried on skin scales, and as it is estimated that an average person sheds one layer of scales per day, there is a large potential for contamination.

Finally, the gowns are not robust, require inspection and mending, and will only survive a limited number of laundry cycles. To a lesser degree the same is true of the 'skin towels' used to drape patients.

Improved fabrics are now available made of non-woven synthetic fibres such as 'Gore-tex' or polyester. A 'Gore-tex' gown can completely abolish 'strikethrough' both of blood and bacteria, and also reduce the numbers of bacteria shed into the air by the wearer; in fact a 'Gore-tex jump-suit' almost completely stops spread of bacteria into the air, but is totally impractical. The current generation of polyester gowns is much more comfortable to wear, and should be cost-effective because of increased durability. Some have impervious panels in patient-contact areas, while others are made of the same material throughout and so are more robust. A similar material can be used for drapes, with the possibility of using adhesives to glue the drapes to the wound edges to prevent washing of the patient's skin bacteria into the wound. However, the use of plastic drapes has been shown to increase wound infection (Cruse and Foord).

The 1980s saw the use of disposable gowns, drapes and tray wraps made from paper. These create a certain amount of dust in the theatre, as well as a disposal problem (large volume of waste). The availability of better man-made fibre re-usable gowns, and of new re-usable materials that can block passage of bacteria for tray wraps, means that the use of paper should decrease. Laundry for re-usable drapes & gowns however is not without hazards. The occurrence of serious but sporadic infections with *Bacillus cereus* after neurosurgery was traced to the contamination of freshly laundered theatre linen. The problem lay in the type of commercial 'tunnel washer' used, in which the water was never properly changed, so that the laundry was rinsed with contaminated water at the end of the wash cycle. If a similar problem is suspected, a simple check is to take an impression of clean linen on to a contact plate; a growth of less than five colonies is regarded as acceptable.

The use of the new materials is logical, but difficult to substantiate in terms of wound infections. No entirely conclusive hard data exist; thus, reports suggesting a reduction in wound infection from 6.4% to 2.3% by the use of new materials are challenged by others showing no difference in the outcomes. Laboratory tests may help to settle the point. It is easy to show changes in dispersal of bacteria into the air, by comparing counts obtained using a slit sampler to measure particles liberated from a subject wearing 'test clothes' inside a 'body box' supplied with filtered air. This apparatus is difficult to come by, however, and a simpler approach is to assess the number of bacterial particles found in an operation wound before skin closure. Wound wash outs with sampling fluid are open to contamination and are messy; biopsies are needlessly invasive, and better samplers include a sterile velvet pad on a backing of silver foil, or a cotton swab. Bacteria are recovered by shaking these samplers in a recovery medium, which is passed through a membrane filter to provide a quantitative count. Using this approach the author found that the counts after cardiac surgery were reduced by 33% by the use of 'Goretex' gowns. An ingenious recent approach, that omits the need for a recovery medium (with possible fragmentation of bacteria containing particles, so leading to higher counts), is to make impressions of the wound using 47 mm-diameter 5 μm cellulose acetate/nitrate membranes. The membranes are then cultured directly on plates of medium containing β-lactamase (to neutralize any prophylactic antibiotics). Colonies are visualized by staining with tetrazolium, and then counted. Such methods help to support use of the new textiles; however, the comfort of the theatre staff remains a major factor in choice of gowns, especially during the long complex procedures which are now commonplace.

Masks come under the 'ritual' heading, as there is little evidence that wearing a mask reduces wound infection rates. The casual '**mask over the mouth**' approach, while stopping the surgeon from spitting into the wound, is actually unhelpful, because the greatest danger is from the staphylococci in the nose. These tend to remain *in-situ* unless the user has a cold, when a 'snort' can release large numbers into the air. However, the use of a mask does prevent the operator from being splashed by the patient's blood, and so for this reason they are likely to continue in use. An appreciable amount of blood may also hit the surgeon's forehead, and masks with clear upwards plastic extensions, or visors are recommended for use when operating on patients with HIV infection.

5.4 PREPARATION OF THE PATIENT FOR SURGERY

5.4.1 Introduction

This section includes general points, but specific details relating to different types of surgery will be found in the relevant chapters. Endogenous infection is much more common than infection from the theatre environment. The causative bacteria may be part of the patient's normal flora (e.g. *E. coli* and *Bacteroides fragilis* from the gut), or they may have been picked up in hospital (e.g. MRSA). Cruse and Foord showed clearly that the longer a patient spent in hospital before operation, the more likely they were to suffer a wound infection. Sometimes this is unavoidable because of serious illness (in itself a possible risk factor). Therefore the shortest possible preoperative stay is essential. The infection risks of both dirty and clean-contaminated surgery can be reduced by antibiotic prophylaxis, but good wound closure technique is very important. Frequently the lead surgeon will leave closure to an assistant, and 'wound closure' nurses have been used. Leaper noted that the wound should not be under tension, and that haemostasis is important, especially if obtained by tying off vessels rather than diathermy; a residual collection of blood is an excellent medium for bacteria. Wound healing is stimulated by hypoxia. The amount and type of suturing is important, and while skin clips have been associated with a reduced infection rate, skin tapes might be considered. Wound drains have been regarded by some as a risk factor for infection, but a recent 'Task Force Report' from the USA concluded that the use of drains was only weakly correlated with infection.

The use of special equipment has been associated with infections in the past, but this is usually countered by antibiotic chemoprophylaxis, again commenced as near the operation as possible (usually with the premedication), and often given as a single dose. Pre-existing infections, particularly of the skin, are also a risk factor for wound infections, and should be dealt with preoperatively if possible.

Infections such as HIV or hepatitis B present a risk to the theatre staff, but would also be a contraindication to transplant surgery where immunosuppression is used or where renal dialysis is required. Carriage of MRSA may also be a problem, especially where a patient is cared for as part of a cohort; for example in a transplant or renal programme, in which they may be a source for cross-infection to other patients. Preoperative screening may be required for such patients.

5.4.2 Preoperative skin preparation

Traditional preoperative shaving has been shown to do more harm than good if it is performed clumsily and/or an appreciable time before the operation, as it creates skin abrasions and allows time for bacterial multiplication. Contaminated shaving brushes have been a source of infections (for example *Pseudomonas* infection in neurosurgery). Hair removal can sometimes be avoided, but if necessary the use of clippers or depilatory creams have been shown to halve the rate of wound infections. If shaving is essential, it should be performed as near the operation time as possible. The number of bacteria on the patient's skin can be greatly reduced by use of showers taken preoperatively using an antiseptic scrub (e.g. chlorhexidine). However, a European study found no difference in the number of wound infections following this procedure.

The application of 0.5% alcoholic chlorhexidine to the patient's skin prior to the incision, kills all transient skin flora, and greatly reduces the number of resident flora, and so is commonly used. An alcoholic solution of povidone-iodine may be preferred for use when spore-bearing bacteria are likely to be present. Care must be taken to reduce the risks of fire or explosions if an alcoholic solution is used, and a diathermy spark can be hazardous.

MASKS

It has become traditional for masks to be worn in the operating theatre by all theatre staff. They are also frequently worn by ward staff for dressings, by midwives at delivery, by laboratory staff, and occasionally by community nurses when doing dressings in the patient's home. There is no evidence that wearing a mask reduces the incidence of postoperative infection in the operating theatre. If masks are to be worn they should be of the type which have a bacterial filter built into them, and fit closely round the mouth and nose. They should be changed after every operation, but this is probably only justified in ultraclean implant operative procedures (see also Chapters 1 and 3).

CAPS, GOWNS AND OVERSHOES

There is little evidence that wearing caps or gowns – and no evidence that wearing plastic overshoes – influences the incidence of postoperative infection. However, these have become part of the traditional rituals in many operating theatres and perhaps are important to ensure that all personnel working in that environment are aware of the special risk to which the patient is being put. Plastic overshoes do not influence the bacterial count of the theatre floor or postoperative infection, and simply putting them on and off may actually increase the incidence of infection by spreading bacteria from the shoes to the hands of the surgeon.

5.4.3 Endogenous risks: preparation of the patient

Man is host to some 10^{14} bacteria of 500 or more species. These organisms mainly reside in the gastrointestinal tract, but other important repositories are the genitourinary tract, the respiratory tract, the skin, and the antra and sinuses of the skull. Normally, we live symbiotically with these bacteria, which are important in the digestion of food and in preventing the colonization of our bodies by other, more pathogenic, species. It is this bacterial load that is brought to the operating table by each patient. Most (95%) postoperative wound infections are endogenous in origin, and much thought should be given to this area of preoperative preparation of the patient (see also Chapter 4).

SKIN PREPARATION

Before undertaking a surgical procedure it is important to try to reduce the bacterial load on the skin through which the incision is to be made. Clearly, it is important not to operate through an area of skin already infected but also distant skin infection, e.g. a boil on some other part of the body, has also been identified as a risk factor for surgical wound infection.

The skin should be prepared before incision, and suitable agents are those containing 60–80% alcohol (ethanol or isopropanol). These work rapidly and evaporate, leaving the skin dry. Iodine or chlorhexidine are added to prolong the antimicrobial effect and to help to identify (by coloration) which area of skin has been prepared. Skin preparation with flammable solutions must be carried out in a way that eliminates this risk.

Aqueous solutions are as effective and may be safer, but a longer time must be allowed for antimicrobial efficiency.

PREOPERATIVE SHAVING

It is customary to shave the surface of the body through which the incision is to be made. Previously, it was normal to shave a wide area around the incision site, but this is no longer considered necessary and may be positively harmful. The **skin should be prepared immediately preoperatively**, and not on the day prior to operation, as this has been shown to increase the risk of infection. This is because microscopic cuts of the skin caused during shaving become infected overnight, converting the clean area into an infected field through which the incision is made. Depilatory creams have been shown to be as effective as shaving in reducing the incidence of infection, but they are not popular with patients.

GASTROINTESTINAL TRACT PREPARATION

The upper gastrointestinal tract, particularly the stomach, is usually sterile in fit, healthy, people because of the acid secretion. However, in patients with gastric malignancy in which achlorhydria is common, bacterial colonization of the stomach is usual, and high bacterial loads may contaminate the tissue at the time of operation. This situation also occurs in patients taking H_2-receptor antagonists or proton-pump inhibitors to prevent peptic ulceration. Where ulcer surgery is performed, stopping these drugs 2–3 days preoperatively will help to sterilize the stomach.

In situations where the small bowel is obstructed, bacterial overgrowth of the luminal contents with faecal organisms rapidly occurs. In this situation, and also for elective colorectal surgery, great care must be taken to minimize contamination of the tissues with the luminal contents from the gastrointestinal tract.

It is normal practice for patients to be administered some form of bowel preparation before colonic and rectal operations where the surgery is for non-obstructive pathology. Whilst this reduces the total bacterial load it may not reduce the risk of infection, which remains high because of the bacterial colonization of the mucus on the colonic mucosa. It is usual practice in the USA for non-absorbable antibiotics to be given orally on the day before surgery to help reduce the bacterial load, but this should be in addition to systemic antibiotic prophylaxis. The value of preoperative oral antibiotics in this situation has been contested, but selective removal or reduction of Gram-negative aerobic bacilli may disturb the synergy known to occur between aerobic and anaerobic bacteria, which may lead to postoperative abscess formation.

WOUND DRESSINGS

The operative wound is sealed within a few hours; leaving the sutured wound exposed to the environment is not a risk factor for infection.

DURATION OF HOSPITALIZATION

Prolonged preoperative hospitalization remains a risk factor for infection. The organisms isolated within hospitals are frequently resistant to many antibiotics, whereas those in the community are sensitive. The longer the patient is in hospital preoperatively, the more likely they are to be colonized by antibiotic-resistant organisms, which increases the risk of infection.

5.4.4　Bacterial load

The number of bacteria contaminating the tissue is an important risk factor for infection. Normal tissue in a healthy adult can cope with a bacterial load of up to 10^5 organisms per gram of tissue, but above this level the risk of infection increases significantly. The influence that the degree of bacterial contamination has on the

risk of postoperative infection has been recognized in the **international classification of wounds** into: **clean**; **clean-contaminated**; **contaminated**; and **dirty**. It is important to realize that the classification of a wound is based on the pathology for which surgery is performed or the conduct of the operation, and not on the incidence of infection or other outcomes postoperatively.

- *Clean wounds:* these are wounds in which there is **no break in the aseptic technique** during surgery, no infection is encountered during the procedure, and no bacterially colonized tract of the body is opened. Such a classification would include operations such as thyroidectomy, varicose vein surgery, prosthetic implant procedures, etc.
- *Clean-contaminated wounds:* an operation would be considered clean-contaminated if one of the bacterially colonized tracts of the body was opened in a controlled fashion, or if there had been some **minor break in aseptic technique** during the operation. Operations in this category would include cholecystectomy, operations on the maxillary antra, gastrectomy, etc.
- *Contaminated wounds:* an operation would be considered contaminated if there had been greater or **uncontrolled spillage of luminal contents** of the gastrointestinal tract, if acute inflammation was encountered, or if the operation was for compound trauma operated upon within 4 hours of the event. Elective colorectal operations would normally fall into this category because of the high bacterial count within the lumen.
- *Dirty wounds:* this category would include all operations in which suppuration was encountered, such as perforation of an intra-abdominal viscus, or compound trauma more than 4 hours after the event.

The evidence that this classification influences the risk of infection is shown in Table 5.1, which reflects the audit of 100 000 operations over a period of some 35 years.

5.4.5　The surgical wound

There are numerous factors relating to the surgical wound which affect the risk of postoperative infection. Many of these factors reflect the degree of surgical

Table 5.1

Classification	Patients	No. Infected	%
Clean	73589	1002	1.4
Clean-contaminated	14018	879	6.3
Contaminated	9085	1211	13.3
Dirty	3308	1310	39.9
Total	100000	4412	4.4

Source: Cruse (1995)

expertise exhibited by the surgeon, whilst others relate to the materials used.

SURGICAL EXPERTISE

Inadequate haemostasis results in a haematoma or seroma forming in the wound; this is an ideal growth medium for bacteria and increases the risk of infection. Similarly, damage to the lymphatic system will allow lymph to collect in the wound and, again, increase the risk.

Sutures applied too tightly, poor dissection or rough tissue handling may devitalize the tissues and cause necrosis with increased risk of infection.

WOUND GUARDS/TOWELS

The use of plastic adhesive sheeting or polythene wound guards have been shown to reduce the bacterial count at the wound edge on completion of the operation, but this has not resulted in a reduced incidence of postoperative infection in those trials that have been completed. Their use cannot be advocated on grounds of reducing infection risks, but they may be useful for securing drapes.

RETRACTORS

Wound-edge retractors are used in many operations. However, the perfusion and oxygenation of the wound edge is often compromised by such retraction, and this is increasingly recognized as a risk factor for infection.

FOREIGN BODIES

A smaller bacterial load is required to cause infection in the presence of a foreign body than in normal tissue. Many organisms can adhere to the surface of the foreign body, secrete a glycocalyx and thereafter be effectively immune from the action of antibiotics. Foreign bodies not only include prosthetic implants such as total hip replacements, aortic grafts, breast prostheses, but must also include non-absorbable sutures, meshes, etc. Infection of a foreign body may present long after the operation, and **surveillance audit** for infection after prosthetic implant procedures should be continued for at least one year.

DRAINS

Drains are a foreign body and, like all foreign bodies, they potentiate infection – particularly in the presence of contamination. The use of drains has been associated with an increased risk of postoperative wound and intra-abdominal infection, and there is some evidence that placing a drain adjacent to an anastomosis may increase

the risk of anastomotic leak. In addition, the tract of the drain provides an easy route of ingress of bacteria from the surface. Hence, whilst drains are necessary in some operations, their use should be minimized and always justifiable.

5.4.6 Immunocompetence

There is at present little that can be done to enhance the immunocompetence of a fit, healthy, person. However, there are many reasons why that immunocompetence can be compromised leading to an increased risk of infection. Of these, probably the most easy to correct is the state of nutrition of the patient, but correction of anergy dependent upon malnutrition has been more difficult to demonstrate.

BLOOD TRANSFUSION

Whole blood transfusion is a risk factor for infection, but controversy continues as to which element of blood is responsible for the immunosuppression. The increased risk of infection was originally demonstrated in colorectal surgery but has been confirmed in other areas. The value of blood transfusion as an immunosuppressant was first realized in the early days of renal transplantation. There is now evidence that blood transfusion increases the risk of tumour recurrence if administered in association with tumour surgery, and that the immunosuppression also has an immediate effect on the body's ability to resist bacterial contamination of the wound or peritoneal cavity.

ASSESSMENT OF IMMUNOCOMPETENCE

Many studies have been undertaken to examine the effect of anergy on postoperative infection and sepsis. American Society of Anesthesiology (ASA) grades III, IV and V, the duration of operation beyond the norm for that operation, and operations in the contaminated and dirty classification are considered to be the three most important factors in the development of postoperative wound infection.

5.5 RISK FACTORS FOR SEPSIS

Twenty years ago, MOF was believed to be the fatal expression of uncontrolled infection. However, it then became apparent that MOF could occur in the absence of infection and frequently followed blunt trauma. Bacterial translocation from the gastrointestinal tract in the haemodynamically-shocked patient was suggested to be the mechanism of post-injury MOF, and this led to the suggestion that selective decontamination of the gastrointestinal tract would reduce the incidence of MOF. This form of therapy, whilst reducing the incidence of nosocomial pneumonia, has not been shown to reduce death from MOF. It is now recognized that SIRS may occur with or without infection as the initiating cause, and the term sepsis is used when there is the same inflammatory response but there has been an identified microorganism which has invaded through a defined portal of entry. More recently, it has been suggested that progression to MOF may be the direct response of severe SIRS consequent upon massive trauma. Alternatively, a more minor trauma may stimulate a moderate SIRS, but a second event, which may be infective, precipitates amplification of the SIRS to produce MOF. Production of nitric oxide (NO) as an intermediary in the inflammatory response at the cellular level has been shown to play a significant adverse role in the amplification of the SIRS.

Much research has been carried out in an attempt to determine which patients are at greatest risk of SIRS and MOF, but infection and severe trauma appear to be the most common precipitating causes. Pancreatitis, abdominal trauma, pulmonary contusion, pelvic fractures, multiple long bone fractures, aspiration pneumonia, sepsis and hypertransfusion are known risk factors for ARDS and MOF. An abdominal trauma index >15 is associated with 18% incidence of ARDS, hypertransfusion with 21%, and pulmonary contusion with 25%. Multiple fractures have been shown to cause ARDS in 48% of cases. There would seem to be little association between head injury and ARDS or MOF. ARDS is a systemic state and part of SIRS, and presents first either because the lungs are more vulnerable to this state or because our ability to measure the onset is more sensitive in relationship to lung function than to other organ dysfunction.

Infections of gut origin would appear to be associated with higher risk of SIRS and MOF than urinary tract infection, whilst multiple sources of infection are associated with a poor prognosis.

5.6 FURTHER READING

American Society of Anaesthesiologists. (1963) *New classification of physical status. Anesthesiology* **24**, 111.

Farber, B.F., Kaiser, D.L. and Wenzel, R.P. (1981) Relationship between surgical volume and incidence of post operative wound infection. *N. Engl. J. Med.*, **305**, 200–204.

Haley, R.W., Culver, D.H., Morgan, W.M. *et al.* (1985) Identifying patients at high risk of surgical wound infection. A simple multivariate index of patient susceptibility and wound contamination. *Am. J. Epidemiol*, **121**, 206.

Health Building Note 26, Operating department. NHS Estates (1988), HMSO, London.

Leaper, D.J. (1995) Risk factors for surgical infection. *J. Hosp. Infect.*, **30** (Suppl. A), 127–139.

Matthews, J., Slater, K. and Newsom, S.W.B. (1985) The effect of surgical gowns made with barrier cloth on bacterial dispersal. *J. Hyg.*, **95**, 123–130.

Scottish Intercollegiate Guidelines Network. (2000) No. 45. *Antibiotic Prophylaxis in Surgery*, July.

Scottish Office Department of Health. (1999) *Hospital acquired infection – a framework for a national system of surveillance for the NHS in Scotland*. Scottish Office, Edinburgh.

Preventing infection of the surgeon and staff

A.M. SEFTON

6.1 PREPARATION OF THE THEATRE STAFF FOR SURGERY

6.1.1 Staff health

Although direct infection of patients from staff during surgery is very uncommon in comparison to the number of operations performed, an infected staff member can present a major hazard. Two possibilities exist, namely infection with: (i) viruses from blood; or (ii) staphylococci from skin. Blood-borne virus infections in patients after surgery are extremely rare, but carry a high publicity profile and are covered more fully in Chapter 9, which in particular considers precautions to be taken with HIV, when the major concern is infection of staff from an HIV-positive patient.

As the concerns about blood-borne viruses have increased and more knowledge becomes available, then Occupational Health Departments receive stricter governmental guidelines. Of the three possible viruses, hepatitis B (HBV), hepatitis C (HCV) and HIV, HBV is of the most concern. This is because the infective dose is the smallest, so the surgeon is likely to acquire the infection from a patient, and can pass it on. The risk may not be negligible. Following the identification of a cardiothoracic surgeon who had performed exposure-prone procedures over 18 months, 95% of the 323 affected patients were tested. Twenty patients (6%) were classified as having acquired hepatitis-B infection in association

with the surgery. Those in whom the surgeon had performed a sternotomy were more at risk of hepatitis than those in whom he had performed vein harvest (17% versus 3%). As efficient HBV vaccines are available, current policy in the NHS is that no surgeon is allowed to work without documentary evidence of immunity to HBV, or if about to be vaccinated, to have no evidence of HBV antigens in the blood. The issue is such that the personnel department may demand to see the antibody test results as a condition of employment. Although bureaucratic, hopefully such an approach should obviate future problems for both surgeon and patient.

Hepatitis caused by HCV has usually been associated with blood transfusion as the infective dose is low (probably 100 to 1000 times less than HBV); thus, healthcare workers are much less at risk. The results of surveys comparing antibodies in healthcare workers with those in the general population have produced results that varied according to the type of test used. Most find no difference, although follow-up of needlestick injuries in Spain revealed a 1.9% seroconversion rate (of 53 employees!), and there is a single report implying transmission of HCV from a cardiac surgeon to six patients, also in Spain. It is impossible to assess the significance of this at present. Transmission to patients must be regarded as extremely rare, and no restrictions should be applied to HCV-carrying surgeons (should any exist) in the current state of knowledge.

HIV infections carry the cachets of both high profile and incurability. The infective dose is again perhaps

1000 times less than HBV, but even so transmission to healthcare workers has been recorded. Most instances have however required a significant dose, as for example inadvertent self injection of contaminated blood from a needle. Therefore the risk for a patient must be negligible; much less than of injury crossing the road or from receiving an injection of penicillin. However, the reported well-known instance of nosocomial infections from the dentist in Florida, together with the traditional concern that 'doctors do not harm their patients' has led to widespread anxiety which was recently justified by the well-documented case of the French surgeon who acquired HIV from a patient, and later transmitted the identical strain during a particularly traumatic operation. Furthermore, while an HIV-positive surgeon might not present any risk to patients from the disease, its possible sequelae of infections, such as tuberculosis, could present a problem. The current procedure for theatre staff who become HIV-positive is to seek advice from the Occupational Health Department, the likelihood being that they would be banned from exposure-prone procedures. In one instance however, a surgeon who used notouch techniques via an operating microscope was allowed to continue operating, in contrast to the surgeon who delayed revealing his condition to such an extent that it led to his being removed from the medical register by the General Medical Council.

Transmissions of staphylococcal infections are much more common than virus infections. Staphylococci may be associated with clinical lesions or merely carried on skin or in the nares. The MRC trial of operating theatres noted 13 occasions when patients had postoperative hip infections with strains of staphylococci carried by staff members, although the obvious conclusion was weakened by the fact that one of the relevant staff carriers was not present at the operation on one patient. Recent papers documented the linking of seven wound infections to an operating theatre assistant with a boil on his arm, and of six cases of mediastinitis caused by the same strain of a methicillin-resistant strain of *Staph. aureus* (MRSA) following coronary artery by-pass surgery to the presence of the same assistant surgeon at all operations. The latter carried the same strain in his nose, and was also subject to allergic rhinitis.

Some 30% or more of the population carry *Staph. aureus* in the nose, and it is only helpful to screen theatre staff when investigating an unexpectedly high incidence of postoperative wound infections. Some carriers may be 'dispersers' of larger than normal numbers of bacteria into the air, but special equipment is required to investigate this and again 'dispersers' are not normally looked for. Males disperse more than females, mainly from the skin on the lower half of the body. Most people disperse increased numbers of bacteria for up to 2 hours after a shower, and upper respiratory tract infections may increase dispersal. Indeed, a recent report described a neonatologist who infected eight infants in the special care baby unit with MRSA, while suffering a rhinovirus infection – a so-called 'cloud adult'.

In practical terms staff should be aware of the potential danger of skin infections, and also of skin disorders such as psoriasis, because staphylococci can multiply in the dead skin, even if unrelated to the disease. The Occupational Health Department should be asked for advice. For diseased skin, treatment may include antibiotics and washing with a chlorhexidine scrub, while local mupirocin, with systemic antibiotics such as rifampicin can be used for eradication of carriage.

6.2 INFECTED PATIENTS AND THE SURGEON

Patients admitted under the care of surgical teams sometimes may be clinically infected with or carrying or incubating dangerous infectious agents such as hepatitis B or C, Human Immunodeficiency Virus (HIV), *Salmonella* spp. or other bacterial or viral gastrointestinal pathogens, *Mycobacterium tuberculosis*, varicella-zoster or various parasites or infestations. It is important to remember that asymptomatic carriers – with no overt signs of disease – can still act as a source of infection for others. Possible sources of infection from these patients include excretions, secretions and blood. Hence, it is important to treat blood and all body fluids from patients as potentially infectious, and avoid contamination with them.

On occasion, a patient might become colonized or infected with a potentially pathogenic organism while in hospital. For example, they may occasionally become colonized and/or infected with the methicillin-resistant *Staph. aureus* or multi-resistant Gram-negative rods. Staff can also become colonized with these organisms and hence a source of spread to other staff members and patients.

If a patient is known to be at special risk of having a certain disease, then extra precautions relevant to that risk should be used, e.g. a patient known to be a chronic carrier of *Salmonella* spp. or indeed any patient with diarrhoea of unknown aetiology, in whom infection cannot be ruled out, should be nursed with 'stool' and/or excretion/secretion precautions (see Chapter 4). Patients known to be carrying blood-borne viruses, e.g. hepatitis B, should be nursed with 'blood precautions', whilst a patient with pulmonary tuberculosis should be nursed in a single room with 'respiratory precautions'.

Samples taken from 'high-risk' patients and their accompanying forms should be labelled with 'danger of infection' stickers when they are sent to the laboratory for testing (consult your local laboratory if in doubt). In the case of HIV testing it is vital that counselling and informed consent should be obtained from the patient prior to screening. This chapter discusses ways of preventing infection in the surgeon pre- and post-exposure to infected patients. Particular emphasis is placed on needlestick injuries, as these occur relatively frequently and are a common source of concern to medical staff, especially if the source is thought to be 'high-risk'.

6.3   NEEDLESTICK INJURIES

In order to minimize the risk of inoculation and other contamination incidents, blood and body fluids from all patients should be treated as a possible source of infection. All members of staff should be immunized against hepatitis B, and should know their immunization status.

Although intact skin is a fairly good barrier against infection, skin with abrasions or lesions is not. Waterproof sealant dressings should thus be applied to any abrasion of the hands, and if a member of staff suffers from eczema for instance, they should wear disposable gloves. Disposable gloves should also be worn if staff are likely to come into contact with body fluids. Similarly, protective gowns, masks and visors should be worn if other areas of the skin on the body and face are at risk of exposure to body fluids. Needles and all sharp instruments should be handled with care. The surgeon must not resheath used needles, nor ask other people to do it for him/her.

6.3.1   Procedure after a needlestick injury or contamination incident

Needlestick injuries/contamination incidents sometimes occur in spite of the staff member having taken all reasonable precautions. In order to ensure optimal management of the injured person, it is important to know what to do and whom to contact in these instances. Exact procedures following a needlestick injury may vary from hospital to hospital, so it is important to know your local guidelines.

If you do have a needlestick injury/contamination incident do not panic. The surgeon should first carry out a personal risk assessment. Is the hepatitis status or HIV status of the patient known? Are they a drug addict? Is the patient jaundiced? The majority of such injuries occur from sources which are unlikely to be at high risk of hepatitis B, hepatitis C, HIV or other blood-borne viruses. Hepatitis B is more infectious than either hepatitis C or HIV: following a needlestick injury from a hepatitis B antigen-positive carrier, up to 30% of subjects may become infected unless they are already hepatitis B immune or undergo an immediate immunization course. Hepatitis B immunization either pre- or post-exposure is extremely effective in preventing infection. The action that an individual should take following a needlestick injury/contamination incident is summarized in Table 6.1.

Table 6.1 *Action to be taken following a needlestick/contamination injury*

1. Immediately after a needlestick/sharps injury, encourage bleeding from the puncture site and wash it thoroughly with soap and water.

2. If eyes or mouth are contaminated, rinse immediately with water.

3. If contamination of intact skin has occurred, wash with large amounts of soap and water.

4. If clothes have been contaminated, remove them immediately and wash the skin.

5. Contact the Occupational Health Department/Virology Department/on-call Virologist/Accident and Emergency Department as specified in the local needlestick injury policy **immediately** after washing the contaminated area. If treatment is required, the earlier it is started the more effective it is likely to be. Post-exposure prophylaxis against HIV should commence within 1 hour after exposure. Let Occupational Health, etc. know the source of the injury – if known.

6. Inform a senior member of your department about the incident.

The exact infectivity of hepatitis C is not known, but seroconversion is thought to be in the range of 1–3% following an inoculation incident from a hepatitis C-positive patient. HIV is the least transmissible of these three viruses. Even in the absence of taking antiretroviral therapy the seroconversion rate following an inoculation injury from a known HIV-positive source is about 0.3–0.4% and following a contact contamination incident (e.g. splashing of mucous membranes with body fluids from an HIV-infected source) it is less than 0.1%.

6.3.2   The role of the Occupational Health, Virologist or Accident and Emergency doctor in viral needlestick injuries

When you contact any of the above following a contamination incident they will perform a risk assessment to ascertain what, if any, further action may be required. For this it is extremely useful if the source of the injury is known, but sometimes this is not the case. Often, if you are seen in either Occupational Health or the Accident and Emergency Unit, they will discuss your care with a medical virologist. You will be asked to provide a blood sample which will be stored. Every effort will be made to maintain confidentiality. If you have been immunized against hepatitis B but do not know your antibody state, some of your blood may be tested to determine your level of antibodies against hepatitis B.

Any further actions will depend on the result of the risk assessment. These may include:

- being given an additional dose of hepatitis B vaccine;
- commencing a course of hepatitis B vaccination;
- administration of hepatitis B immunoglobulin;
- commencing an anti-HIV starter pack.

If the source of the inoculation incident is known, Occupational Health, the medical virologist or the Accident and Emergency Department will ask the 'source's' medical team to try and obtain consent for the patient's blood to be tested for carriage of hepatitis B, hepatitis C and HIV. Negative results for these tests will greatly reassure the injured member of staff, especially if the source is thought to be at high risk for HIV. The patient, however, is at liberty to refuse such a request (in which case it may be necessary to assume a positive result). Specific advice on management of the injured member of staff will be offered as appropriate. Management of needlestick injuries with respect to hepatitis B is summarized in Table 6.2.

For needlestick or contamination injuries where the source is either known or strongly suspected of being HIV-positive, there is some evidence that giving anti-retroviral treatment to the injured person reduces the risk of their subsequent seroconversion. It should be considered where there has been percutaneous injury, exposure to broken skin or exposure of mucous membranes to blood or high-risk body fluids. For optimal efficacy **the first dose of anti-retroviral treatment should be commenced within 1 hour post-injury**: however, it should still be considered if this time interval has passed. Until recently, zidovudine was given as monotherapy post-needlestick injuries from such HIV patients, but combination therapy appears to be more effective at suppressing viral replication and is now used. If anti-retroviral therapy is commenced the staff member will be referred as soon as possible to a specialist for follow-up, including counselling and drug monitoring if he/she decides to stay on therapy (which is usually given for one month). Every endeavour will be made to obtain consent to test the source for HIV.

The combination of drugs currently recommended for post-exposure prophylaxis against HIV in the UK is zidovudine + lamivudine + indinavir. All three drugs are usually taken for 4 weeks. As with any drug regimen, factors such as pregnancy, interaction with other medicines and possible allergy should be taken into account when prescribing them, as also should be the views of the affected healthcare worker.

Any member of the medical staff who thinks that they may have been exposed to HIV or hepatitis B – either occupationally or otherwise – has an obligation to inform their Occupational Health Department. The Occupational Health Doctor or his/her deputy will advise them about the need for screening and whether or not they require to modify their working practices prior to obtaining the results of primary and follow-up screening tests for hepatitis B and HIV.

Table 6.2 *Specific management of staff post-inoculation incidents regarding risk of hepatitis B infection*

Vaccination status of staff regarding anti-HBs level	Hepatitis status of source	Management of staff
Vaccinated in last year. Known to have good antibody levels	+ve or −ve	No booster required. Reassure
Vaccinated. Known to have low antibody level	+ve	Give hepatitis B vaccine booster within 48 hours
Not vaccinated	Unknown	Start accelerated hepatitis vaccine course (0,1,2 months ± dose at 12 months ± Give hepatitis B immunoglobulin. Test source if possible
Non-responder to vaccine	i) Unknown	i) Test source as soon as possible, then act as appropriate
	ii) Negative	ii) Reassure staff
	iii) HbsAg-positive	iii) Give hepatitis B immunoglobulin as soon as possible (certainly within 48 hours) + further dose 1 month later

6.4 OTHER INFECTIONS TRANSMITTED FROM PATIENT TO STAFF

6.4.1 *Mycobacterium tuberculosis*

Tuberculosis (TB) is spread by inhalation of droplets containing tubercle bacilli. A patient is described as having 'open pulmonary TB' if acid-fast bacilli are seen in direct microscopic examination of their sputum: he/she may remain infectious during the first 14 days of their treatment, even if the organism is fully susceptible to standard anti-tuberculous therapy. If infection is caused by multi-drug-resistant TB, the period of infectivity will be much longer: fortunately this is rare in the UK.

The patient should thus be nursed in a sideroom with the door closed. If the patient has an uncontrollable cough, he/she should wear a mask when other people are in the room. Protective clothing is only required for staff members if hands or clothing are likely to be contaminated by respiratory secretions. Contact tracing of staff will be performed following a case of open pulmonary TB on the ward. In the UK, children routinely receive the BCG vaccine which currently is thought to provide fairly good protection in this country against infection by *M. tuberculosis*. However, in some other parts of the world it is found to be less effective or even ineffective, and so is not given.

If at operation a surgeon finds a surgical lesion which is likely to contain tubercle bacilli, the possibility of spread to staff and patients should be considered. The first concern is to contain the infected tissue or pus into a secure container. After completion of the surgery the theatre will require thorough cleaning and decontamination of any surfaces likely to have been contaminated. No further patients should be operated on in that theatre until the control of infection doctor is satisfied that all appropriate steps have been taken.

A decision should be made as to whether or not chemoprophylaxis should be administered to the staff exposed during the operation. This assessment should be carried out by someone able to assess the risk which depends on the degree of risk from the lesion, the degree of exposure, the immune status of the person and other factors. The minimum course of chemoprophylaxis is three months' duration and this should be started within 3–4 days if a decision is made that this is necessary.

WHAT ARE MASKS FOR?

There are two sorts of mask. One type is designed to prevent contamination of the environment and patients from the sprayed oral flora from attendants' mouths. This does not create a hazard during normal conversation but coughs and sneezes can expel numerous bacteria into the environment or over a patient. If there is an open operation wound or invasive device even organisms of low pathogenicity can give rise to inflammatory response. For this reason simple masks to deflect such spray of oral flora are commonly used by operating theatre staff. Cotton or paper masks become moistened by breath and eventually become pervious and thus a poor barrier to oral flora. For this reason cellophane sheets are often inserted into the mask to ensure it remains impervious.

The second type of mask is 'protective', to prevent airborne particles containing bacteria from colonizing the upper respiratory passages of health attendants. They can also offer protection from blood sprays carrying viruses such as Hepatitis B and C and HIV. Bacteria such as *Myco. tuberculosis* and multi-resistant *Staph. aureus* are examples of such risks when operating on patients known or suspected to be harbouring these organisms.

PROTECTIVE MASKS

Protective masks are more complex than deflector masks. They must be close fitting to prevent particles reaching the mucous membranes; yet they must allow free passage of air. Filters of varying degrees of complexity are used in these masks. They are graded on the basis of how fine the filter is but for most areas of a hospital the lowest grade of filter is all that is required.

Most of the debate about whether or not masks should be worn fails to distinguish between these two different types of mask. One daily sees inappropriate use of masks in hospitals because the first question – what is the mask for? – is not asked. Flimsy paper masks are used by nurses dressing wounds infected by MRSA. Theatre staff sweat with tight fitting filter masks while attending to a herniorrhaphy. Both of these are unsuitable usage. The availability of masks is limited so that a choice often is not available even if the right question is asked.

6.4.2 Gastrointestinal pathogens

Gastrointestinal pathogens are spread by both the faecal and oral routes. Chronic carriers of *Salmonella* spp. and any case of gastroenteritis or suspected food poisoning on the ward should be treated as potentially infectious. Two or more associated cases should be treated as an outbreak and the Infection Control Team alerted. Staff with diarrhoea and/or vomiting should not work. Ideally, any patient carrying a stool pathogen should be nursed in a sideroom. Staff must pay particular attention to handwashing (see Chapter 5) when dealing with these patients, and wear disposable gloves and a plastic apron when in contact with their stools.

6.4.3 Methicillin-resistant *Staphylococcus aureus* (MRSA)

This is a *Staph. aureus* which is resistant to penicillin, methicillin, flucloxacillin, cloxacillin and other β-lactam antibiotics such as the cephalosporins and the carbapenems. The organism commonly shows multiple resistance to other antibiotics. Direct contact, usually by hands, is the commonest mode of transmission. Staff may occasionally become colonized or infected with the MRSA, and if this occurs their management should be discussed by the Infection Control Team on an individual basis. Depending on their circumstances, such staff members may be required to be off work until they have been cleared. Good nursing/hand hygiene techniques minimize the risk of transmission of MRSA. Staff with severe eczema of the hands are particularly likely to become colonized with MRSA.

6.4.4 Varicella-zoster virus (VZV) infection

Chickenpox is the clinical manifestation of primary infection with VZV. Following the primary infection the virus becomes latent and may be reactivated later, resulting in **shingles**. The virus is carried in the respiratory tract and in the skin lesions, and hence it can be spread both by the air-borne route and by direct contact with skin lesions. Anyone who has not had chickenpox and is in contact with VZV from about 24–48 hours before the spots appear until after they are all crusted is at risk of infection. Ideally, all medical/nursing staff should have their VZV status checked by antibody determination prior to starting employment. If a non-immune member of staff comes into contact with someone with VZV infection – either at home or work – they should seek advice from the Occupational Health Doctor/Consultant Virologist as soon as possible to ascertain whether or not they should remain at work: this is particularly important if they are in close contact with immunosuppressed individuals.

Any patient with VZV infection should be nursed in a sideroom to prevent cross-infection, and the Infection Control Team should be informed. Non-immune staff, patients or visitors should not enter the room while the patient remains infectious. Further details on management will be available from every hospital's Infection Control Manual, Infection Control Doctor or Clinical Virology Department.

6.4.5 Infestations

Examples of infestations which might be seen in patients are scabies and louse infections. **Scabies** is a contagious disease caused by the mite *Sarcoptes scabei*.

The female scabies mite burrows into the skin to lay eggs, and a pruritic rash, which is allergic in nature, follows about 4–6 weeks later. Scabies is spread by direct skin-to-skin contact, so if a patient is thought to have scabies, then gloves should be worn when examining them and a specialist should be asked to both confirm the diagnosis and advise on treatment.

Humans can be infected by the **head louse**, the **body louse** or the **pubic louse**. Initially, the lice may not be visible to the naked eye. Transmission is by close contact. The local Infection Control Manual should contain a decontamination policy for these organisms. Ideally, to confirm a diagnosis a louse should be caught and sent it to the microbiology laboratory for identification.

6.5 CONCLUSIONS

'Prevention is better than cure'. Good nursing practices, especially care in dealing with all body fluids, keeping sideroom doors shut on patients in standard isolation and meticulous hand hygiene will help to minimize the spread of infection from patient to staff, or from patient to patient. Common sense, close liaison with the Infection Control Team and adherence to local infection control policies are also important in this respect.

6.6 FURTHER READING

Guidelines on Post-Exposure Prophylaxis for Health Care Workers occupationally exposed to HIV. DoH document, UK Health Department, June 1997.

Guidance from the UK Chief Medical Officers' Expert Advisory Group on AIDS. (2000) *HIV post-exposure prophylaxis.* UK Health Department, July.

Haiduven, D.J. (2000) Planning a hepatitis C postexposure management program for health care workers. Issues and challenges. *AAOHN J,* **48**(8), 370–375.

Harrison, J., Woodhouse, J. and Dowson, A.J. (1999) The management of occupational health by NHS Trusts in the north of England. *Occupational Medicine,* **49**(8), 525–533.

Poole, C.J.M., Harrington, J.M., Burge, P.S. and White, A.C. (2002) Guidance on standards of health for clinical health care workers. *Occupational Medicine,* **52**, 17–24.

Scoular, A., Watt, A.D., Watson, M. and Kelly, B. (2000) Knowledge and attitudes of hospital staff to occupational exposure to bloodborne viruses. *Commun. Dis. Public Health,* **3**(4), 247–249.

Stevens, A.B. and Coyle, P.V. (2000) Hepatitis C virus: an important occupational hazard? *Occupational Medicine,* **50**(6), 377–382.

Your local Trust's/hospital infection control manual.

Litigation related to surgical infection

E.M. COOKE

7.1 INTRODUCTION

The prevention of sepsis is associated with many quality assurance aspects of surgical care, and litigation related to surgical infection is inextricably related to litigation related to other aspects of surgery. Such litigation is often, although not always, part of a general discontent on the part of the patient with the care he/she has received. For these reasons, some of what is included may appear at first sight to go beyond the remit of this chapter. However, it is hoped that it will become apparent that this is not in fact the case.

7.2 PRESENT POSITION

7.2.1 Levels of litigation

There has in recent years been a considerable increase in levels of litigation in relation to medical malpractice. For example, one defence organization reports that claims costs continue to increase, on average, by approximately 15% each year. The situation in the UK is now such that it would be unusual for a surgeon to reach the end of his/her professional life without personal experience of litigation, and some surgeons will find that at any one time they are involved in several cases. There is no evidence that this trend is likely to change. The possibility of litigation is therefore an important part of surgical practice and should be treated as such. At the same time it is highly desirable that 'defensive medicine', which may not be in patients' best interests, is avoided.

Achieving this objective involves active consideration of all aspects of surgical practice, and it is worth bearing in mind that avoidance of litigation may have a useful role in maintaining and raising standards and as part of risk management and quality assurance processes.

7.2.2 Medical indemnity

The situation as regards medical indemnity varies from country to country. There are, however, some aspects which are of general importance. The terms of the indemnity must be clearly understood. Often it is only for the treatment of patients although the UK defence organisations also offer advisory services and the benefits of membership of those organisations are discretionary or combine an insurance contract with access to discretionary benefits. Indemnity may also be related either to the time at which the claim was first made or to the time the event which led to the litigation occurred ('claims made' or 'claims incurred'). It is worth remembering that claims may not arise until a long time after the event and a claim may, in fact, first be made against a deceased practitioner's estate.

Currently in the UK work carried out in the Health Service will be indemnified by the Trust hospital as long as the work is part of the surgeon's contract. Work outside that contracted for would not normally be indemnified. The benefits of membership of the three UK medical defence organizations include private practice, the subscription rate depending on the speciality and the income generated.

As mentioned, the defence organizations also offer advisory services to the medical profession, and these form an important part of their work.

Family doctors in the UK are responsible for arranging their own indemnity for all aspects of their work. As some minor surgical procedures are carried out by general practitioners many of the problems in relation to litigation and surgery apply to them also.

7.3 FUTURE DEVELOPMENTS

As has been stated, there is little evidence that levels of litigation are likely to fall. However, in most countries litigation is slow and costly with the costs falling on the medical profession (and insurers) and on claimants or the tax-payer in the UK if the claimant has state funding. This situation has prompted a search for more rapid and cost-effective mechanisms. Proposed solutions have generally involved either the streamlining of the existing system or the development of a quite different approach, such as 'no fault' compensation. The Woolf reforms introduced from April 1999 provide for a strict timetable with a pre-action protocol and active court management after proceedings have been served. The pre-action protocol requires considerable exchange of information and allows many more claims to be resolved without litigation. It is too early to assess the full impact of these reforms, but they are already having an effect on the way in which cases are being conducted and have increased the speed of many.

The cost of litigation has increased and the NHS Litigation Authority's total liabilities are now recognized to be significant. Consideration continues to be given to the use of structured settlements instead of lump sum payments but most awards tend to be as lump sums. The Government is considering clinical negligence procedures in the NHS.

7.4 AVOIDANCE OF LITIGATION (see Table 7.1)

7.4.1 Relationships with patients

An essential part of avoiding litigation is the development and maintenance of good relationships with patients. This involves particularly a careful discussion of the risks of a procedure and an explanation of what has happened when things do not turn out as well as had been hoped. It should be remembered that embarking on litigation which is not justified and which is unlikely to be successful can be highly damaging to a patient. An expression of regret at an undesirable result is not an admission of liability, and this should be made clear. However, such a statement may reassure a patient that his or her anxieties are taken seriously.

Table 7.1 *Measures to reduce litigation*

1. Remember the possibility of litigation.
2. Explain the nature of a proposed operation carefully, and its possible risks.
3. Keep good records.
4. Explain and express regret for an undesirable consequence.
5. Maintain good interpersonal relationships in the work environment.
6. Always arrange appropriate cover and hand-over arrangements.
7. Ensure adequate standards of infection control.
8. Know the infection hazards in the perioperative environment.
9. Ensure that the procedure is performed to the appropriate standard.
10. Ensure that any procedure is justified.
11. Ensure that antibiotic use is correctly managed.
12. Use modern communication methods (e.g. mobile phones) circumspectly, preserving confidentiality.

7.4.2 Relationships with colleagues

Maintenance of good working relationships with colleagues of all grades and in a variety of disciplines is important in producing a working environment in which mistakes are minimized, and in particular in which appropriate **cover and hand-over arrangements** can be implemented. Modern surgery requires input from people with many different skills. No single person can be responsible for all aspects of modern surgical practice, and definition of the responsibilities of different members of the team is important (see below).

7.4.3 Responsibilities of the surgeon

It is not possible for the surgeon to be personally responsible for all aspects of infection control in the hospital in which he or she works. Other people will be expert in sterilization, disinfection, theatre ventilation, isolation procedures, surveillance of hospital-acquired infection, and other aspects of infection control (see Chapter 2). However, the surgeon does have a responsibility to ensure that all relevant aspects are being addressed and are satisfactory. This can be done either by discussions with the Infection Control Doctor (ICD) or through the Hospital Infection Control Committee (HICC). Records of the discussions with the ICD or minutes of the HICC should be comprehensive. Inadequacies of the systems in operation should be reported appropriately, and if not rapidly corrected the Chief Executive should be informed, with a clear indication of the possible consequences of failure to correct the fault.

7.4.4 Records

As has been indicated, many medicolegal cases will come to court many years after the event, and reliance on memory will not be possible. **Mounting a good defence** is often critically reliant on the contemporaneous patient records and too frequently these are inadequate. It is especially important that an appropriately worded consent form is used and a careful note made of the information provided to the patient about the drawbacks of an operation. Too often, for example, a surgeon feels confident that he warned a man about to undergo sterilization of the dangers of late recanalization, but as no note was made it later becomes difficult to resist a claim.

If inadequate notes have been made and an untoward event occurs, any additions must be dated and clearly marked that they were added later. Such notes near to the event are useful as they record recent memory, but there must be no risk of them being confused with the original record.

Good records should be made of discussions about services and facilities and copies of letters kept. Although many people find this difficult, a brief note of telephone calls of any significance should be kept and a notebook by the telephone for this purpose is useful. However, important clinical advice may now be given using mobile phones and a particularly rigorous discipline is required to keep a note of such calls. Patient confidentiality must also be carefully considered if mobile phones are used in public places.

7.4.5 When not to operate

One of the most difficult decisions is not to operate, and this may become necessary in a number of circumstances. If an operation is not in the best interests of a patient, then pressure from the patient must of course be resisted and the situation is clear. Also clear is the situation in which there is a temptation to use a technique in which the surgeon is not fully trained or experienced. To do this may have serious medicolegal consequences. More difficult may be the decision not to operate because conditions are inadequate. A serious well-documented attempt to get things corrected is necessary, as is an assessment of the consequences of not operating. Under these circumstances the advice of a defence organization is essential. A surgeon may also find it very supportive to have external advice if he/she feels that age, sickness or other personal factors have impaired his or her ability and is doubtful whether to continue to operate.

7.5 HANDLING LITIGATION

7.5.1 Reasons for litigation

Many of the aspects of handling litigation have already been mentioned as part of the discussion of methods of avoiding litigation, and indeed the two form a continuum, as clear evidence provided early that all reasonable steps have been taken to prevent untoward events will often prevent litigation going forward. Litigation in relation to infection is, as has been mentioned, often part of a general discontent with the outcome of surgery, the infection being regarded as 'the last straw', although on occasion quite unexpected consequences of infection may occur and be significant in their own right. Septicaemia and endocarditis are obvious examples of the latter.

7.5.2 Early advice

If, in spite of all attempts to avoid litigation a surgeon becomes involved, an important approach is to contact a defence organization at a very early stage. This is advisable even if the defence organization is not providing the indemnity, as the advisory service will be valuable. Decisions taken and statements made in the earliest stages of a prolonged action can have a profound effect on what happens later.

7.5.3 Types of defence

In many cases of infection following surgery the defence will be related to the process, the outcome, or both.

PROCESS

It is enormously helpful to be able to demonstrate that the surgery was performed in a totally suitable way. Aspects to be considered include the training and experience of the surgeon and his assistants, and the environment in which the surgery was performed. It is important to remember that the standard that is being aimed at, as regards defence against litigation, is not that in the best institution in the world, but that which is regarded as acceptable by a responsible body of fellow practitioners in the country in which the event occurred. It is also worth noting that the impression given to the patient is quite significant. The relationship of standards of ward cleaning to infection rates is difficult to assess, but people find it hard to accept that a ward which looks dirty is not also unhygienic and therefore predisposes to sepsis.

Evidence of well-established infection control arrangements, i.e. the Infection Control Team and the Infection Control Committee, as described elsewhere in this book (see Chapter 2), is also essential.

OUTCOME

The advantage of some information on infection rates in a hospital for providing a defence against litigation cannot be over-emphasized. Anecdotal evidence is not likely to carry much weight unless it can be substantiated by well-kept records. However, if records have not been kept there is good evidence in the medical literature about infection rates following many forms of surgery and this literature can be cited. Development of infection in itself is not evidence of negligence, although if infection rates following a particular procedure are known to be significant the question will arise as to whether the patient should have been informed of this as part of the consent procedure. The argument that, for example, 5% of patients undergoing a particular type of operation develop infection is a powerful one. It is also helpful to be able to demonstrate that there was no outbreak of infection, for example with MRSA or group A streptococci, on the surgical unit at the time. The records of 'alert organisms', i.e. those organisms likely to cause outbreaks, which are kept by most UK hospitals, may be very helpful.

Participation in local and national schemes to study infection rates indicates that a hospital is taking infection control seriously, and some schemes provide data showing the situation of that hospital in relation to similar ones. Essentially, the more evidence that can be provided that a particular institution has infection rates within an acceptable range, the easier the defence.

ANTIBIOTIC USAGE

The failure to administer appropriate antibiotics is often cited by plaintiffs as a reason for the develop-

ment of, or failure to cure, an infection. Prophylaxis should follow accepted methods and (if not) reasons for local variations should be clear and adequate. Treatment of difficult infections should be discussed with the hospital microbiologist and appropriate specimens always taken. If patients are sent home with an infection, clear advice on antibiotic treatment while at home must be given and appropriate follow-up arrangements made.

7.6 CONCLUSIONS

In an increasingly litigious society it is essential that surgeons take appropriate steps to avoid litigation and to be able to defend themselves when it occurs. However, most of what needs to be done is part of good surgical practice and, if seen in this light, becomes less irksome and indeed can be viewed positively as part of maintaining and raising standards of patient care.

7.7 FURTHER READING

Dyer, C. (2000) Patients, but not doctors like mediation for setting claims. *British Medical Journal*, **320**, 336.

Rubinstein, E. (1999) *Journal of Hospital Infection*, **43**, 165–167.

Scheckler, W.E. (2002) Healthcare epidemiology is the paradigm for patient safety. *Infection Control and Hospital Epidemiology*, **23**, 47–51.

Website www.the-mdu.com

PART II

Specific chapters

8

Infections in intensive care units

S. MEHTAR

8.1 INTRODUCTION

Intensive care units (ICU) are clinical areas with a concentration of acutely ill patients who are dependent upon specialized medical care. Some of these patients may have undergone surgery, but all of them would have had invasive devices such as urinary catheters and intravenous devices inserted as part of their clinical management. Patients requiring assisted mechanical ventilation require further invasive devices such as endotracheal tubes and nasogastric tubes.

The risk of colonization leading to infection with multiply antibiotic-resistant bacteria and fungi, is at least 20% greater than in ordinary hospital wards; moreover, the sources and incidence of infection increase with the length of stay in the ICU.

8.2 SOURCES OF INFECTION

The sources of infection are:

- Endogenous: these are infections which arise from within the patient's own flora, particularly when antibiotics have been prescribed and antibiotic-resistant bacterial colonization has occurred.
- Exogenous: these infections are introduced from external sources such as the hands of staff, or invasive devices.

8.3 RISK FACTORS

The risk of acquiring an infection depends on several factors, including: (i) the source of infection; (ii) the immune status of the patient (host); and (iii) the 'environment' in the ICU. The latter includes such items as facilities, bed spacing, the number of staff, the number of invasive devices, the state of cleanliness or sterility of such devices, and the infection control measures practised. In addition, direct patient management, including technique for insertion of devices, assessment of the clinical state of the patient, and antibiotic usage, are recognized as risk factors for infection. However, many factors are directly attributable to the patient's own ability to resist infection, as discussed in the next section.

8.4 THE PATIENT

Factors which are predominantly patient-associated include the immune status of the patient and his/her host defences; especially clinical state, age and concomitant disease, effect of surgical operation, life-saving drug therapy, colonization with hospital pathogens and reduction in defences due to invasive devices. All of these deserve special discussion, as follows.

8.4.1 Immune status

This is a critically important factor. It is discussed extensively elsewhere in this book and will not be described at this point.

8.4.2 Clinical state

The sicker the patient, the more intensive the treatment, and in the ICU this is interpreted as more invasive devices, both in numbers and in frequency. The length of stay in the ICU is also longer and the prospects of colonization (and thus infection) increase. In order to provide appropriate medical attention to patients in the ICU, the staff dealing with these patients have to touch or handle the patient and his/her invasive devices and environment more frequently than in a surgical ward. It is estimated that the number of contacts with a patient in a surgical ward is eight to ten times a day, whereas in the ICU this may increase four- to five-fold. Each patient contact carries with it a risk of transmission of pathogens from the hands of the staff, particularly when several patients are dealt with by one member of staff. Cross-infection is inevitable, but this can be reduced by vigilant hand disinfection between each patient contact using an alcohol rub if there is no organic contamination, and thorough hand washing with a suitable disinfectant such as chlorohexidine if there is.

Some patients are admitted to an ICU in such a critical condition (e.g. after multi-organ high-speed injury or overwhelming sepsis with associated shock) that survival is very unlikely, regardless of the standard of infection care. Great advances have been made, however, in the treatment of severe burns, to which the prevention or limitation of infection has been the most important contribution (see also Chapter 13).

8.4.3 Age and concomitant disease

The age of the patient and concomitant diseases such as **hypertension**, **diabetes mellitus**, **carcinoma** and **chronic lung disease** are relevant to clinical outcome and increase the risk of postoperative infection. The older the patient, the greater the chances of a unfavourable outcome.

8.4.4 Effect of surgical operation

Surgical patients are at further risk depending upon the type of operation, and the duration of both the surgery and anaesthesia. Patients undergoing intra-abdominal surgery where peritonitis is present at the time of surgery are generally more susceptible to postoperative infection. By admitting such patients to the ICU, the risk of colonization and thus, infection, increases.

The prognosis depends on the severity of the acute episode of infection, underlying chronic disease and complications associated with infection. In surgical ICU patients, infection rates of 3.2 per 100 admissions were recorded in one study, with a fatality rate of 35% at 28 days after the onset of sepsis. The in-house mortality rate was 43%. The predictors of mortality include:

(i) previous antibiotic therapy; (ii) hypothermia; (iii) mechanical ventilation; and (iv) APACHE II score at the onset of sepsis.

8.4.5 Life-saving drug therapy

Patients in the ICU require aggressive management strategies, and both steroid therapy and non-steroid drugs are an integral part of the management. The sicker the patient, the more chances of receiving steroids, and by lowering the immune defences these inherently carry an increased risk of colonization followed by infection.

Antibiotic therapy in the ICU is another risk factor. It may be extremely difficult to differentiate between colonization and infection. Colonization is the isolation of bacteria or fungi from a clinically relevant site such as the endotracheal suction or sputum, urine or wound in the absence of clinical signs or symptoms. In seriously ill patients it is difficult to assess whether the isolated pathogens are causing disease or not. The situation is also confounded by the administration of steroids and other non-anti-microbial agents which may suppress the clinical signs such as fever ($>38°C$ or more) and depress a raised white blood cell count ($>12\,000\ \mathrm{mm}^{-3}$). Another factor is that during the immediate postoperative period, pyrexia is common and is difficult to differentiate from an infective process.

The choice of antibiotic(s) is usually empirical and therefore, has a wide spectrum to cover staphylococci, streptococci, enterobacteriaceae, *Pseudomonas* spp., *Acinetobacter* spp. and anaerobes. The effect is two-fold: first, the patient's susceptible flora is replaced by more antibiotic-resistant bacteria; and, second, there is further suppression of the immune system in an already seriously ill patient. Some antibiotics have further untoward effects such as increased bleeding, diarrhoea and jaundice. All of these contribute to worsening the patient's condition. Antibiotics must be used with careful consideration and caution, and should be clinically appropriate. Antibiotic policies for the ICUs should contain clear indications for use in different clinical conditions. Frequently, several organs are affected in the same infective episode and this should be taken into consideration when prescribing antimicrobial therapy.

8.4.6 Colonization

It is inevitable that patients admitted to the ICU become colonized after a certain period of time. There

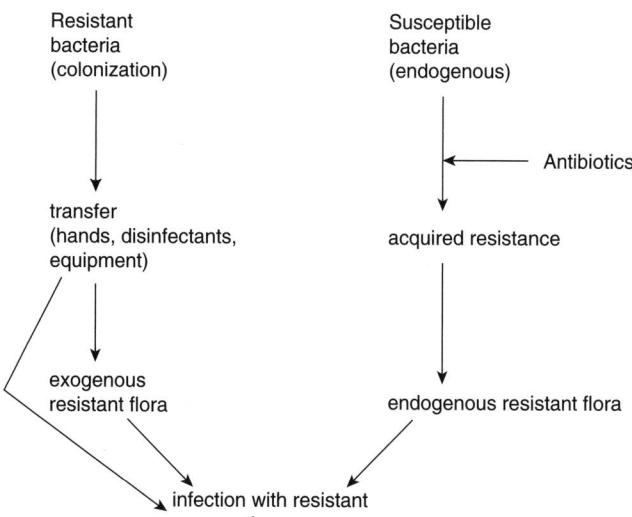

Figure 8.1 *Acquisition of antibiotic-resistant flora leading to infection in ICU patients.*

is a colonization risk relationship between the length of stay on the ICU, number of invasive devices and the use of life-saving drugs such as steroids. Moreover, the rate of colonization has been shown conclusively to play a significant part in this process. Colonization occurs in the gut, via the oropharageal route and is the most likely source of endogenous infection, particularly under antibiotic pressure (Figure 8.1). These bacteria are then introduced to the sites of infection either by the hands of the staff or via the medical equipment used on patients.

When colonization becomes infection is dependent on the individual patient (host), and clinical parameters have to be taken into account before such a decision is reached. The difference between colonization and infection should be clearly defined as far as possible, and it is advisable not to treat colonization in the absence of clear clinical parameters because inappropriate antibiotic use can have serious consequences not only for the patients concerned but also for other patients on the ICU; the promotion of resistant strains is particularly to be feared.

8.4.7 Invasive devices

The presence of foreign bodies such as endotracheal tubes, nasogastric tubes, urinary catheters, etc. reduces the local site immunity of the patient and increases the risk of colonization and infection. The normal ciliary mechanisms cannot function in the presence of an endotracheal tube, and the accumulation of secretions inevitably becomes colonized (see below). Similarly, the presence of nasogastric tubes and urinary catheters have a suppressive effect on the local humoral defences which increases the risk of colonization and infection.

8.5 THE ENVIRONMENT

The ICU environment is influenced by the following (all of which have implications for infection):

- The number of beds and the type of patients
- Clinical equipment
- Non-clinical equipment
- Pathogens
- Staff

Colonization of the environment in an ICU is inevitable (see Section 8.4.6). Moist reservoirs, particularly humidifiers for respirators, handwash basins and sinks, sluices and waste disposal areas, are very often found to be colonized with multiply antibiotic-resistant bacteria. Most of these bacteria are Gram-negative and are ubiquitous. *Pseudomonas aeruginosa, Acinetobacter* spp. and other non-fermentors are frequently found in the environment. The potential to cause infection is when these Gram-negative bacteria are introduced inadvertently into a vulnerable patient either via the hands of staff or via inadequately processed clinical and non-clinical equipment.

Currently, it is rare to find ICUs dedicated to each speciality, and most units contain a mixture of seriously ill medical and surgical patients who may require short- or long-term attention. Most ICUs will contain between six to twelve beds and have a common staff, a situation which has both advantages and disadvantages.

ADVANTAGES

Surgical and non-surgical patients require varying degrees of attention, and so the sicker patients in both groups may be given more attention if necessary. Also, it is considered by management to provide better usage of staff skills. However, the entire unit is under the supervision of a medical specialist who will liaise and consult with the relevant specialities on appropriate management, and any changes in the day-to-day management of the unit can be channelled through one person. Specialist management of ventilation, etc. will be based on protocols which should provide the best medical care under the given circumstances. Clinical equipment can be used to maximum benefit and be shared between patients.

DISADVANTAGES

Patients admitted to different parts of the hospital may have had varying lengths of stay in hospital before being admitted to the ICU, and hence bring with them hospital pathogens acquired from the previous wards. Another problem is that highly specialized support nursing may be required, for example when dealing with patients from oncology or paediatrics – an expertise which may be lacking in the ICU. If communication breaks down between the medical team in charge of the ICU and the admitting team, then the management of the patient suffers. Sharing of equipment also has its own risks if decontamination and sterilization processes are not adequate.

8.6 DESIGN AND LAYOUT

The ICU should be designed such that the main ward area has adequate space between beds (3 m) to allow for easy movement of staff and equipment. Where possible, isolation cubicles should be present to segregate infectious patients. There must be adequate handwashing facilities provided which are well spaced in the ward. Hand decontamination facilities (alcohol rub) should be available next to each patient's bed and at the entrance to the unit. Ventilation on the unit should be adequate to maintain comfortable working conditions. In some units, six to eight air changes per hour are provided by an air handling unit. This may be appropriate where a specialized ICU is linked to other complexes such as an operating suite or a burns unit. In a general unit, normal air from outside is adequate provided that there is minimal dust in the atmosphere, no building works are being carried out, and main roads or traffic are far from the unit. There should be no sewage or waste pipes laid above the patient area in the ICU. All pipes should run along the wall and away from the ventilation ducts. This is to prevent contamination of the main ICU ward and patients in case of an accident.

The sluice and dirty areas should be segregated, and there should be no through traffic via these areas. All equipment in these areas should be cleaned thoroughly and stored dry. Clean and dirty equipment should be stored separately and disposable equipment stores should be kept well ventilated and dry. There should be no environmental moisture or water traps. Servicing of respiratory equipment should ideally be carried out in a separate room, and appropriate protocols should ensure regular cleaning and maintenance of such equipment.

8.6.1 Protective clothing

There is no advantage to changing into special clothing before entering the ICU. However, white coats should be removed and the hands thoroughly decontaminated before patient contact. There is no need for overshoes or head gear, but well-fitting latex disposable gloves and a plastic apron should be worn for each patient procedure and discarded immediately afterwards. Hands must then be washed and dried thoroughly before attending the next patient. While gloves should only be worn when indicated, such as during an invasive procedure, the rules should be strongly adhered to. In some countries there have been suggestions that the gloves be decontaminated with alcohol rub while still worn by the staff. This is not practical or recommended for intensive care units. Hand hygiene has to be paramount. It is not good practice to attend several patients with the same pair of gloves or plastic apron as these can transfer pathogens; it should not be allowed.

8.7 THE EQUIPMENT

8.7.1 Respirators

One of the most common source of pathogens in the ICU, especially *Pseudomonas aeruginosa* and *Acinetobacter* spp., is poorly cleaned respirator equipment which is stored in an inappropriate environment. It is now customary to install inspiratory and expiratory filters to the main respirator, and this is usually provided by the manufacturer. Should such filters not be present, then external filters should be installed. The manufacturer should also provide information on decontamination procedures for newly purchased equipment, and this should be verified by the Infection Control Team (ICT).

Patient circuits are now fitted with self-humidifying respiratory filters (disposable) which are used with each individual patient circuit and changed frequently (every 72 hours or weekly if the patient is on long-term ventilation, depending on the local unit protocol). This alleviates the need for external humidification and thus reduces the risk of colonization from water-loving Gram-negative bacteria such as *Pseudomonas* and *Acinetobacter* spp. Where disposable filters are not available, the humidifiers should be sterilized by heat and filled with **sterile** distilled water (as stated elsewhere in the book, distilled water is not sterile unless it is sterilized) which should be changed every 48 hours. Topping up with distilled water after 48 hours leads to colonization, as is inevitable when a circuit is constantly being broken.

Patient breathing circuits may be either disposable or reusable. Disposable circuits are expensive and may be used for a week for one patient provided that humidifying filters are used. Reusable circuits require disinfection at 80–90°C for 1 minute to render them safe for use. Vegetative forms of bacteria are eliminated, but killing of spores and tuberculous bacilli requires steam sterilization. Soaking in disinfectants is not advised; this procedure leads to inadequate, uncontrolled decontamination, allows for contamination of the circuits by multiply antibiotic-resistant bacteria, and may cause chemical irritation to the patient if the circuits have not been rinsed properly.

The main body of the respirator should be cleaned regularly. All the parts should be removed and cleaned thoroughly with warm water and detergent only. The filters will protect the main ventilation circuits. However, in the case of gross contamination, a suitable disinfection method suggested by the manufacturers or the IC Team should be considered.

8.7.2 Endotracheal tubes and suction

An integral part of mechanical ventilation is the insertion of an endotracheal (ET) tube. Most ET tubes these days are disposable and made of material which causes minimum friction and strictures. Although not recommended, if ET tubes are recycled, heat disinfection is sufficient (see Respirators). Soaking in disinfectants is not only toxic to the patient but also does not guarantee disinfection or sterility. The presence of an ET tube suppresses local defences and, in combination with mechanical ventilation, increases secretions in the bronchi which have to be removed periodically by suction. The process of introducing ET tube suction catheters has several problems.

First, the suction catheter has to be sterile. In some units the catheter is kept for 24 hours if used on the same patient, the following sequence being used. After suction the catheter is stored in its sleeve until the next time; before suction, the catheter is wetted with sterile saline which is poured into a sterile bowl lying next to the patient. The open bowl can become colonized and may be a source of potential pathogens such as *Pseudomonas* and *Acinetobacter* spp. and other Gram-negative bacilli. These are then introduced into a moist ET tube. It can be readily seen that this sequence is hazardous and is sub-optimal.

Second, the process of suction may be carried out with the introduction of saline to ease the extraction of secretions, particularly in patients who have been on ventilation for less than 48 hours. Also, hyperinflation of the lung to ease aspiration was considered useful in the past. Both of these methods create extension of infected material to previously uncontaminated regions of the tracheo-bronchial passages.

The use of a disinfectant spray or aerosols to clean bronchial catheters is also to be deplored, as they increase infection risk, particularly the latter. Moreover, staff carrying out the procedure may get sprayed and covered with aerosol particles that contain colonizing pathogens. Particles may also travel to the patient in the adjacent bed. Endotracheal suction should be carried out with care and best practice dictates that in addition to a sterile suction tube, protective clothing such as gloves and impermeable clothes cover (plastic aprons) should be worn. Finally, when ET tube secretions are sent for microbiological culture, the results may be misleading. Colonizing pathogens may not necessarily be causative of respiratory tract infection; any antibiotic therapy that is instituted on the basis of the result should be considered very carefully to avoid inappropriate prescribing.

8.7.3 Urinary catheters

Disposable sterile urinary catheters of an appropriate size attached to a closed drainage system are preferred. Calibration containers to assess fluid balance are attached to the circuit and should not be opened unnecessarily. The urinary drainage bag should be part of the closed circuit and should be fitted with a non-return valve and a tap that can be easily manipulated to empty the urine contents. The bag should always be below the level of the pelvis, but raised from the floor on a stand or an attachment to the bed of the patient. A clean dry jug should be used to empty each urinary bag; communal urinary jugs for emptying a series of bags should not be allowed as it leads to cross-contamination.

8.7.4 Intravenous devices

All patients on the ICU will have a peripheral intravenous device (IVD) at some time during their stay. Most patients will also require a central venous catheter (CVC) for monitoring pressure and administering large quantities of drugs and fluid which peripheral lines cannot cope with. Some patients may be on total parenteral nutrition (TPN) where there has been extensive loss of bowel either due to surgery or infarct and enteral nutrition via a nasogastric tube is inadequate. IVDs are a common source of infection, particularly CVCs and TPN lines. These have to be maintained meticulously by frequent visual inspection. The line sites must be inserted under strict asepsis with minimum trauma, i.e. by an attendant with the required skills and experience. The site must be kept dry and inspected visually at frequent intervals. Any signs of redness or swelling should be taken seriously. In most situations the clinical condition demands the maintenance of a CVC, and therefore immediate removal may not be appropriate. It is therefore likely that antibiotic therapy will be considered. However, if no change in the clinical picture occurs within 48 hours, replacement of the CVC and transfer to the opposite side should be considered under antibiotic cover.

8.7.5 Nasogastric tubes

Patients on mechanical ventilation require the insertion of a nasogastric tube to prevent regurgitation. Nasogastric tubes are also used for enteral feeds; these should be fine bore, disposable and made of a non-reactive material. **Red rubber tubes are no longer acceptable** because they cause irritation and oesophageal strictures.

One consequence of nasogastric tubes is sinusitis associated with bacteria colonizing the throat and upper respiratory tract of the patient. This is often missed as one of the infective causes, and should be borne in mind when dealing with such patients.

8.7.6 Wound dressings

Strict asepsis and a no-touch technique should be used when dealing with a wound site, including the IV catheter insertion site. Any type of dressing in direct contact with an open wound should be sterile. The dressings used should be packed and sterilized individually, the remaining pack to be discarded at the end of a dressing.

Dressing trolleys which carry multiple-use disinfectant bottles, jars of cotton wool either stored dry or containing a skin disinfectant should not be permitted as these are frequent sources of multiply antibiotic-resistant bacteria found in the environment and lead to contamination of the wound site. Disinfectants if required, should be packed in single-use sachets or small containers which hold up to 50 ml of fluid. The remainder should be discarded at the end of the dressing.

8.8 NON-CLINICAL EQUIPMENT

Bed-pans, urinal jugs and other non-clinical equipment should be **cleaned thoroughly**, then **heat disinfected** at a minimum temperature of 90°C for 1 minute or 80°C for 3 minutes and finally **dried thoroughly** between each patient use. It is advisable that a bed-pan disinfector be installed in the sluice area and be maintained regularly to ensure safe disinfection. This also reduces the amount of manual handling by the staff who may inadvertently carry pathogens on their hands to the patients.

There is no need for environmental disinfection of the rooms unless specified by the Infection Control Team, for which a possible indication may be an infection outbreak. Regular cleaning with warm water and detergent

Table 8.1 *Types of pathogens likely to be present in patient sites in the ICU (these may not necessarily be causing disease)*

Site	Primary pathogens	Secondary pathogens
Urinary tract	*Escherichia coli, Klebsiella pneumoniae, Proteus mirabilis* Coagulase-negative staphylococci, enterococci	*Pseudomonas aeruginosa, Enterobacter* spp. *Acinetobacter* spp. *Candida albicans* Enterococci
Upper respiratory tract	*Staph. aureus*, streptococci, Gram-negative bacilli	As above Methicillin-resistant *Staph. aureus* (MRSA)
Lower respiratory tract	*Streptococcus pneumoniae Haemophilus influenzae, Staphylococcus aureus* Gram-negative bacilli (rare)	*Klebsiella pneumoniae Pseudomonas aeruginosa Acinetobacter baumanii Candida albicans Staph. aureus* (MRSA) Enterococci Anaerobic bacteria
Device-associated	None	Coagulase-negative Staphylococci Diphtheroids Gram-negative bacilli
Wound (trauma, post-surgical)	*Staph. aureus* Coagulase-negative staphylococci enterococci Gram-negative bacilli anaerobes	*Pseudomonas aeruginosa, Enterobacter* spp. *Acinetobacter* spp. *Candida albicans* Enterococci

is quite sufficient, and the environment should be kept completely dry.

8.9 STAFF

The staff working in the ICU must be adequately trained and frequently updated on the latest developments. Frequent visits by the Infection Control Team is necessary not only for them to be available for appropriate clinical advice but also to educate and inform the staff. Training in handwashing and disinfection, dealing with equipment, patient procedures and keeping of appropriate records is a vital part of staff education. Junior doctors should be also advised on procedures and management of patients, particularly antibiotic usage. An infection manual relevant to local needs should be available, and staff should be familiar with its principal directives.

8.10 PATHOGENS

Pathogens encountered in the ICU may be primary pathogens isolated from patients who have been admitted directly from the community or who have been in hospital for less than 48 hours (Table 8.1)

Secondary infecting or colonizing pathogens are those which have been acquired in the ICU and usually reflect the resident flora of the unit or newly emerging antibiotic resistance. The sensitivity patterns differ particularly amongst the Gram-negative population, and therefore antibiotic requirements can change quickly. It is beyond the scope of this chapter to provide details of antibiotic therapy, but local antibiotic policies should take into consideration the effect on the ecology of the ICU.

8.11 FURTHER READING

Bergogne-Bérézin, E. (2001) Guidelines on anti-microbial therapy for prevention and treatment of infections in the intensive care unit. *Journal of Chemotherapy,* **13**, 134–149.

Brun-Buisson, C., Doyon, C., Carlet, J. and French Bacteraemia Study Group. (1996) A multi-centre prospective survey in ICUs and wards of 24 hospitals. *American Journal of Critical Care Medicine,* **154**, 617–624.

Emori, T.G. and Gaynes, R.P. (1993) An overview of nosocomial infections including the role of the microbiology laboratory. *Clinical Microbiology Reviews,* **6**, 428–442.

Markowitz, P., Woolf, M., Djedaini, K. *et al.* (2000) Multicentre prospective study of ventilator-associated pneumonia during acute respiratory distress syndrome. *American Journal of Respiratory Critical Care Medicine,* **161**, 1942–1948.

Pittet, D. and Horbarth, S.J. (1998) The Intensive Care Unit. In *Hospital Infections,* J.V. Bennett and P.S. Bradman (eds). 4th Ed., Lippincott-Raven, Philadelphia, pp. 382–402.

Pittet, D. and Wenzel, R. (1995) Nosocomial bloodstream infections; secular trends in rates, mortality and contribution to total hospital deaths. *Archives of Internal Medicine,* **155**, 1177–1184.

Vincent, J.L., Bihari, D., Suter, P.M. *et al.* (1995) The prevalence of nosocomial infection in intensive care units in Europe: the results of the EPIC study. *Journal of the American Medical Association,* **274**, 639–644.

Vincent, J.L. and Preiser, J.C. (1999) Management of critically ill patients with severe sepsis. *Journal of Chemotherapy,* **11**, 524–529.

Blood transfusion infections

A.D. KITCHEN AND J.A.J. BARBARA

9.1 INTRODUCTION

All blood transfusions carry an associated, albeit small, risk. In recent years the risk of transmission of infectious agents has been especially highlighted. There is no doubt that blood transfusion is a potentially effective route of infection, the results of which can lead to serious consequences, not only for the patients concerned, but in some cases also for the close contacts of that individual.

Although blood transfusion services recognize the risks and actively strive to ensure that the blood supply is both safe and plentiful, rare instances of transmission of infection by blood transfusion can occur, despite the rigorous screening procedures that are in place.

In most transfusion services the safety of the blood supply relies upon two levels of screening. First, the **donor** and second, the **donation**. Blood donors are screened by questioning and visual inspection, whilst blood donations are screened by *in-vitro* diagnostic tests.

9.2 BLOOD DONORS

The concept of voluntary, non-remunerated donation of blood units is central to safe blood. *In-vitro* diagnostic tests may not detect every potentially infectious unit (for reasons that will be considered later on), but their effectiveness can be increased by careful preselection of blood donors prior to donation. It is generally accepted that those individuals who give their blood voluntarily, without coercion or expectation of reward, are the safest donors. The key issue of donor selection is to assess whether a donor is at 'high' or 'low' risk, i.e. whether the donor is likely or not to have been exposed to certain transfusion-transmissible infectious diseases and is therefore likely to be infected and thus potentially infectious at the time of donation.

Donor selection is thus a vital process that seeks to ensure that donors are low-risk individuals who have not been exposed to certain infectious diseases, have no underlying chronic conditions that may result in illness in the recipient of the blood, and for whom donation would not be contraindicated as a health risk to themselves. This selection procedure comprises: (i) the predonation presentation of specific information to donors enabling donor self-referral of individuals with apparent risk factors; (ii) a brief visual examination of each donor to look for any obvious signs and symptoms of disease, illness or behaviour; and (iii) direct questioning prior to the actual donation. Donor education is a prerequisite of this process. Donors need to be educated to understand the concept of high-risk behaviour and its hazards, and the need for honesty in their response to predonation questioning. The importance of good donor selection must not be underestimated. It is a relatively inexpensive procedure that is the first stage in the screening procedures used to ensure a safe blood supply – a safer donor provides a safer donation.

Laboratory testing however, is still the mainstay of blood screening. Whilst donor selection is a broad process, laboratory testing is very specific, and applied to identify those donations, and thus donors, infected with certain infectious agents.

9.3 INFECTIOUS AGENTS TRANSMITTED BY BLOOD TRANSFUSION

The number of infectious agents transmitted by blood transfusion is not particularly large, but includes viruses, bacteria and protozoa and, possibly, prions. Most importantly, a number of these viruses can cause severe disease for which effective treatment is not always available. The particular infectious agents in any donor population are dependent upon the infectious agents prevalent in the general population from which it is drawn. Globally, these tend to be the same agents, although there may be regional variations. This implies selective screening for certain agents that are present normally in the population and which are only likely to give rise to significant disease in certain recipient groups. It is accepted that all donated blood should be screened for: antibodies to the human immunodeficiency viruses $1 + 2$ (anti-HIV $1 + 2$); hepatitis B virus surface antigen (HBsAg); antibodies to hepatitis C virus (anti-HCV); and serological evidence of syphilis infection. In addition, some countries screen blood for antibodies to the human T-cell leukaemia viruses (anti-HTLV I + II), antibodies to hepatitis B virus core antigen (anti-HBc) or antibodies to *Trypanosoma cruzi*, the causative agent of Chagas' disease. Finally, selected donations may also be screened for antibodies to human cytomegalovirus (anti-HCMV), or evidence of malaria. In Japan, screening of donors for parvo-virus B19 antigen has recently been introduced.

As well as specific bacterial infections such as syphilis, there is also the potential for bacterial contamination of blood and products. The growth of contaminating bacteria in blood and products is potentially fatal due to the build-up of toxic bacterial waste products resulting in septic shock. The prevention of such contamination is dependent upon cleanliness during the collection, processing and storage of blood and is an area that will not be discussed any further in this text.

This chapter will discuss the major infectious agents transmitted by transfusion, but from a largely transfusion microbiology standpoint, will focus on important issues in the screening of donated blood for these agents.

9.4 THE 'WINDOW PERIOD' OF INFECTION

Unfortunately, with most infectious agents, there is a clearly defined period following infection – the 'window period' – during which infection may not be detected by routine serological screening tests, although the individual may be infectious. Following infection with any infectious agent there is an incubation phase during which the agent proliferates and the infection establishes, although markers of this infection may not be readily detectable. The length of this period varies tremendously depending upon the infectious agent, the individual and the particular marker used to detect the agent. Subsequently, the response of the immune system to the infection becomes detectable as antibodies against the agent appear (seroconversion). Sophisticated and expensive testing for viral nucleic acid (or for hepatitis C core antigen) to practically eliminate the 'window period' risk is increasingly becoming routine.

9.5 HEPATITIS B VIRUS (HBV)

Detection of HBV infection in donated blood is best achieved by screening for HBsAg, and this is universally accepted. HBsAg is the first marker to appear in the bloodstream, and generally persists throughout the period of infectivity. The other markers of HBV infection are of use in confirming infection and determining the type and stage of infection, but apart from anti-HBc they have no value in routine blood screening. Detection of HBV DNA may be beneficial in assessing the individual's status, but again this has limited value for blood screening as the techniques are not yet suitable for mass screening and DNA levels can fall to below detectable levels, but with infectivity remaining. The sensitivity and specificity of HBsAg assays is generally good, with sensitivities increasing continuously, and currently being as low as 0.1 IU ml^{-1}. Anti-HBs is a protective antibody which usually appears shortly after the disappearance of HBsAg, although there are some individuals in whom there is an extended delay before its appearance, and this marks the resolution of infection. Titres may decline over extended periods, but recovery from acute infection does normally confer lifetime protection.

9.5.1 Anti-HBc screening

For many years the subject of anti-HBc screening of donations has been discussed. Before specific anti-HCV screening became possible, anti-HBc screening was considered to be a possible way of reducing the number of cases of posttransfusion non-A,non-B hepatitis (PTNANBH) then seen in large numbers. The identification of the hepatitis C virus (HCV) and the advent of anti-HCV screening have now demonstrated that this particular strategy had no significant value in the prevention of PTNANBH.

However, it is now realized that the main value of anti-HBc screening is to identify that very small number of donors who are either resolving an acute infection or clearing a chronic infection, and are apparently HBsAg negative on screening, but who may still have a low-level viraemia and be infectious. The latter group have been called 'tail end carriers'. In such individuals anti-HBc may be the only detectable circulating marker of infection, and thus would only be detectable by anti-HBc screening. This situation could explain cases of post-transfusion HBV reported resulting from transfusion of donations screened as HBsAg-negative where the patient does not appear to have other risks or sources of infection (see below). A major problem with anti-HBc screening is to then identify those donors who possess only anti-HBc and distinguish them from those who are naturally immune following infection earlier in life. Many anti-HBc screening tests have relatively poor specificity, and there are also problems confirming initial anti-HBc reactivity. Even if anti-HBs is also subsequently detected, it is generally agreed that those donors with low-level anti-HBs (usually <100 mIU ml^{-1}) cannot be considered to be sufficiently immune to be suitable as donors. Whilst there is no doubt that there may be a small number of individuals who may be infectious and have only anti-HBc detectable, in non-endemic areas this is likely to be a very small number. Currently, some countries do screen all donations for anti-HBc, although most do not. At present, however, the value of anti-HBc screening remains a subject for debate. However, if nucleic acid testing (NAT) for HBV DNA were introduced, it would be inconsistent not to also introduce anti-HBc.

9.5.2 HBV Mutants

Currently, two groups of HBV mutants have been identified: the pre-core mutants; and the surface antigen mutants. The pre-core mutants have a normal HBsAg expression but have missing or altered HBeAg expression. These mutants currently are not thought to present any threat to the blood supply because HBsAg expression is normal and blood screening would therefore not be compromised. However, the HBsAg mutants (originally termed 'vaccine escape' mutants) are of concern to blood screening as HBsAg expression is altered such that some assays may fail to detect certain HBsAg mutant forms. This is most likely where the assays use monoclonal antibodies either on the solid phase or in the conjugate if these antibodies are specific for the 'a' determinant of HBsAg (which is the usual missing or altered protein of the HBsAg mutants). Assays using polyclonal antibodies are less likely to fail to detect HBsAg mutants as their reactivity is broader and usually encompasses other

epitopes on the HBsAg molecules. Studies so far have found that most HBsAg assays from reputable international manufacturers do detect the majority of the HBsAg mutants available for study. In addition, anti-HBc is positive in infection with HBV mutants.

9.6 HEPATITIS C VIRUS (HCV)

Infections with the hepatitis C virus (HCV) have been recognized for many years, but the virus has only been cloned and characterized in the past 10 years. The virus is transmitted parenterally, including intimate contact, although debate continues about the risk of transmission through sexual contact; the routes of infection are essentially the same as for HBV. The virus is an enveloped RNA virus that has been classified as a separate genus within the flavivirus (flaviviridae) family. This has been deduced from the structure of the RNA and specific sequences within it. Although much is now known about the virus, the virus itself has still not been isolated as an intact virion. Current knowledge about HCV and the diagnostic assays that are at present available, have all arisen from the isolation of the complete viral genome from human plasma, and the *in-vitro* expression of the genome and subsequent characterization of the proteins expressed. The humoral immune response to HCV appears to be relatively weak, the antibodies are not present at high titres, and the reactivity against the currently identified individual epitopes is variable. There is no doubt that the identification of HCV and the introduction of anti-HCV screening of blood donations has been a significant step in the prevention of cases of PTNANBH and thus an increase in the safety of the blood supply.

9.6.1 Screening blood donations for HCV

Currently, blood donations are only screened for anti-HCV. Screening for HCV RNA is currently in place in developed countries, usually on pools of, e.g. 48 samples. However, in England and Wales the yield of confirmed positives detected by nucleic acid testing (NAT) is only 1 in 1–2 million. A major problem that faced transfusion services and laboratories at the start of anti-HCV screening was the generally poor specificity of anti-HCV screening assays. A second problem was, and still is, confirmation of the screening results. Again, because of the way in which anti-HCV screening has developed, the 'confirmatory assays' currently available commonly incorporate the same basic antigens as used in the screening assays, although presented in a different format.

Donors with indeterminate HCV serology are another major problem associated with anti-HCV screening. A number of individuals are found to be positive on screening, but, when subsequently tested by a 'confirmatory assay', are neither clearly positive or negative. They show some apparent anti-HCV reactivity, but insufficient to differentiate true HCV infection from non-specific reactivity. Depending upon the donor population and the prevalence of HCV, up to 30% of repeatedly screen-reactive donors may be classified as HCV indeterminate. The problem with HCV indeterminate results is that, within the large number of non-specific false-positive results, some may actually indicate true HCV infection, either recent seroconversion when the antibody response has not yet developed fully, or at the other extreme, resolved previous acute or chronic infection. Although, because they give positive screening results, such donations are unlikely to be transfused, there is a concern that any donors who may be (or may have been) truly infected with HCV should be referred for appropriate clinical management. Thus, a number of studies are currently being performed to try to identify, as reliably and quickly as possible, donors with uncertain HCV serology but who may be truly infected.

Since the introduction of anti-HCV screening, a number of confirmed cases of transmission of HCV by confirmed anti-HCV-negative blood donations have been reported. These cases have been caused by donations collected from viraemic but anti-HCV-negative donors, most probably in the acute phase of infection, who would not routinely be identified by serology. Such 'window period' individuals remain a problem for transfusion services, especially when many cases of HCV infection are asymptomatic and risk factors may not be readily identifiable. The extent of the problem of transmission of HCV by 'window period' donors is also largely unknown, as the cases reported may just represent the tip of the iceberg, being identified by chance rather than because of clinical concerns and subsequent investigation.

Assays to detect HCVAg (e.g. in the window period) are now available and detect 85–90% of those infected individuals by NAT on single samples.

9.7 HUMAN IMMUNODEFICIENCY VIRUSES (HIV 1 + 2)

The human immunodeficiency virus (HIV) is transmitted by the parenteral route, mainly by: (i) sexual contact; (ii) mother-to-infant transmission; (iii) blood transfusion; or (iv) IV drug use. Although transmission by blood transfusion is a particularly effective means of transmission, it is largely preventable by the appropriate donor selection and donation screening.

Following infection with HIV, seroconversion occurs usually 1–3 months later. Prior to seroconversion, virus can be detected in the bloodstream, and viral RNA and DNA can be detected in the lymphocytes. In addition, HIV p24 Ag can be detected 1–2 weeks before seroconversion. This antigen is viral core antigen and is one of the most abundant proteins produced by infected cells. As the antibody levels rise, the level of p24 Ag declines as the Ag is bound by antibody. Although not directly detectable by normal methods, Ag production does persist during the majority of the period until AIDS develops.

9.8 SCREENING BLOOD DONATIONS

The vast majority of blood donations are screened for HIV infection using anti-HIV assays. In some countries, however, additional testing is performed using HIV p24 Ag assays. In the vast majority of cases, anti-HIV screening will identify HIV-infected blood donations and prevent cases of post-transfusion HIV infection. Although screening was initially only for anti-HIV 1, the emergence of HIV 2 meant that the anti-HIV assays had to incorporate specific HIV 2 antigens, and the emergence of HIV 1 subtype O has resulted in the additional incorporation of specific subtype O antigens in assays.

9.8.1 HIV p24 Ag screening

Late in 1995, the US Food and Drug Administration (FDA) mandated that HIV p24 Ag testing of blood donations should start in the USA, in addition to anti-HIV 1 + 2 testing. In a similar way to screening for HCV nucleic acid, the intention is to decrease the 'window period' in an acute infection during which a potentially infectious but anti-HIV 1 + 2-negative donation could be donated. However, in the case of HIV the situation is far more complicated as, although closing the 'window period' by a few days, there still remains a small risk of transmission from donors who are viraemic but p24 Ag- and anti-HIV-negative. Screening for HIV DNA in addition would reduce the 'window period' by perhaps one or two days more, whilst screening for pro-viral RNA would reduce it by about another week. Thus, screening for HIV RNA would actually be more beneficial than screening for p24 Ag, although, like HCV, such molecular mass screening is currently not possible. It has been calculated that, in the USA, the introduction of p24 Ag screening may prevent up to 10 cases of transmission per year, but at a cost of about US$100 million. Whether p24 Ag screening will have any significant effect on the safety of the blood supply in the USA is, as yet, uncertain, but this will be watched with interest.

Recently a range of sensitive assays that can simultaneously detect anti-HIV and/or HIVAg have become available.

9.8.2 HIV 1 subtype O

In May 1994 reports were published of a new subtype of HIV 1, subtype O. Although there are many subtypes of HIV 1, this one was of particular concern, as some of the then current screening tests did not detect all examples of the new subtype. The subtype was first identified in one country in West Africa, but has now been identified (albeit in very small numbers) in several other countries. The identification of a number of examples of HIV 1 subtype O enabled a panel of samples to be put together and commercial assays to be tested against the panel. A small number of tests detected only a few of the samples, whilst most tests detected 60–90% of samples. Interestingly, most of the assays detected subtype O through cross-reactivity with HIV 1. However, most commercial assays used for blood screening have now been modified to be able to detect all examples of subtype O; whilst cross-reactivity is still utilized by some assays, the majority of modifications have included specific subtype O antigens. Although a theoretical problem for transfusion services, cases of subtype O are very rare and most assays will be able to detect most examples.

9.9 HUMAN T-CELL LEUKAEMIA VIRUSES (HTLV I + II)

The human T-cell leukaemia virus I (HTLV I) was the first human retrovirus identified. The virus is potentially oncogenic causing adult T-cell leukaemia and lymphoma (ATLL or ATL), and tropical spastic paraparesis (TSP), also known as HTLV I-associated myelopathy (HAM). A second virus, HTLV II, has also been identified in specific groups of individuals, for example intravenous drug users, although no disease has yet been clearly associated with this virus. The viruses are distributed worldwide, but are concentrated in certain specific areas and countries, mainly in the tropics. Even within countries, particular areas may have higher prevalences of HTLV.

Most infections with HTLV I are asymptomatic and remain so. However, there is a small risk that disease may develop any time up to 40 years after infection. ATLL can present as an acute leukaemia of CD4+ lymphocytes, most often between the ages of 30 and 50 years. Death usually occurs within a year of the onset of symptoms. TSP is a progressive disease involving the degeneration of neurones in the spinal cord, leading to gradual paralysis of the lower limbs. The virus is virtually always cell-associated, being present in CD4+ lymphocytes, and is transmitted in these cells parenterally via blood or semen, or from mother to infant via breast milk. Blood transfusion is another potential route of infection. Early studies demonstrated transfusion transmission, but not via cell-free products such as plasma.

9.9.1 HTLV serology

Following infection with HTLV I there is an incubation period from 30–90 days before seroconversion, before which viral RNA can be detected in lymphocytes. At seroconversion, antibody to HTLV appears and this is the major target for the diagnosis of HTLV infection. After seroconversion the antibody generally persists for life, even if clinical disease subsequently develops later in life. The serological response to HTLV I and HTLV II are very similar, and specialized tests are needed to be able to discriminate reliably between HTLV I and HTLV II.

9.9.2 Blood screening for HTLV

The potential significance of blood transfusion as a route of transmission of HTLV has meant that, in a number of endemic countries, screening of donations has been carried out for some time. Screening has also been introduced in some non-endemic developed countries with mixed populations. In several other countries debate continues over the need and value of screening donations.

Blood donations are screened for an indication of current or previous HTLV I/II infection by screening for antibody against the viruses – anti-HTLV I + II. There are now a few good anti-HTLV screening assays commercially available which have good sensitivity and specificity. In addition, suitable serological confirmatory assays are now available, but NAT for genomic detection is sometimes needed to help clarify unresolved serology.

9.10 HUMAN CYTOMEGALOVIRUS (HCMV)

Human cytomegalovirus (HCMV) is a member of the herpesvirus family, a group of DNA viruses that are widespread in the general population and characterized by their ability to give rise to persistent latent infections. The virus is the largest of the herpesviruses, and has the largest genome of any known virus. HCMV is globally the most common virus to be transmitted *in utero*, affecting up to 2.5% of all live births, and causing serious disease in symptomatic individuals. Globally between 40–90% of adults are infected with HCMV, the prevalence usually increasing with age from late childhood onwards, although in endemic areas the prevalence can reach 90% in young adults. HCMV has been recognized for more than 25 years as a potentially serious complication of blood transfusion, but only in certain patient groups. Infection in healthy immunocompetent individuals is usually asymptomatic (any symptoms resembling a mild, glandular fever-like illness), and is essentially clinically insignificant unless occurring in a pregnant woman.

The virus is transmissible by the parenteral route, and during acute infection may be present in most body fluids. During acute infection the virus infects circulating leukocytes, and eventually may persist latently in those cells. In addition, latent infection has been demonstrated in the endothelial cells lining the walls of blood vessels.

As the acute infection resolves, specific circulating antibody to CMV appears. However, because of the latency this anti-HCMV does not eliminate the virus from white cells and serves to identify potentially infectious donors. Following acute infection, it is quite possible that later on an individual may undergo another acute infection, either due to reactivation of latent virus or reinfection from an external source. This is not thought to be a serious problem in immunocompetent individuals, but it can be serious in the immunocompromised. Many such patients, for example leukaemia and transplant recipients, may face serious illness from HCMV. In previously infected donors, it is the latent virus in the transfused leukocytes that is thought to reactivate and give rise to post-transfusion HCMV infection. Leukodepletion (LD) of blood products was subsequently shown to prevent HCMV transmission from seropositive donors but definitive prospective studies to demonstrate the equivalence of LD to anti-HCMV screening are not yet available.

9.10.1   Blood screening for HCMV

HCMV-infected blood donors are identified by screening for anti-HCMV. Unfortunately, as discussed above, the presence of anti-HCMV does not mark immunity, but rather indicates previous infection and thus a donor with latent and potentially infectious virus. Therefore, only donations from donors who have not been infected with HCMV are suitable for transfusion to immunocompromised patients. Anti-HCMV screening of donations is selective, with only a proportion of donations needing to be screened for HCMV, and the anti-HCMV-negative donations identified are then restricted for issue to those patients who need anti-HCMV-negative blood.

9.11   SYPHILIS

The spirochaete *Treponema pallidum* is the causative agent of syphilis. Following initial infection, the course of infection can follow several stages leading to primary, secondary and tertiary syphilis. All parts of the body may be involved, giving rise to a wide variety of clinical symptoms. At 1–2 months after infection the characteristic lesions normally disappear and the infection becomes latent. Tertiary syphilis may then present anytime from 5 to 40 years after the primary infection. At this stage there is usually involvement of the central nervous system (CNS) with the potential for serious brain damage.

Because treponemes are released into the bloodstream as part of their life-cycle, there is the potential for transmission by transfusion. They are particularly fragile but can be transmitted by transfusion if they are present in the donation. However, because they are very heat-sensitive, storage at 4°C soon destroys the organism; it is generally held that any spirochaetes present in the pack would be destroyed within 72 hours of storage at 4°C. As spirochaetes can be seen only for short periods during infection, identification of infected individuals relies upon serology. Blood is therefore screened either using non-specific cardiolipin-based tests, or for the presence of specific antibody to *T. pallidum*, as evidence of current or previous infection with *T. pallidum*. All positive donations are normally considered to be infectious and not transfused. Although the vast majority of cases of syphilis identified in blood donors are due to 'old' infections that have been treated successfully and present no risk of transfusion transmission, cases of recent primary acute syphilis are occasionally identified. However, syphilis screening of donated blood has also been considered to have value as a 'lifestyle' indicator, as individuals exposed to syphilis may also have been exposed to other sexually transmitted diseases (such as HIV) and therefore should not donate.

9.11.1   Non-specific screening tests for syphilis

The Venereal Disease Research Laboratory (VDRL) and Rapid Plasma Reagin (RPR) tests are still used frequently in many countries. Both tests are rapid tests based upon mixing a suspension of cardiolipin, lecithin and cholesterol (VDRL antigen) with test serum; clumping of the cardiolipin indicates a positive result. Although such non-specific cardiolipin tests may give rise to a high number of false-positive reactions, they are diagnostically useful because in treated acute infections anti-cardiolipin titres fall and the tests become negative.

9.11.2   Specific screening tests for syphilis

These screening tests detect specific antibody to *T. pallidum* and include a number of different assay formats. The most commonly used test, and the most suitable for the mass screening of blood donations, is the *Treponema pallidum* haemagglutination assay (TPHA) which is based upon the agglutination of non-human red cells coated with treponemal antigens. A number of enzyme immunoassays (EIAs) are now available, but in many countries the cost of these, when faced with the significantly cheaper TPHA, is prohibitive.

9.12 POST-TRANSFUSION INFECTIONS, MONITORING AND INVESTIGATION

Unfortunately, instances of post-transfusion infection (PTI) do still occur, although only rarely in the UK and other countries with well-developed healthcare systems, but more frequently in countries with poorly developed healthcare systems. The major problem in understanding the precise basis of PTI is the failure to identify all cases, and the lack of detailed and accurate information about many of those cases actually identified. In the same way that donors present as asymptomatic carriers, infected patients – even those receiving large amounts of blood or blood products – may remain asymptomatic throughout the course of infection. It is possible that some patients subsequently develop symptoms after discharge which, depending upon their severity and the patient's general condition at the time, may never be identified by the patient as unusual or unexpected, and even if they were to be, they still may never be reported. Even in cases where the recipient is symptomatic it can still be difficult to identify symptoms when there is an underlying active disease process or the recipient is recovering slowly from the condition or situation that necessitated transfusion, as some or all of the symptoms may be masked. Thus, without prospective monitoring of all transfused patients it is easy to see how cases of PTI can, and do, go unidentified. The significance of this should not be underestimated as such undiagnosed PTIs can result in the further spread of infection to previously uninfected individuals such as household contacts, partners and carers, including professional hospital staff. Indeed, cases of suspected PTI, although subsequently shown to be nosocomial, have been identified only because the partner of the recipient subsequently developed symptomatic infection after asymptomatic infection in the recipient.

Although a case of PTI may go unnoticed by clinical diagnosis, diagnosis can be made on the basis of *in-vitro* testing. Full viral serological profiles can be expensive, and requiring or even requesting a full profile on all transfusion recipients would soon cripple laboratory systems. In addition, clearly the vast majority of recipients are not exposed to any infectious agents in the transfused blood, and the testing will simply confirm this. Perhaps the single most appropriate test to perform however, is to look for raised liver enzyme levels, most usually alanine aminotransferase (ALT), as presumptive evidence of liver damage which, in the absence of other good cause, may be due to viral infection. Although there are many reasons why ALT levels may be raised (viral infection being just one of them), testing has the value of being cheap and simple and therefore a good first-level screen no matter how non-specific it may be. ALT screening is the basis of a number of studies on PTI where potential cases were first identified in this way, the serological profiles then being monitored on patients with raised ALT levels.

All cases of possible PTI identified should be followed-up as far as possible to confirm PTI as the actual source of the infection identified. Once a possible case has been identified, the transfusion centre supplying the particular hospital with blood and products must be informed as soon as possible. An investigation would be needed to identify an infectious or potentially infectious donation amongst those supplied and transfused, and then to find a reason for the failure to identify the donation when the blood was screened. Such investigations are important, even if the cause of infection seems to be clear, to both transfusion services and to the clinical users of their blood and products. The subsequent enquiry should involve both the transfusion centre/ service and the clinical infection control system. Although PTI was the initial assumption, other risk factors must be eliminated. In many cases transfusion was subsequently found not to be the source of the infection, as another route was involved. Such other routes are many and varied, and include: (i) risk associated with the recipient's behaviour, lifestyle or origin; (ii) nosocomial transmission from other patients or clinical care staff; or (iii) from unsterilized or not fully sterilized instruments or equipment. It is important to try to determine if the patient was or had been infected before the transfusion, and indeed – if nosocomial transmission is to be ruled out – before admission. Depending upon the circumstances of admission, at least a pretransfusion blood sample should be available, for red cell serology and cross-matching, etc., and the initial status of the patient determined.

At the same time, follow-up samples from the donors or stored archive samples from the implicated donations can be retested by the transfusion centre in an attempt to identify a potentially infectious donation. This may be due to a donor being in the 'window-period' of infection, or being chronically infectious but undetectable by routine tests. Extremely rarely, test or clerical errors may be revealed, although current automation and computerization of testing makes this very unlikely. Normally the routine tests previously applied to the donations for the particular infectious agent concerned should be repeated and the results assessed before any additional investigations are instigated; this assessment needs to be made together with the results of the initial enquiries at the hospital. If no other cause or potential cause of the infection can be identified, and none of the implicated donations has any evidence of infection following retesting, then further testing of the donation archives may be needed together with more detailed investigations at the hospital. Additional testing of archive samples can include sensitive molecular techniques to identify those individuals in the 'window period' of an infection, at which stage the routine serological screening tests performed will be unable to identify them. Additional investigations at the hospital may include looking for other similar cases, not necessarily transfusion-related, and common factors between patients such as nursing and medical staff, invasive procedures performed, recovery ward, etc. Whilst there will always be a number of cases where no specific route of infection can be identified (even after exhaustive investigations), most cases can be traced back to their origin, whether it be genuine PTI or another cause. The large number of instances of infection in healthcare workers, in some cases preventing them from continuing in their chosen profession, testify to the need to be able to document clearly the routes of infection in all patients who develop infections following clinical interventions.

Over the past few years, a national initiative to report confidentially and collate all potential 'serious hazards of transfusion' (SHOT) has been launched with the aim of producing more accurate statistics relating to post-transfusion complications, including those pertaining to infection. This scheme (and similar ones in other countries) reveal that, with all the current safety measures in place, (symptomatic) microbial complications constitute only a small proportion of complications. Of these, the major component is due to bacterial transmissions.

9.13   BACTERIA

The residual risk of viral infection transmitted by transfusion can be calculated from data on seroconversion rates in 'repeat' donors and compared with actual incidence detected by NAT positivity in the 'window period' prior to detectable antibody formation. In developed countries such as England, this risk is now extremely low (Table 9.1). In contrast the risk of bacterial transmissions and complications, although also low in absolute terms, is relatively high in comparison with viral transmissions, as revealed in the SHOT reports. In part this is due to the rapid manifestation of bacterial complications compared with the often chronic nature of adverse viral effects. Table 9.2 analyses microbial, as a percentage of total, 'serious hazards' reported annually in the SHOT scheme in the UK, the bacterial as a percentage of the total microbial and the percentage of bacterial transmissions that are fatal.

Fortunately, transfusion practitioners are at last recognizing the significance of bacterial transmission and several interventions such as improved skin cleansing (and monitoring) of the venepuncture site, diversion of the first 20–30 ml of the blood donation into a separate pouch and options for semi-automated bacterial screening (of platelets in the first instance) are either in place, or are being introduced in several countries. The impact of Pathogen Indication systems, as they become available, remains to be seen.

Table 9.1 *Calculated microbial risk from blood transfusion in England*

Risk of releasing an infected donation into the blood supply in England[1]	HIV[2]	HBV[3]	HCV[4,5]
1 in x million donations released (*range with low and high yielding parameters for tests*)	5.2 (5.0 to 5.5)	0.12 (0.06 to 0.25)	2.7 (2.5 to 2.9)

[1] Risk of donation during marker negative window periods (including HbsAg negative period at tail-end of HBV carriage), and of erroneous release of positive donations, using observed frequencies of infections in donations collected in England, 1996–1998.
[2] With HIV Ab&Ag combined assays in use (i.e. without NAT for HIV).
[3] With HbsAg assays in use (i.e. without anti-HBc assays, or NAT).
[4] With anti-HCV and pooled NAT for HCV RNA in use (NB. assuming no NAT failures).
[5] 'NAT-only' positives in 8 million donations to end February 2002.

Table 9.2. *SHOT report (UK) 01/10/1996 to 30/09/2001*

Report year	All reported adverse events	Microbial (%)	Bacterial	Bacterial as % of microbial	Fatal bacterial	% of bacterial fatal
1996/97	169	8	3	38	0	0
1997/98	196	3	1	33	1	100
1998/99	255	9	6	67	2	33
1999/00	293	6	5	83	2	40
2000/01	315	6	4	67	1	25
Totals	**1228**	**32 (2.6%)**	**19**	**59**	**6**	**32**

Source: SHOT, data at 21/02/2002

9.14 VARIANT CREUTZFELDT-JAKOB DISEASE (vCJD)

The recognition of the prion disease variant Creutzfeldt-Jakob disease (vCJD) as the human form of bovine spongiform encephalopathy (BSE, or 'mad cow disease') and the demonstration of prion infectivity in the blood of infected animals has raised the (as yet unproven) possibility of potential transfusion transmissibility. Despite the lack of evidence of transfusion transmissibility of vCJD and the unknown extent of the epidemic in humans, any possibility of a transfusion risk has enormous implications and has to be taken very seriously. To this end a range of major interventions aimed at (potentially) reducing any (potential) vCJD risk to the blood supply have been implemented. These include: stricter donor selection regarding possible prion exposure, replacing plasma for fractionation from UK donors with plasma purchased from countries free of BSE/vCJD and pre-storage leucodepletion of all UK blood components. Despite efforts worldwide, a specific practical test to screen blood donors for vCJD or prion disease is not yet available although 'indirect' tests for surrogate markers are offering some promise.

9.15 PATHOGEN INACTIVATION

Several commercial systems to effectively inactivate a range of micro-organisms in blood components are becoming available. As yet, validation and operational evaluations within Blood Services have not been undertaken. Most work has been reported using psoralens which inactivate a wide range of viruses (intra- and extra-cellular), bacteria, parasites and white blood cells by intercalation in DNA (and RNA loops) and the blocking of nucleic acid replication. A system for microbial inactivation by psoralen in platelet preparations has been launched. The tactical and strategic impact of such a product on microbial safety approaches in blood transfusion remain to be seen but really 'daring' changes in strategy are unlikely to be forthcoming until inactivation systems for all components of blood become available.

9.16 APPROPRIATE USE OF BLOOD

A important final issue, although of more critical significance in countries with less highly developed healthcare systems, is the appropriate use of blood. There is no doubt that in the past many patients have been transfused when infusion of a suitable volume replacer/expander would have given equal clinical benefit, but without the risks of transfusion. The use of protein solutions, colloids and synthetic volume expanders should be encouraged where simple and rapid volume expansion is needed and haemoglobin levels are not low or would not be compromised. This serves two purposes: (i) it minimizes unnecessary exposure of patients to human material; and (ii) it minimizes wastage of donated blood – a precious resource which most countries cannot afford to waste.

At this point the subjects of **autologous transfusion** and **blood salvage** need to be considered. Both of these procedures clearly minimize exposure to foreign material and also simplify cross-matching, etc. There are however, many instances where neither is possible and where homologous transfusion is an essential part of modern medicine. However, equally there are many instances where either can be applied and with significant benefits to the patient, clinician and transfusion service.

Autologous transfusion has had an increasing band of supporters over the past few years, but has not yet become as widespread as many first thought it would. There are a number of reasons for this, including the uncertainty and unpredictability of hospital workloads and increasing numbers of individuals on long-term transfusion support. The logistics of healthcare in many countries have meant that elective surgery – probably one of the main stimuli for autologous blood transfusion – does not always follow the planned schedules and may have to be postponed, possibly resulting in the expiry and wastage of the pre-deposited blood. Additionally, there will be a number of potentially suitable individuals but from whom the collection of blood is clinically contraindicated, for example the elderly. Patients on long-term transfusion support can account for up to one-half of the recipients of donated blood in many countries, and for such individuals autologous transfusion is clearly inappropriate.

9.17 ACKNOWLEDGEMENT

We are grateful to Dr Kate Soldan for assistance in the risk evaluations.

9.18 FURTHER READING

Barbara, J. and Muller, J.Y. (1994) The side effects of blood transfusion: transmissible infections. In *Transfusion Medicine: a European Course on Blood Transfusion*, ed. W. van Aken and B. Genetet, Centre National d'Enseignement à Distance, Vanves, 274–311.

Barbara, J.A.J. (2002) Transfusion-transmitted infections. *Transfusion Alternatives in Transfusion Medicine*, **1**, 42–47.

Kitchen, A.D. and Barbara, J.A.J. (1994) Transfusion-transmitted non-viral infections. *Curr. Opin. Infect. Dis.* **7**, 493–498.

Mollison, P.L., Engelfriet, C.P. and Contreras, M. (1993) Infectious agents transmitted by transfusion. In *Blood Transfusion in Clinical Medicine*, 9th edition. Blackwell Scientific Publications, Oxford, 710–785.

Serious Hazards of Transfusion (SHOT) Annual Reports. SHOT Office, Manchester, UK.

Principles of antibiotic prescribing for prophylaxis and treatment

P.G. DAVEY AND E.W. TAYLOR

10.1 INTRODUCTION

Surgeons need antibiotics. Antibiotics are one of the reasons why the whole practice of surgery has changed in the past 50 years. In some cases antibiotics have reduced the need for surgery, for example in the management of tuberculosis or in peptic ulceration now known to be related to infection with *Helicobacter pylori*. Antibiotics have eased the treatment of abdominal sepsis, cholecystitis and urosepsis. Antibiotics have enabled surgeons to carry out extensive advances in technique and support new fields of implant and transplant surgery. Helped by antibiotics and other control measures there is no place that the modern surgeon fears to tread. Unfortunately the continuance of this current state of affairs depends on continued improvement in the ways in which all doctors use antibiotics, including abstaining from antibiotics when they are not indicated. The correct choice of agents, the correct choice of dosage and the duration of therapy are all critical in obtaining the best results from antibiotic therapy and preservation of the efficacy for future use. Antibiotics are only a part of the armamentarium to prevent acquisition of infection, but are a key part.

Surgical use of antibiotics is almost equally divided between therapeutic and prophylactic use, whereas in almost all other types of medical practice the overwhelming use of antimicrobial agents is for therapy; chemoprophylaxis is of limited value.

This chapter concerns general principles of use of antibiotics. Most organ-specific chapters of this book will have a section on the indications and choice of anti-infectives. The chapter will also contain basic information on those antibiotics that are most commonly used in surgical practice. The nature of the infecting organisms and the range of antimicrobial agents available have changed quickly over recent years so that when faced by an out-of-the-ordinary infection, or one which is rarely encountered, it is worth seeking specialist advice.

10.1.1 Antibiotics and chemotherapy

What distinguishes antibiotics and chemotherapy from antiseptics is that they are selective against microbial targets, rather than mammalian targets, and can be given systemically. Antibiotics are derived from biological sources whereas chemotherapeutic agents are chemicals and both types of antimicrobial have activity against microbes in low concentrations. Chemotherapy started over 100 years ago with dyestuffs active against protozoa and anti-treponemal agents such as salvarsan and later by sulphonamides. Antibiotics started with penicillium extracts in the 1940s and most of the other antibiotic classes were discovered over the next 10 years. These are still the mainstay of infection therapy. The vast majority of infection can be treated by antimicrobial agents such as penicillins, macrolides, tetracyclines, aminoglycosides (antibiotics), trimethoprim, quinolones and metronidazole (chemotherapeutic agents) discovered 40 years ago. Analogues of many of these compounds have been developed as resistances to antimicrobials have developed. Resistance is more common in organisms affecting persons already critically ill in intensive care units, cancer and transplant units. Patients with relatively normal immunological defences and unexposed to multi-resistant bacteria do not fall into the highly vulnerable group where antibiotic resistance is a serious limitation of therapy. The majority of patients undergoing surgery present little difficulty in treatment of infection and effective chemoprophylaxis is straightforward.

10.1.2 Micro-organisms in surgical infections

Antibiotics are directed against microbes, of which there are many different varieties. The bacteria that most concern the surgeon are:

1. The normal flora of the non-infected patient coming into hospital.
   Skin: coagulase-negative staphylococci, (occasionally *St. aureus*) corynebacteria, viridans streptococci and clostridial spores and other anaerobes in the perineum/buttocks.
   Mouth: Gram-positive cocci, anaerobes, candida.
   Small and large bowel: enterobacteriaceae, anaerobes, enterococci.
   Nasal mucosa: *Staph. aureus*.
   Vagina: enterobacteriaceae, anaerobes, group B streptococci.
2. The patient being admitted with infection.
   Skin infection: *Staph. aureus*; beta-haemolytic streptococci.
   Infected skin ulcer: as above plus anaerobes, enterobacteria and *Pseudomonas*.
   Urinary tract infection: predominantly Enterobacteria.
   Cholecystitis: enterobacteriaceae; enterococci.
   Peritonitis/abdominal abscess: enterobacteriaceae; anaerobes.
   Organism-specific infections: tuberculosis, actinomycosis; typhoid fever; salmonellosis, etc.
3. The inpatient acquiring an infection in hospital.
   Resistant *Staph. aureus*; resistant enterobacteriaceae; pseudomonads, Acinetobacter, other non-fermenting rods, resistant corynebacteria, enterococci, candida species.

In surgical practice there is often a mixture of bacteria involved in infection, so selection of an appropriate agent or combination of agents is important. One should always consider the presumptive organisms against which treatment is directed, whether for chemoprophylaxis or therapy. For chemoprophylaxis all antibiotics are given against presumptive organisms; therapy against infection present on entry to the hospital is almost always presumptive or 'best guess', based on a clinical diagnosis until bacterial cultures are available.

For the uninfected patient undergoing surgery the main threats are from the patient's own normal flora. Careful measures are taken to protect the patient from the normal flora of the attendants and from hospital pathogens. The normal flora of patients in hospital begins to change after a few days' stay. Coagulase-negative staphylococci are ubiquitous in hospital and antibiotic-resistant clones circulate in the hospital; a high proportion of hospital staff become colonized with such clones replacing the strains which are normally susceptible to many classes of antibiotics. Should the patient undergo operation within two days of admission, their colonizing staphylococci on the skin will be methicillin-susceptible and the Gram-negative bacteria in the gastrointestinal tract predominantly susceptible to antibiotics such as co-amoxiclav or cefuroxime. After about a week many antibiotic-resistant bacteria colonize the intestine.

Infections arising in hospital are much less predictable in aetiology but epidemiological and microbiological evidence is frequently present to guide therapy. Presumptive therapy is sometimes necessary in patients with sudden onset of severe infection but cultures and susceptibility testing of significant isolates of bacteria is essential for precise therapy.

10.2 ANTIBIOTIC RESISTANCE

The use of the word 'resistance' is best reserved for its strict microbiological meaning. Some antibiotic resistance is natural in bacteria. For example, *E.coli* is resistant to penicillin G because it has an outer coat which prevents access to the target and *Klebsiella* are resistant to amoxycillin because of a β-lactamase which destroys penicillins. Some antibiotic resistances are acquired; in the normal state the bacterial species may be fully susceptible but a change in genetic structure can occur by mutation or importing of resistance genes from other sources. *Staph. aureus* in its natural state was penicillin-susceptible, but soon acquired genes enabling strains to produce beta-lactam enzymes which destroy penicillin. Over 90% of *Staph. aureus* isolates are now penicillin-resistant

Resistance in microbiological terms is defined by a known mechanism by which the bacteria are able to avoid the antibiotic action. The quantitative measure of resistance or susceptibility is the minimum concentrations of antibiotic needed to inhibit the organisms. If the minimum inhibitory concentration (MIC) is not exceeded by the concentrations of antibiotics reached in the infected site, the antibiotic will have minimal or no effect.

In clinical practice the patient may be able to rebuff the organism even if the organism is resistant to the antibiotic. If this happens it will be due to the patient's own defence and repair mechanisms – a natural or spontaneous cure rather than an antibiotic-assisted use. It stems from this that patients with impaired immunological defences require more help with infection than those with normal 'host defence resistance' to infection. Resistance of patients to infection is clearly different from resistance of bacteria to antibiotics. Patients with poor host defences may be vulnerable to infection even with organisms of low pathogenicity (such as enterococci), regardless of whether the organisms are susceptible or resistant to antibiotics. A resistant infection (i.e. one failing to respond to fully active antibiotics) is better termed 'refractory'. An infection may be refractory even if the organism is fully susceptible. The infection may be such that it cannot be resolved by antibiotics alone, e.g. the infected area may need to be drained.

The term 'sensitive' is also used in two contexts with antibiotic use and can lead to misinterpretation unless more specific words are used. A bacterium is susceptible to an antibiotic. A patient is hypersensitive to an antibiotic.

10.2.1 Mechanisms or antibiotic resistance

ACQUIRING ANTIBIOTIC-RESISTANT BACTERIA

Exposure of bacteria to antibiotics can result in a patient acquiring bacteria resistant to those antibiotics. This may occur in several ways.

Antibiotics and the normal microbial flora of patients

1. Outpatients. The normal flora are mainly antibiotic susceptible, with some naturally-resistant species present in gastrointestinal tract, mouth and skin. Antibiotic therapy leads to reduction of the normally susceptible flora to antibiotics. Strains in normal flora that are naturally resistant to antibiotics grow up and replace the normal flora. Some of these may be pathogens
2. Hospital inpatients. While in hospital the patient is exposed to hospital microbial flora, e.g. staphylococci from air or skin; enterobacteriaceae from food or bowel. Antibiotic therapy leads to reduction of normal flora and growth of endogenous resistant flora as above. Antibiotic-resistant strains from the hospital also colonize the patient. Many of these bacteria, e.g. *Staph. aureus* or *Cl. difficile*, are potential pathogens.

All antibiotics have an adverse effect on the normal bacterial flora of patients, and it has taken a long time for the importance of this simple fact to be

understood. The consequences include replacement of the normal flora by pathogens such as *Clostridium difficile*, yeasts or *Pseudomonas aeruginosa*, and in-situ selection of drug-resistant bacteria from the normal flora.

The problem of *C. difficile* colitis is increasing exponentially in some hospitals (Figure 10.1). In this review of 201 cases, the most frequent indication for antibiotic use was surgical prophylaxis, and surgical patients accounted for 55% of the total cases.

The problem of antibiotic resistance in hospitals is also increasing inexorably. In 1996, the Centers for Disease Control and the National Foundation for Infectious Diseases published a set of strategic goals to help hospitals to control the problem, which included five strategies to optimize the prophylactic, empiric and therapeutic use of antimicrobials in the hospital (see Further reading). These strategies are to:

- optimize antimicrobial prophylaxis for operative procedures;
- optimize the choice and duration of empiric antimicrobial therapy;
- improve antimicrobial prescribing practices by educational and administrative means;
- establish a system to monitor and provide feedback on the occurrence and impact of antibiotic resistance; and
- define and implement institutional or healthcare delivery system guidelines for important types of antimicrobial use.

10.2.2 Effects of antibiotics on pathogenic bacteria

The objective of giving antibiotics to the patients is to affect the pathogen causing the diseases. Changes of antibiotic susceptibility in the bacteria causing the

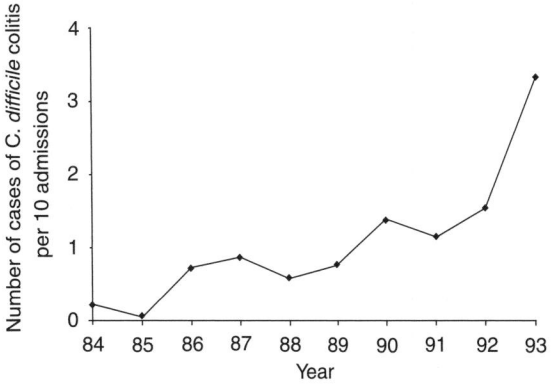

Figure 10.1 *Increase in the annual incidence of* Clostridium difficile *colitis at two hospitals in Oregon from 1984–1994. There were a total of 201 cases. Redrawn from data in Jobe* et al., American Journal of Surgery, **169**: 480–483.

infection are not usual but there are certain antibiotic/bacteria combinations that are at particular risk of producing resistant pathogens. For example, *Staph. aureus* can mutate in a single step to high resistance to rifampicin so should never be treated using rifampicin alone. If in special circumstances rifampicin is needed for a staphylococcal lesion, it should be accompanied by another agent to which it has been confirmed to be susceptible, e.g. trimethoprim, fusidic acid. A *Staph. aureus* population always contains a number of organisms intrinsically resistant to quinolones and these usually grow up when the susceptible strains are killed. Lesions such as surgical site infections that contain a high number of bacteria should not be treated by quinolones. Even when combined with other antistaphylococcal agents, failure due to resistant organisms is usual. An exception may be in staphylococcal lesions in bone, which have a low number of organisms.

Some species of Gram-negative bacteria with a chromosomal enzyme may be switched-on (induced) to produce this enzyme at a high level when exposed to beta-lactam antibiotics. When treating *Pseudomonas*, *Serratia* and *Enterobacter morganella* with cephalosporins, an overgrowth of resistant cells may occur. These may be producers of chromosomal enzyme and a change of therapy is necessary.

10.3   KEY POLICIES: PROPHYLAXIS AND TREATMENT

10.3.1   Prophylaxis

The aim of prophylaxis is to prevent infection from occurring. In surgery, the term can only logically be applied to clean or clean-contaminated wounds because, if the wound is frankly contaminated or dirty at the time of surgery, then infection has already occurred, or is highly likely to have occurred. Therefore administration of antibiotics at the time of contaminated or dirty surgery is treatment of established, or incipient infection, and not prophylaxis.

10.3.2   Indications for prophylaxis

The strongest evidence for the effectiveness of prophylaxis in elective operations concerns colorectal surgery, in which prophylaxis also reduces the risk of peri-operative mortality, and in prosthetic joint surgery, in which it reduces the risk of infection of the prosthetic joint. These are now regarded as mandatory indications for peri-operative prophylaxis. There is continuing debate about prophylaxis for other clean and clean-contaminated surgery, and surveys have documented practice variation

amongst UK surgeons. There are two requirements to inform the debate about prophylaxis:

1. Evidence that prophylaxis reduces the risk of postoperative infection.
2. Quantification of the risk of mortality or morbidity from postoperative infection in defined patient groups.

Applying these two criteria, operations can be divided into three categories (the examples given are intended to be illustrative, not exhaustive):

*   Prophylaxis is mandatory: all surgeons should administer prophylaxis where there is
    *   (a)   Evidence from at least two randomized, controlled trials that prophylaxis reduces the risk of postoperative infection.
    *   (b)   The risk of mortality or major morbidity resulting from postoperative infection is sufficiently high to justify prophylaxis in all patients. Examples are colorectal surgery and surgery involving the insertion of prosthetic devices.
*   Prophylaxis is recommended: prophylaxis should be given to the majority of patients where there is
    *   (a)   Evidence from at least two randomized, controlled trials that prophylaxis reduces the risk of postoperative infection.
    *   (b)   The risk of major morbidity is sufficiently high to justify prophylaxis in most patients, but a case can be made for omitting prophylaxis in some (e.g. for surgeons with low infection rates, or for defined patient groups who have a low risk of infection or do not wish to receive prophylaxis). Examples are cholecystectomy, hysterectomy, Caesarean section and gastric surgery.
*   Prophylaxis is controversial: i.e. can be given for selected patients exercising clinical judgement. Either:
    *   (a)   There is evidence from at least one randomized, controlled trial that prophylaxis reduces the risk of infection, but most surgeons consider the risk of morbidity or mortality from postoperative infection to be too low to justify prophylaxis. Examples are repair of inguinal hernia and breast surgery.

    Or:
    *   (b)   The risk of morbidity or mortality from postoperative infection is high, but there is no evidence from randomized, controlled trials to show that prophylaxis reduces the risk of infection. Examples are laminectomy and spinal fusion without implant.

Local policies about indications for prophylaxis should clearly identify which operations are indications for prophylaxis, and whether prophylaxis is mandatory (all patients must receive prophylaxis) or recommended in defined patient groups (in which case the policy must clearly state the criteria for omitting prophylaxis).

10.3.3 General principles of prophylaxis

Having defined the indications for prophylaxis, there are three general principles of prophylaxis which should be applied across all operations:

1. The first dose of prophylaxis should be given within 2 hours of the start of the operation (and preferably just before the incision is made; see below).
2. The total duration of prophylaxis should not exceed 24 hours.
3. Indications for additional doses should be clearly specified, and may include additional doses administered in theatre if the operation exceeds a specified length, or additional doses to be administered postoperatively.

TIMING OF THE FIRST DOSE

The aim of prophylaxis is to ensure that there is an effective concentration of antibiotic in the wound while it is open and at risk of bacterial contamination. Giving the drug too early may reduce effectiveness because drug concentrations in the wound are beginning to decline to ineffective levels when the incision is made. On the other hand, experimental evidence from animal models has suggested that a delay in the administration of antibiotics after the incision was made also reduced the effectiveness of prophylaxis. A large clinical study has clearly shown the importance of timing of the first dose of prophylaxis (Figure 10.2), and it is now clear that the best time to administer the first dose of i.v. prophylaxis is just before the incision is made, at the time of induction of anaesthesia. There is increasing interest in the use of orally administered prophylaxis, but if this route is used then the first dose should be administered about 2 hours before surgery, in order to ensure adequate absorption of the drug from the gut. However, many surgeons and anaesthetists are reluctant to advise oral administration close to a surgical procedure.

ADDITIONAL DOSES OF PROPHYLAXIS

There is no evidence to support the continuation of prophylaxis beyond 24 hours after a clean or clean-contaminated operation. However, if the operative field is dirty, or becomes heavily contaminated during the operation, then the duration may be prolonged beyond 24 hours (but this is treatment of confirmed or incipient infection, and not prophylaxis).

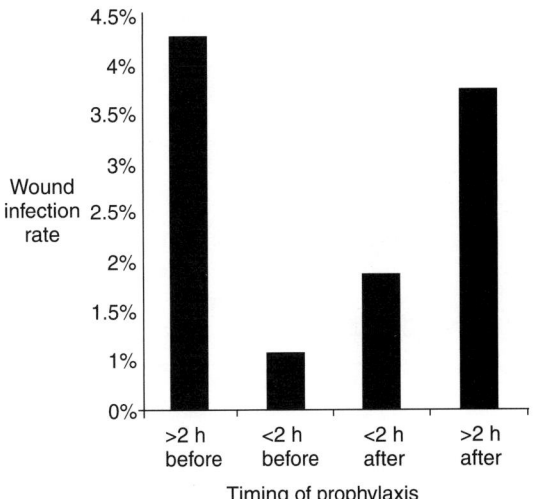

Figure 10.2 *The relationship between timing of the first dose of i.v. antibiotic prophylaxis and the risk of wound infection in 2847 patients undergoing clean or clean-contaminated surgical procedures at a large community hospital. Redrawn from data in Classen et al., New England Journal of Medicine 1992,* **326***: 281–286.*

There is growing evidence to support the use of a single, peri-operative dose of prophylaxis for most operations. The aim of additional doses should be to continue the period of effective protection of the wound while it is vulnerable to bacterial contamination. Consideration should therefore be given to administration of additional intra-operative doses if the prophylactic drug is rapidly excreted (serum half-life 1–2 hours) and the duration of surgery exceeds 2 hours. It is extremely doubtful that any additional benefit is achieved by administration of additional doses at 8 hours or 16 hours after the start of surgery.

10.4 TREATMENT OF SUSPECTED OR ESTABLISHED INFECTION

Prescribing an antibiotic always requires reconciliation between two opposing aims to ensure that:

- patients with bacterial infection receive effective antibiotic treatment as rapidly as possible; and
- antibiotics are not prescribed to patients who do not have bacterial infection.

10.4.1 Early effective antibiotic treatment for patients with bacterial infection

Effective antibiotic prophylaxis depends on administration within a window of opportunity (Figure 10.2), in

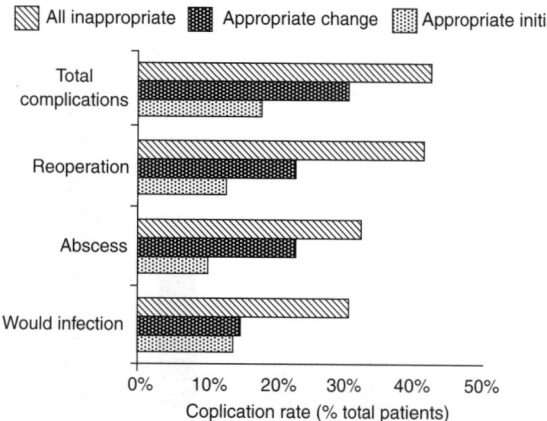

Figure 10.3 *Outcomes of antibiotic treatment for 480 patients with community-acquired bacterial peritonitis treated at five hospitals in Albuquerque, New Mexico. Antibiotic treatment was classified as appropriate if the drug(s) were active against all of the pathogens isolated from peritoneal cultures. Patients with appropriate treatment were further subdivided according to whether the right drugs were selected at the time of surgical débridement ('appropriate initial') or treatment was changed only after the results of peritoneal cultures became available ('appropriate change'). 'All inappropriate' indicates patients whose treatment was not changed despite the fact that peritoneal cultures grew pathogens resistant to the antibiotics they were receiving. 'Total complications' indicates patients who had at least one complication; some patients had multiple complications. Redrawn from data in Mosdell* et al., Annals of Surgery 1991, **214**: 543–549.*

many cases at the time of surgical debridement. The same also applies to antibiotic treatment of established infection (Figure 10.3). This figure contrasts the outcomes of treatment in patients with bacterial peritonitis according to whether or not they received appropriate treatment. The complication rate was clearly highest for patients who never received appropriate treatment, and lowest for patients who received appropriate treatment at the time of surgical debridement. Changing antibiotic treatment according to the results of bacterial cultures improved outcome ('Appropriate change' versus 'All inappropriate'), but the complication rate was still higher than in patients who received appropriate antibiotic treatment at the time of surgical debridement ('Appropriate initial').

Why was appropriate antibiotic treatment more effective when it was started at the time of surgical debridement? There are two likely explanations. The first is that antibiotics work best against rapidly dividing bacteria and are relatively ineffective once abscess formation occurs (Table 10.1). The second is that ineffective treatment results in uncontrolled systemic effects of sepsis, which further compromises patient outcome.

A further important message is contained in this study. Patients who received appropriate antibiotic treatment at the time of surgical debridement still had a

Table 10.1 *Reasons why antibiotic efficacy is reduced against bacteria in abscesses*

- The walls of an abscess act as a barrier to diffusion of antibiotics
- The bacteria within abscesses are growing slowly, which reduces the activity of all antibiotics
- The physical environment in an abscess further reduces the activity of antibiotics. For example:
  – Low pH reduces the activity of macrolides and quinolones;
  – Low pO_2 reduces the activity of aminoglycosides;
  – Debris in pus contains fragments of cell wall and nucleic acids; these are the target sites for antibiotics, and therefore the drugs bind to these fragments and are inactivated.

19% complication rate; conversely, patients who continued to have inappropriate antibiotic treatment had a 44% complication rate, and therefore the majority (56%) of patients who received inappropriate antibiotics had no complication. These data were collected over a period of 3 years in five hospitals. The individual surgeon treats too few cases of surgical peritonitis to assess the appropriateness of his/her antibiotic treatment based on clinical outcome, and may well be lulled into a false sense of security, despite prescribing less than optimal antibiotic treatment. An overview of an individual surgeon's prescribing habits by a microbiological colleague should be welcomed. However, regularly obtaining adequate intra-operative specimens for microbiology will provide the surgeon with information which can be used to assess the appropriateness of local antibiotic policies.

10.4.2 Reducing antibiotic prescribing to patients who do not have bacterial infection

The importance of early appropriate treatment of patients with bacterial infection is balanced by the need to minimize antibiotic prescribing to patients who do not have bacterial infection. Less than 25% of patients with postoperative fever have bacterial infection, so how can the surgeon identify those patients? Assessment of the systemic inflammatory response is important. A temperature of > 38 °C and/or the presence of tachycardia, tachypnoea or a high white blood cell count increase the probability of bacterial infection. Nonetheless, only about 50% of patients with all four systemic inflammatory response syndrome (SIRS) criteria actually have bacterial infection. Given the consequences of delaying appropriate antibiotic treatment in surgical sepsis (see Figure 10.3), it is better to start treatment promptly, knowing that most patients treated do not have bacterial infection. However, the need for antibiotics should be re-evaluated after 48–72 hours, when the results of microbiological and other tests are available. Treatment should be stopped if the patient does not have confirmed bacterial infection. There is no need to complete an arbitrarily defined 'course of antibiotics' if the patient does not in fact have a bacterial infection.

10.5.1 Comparison of dosage routes

The advantages of oral administration of antibiotics in comparison with parenteral administration by intravenous (i.v.) or intramuscular (i.m.) injection can be summarized as follows:

- Oral formulations are up to ten-fold cheaper than equivalent i.v. formulations.
- Parenteral administration requires additional consumables (needles, syringes, i.v. cannulae, giving sets) for preparation or administration, i.e. more expense and time expanded.
- I.V. vials do not always conform exactly to the prescribed dose, resulting in drug wastage which is further exacerbated by disposal of vials which have been prepared incorrectly.
- Oral administration is safer than i.v. administration, avoiding the hazards of contamination by bacteria or particles, the preparation of infections in incompatible infusion fluids, and phlebitis or infection at the i.v. injection site.
- Parenteral administration requires more staff time for preparation and administration. Moreover, the hazards of i.v. drug administration mean that additional time is consumed by training of staff and audit of procedures.

An audit in Dundee showed that over 5000 i.v. antibiotic injections are administered annually on a 40-bed surgical unit. The cost of equipment used in preparation and administration of i.v. antibiotics ranged between 36p to £1.33 for bolus injections, and from £1.90 to £2.55 for infusions. Estimated annual costs for equipment and discarded doses for a 40-bed surgical ward were between £6 206 and £19 509. Moreover, 86–95% of patients could have taken oral drugs.

10.5.2 Absorption of oral drugs

The advantages of oral drug administration are balanced by concerns about the reliability of absorption of oral drugs. Moreover, there is no oral formulation for some parenteral drugs, so that oral therapy may mean changing the drug as well as the route of administration. It is useful to consider two questions in assessing the oral alternatives to i.v. therapy:

1. Is the oral alternative a different formulation of the same drug, or must a different drug be selected for oral treatment?
2. How reliable is absorption? Specifically, is > 50% of an administered dose absorbed?

Oral alternatives will fall into four groups according to the answers to these two questions:

- Oral formulation is the same drug as would be administered i.v., and has > 50% oral absorption.
- Oral formulation is a different drug, and has > 50% oral absorption.
- Oral formulation is the same drug, but has unreliable (< 50%) absorption.
- Oral formulation is a different drug, and has < 50% absorption.

There is no dispute that the best option is to have a reliably absorbed oral formulation of the same drug, and therefore that the worst option is a different drug which is unreliably absorbed. However, there is debate about the ranking of the intermediate alternatives. The antibiotic policies at Dundee Teaching Hospitals Trust are based on the firm belief that reliability of absorption has priority, and therefore a different drug which is reliably absorbed is preferable to an unreliably absorbed formulation of the same drug.

10.6 ADVERSE EFFECTS OF ANTIBIOTICS

Antibiotics are substances that are produced by one living organism and which kill or inhibit the growth of another living organism. Almost all antibacterial drugs are true antibiotics, or semi-synthetic derivatives of true antibiotics.

10.6.1 Allergy to antibiotics

The natural origin of antibiotics may explain why allergy to these drugs is more common than to other drug types, but this may be due also to the large number of people who are exposed to therapeutic antibiotics. Type 1 immediate hypersensitivity reactions have been reported for most antibiotics, and it is essential that patients are asked if they have a history of allergy before an antibiotic is prescribed.

PENICILLIN ALLERGY

The most commonly prescribed antibiotics in hospital belong to the β-lactam class (characterized by the carbonyl-imido grouping, CONH), which includes penicillins, cephalosporins, carbapenems and monobactams. It is therefore essential that the prescriber knows about penicillin allergy in detail. Approximately 3% of patients will have a reaction suggestive of allergy after a single injection of penicillin, 0.2% will have a full-blown anaphylactic reaction, and 0.05% will have a fatal reaction.

If a patient has had a full anaphylactic reaction to penicillin, or a reaction that includes signs of respiratory obstruction (facial swelling, laryngeal oedema, bronchoconstriction), there is no question that they are allergic to penicillin and should not receive penicillin again. However, if the patient has a history of rash after penicillin treatment then the situation is not so clear-cut. Long-term follow-up of patients who gave a history of a rash associated with penicillin therapy showed that about half were re-exposed to penicillins within 5 years but, fortunately, only 6% of these people had an adverse reaction to penicillin. The problem is that a rash is a common sign of infection; therefore a rash associated with penicillin therapy is more likely to be caused by the infection than the drug. Moreover, some infections predispose the patient to drug reactions. The most famous example is the reaction to aminopenicillins (ampicillin/amoxycillin) which occurs in 90% of patients with infectious mononucleosis. Such a patient is not allergic to ampicillin, and would not have a reaction if re-exposed to ampicillin after recovery from infectious mononucleosis. Infection with the HIV virus also increases the probability of reaction to antibiotics, especially to co-trimoxazole and it is likely that other infections can also alter the body's reaction to antibiotics.

True immediate, IgE-mediated hypersensitivity produces a characteristic urticarial rash (Figure 10.4b) which is quite different from the ampicillin rash in infectious mononucleosis (see Figure 10.4a). Urticaria causes a weal and flare reaction, very similar to the rash produced by a nettle sting, with intense inflammation and itching. In contrast, the ampicillin/infectious mononucleosis rash is macular. If a patient has an urticarial rash after receiving an antibiotic they should be assumed to be truly allergic and should not receive that antibiotic again.

CROSS-REACTION BETWEEN β-LACTAM ANTIBIOTICS

The foregoing discussion about penicillin allergy explains why there is so much confusion about the risk of cross-reaction to cephalosporins in patients who are said to be allergic to penicillin (which some immunological investigations have put as high as 50%). Most clinicians are highly sceptical, and will cite numerous instances of patients who have tolerated cephalosporins despite a history of allergy to penicillin. However, if only 6% of patients with a history of rash associated with penicillin are allergic, then even if there is 50% cross-reaction to cephalosporins, only 3% of patients with a history of penicillin rash will react to cephalosporins.

PRACTICAL PRESCRIBING ADVICE

If a patient has a history suggestive of true penicillin allergy, they should definitely not receive cephalosporins or other β-lactams (Figure 10.4). If the patient's history is a non-specific rash associated with penicillin, the chances are they are not allergic to penicillin, never mind to cephalosporins. Nonetheless, there is usually an effective alternative to β-lactams, and it would be best to select a suitable alternative. If β-lactam therapy is thought to be clinically essential in a potentially allergic patient then a test dose may be given, but only with full resuscitation facilities at hand, including an experienced anaesthetist capable of

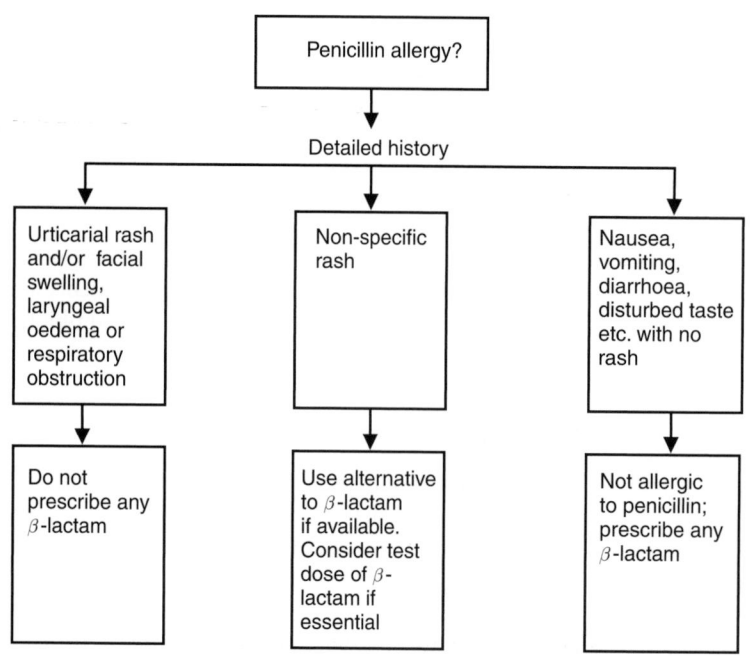

Figure 10.4 *Flow chart for management of a patient with suspected penicillin allergy. Administration of a test dose should only be undertaken with full resuscitation facilities at hand, including an experienced clinician capable of intubating a patient with acute laryngeal oedema.*

Table 10.2 *Key components of a policy for prophylactic and therapeutic antibiotics in surgery*

Prophylaxis

- General principles of prophylaxis:
  - The first dose must be administered within 2 hours of the start of surgery, preferably at induction of anaesthesia immediately before surgery
  - A second intraoperative dose may be required if the operation lasts >2 hours
  - Prophylaxis should not be continued for >24 hours after surgery
- Define the procedures which require prophylaxis
- Choice of drug, based on susceptibilities of the most likely pathogens
- An alternative drug for patients with allergy if the first choice is a β-lactam

Treatment

- General principles of treatment
  - Early appropriate antibiotic treatment of surgical sepsis is important
  - Appropriate treatment can only be defined with local microbiological information from previous cases
  - Record initial signs of sepsis (SIRS) and resolution of signs in the clinical notes
  - Stop treatment early if bacterial infection is not confirmed
- List the bacteria most likely to cause common infections
- Choice of drug, based on susceptibilities of the most likely pathogens
- An alternative drug for patients with allergy if the first choice is a β-lactam
- Clinical information to be recorded in the notes and tests to be performed:
  - General signs of sepsis (SIRS)
  - Specific signs (e.g. chest signs and chest infection for respiratory infection)
  - Instructions for obtaining microbiology specimens and transportation to the laboratory (e.g. refrigerate urine specimens, incubate blood cultures)
- Criteria for changing patients from i.v. to oral route

intubating a patient with laryngeal oedema. Test doses should also be considered for patients with recurrent infections (e.g. chronic osteomyelitis or underlying immunosuppression) and a questionable history of allergy to penicillin. A test dose of penicillin administered when the patient is relatively well, between infections, may avoid difficult decisions when the next infection occurs.

10.7 NOTES ON ANTIBIOTICS COMMONLY USED BY SURGEONS

The range of antibiotics available is very wide and several classifications have been made. Some antibiotics need to be well known by surgeons; other are best left to specialists.

10.7.1 Classification of antimicrobials

The following list of agents is based on microbiological activity and is perhaps the most useful clinically. The table shows the great range of antimicrobials in use. The ones of greatest value in surgery are:

ACTIVE AGAINST GRAM-POSITIVE AND GRAM-POSITIVE COCCI AND GRAM-POSITIVE BACTERIA

Penicillin, flucloxacillin, macrolides, lincosamines, ketolides, oxazolidinones and fusidic acid. Vancomycin. Lincosamines and vancomycin are not active against *Neisseria.*

ACTIVE MAINLY AGAINST GRAM-NEGATIVE RODS

Ampicillin and piperacillin with/without beta-lactamase inhibitors, aminoglycosides, quinolones.

BROAD-SPECTRUM

Cephalosporins, carbapenems, trimethoprim, new quinolones (post-2000).

ANAEROBES

Metronidazole.

ATYPICAL BACTERIA, MYCOBACTERIA, VIRUSES, FUNGI

These have their own specialized antimicrobials.

10.7.2 Compounds of special importance to most surgeons

These include β-lactams, aminoglycosides, quinolones, glycopeptides and imidazoles

THE β-LACTAM ANTIBIOTICS

The β-lactam group is complex with three main sub groups: penicillins, cephalosporins and carbapenems. So many different penicillins and cephalosporins have been developed that most bacterial infections encountered by surgeons can be managed with β-lactam antibiotics.

Penicillins and beta-lactamase inhibitors

The spectrum of benzyl penicillin against bacteria in their natural state, i.e. pre-antibiotic state, is wide. Resistance due to difficulty in crossing the outer membrane of Gram-negative bacteria was reduced to some extent by ampicillin/amoxycillin and more effectively by piperacillin. The problem of resistance by alteration of the targets in the bacterial cell was resolved by a higher dosage or combination with aminoglycosides for some bacteria. β-lactamases, especially those of staphylococci, were resolved by enzyme-stable penicillins like methicillin, flucloxacillin and many others.

β-lactamases are highly prevalent and occur in many different bacteria. β-lactamase inhibitors developed in the 1970s have prolonged the valuable activity of many beta-lactams for the past 30 years. β-lactamase inhibitors are also penicillins with feeble antimicrobial activity against most bacterial species. (There are some important exceptions; see below.) Clavulanic acid is an early carbapenem, sulbactam and tazobactam are penicillanic acid sulphones. They are combined with amoxycillin, ampicillin or piperacillin respectively. These three compounds combined with penicillins or cephalosporins are now at least as widely used as the partner penicillins.

They are particularly valuable for surgeons because not only do they provide against many enterobacteriaceae with β-lactamases but also are active against Bacteroides enzymes and, in the case of the penicillanic acid sulphones, are also active against Acinetobacter. All are used both for chemoprophylaxis and treatment.

Cephalosporins

The cephalosporins were only developed because of their stability to staphylococcal penicillinase. The early cephalosporins were excellent for staphylococci but were destroyed by Gram-negative β-lactamases and were also unable to penetrate Pseudomonas and other non-fermenting Gram-negative rods. Oral cephalosporins and cefuroxime were able to withstand the prevalent β-lactamases of the 1970s but when the spectrum of activity of β-lactamases gradually enlarged the successive waves of cephalosporins such as cefotaxime, ceftriaxone, ceftazidime also became prey to the extended-spectrum

β-lactamases (ESBLs). In most northern European countries the prevalence of these enzymes is low except in Klebsiella species and in some intensive care units. A second type of β-lactamase provides problems for cephalosporins and to a lesser extent penicillins. These are enzymes present in a few important hos-pital pathogens such as Pseudomonas, Serratia and Enterobacter. The enzymes are not transferable and are expressed in small amounts by genes located on the chromosome. Unfortunately exposure to cephalosporins or carbapenems induces the organism to produce this chromosomal enzyme at high levels and resistant organisms appear during therapy. The latest cephalosporins, cefepime and cefpirome, show better stability to chromosomal enzymes than do previous cephalosporins but unfortunately they are more easily destroyed by the prevalent transferable β-lactamases.

Two cephalosporins, ceftazidime and cefaperazone, are active against Pseudomonas as well as other enterobacteriaceae and are the preferred cephalosporins when Pseudomonas is a potential pathogen. Like cefepime, cefoperazone is slightly labile to transferable enzymes and is combined with an inhibitor – sulbactam – to counteract this. All three inhibitors are active transferable β-lactamases, including ESBLs, but have negligible inhibitory effect on the chromosomal enzymes.

One interesting group of cephalosporins are the 7-alpha-methoxy cephalosporins (or cephamycins): cefoxitin and cefotetan. These are active against enterobacteria and Gram-negative anaerobic bacteria such as Bacteroides and Prevotella. In many countries they are widely used as single agent chemoprophylaxis for abdominal surgery.

Penicillins enjoy one advantage in surgical infection over cephalosporins and that is the activity against Enterococcus faecalis, the commonest enterococcus in human infections. The wide use of cephalosporins may play a role in the increasing prevalence of enterococcal infections in hospital.

The carbapenems

In some ways the carbapenems are the ultimate β-lactam antibiotics with activity against most of the bacteria involved in surgical infections – enterobacteriaceae, anaerobes, Pseudomonas, staphylococci and Acinetobacter. Two compounds are presently in use – imipenem and meropenem – and are certainly useful agents. However, in the intensive care units where these agents are widely used resistant bacteria emerge. They usually arise in patients already suffering from severe underlying disease undergoing invasive procedures and the organisms can spread rapidly in intensive care units. Rarely, if ever, should imipenem or meropenem be used as antibiotics of first resort. Initial presumptive therapy in surgical patients in such critical units should be with less broad spectrum antibiotics such as ceftazidime or piperacillin-tazobactam, with or without gentamicin. Several new carbapenems with properties different from imipenem/meropenem are now appearing for approval.

AMINOGLYCOSIDES

Gentamicin is rapidly bactericidal for most Gram-negative rods including *Pseudomonas*. Unfortunately it affects glomerular function and even in patients with normal renal function after 5–7 days of therapy accumulation occurs and blood levels start to rise. This effect is reversible when treatment is discontinued, but the high level in the blood produces permanent damage to the cochlea with loss of hearing of unsteadiness. If aminoglycosides are used, steps should be taken to avoid these side-effects. Therapeutic drug monitoring is needed in persons with pre-existing renal impairment or aged 45 and over, and advisable in persons under 45. Only short courses should be necessary. Pharmacodynamic studies indicate that one dose a day of 2–7 mg/kg is more effective than doses divided throughout the day.

QUINOLONES

The early quinolones were used for urinary infection only. The arrival of the fluoro-quinolone, ciprofloxacin and ofloxacin, has led to their use in a much wider range of infections, both in the community and in hospital. Ciprofloxacin, a long awaited oral treatment for pseudomonas infection, is apparently the second most-widely used agent after ampicillin/amoxycillin (with or without inhibitor). The surgical uses are in urology, orthopaedics, sepsis, and hospital-acquired infection. Newer quinolones than ciprofloxacin and ofloxacin will inevitably lead to an even more widespread use in respiratory infections and skin infection. The fear, of course, is resistance. Some organisms are highly susceptible, e.g. *N. gonorrhoeae* and *E.coli*, but even here resistance is becoming a problem, both in the community and in the hospital. Some organisms such as *Staph. aureus* and *Ps. aeruginosa* are of medium susceptibility and resistant variants are commonly produced. Resistant variants arise fairly quickly in patients with *Staph. aureus* and the indication for quinolones are currently few. Ciprofloxacin may be helpful in invasive systemic infections with *Pseudomonas aeruginosa* and unobstructed urinary tract infection, but in complicated lesions with pus, resistant strains may appear rapidly. The new quinolones appearing since 2000 have increased anti-Gram-positive activity; this is mainly of value against *Streptococcus Pneumoniae*. Acquisition of quinolone resistance by staphylococci is likely to remain a problem.

GLYCOPEPTIDES, VANCOMYCIN AND TEICOPLANIN

Although vancomycin has been used clinically for 40 years, acquired resistance to it is rare. This is due in part to the limited indications for the uses of glycopeptides, the need for therapeutic drug monitoring and for careful slow intravenous infusion of vancomycin. Vancomycin is the more active of the two glycopeptides against staphylococci and is less active against enterococci than teicoplanin. The widespread use of glycopeptides since the 1980s stems from the high prevalence of methicillin resistance in staphylococci in hospitals. The appearance of enterococci resistant to glycopeptides and, more recently, of staphylococci with diminished susceptibility is a cause for concern and therapy with glycopeptides should only be used when there is very good cause. Vancomycin should not be used for chemoprophylaxis except when operation is necessary in a patient known to have MRSA in an infected lesion in the heart or in a prosthesis. Much effort has been expended to find antibiotics other than glycopeptides for treatment of MRSA because there is no other dependable choice at this time among the well-established antimicrobials. Glycopeptide resistance in *staph. aureus* would create major therapy problems. Resistant enterococci cause treatment problems for patients in some highly specialized units in hospital; MRSA are much more prevalent.

METRONIDAZOLE AND RELATED IMIDAZOLES

Metronidazole was introduced for treatment of protozoa (trichomonas and amoebae) and the activity against anaerobes only became prominent in 1972 when the activity against bacteroides was reported. Anaerobic bacteria have not become resistant to metronidazoles and because it can be given orally, parenterally and per rectum its place in chemoprophylaxis and therapy is still secure. Metronidazole only acts against strict anaerobes and is not active against streptococci of the *milleri* group which are also involved in intra-abdominal sepsis, nor against enterococci. Metronidazole is active against *Cl. difficile* and should be used as initial therapy for pseudomembranous colitis in order to spare use of vancomycin.

One important side effect is peripheral neuropathy, but this only appears with high dose and prolonged course so is not seen with chemoprophylaxis.

10.8   FURTHER READING

Antibiotic Prophylaxis in Surgery. *Scottish Intercollegiate Guidelines Network*, July 2000.

Davey, P. and Nathwani, D. (1996) Antibiotic policies. In: *Antibiotics and Chemotherapy*, (ed. F. O'Grady, H. Lambert, R.G. Finch and D. Greenwood). Churchill Livingstone, London.

Davey, P., Dodd, T., Kerr, S. and Malek, M. (1990) Audit of iv antibiotic administration. *Pharm. J.*, **30**, 793–796.

Goldmann, D.A., Weinstein, R.A., Wenzel, R.P., Tablan, O.C., Duma, R.J., Gaynes, R.P., Schlosser, J. and Martone, W.J. (for The Workshop to Prevent and Control the Emergence and Spread of Antimicrobial Resistant Microorganisms in Hospitals) (1996) Strategies to prevent and control the emergence and spread of antimicrobial-resistant microorganisms in hospitals. A challenge to hospital leadership. *JAMA*, **275**, 234–240.

Gorbach, S.L., Condon, R.E., Conte, J.E., Kaiser, A.B., Ledger, W.J. and Nichols, R.L. (1992) General guidelines for the evaluation of new anti-infective drugs for prophylaxis of surgical infections: evaluation of new anti-infective drugs for surgical prophylaxis. *Clin. Infect. Dis.*, **15**(Suppl.1), S313–S338.

Graff-Lonnevig, V., Hedlin, G. and Lindfors, A. (1988) Penicillin allergy – a rare paediatric condition? *Arch. Dis. Child.*, **63**, 1342–1346.

Kaiser, A.B. (1986) Antimicrobial prophylaxis in surgery. *N. Engl. J. Med.*, **315**, 1129–1137.

Nichols, R.L. (1994) Antibiotic prophylaxis in surgery. *Curr. Opin. Infect. Dis.*, **7**, 647–652.

Pestotnik, S.L., Classen, D.C., Scott Evans, R. and Burke, J.P. (1996) Implementing antibiotic practice guidelines through computer-assisted decision support: clinical and financial outcomes. *Ann. Intern. Med.*, **124**, 884–890.

Privitera, G., Scarpellini, P., Ortisi, G., Nicastro, G., Nicolin, R. and de Lalla, F. (1991) Prospective study of Clostridium difficile intestinal colonization and disease following single-dose antibiotic prophylaxis in surgery. *Antimicrob. Agents Chemother.*, **35**(1), 208–210.

Schein, M. and Wittmann, D.H. (1993) Editorial: antibiotics in abdominal surgery: the less the better. *Eur. J. Surg.*, **159**, 451–453.

Solomkin, J.S., Meakins, J.L., Allo, M.D. *et al.* (1984) Antibiotic trials in intra-abdominal infections. A critical evaluation of study design and outcome reporting. *Ann. Surg.*, **200**, 29–39.

Solomkin, J.S., Reinhart, H.H., Dellinger, E.P., Bohnen, J.M., Rotstein, O.D., Vogel, S.B., Simms, H.H., Hill, C.S., Bjornson, H.S., Haverstock, D.C., Coulter, H.O. and Echols, R.M. (1996) Results of a randomized trial comparing sequential intravenous oral treatment with ciprofloxacin plus metronidazole to imipenem/cilastatin for intra-abdominal infections. *Ann. Surg.*, **223**(3), 303–315.

Widdison, A.L., Pope, N.R.J. and Brown, E.M. (1993) Survey of guidelines for antimicrobial prophylaxis in surgery. *J. Hosp. Infect.*, **25**, 199–205.

Infections in transplanted and other immunocompromised patients

J.P. BURNIE, B.L. OPPENHEIM AND T.G. WREGHEITT

11.1 INTRODUCTION

Certain infections caused by several viruses and micro-organisms are more severe and more frequently encountered by immunocompromised patients. These patients fall into well-defined categories, each of which carry their own risk of infection:

- solid organ transplant recipients;
- bone marrow transplant recipients;
- patients with haematological malignancies;
- patients with HIV/AIDS;
- patients receiving chemotherapy;
- patients with immunodeficiency syndromes; and
- elderly patients.

Transplant patients need to receive immunosuppressive drugs in order to prevent the rejection of donor organs or bone marrow. There are several immunosuppressive drugs and antibody preparations which may be used singly or in combination, each of which functions by suppressing various components of the T-cell immune function. Different regimens are used for induction and maintenance therapy, and for treating rejection episodes.

Immunosuppressive agents include:

- azathioprine;
- prednisolone;
- steroids;
- cyclosporin A;
- FK506;
- ATG/ALG; and
- OKT3.

Azathioprine and steroids inhibit the cell division of all elements of the immune system, and also inhibit cytokine production. Cyclosporin A inhibits the synthesis of interleukin-2 by T cells, while ATG/ALG inhibits T-cell function. OKT3 is a murine monoclonal antibody directed against the CD3 molecule known to be associated with the T-cell receptor for antigen recognition.

Some immunosuppressive agents (e.g. azathioprine, ATG and OKT3) affect (increase) the severity of virus infections (especially herpesviruses) more than others (e.g. cyclosporin A), and antiviral prophylaxis or treatment may be required if these drugs are used.

Some viruses (e.g. cytomegalovirus [CMV] and HIV) are themselves immunosuppressive. The frequency of CMV-specific cytotoxic T cells is lower in immunocompromised patients, and recovery from CMV disease in transplant patients has been correlated with directly measurable cytotoxic T cells in the blood.

The factors listed in Table 11.1 make transplant patients particularly vulnerable to infection, and the vast majority of them will encounter at least one infection in the post-transplant period. The timing of the infection can give some clue as to the nature of the infecting agent, although there is considerable overlap. In general, infections occurring within the first month post-transplant

Table 11.1 *Factors contributing to infection following transplantation*

- Underlying disease, e.g. renal failure, cystic fibrosis
- Trauma of major surgery
- Immunosuppression
  - routine
  - for episodes of rejection
- Introduction of organisms via donor organ
- Graft-versus-host disease in allogeneic bone marrow transplant (BMT)
- Some infections (especially CMV) are in themselves immunosuppressive

Table 11.2 *Most common sites of bacterial infection post-transplantation*

Type of transplant	Site(s)
Kidney	Urinary tract
Heart	Lung, sternal wound
Heart-lung and lung	Lung
Liver	Abdomen
Bone marrow transplant	Pyrexia of unknown origin, central line

either result from transplanting an infectious agent present in the donor tissue, from reactivation of latent herpes viruses or occur as postoperative infections not dissimilar from those occurring in other surgical patients. The period spanning 1 to 6 months post-transplant is typically the time of greatest immunosuppression, and a wide variety of opportunistic infections can occur. Following this time period, the post-transplant patient remains susceptible not only to typical community-acquired infections, but also to a wide range of the more chronic viral, fungal and mycobacterial infections.

The bone marrow transplant (BMT) recipient differs somewhat from patients receiving solid organ transplants in that the conditioning regimen results in profound neutropenia and immunosuppression during the immediate post-transplant period, and this renders these patients susceptible to a wide range of opportunists. Graft-versus-host disease may occur in allogeneic BMT recipients, and this is highly immunosuppressive both on its own and by virtue of the management of the condition which often involves high-dose steroids as well as other immunosuppressive agents.

11.2 SOLID ORGAN TRANSPLANT RECIPIENTS

There are four main categories of solid organ transplant recipients:

- heart-lung and lung;
- heart;
- liver; and
- kidney.

Some infections (e.g. CMV) cause problems in all these patient groups, but the relative prevalence and severity of infections vary between these groups, and these will be considered separately.

11.2.1 Heart-lung and lung transplant recipients

Bacterial infections are the most common cause of morbidity in the early postoperative period (Table 11.2). The main site of infections is the chest, with bacterial pneumonia predominating. Pulmonary infections are purported to occur in more than 60% of lung transplant recipients, and are the most common cause of death in this patient group. As well as immunosuppressive therapy, local factors seem to play an important role in favouring infections of the lung. These include impaired mucociliary clearance in the transplant lung, ablation of the cough reflex below the tracheal anastomosis, severed tracheobronchial lymphatics and an altered bronchial circulation.

The predominating infecting organisms are Gram-negative rods, particularly *Pseudomonas aeruginosa*, and *Staph. aureus*, and, in some cases, more than one organism is involved. The infection may be associated with organisms colonizing the donor, and cultures taken from the donor trachea at harvest may be helpful in directing antibiotic therapy.

PNEUMOCYSTIS INFECTION

Pneumocystis carinii pneumonia (PCP) is well described in the settings of both solid organ and bone marrow transplantation, but the highest incidence is found in heart-lung transplant recipients.

The typical presentation is of a pneumonitis with shortness of breath, fever, and a non-productive cough. Impaired oxygenation is the most frequent laboratory finding, and this often appears out of proportion to the clinical features. Rapid diagnosis, usually with bronchoscopy (but if necessary also with biopsy), is essential for successful treatment. The treatment of choice for PCP is high-dose co-trimoxazole.

PCP is not commonly seen because of the widespread use of co-trimoxazole prophylaxis, but must always be considered because of problems with compliance or tolerability of this drug.

CYTOMEGALOVIRUS (CMV)

These patients are at greatest risk of severe herpesvirus infections, of which CMV is the greatest problem. CMV infection may be acquired with the donor organ. Some 80% of CMV antibody-negative patients acquiring an organ from a CMV antibody-positive donor will be infected, and in the absence of antiviral prophylaxis or treatment most patients will have severe CMV disease and some will die (Table 11.3). Most of the CMV antibody-positive patients will either experience reactivation of their own latent CMV or they may be re-infected by CMV from the donor organ or blood donors. Most of these patients will be symptomatic, many will have severe disease, and some will die unless antiviral prophylaxis or treatment are given.

There are several means by which the impact of CMV disease can be reduced in these patients by:

- providing CMV-negative organs for CMV negative recipients;
- giving prophylactic antiviral therapy to patients at risk of severe CMV disease; and
- giving pre-emptive antiviral treatment to patients at risk of severe CMV disease when CMV infection is detected but **before symptoms develop**.

All potential organ recipients and donors should be screened for CMV status before transplantation so that whenever possible organs from CMV-negative donors can be given to CMV-negative recipients. At least two assays should be used for this purpose (ELISA, latex agglutination, CFT) so that the results can be verified. There will be some patients who, because of their rare blood group or other factors, remain on the waiting list much longer than others, waiting for a suitable CMV-negative donor organ to become available. Some will die on the waiting list, and for this reason attempts should be made to select CMV-negative donors for CMV-negative recipients. However, if this is not possible within an appropriate time, rather than denying the chance of a transplant to these CMV-negative recipients, they should be given organs from a positive donor but given antiviral prophylaxis from the time of transplantation.

Since CMV-positive heart-lung and lung transplant recipients also have a high risk of developing severe CMV disease, these patients should also receive prophylactic antiviral treatment from the time of transplantation.

Several antiviral agents have been shown to have some effect in reducing the impact of CMV infection and disease in solid organ transplant recipients, including ganciclovir, aciclovir, valaciclovir, famciclovir and high-titre CMV immunoglobulin.

Most studies have been carried out with aciclovir and ganciclovir, both of which have been shown to have some effect, especially in CMV-positive patients. However, to date there are no confirmed data which have shown a significant effect on the incidence or severity of primary donor-acquired CMV infection in solid organ transplant recipients. Most trials have used oral aciclovir or ganciclovir for 3 months, or intravenous ganciclovir for 1 month after transplant. New data on the efficacy of oral ganciclovir given for 3 months appears promising. CMV reactivation/reinfection in heart-lung and lung recipients is drastically reduced by this regimen, which also has had some beneficial effect on the severity of primary donor-acquired CMV disease in these patients.

For those patients who develop CMV infection or disease despite receiving antiviral prophylaxis, there are several means of diagnosing infection:

- virus culture;
- DEAFF (detection of early antigen fluorescent focus);
- leucocyte antigen staining;
- PCR (polymerase chain reaction); and
- antibody detection.

Virus culture is relatively slow; CMV takes 1–3 weeks to produce a cytopathic effect in fibroblast cells, which is not useful for the clinical management of infections. The DEAFF test is a modified culture test in which virus is grown in fibroblast cells for 24–48 hours, after which then the fixed cell sheet is stained with a fluorescein-labelled monoclonal antibody against either CMV early or immediate-early antigens. This test, although relatively insensitive (compared with PCR) is more useful for the clinical management of patients, especially if histopathology biopsy results are not available. The detection of virus in

Table 11.3 *CMV infections in Papworth heart-lung and lung transplant recipients not receiving antiviral prophylaxis*

CMV antibody status of organ		Patients with primary CMV infection (%)	Patients with CMV reactivation or reinfection (%)	Infected patients with CMV disease (%)	Infected patients who died from CMV disease (%)
Donor	Recipient				
Positive	Negative	88	–	96	38
Negative	Negative	5*	–	30	0
Positive	Positive	–	79	64	5
Negative	Positive	–	71	56	0

*Not all patients received CMV-negative blood.

blood can be correlated with CMV disease. The leucocyte antigen test detects CMV in leucocytes, and has been shown to be useful in clinical management of patients. There are several kinds of PCR which have been developed for detecting CMV DNA in specimens from transplant patients. Most studies have utilized plasma or leucocytes for detecting CMV DNA. One of the problems with PCR is that potentially it is very sensitive; hence, there is a need to adjust the sensitivity of PCR assays so that the results obtained discriminate between those patients with CMV disease (or who are likely to develop CMV disease) and those without disease (or who are not likely to develop it).

Intravenous ganciclovir (5 mg kg^{-1} twice daily) is the antiviral drug of choice for treating CMV infections in heart-lung and lung transplant recipients. On the rare occasion that this drug is not well tolerated, foscarnet should be used. It should be noted that oral ganciclovir is not suitable for treating CMV infections (it is currently licenced only for maintenance therapy in AIDS patients with retinitis).

HERPES SIMPLEX VIRUS (HSV)

Herpes simplex virus (HSV) can be a significant cause of morbidity and mortality in heart-lung and lung transplant recipients. Approximately 60% of patients have experienced previous HSV infection at the time of transplantation; they are at risk of reactivation of HSV usually in the first few weeks after transplantation, as a result of immunosuppression. Some of these HSV antibody-positive patients will not experience HSV reactivation, although approximately 30% will have either herpes labialis, genital herpes or HSV skin eruptions of varying severity in the absence of antiviral prophylaxis, and a few patients will experience fatal HSV pneumonia.

Primary HSV infection is very rare in transplant patients, the infections almost always occurring as a result of HSV reactivation. Symptomatic HSV infection can be eliminated or drastically reduced in severity by giving oral aciclovir prophylaxis (200–400 mg twice daily) to HSV antibody-positive heart-lung and lung transplant recipients.

HSV infection may be diagnosed by visualizing herpesvirus particles in vesicle fluid by electron microscopy, or by virus culture or PCR. HSV respiratory infection can be diagnosed by virus culture or PCR of lung biopsy or bronchoalveolar lavage. HSV antibody detection, while useful for determining those patients likely to experience HSV reactivation after transplantation, is not useful for diagnosing HSV infection. Patients with HSV reactivation do not always produce a rise in HSV antibody titre.

VARICELLA-ZOSTER VIRUS (VZV)

Primary varicella-zoster virus (VZV) infection (chickenpox) is often severe in solid organ transplant recipients, frequently manifesting as haemorrhagic chicken pox, which is usually fatal. The treatment of choice is i.v. aciclovir (10 mg kg^{-1} three times daily for at least 10 days). For this reason, solid organ recipients should be tested for VZV antibody when they are being assessed for suitability for transplantation. VZV antibody-negative transplanted patients should be made aware of the risk of chickenpox infection. If they come into contact with chickenpox, shingles or zoster they should report this immediately and receive prophylactic zoster immune globulin (VZIG; adult dose 1000 mg) and/or prophylactic oral aciclovir (800 mg four times daily for 2 weeks).

VZV reactivation, resulting in zoster occurs in approximately 20% of VZV antibody-positive patients in the first few weeks after solid organ transplantation. Most infections are mild, but some may be severe. Mild cases can be treated with oral famciclovir (750 mg daily for 7 days) or valaciclovir (3 g daily for 7 days). Severe cases should be treated with intravenous aciclovir (10 mg kg^{-1} three times daily). Patients receiving antiviral prophylaxis for potential HSV infection are less likely to experience zoster after transplantation.

VZV infections can be diagnosed by a number of different means. In those transplant centres with access to an electron microscope (EM), vesicular fluid can be examined in the search for herpesvirus particles. Since immunocompromised patients usually produce increased amounts of virus in vesicular fluid, EM diagnosis is usually very sensitive. However, since all herpesviruses are identical under EM examination, clinical evaluation of herpesvirus lesions is important since HSV vesicular lesions will also have herpesvirus particles. VZV can be grown in cell culture but usually takes 7–14 days to grow (compared with HSV, which usually grows in 2–10 days). Infection can also be diagnosed by the demonstration of a significant VZV antibody rise or by detection of VZV DNA by PCR.

EPSTEIN–BARR VIRUS (EBV)

Epstein–Barr virus (EBV) infection is common in transplant patients, and 90–95% of them have already experienced infection at the time of transplantation. Most patients have EBV reactivation which is most commonly detected in the first 6 months after transplantation but can occur at any time. Patients do not experience glandular fever, commonly associated with EBV infection in immunocompetent persons. Symptoms are usually nonspecific (e.g. fever, malaise, flu-like symptoms). Some patients will have lymphoproliferative disease or lymphoma, but these manifestations are more prevalent in heavily immunosuppressed patients.

Primary EBV infection is seen in EBV antibody-negative patients who receive organs from EBV antibody-positive donors. Glandular fever is seldom seen in these patients, who usually have the non-specific symptoms seen in patients with EBV reactivation (see above). Infection is more severe in children.

Although clinical trials have not been conducted, aciclovir is thought to have some effect in modulating the symptoms associated with EBV infection.

EBV infections may be diagnosed serologically (EBV seroconversion, antibody rise) or by demonstration of EBV DNA by PCR.

OTHER VIRUSES

There are few other viruses which are associated with infections in heart-lung and lung transplant recipients associated with increased severity. However, adenoviruses are associated with more severe symptoms in solid organ transplant recipients. These viruses are associated with a range of symptoms from maculopapular rashes, conjunctivitis, respiratory symptoms and gastroenteritis. Infection can be diagnosed by virus culture, antibody rise or EM (gastroenteritis).

TOXOPLASMA GONDII

T. gondii is only ever a problem when primary infection is acquired with the donor organ. Some 60% of *T. gondii* antibody-negative patients given a *T. gondii* antibody-positive organ will have *T. gondii* infection after transplantation. Most infections will be symptomatic, and some may be severe or fatal. Infection can be prevented by co-trimoxazole or pyrimethamine prophylaxis. *T. gondii* reactivation is rare after transplantation and is seldom symptomatic.

11.2.2 Heart transplant recipients

Although cardiac transplant recipients usually experience less frequent or severe infections than heart-lung and lung recipients, infections are still a major cause of morbidity in this group.

Bacterial infections are a particular problem in the early post-transplant period, and are similar in nature to those found in any patient undergoing cardiovascular surgery. Bacteraemia is common and is often found in association with intravascular catheters. The **lungs** are

another important site of infection, and although most infections occur soon after transplantation, bacterial pneumonias continue to occur sporadically in later months. Causative organisms are generally similar to those found in other hospital-acquired infections, namely *Staph. aureus* and Gram-negative rods, but more unusual organisms such as *Legionella pneumophila* are well described and must be considered.

Sternal wound and mediastinal infections are important complications in this setting, and can be extremely difficult to eradicate. *Staph. aureus*, Gram-negative rods and polymicrobial infections are the most common, and methicillin-resistant *Staph. aureus* can create particular management problems. Surgical drainage is vital to the success of treatment of mediastinal sepsis and needs to be combined with long-term antibiotic treatment.

Other nosocomial infections such as urinary tract infections are similar to those found in other postoperative patients. Heart transplant recipients do not appear to be particularly at risk for the development of infective endocarditis.

CYTOMEGALOVIRUS (CMV)

The most severe infections are seen in CMV antibody-negative patients receiving organs from CMV antibody-positive donors (Table 11.4). Infection and disease incidence is severe enough to justify prophylactic antiviral treatment (see also Section 11.2.1).

Infection acquired from blood is much less severe and can be eliminated by use of CMV-negative blood. Although CMV disease does occur in CMV antibody-positive recipients, antiviral prophylaxis is not justified. Symptomatic infections can be treated with ganciclovir.

HERPES SIMPLEX VIRUS (HSV)

HSV infection (always reactivation) occurs in approximately 80% of HSV antibody-positive heart transplant recipients during the first few weeks after transplantation if they are not receiving prophylactic antivirals. Infections are usually not severe and can be treated with either oral or intravenous aciclovir (depending on the severity).

Table 11.4 *CMV infections in Papworth heart transplant recipients not receiving antiviral prophylaxis*

CMV antibody status of organ		Patients with primary CMV infection (%)	Patients with CMV reactivation or reinfection (%)	Infected patients with CMV disease (%)	Infected patients who died from CMV disease (%)
Donor	Recipient				
Positive	Negative	71	–	69	8
Negative	Negative	4*	–	5	0
Positive	Positive	–	67	22	0
Negative	Positive	–	45	14	0

*Not all patients received CMV-negative blood.

VARICELLA-ZOSTER VIRUS (VZV)

Primary VZV infection (chickenpox) can be severe or fatal in heart transplant recipients. All patients should be screened for VZV antibody at assessment, and VZV antibody-negative patients should be advised to avoid contact with chickenpox or zoster after transplantation. Zoster-immune globulin and/or aciclovir prophylaxis can be given to susceptible patients exposed to VZV infection.

Approximately 10% of heart transplant recipients experience zoster during the first few weeks after transplantation. Symptoms are usually not severe and can be treated with either oral or intravenous aciclovir (depending on the severity).

EPSTEIN-BARR VIRUS (EBV)

Most heart transplant recipients experience EBV infection after transplantation. Since approximately 90% of adult patients have had EBV infection before transplantation, very few primary infections occur afterwards. Almost all of these infections are transmitted by the donor organ. EBV reactivation can occur at any time after transplantation, but is most common during the first 6 months. Typical glandular fever-like symptoms are seldom seen; patients usually have non-specific symptoms such as fever, headache and malaise. Some patients (3% in the Papworth series) will develop EBV-associated lymphoma, and a few will develop lymphoproliferative syndrome (the incidence depends on the amount of immunosuppression received).

OTHER VIRUSES

With the exception of adenoviruses, there are no viruses which are associated with increased symptoms in heart transplant recipients. Severe respiratory adenovirus infections are almost always confined to patients less than 20 years of age. There is no treatment available other than by reducing immunosuppression.

TOXOPLASMA GONDII

T. gondii infection is only a problem if acquired from the donor organ. If prophylactic antibiotics are not used, 60% of *T. gondii* antibody-negative patients receiving organs from *T. gondii* antibody-positive donors will acquire primary infection. Symptoms always include fever, and may also include myocarditis, encephalitis and pneumonia. With the current use of co-trimoxazole prophylaxis for *Pneumocystis carinii*, primary donor-acquired *T. gondii* infection is not seen. We have shown that, in the absence of co-trimoxazole prophylaxis, a 6-week prophylactic course of pyrimethamine (25 mg per day) reduces infection and prevents symptoms.

Reactivation of *T. gondii* infection in *T. gondii* antibody-positive patients rarely occurs (<1%) and is seldom symptomatic. Co-trimoxazole prophylaxis will prevent *T. gondii* reactivation.

11.2.3 Liver transplant recipients

Infection is a major problem following liver transplantation, with up to two-thirds of transplant recipients suffering a serious infection. The reasons for particular problems with infection in this setting are largely attributable to technical aspects of the transplant operation, and the fact that patients are often extremely ill at the time of the procedure.

In common with other types of transplant, it is useful to consider three separate periods of risk for infection.

In the **first month post-transplant**, postoperative and nosocomial infections due to bacteria and *Candida* spp. are the main problems.

During the period **between 1 and 6 months post-transplant**, the duration of immunosuppresive therapy has been prolonged enough to cause marked depression of cell-mediated immunity, and it is at this stage that reactivation syndromes may result in clinical illness and infections due to unusual organisms such as *Pneumocystis carinii*, *Aspergillus* spp. and *Listeria monocytogenes* may be seen.

Beyond 6 months, infections become far less common, but recipients remain susceptible to commnity-acquired infections such as influenza and pneumococcal pneumonia.

BACTERIAL INFECTIONS

These are particularly common in the early post-transplant period, with reported rates ranging from 50% to more than 70%. The types of infections which occur are typical of those found following major abdominal surgery, and include intra-abdominal infections, wound infections, pneumonia, urinary tract infection, central line-associated infection and primary bacteraemia.

Intra-abdominal infections are the most important. These include liver abscesses, cholangitis, peritonitis and abdominal abscesses, and a wide variety of bacteria are capable of causing these infections. In most series the aerobic Gram-negative rods such as *E. coli* and *Pseudomonas aeruginosa* predominate, followed by enterococci, staphylococci and streptococci. The type of antibacterial prophylaxis used will influence both the pattern of infecting organism and the antibiotic susceptibility profile.

VIRUS INFECTIONS

Most virus infections in these patients are similar to those experienced by heart recipients, due to a similar immunosuppressive regimen. However, in addition, liver transplant recipients are more likely to be infected with one of the hepatitis viruses (and to be transplanted as a result of chronic viral disease). A few patients receive liver transplants as a result of fulminant hepatitis A infection, but they rarely have a recurrence of hepatitis A virus disease in their transplanted livers.

An increasing proportion of patients are receiving liver transplants as a result of chronic HCV disease. A significant proportion will experience reinfection of their transplanted liver, some with fatal consequences in the first few years after transplantation. Interferon and ribavirin may be used to treat HCV infections, but most responders relapse after treatment is stopped. The optimum duration of treatment is yet to be determined in clinical trials.

Some liver transplant patients are transplanted as a result of severe HBV liver disease (cirrhosis, HCC). Patients who are HBeAg-positive and HBV DNA-positive at the time of transplantation have a high frequency of HBV recurrent disease, resulting from reinfection of their transplanted liver. Hepatitis B immune globulin (HBIG) prophylaxis in these patients is seldom effective in preventing recurrent HBV liver disease. By contrast, patients who are anti-HBe positive and/or HBV DNA negative at the time of transplantation and who receive long-term HBIG prophylaxis are likely not to reinfect their transplanted livers.

TOXOPLASMA GONDII

Some 20% of *T. gondii* antibody-negative patients who receive organs from *T. gondii* antibody-positive donors will experience primary infection if co-trimoxazole or pyrimethamine prophylaxis is not given.

11.2.4   Kidney transplant recipients

During the early post-transplant period, the major causes of infection are bacterial and relate to wound, pulmonary, urinary tract and intravenous line-related infections.

Urinary tract infection (UTI) is particularly important and, indeed, many bacteraemias occurring in kidney transplant recipients originate from this site. The reported incidence of UTI in this setting varies widely in different series. What is now becoming clear is that UTIs in the early post-transplant period can have serious consequences such as pyelonephritis, bacteraemia and activation of rejection. UTIs remain common for months to years after transplant, but these late infections appear to have a more benign course with little effect on graft function or overall mortality. Organisms causing UTIs in this setting do not differ significantly from those seen in other hospitalized patients, and include Gram-negatives such as *E. coli*, *Klebsiella* spp. and *Pseudomonas aeruginosa*, as well as enterococci and candida.

In addition to the usual nosocomial pathogens, kidney transplant recipients have also been reported as being particularly susceptible to a number of rather unusual opportunists such as *Listeria monocytogenes*, *Nocardia* spp. and mycobacteria.

There does appear to be a particular association between **nocardiasis** and kidney transplantation, although it has been noted to occur in a variety of immunosuppressed patients, including heart and liver transplant recipients. The species responsible for most human cases in *Nocardia asteroides*, a branching Gram-positive bacterium which is widespread in the environment. Presentation of infection is extremely variable, but since the respiratory tract is the normal portal of entry, pulmonary infection is the most frequent manifestation. Signs and symptoms include fever, weight loss, cough, shortness of breath and chest pain. In some patients the infection can disseminate, and the commonest sites of dissemination are the central nervous system and the skin. Early diagnosis is the key to successful treatment and, depending on the site of infection, bronchoscopy and/or biopsy may be required. A variety of antimicrobials have been used for the treatment of nocardiasis, but trimethoprim/sulfamethoxazole (co-trimoxazole) seems to be emerging as the regimen of choice. Treatment normally needs to be continued for prolonged periods.

Mycobacterial infections are not common in solid-organ transplant recipients, but they have been described in this setting. Of particular interest is the occurrence of non-tuberculous mycobacterial strains such as *M. haemophilum*, *M. chelonei* and *M. fortuitum*. *M. tuberculosis* infection is most often due to reactivation disease, and there have been reports in the literature of possible transmission of infection via the transplanted kidney. Although the lung is still the most common site of infections, extrapulmonary and disseminated infections have been frequently described.

VIRUS INFECTIONS

Most virus infections in these patients are similar to those experienced by heart transplant recipients (see 11.2.2).

TOXOPLASMA GONDII

Less than 1% of *T. gondii* antibody-negative patients who receive organs from *T. gondii* antibody-positive donors will experience primary infection, even if co-trimoxazole or pyrimethamine prophylaxis is not given.

11.3   BONE MARROW TRANSPLANT RECIPIENTS

11.3.1   Infections

A bone marrow transplant (BMT) involves the intravenous infusion of bone marrow, obtained either from a related or a matched unrelated donor (allogeneic

BMT) or taken previously from the recipient's own marrow (autologous BMT). Peripheral blood stem cell transplants (PBSCT) are increasingly being performed, and this involves infusion of peripheral blood stem cells which have been mobilized using haemopoietic growth factors. Prior to BMT or PBSCT infusion, the recipient's own haemopoietic system is ablated by a conditioning regimen involving either chemotherapy alone or a combination of chemotherapy and radiotherapy.

There are a number of reasons why the infectious complications following BMT differ somewhat from these associated with solid organ transplants. The actual process of BMT is simple and does not involve any surgery, so that surgically induced infections are not a problem. The conditioning regimen renders patients profoundly neutropenic, so that the early post-BMT period until engraftment is characterized by neutropenic sepsis. Finally, allogeneic BMT recipients may develop graft-versus-host disease (GVHD) which both in itself and because of the drugs used to treat it, is highly immunosuppressive.

For convenience, infections following BMT have been categorized as occurring: (i) early (within 30 days); (ii) intermediate, i.e. during the second and third month post transplant; and (iii) late (90 days to several years after BMT).

Infections occurring during the first month after BMT are typical of all infections during neutropenia. The most common presentation is with a fever but no localizing signs. Bacteria causing infections at this stage are most commonly Gram positive, particularly coagulase-negative staphylococci in association with central venous catheter infections, and the viridans streptococci which appear to be a particular problem in patients with mucositis. Gram-negative bacteria also cause problems in the neutropenic host. A wide variety of Gram-negatives can be involved, but of particular concern are infections due to *Pseudomonas aeruginosa*, which can be associated with necrotic skin lesions known as **ecthyma gangrenosum**.

During the second and third months post transplant the patient remains profoundly immunosuppressed, although engraftment has usually occurred by this time. This is also the time period during which acute GVHD may occur, and this adds to the immunosuppression. During this stage viral and fungal infections are a particular problem. *Pneumocystis carinii* pneumonia is not a common problem in BMT recipients because of widespread acceptance of the need for prophylaxis. However, it must be considered in a patient with pneumonitis because of the possibility of failure of compliance with co-trimoxazole.

During the late post-transplant period, community-acquired infections, such as chest infections due to *Streptococcus pneumoniae* and *Haemophilus influenzae*, may occur.

11.4 AUTOLOGOUS GRAFT RECIPIENTS

VIRUS INFECTIONS

A few patients will experience CMV infections, but these are not usually serious or life-threatening. Some patients will have HSV reactivation infections, and some may require treatment with acyclovir. These patients may also have other infections (i.e. VZV) which are more prevalent and problematic in T-cell-depleted patients.

11.5 ALLOGRAFT RECIPIENTS

VIRUS INFECTIONS

A high proportion of patients will experience severe or life-threatening CMV infections of which pneumonitis is the most serious complication. Prophylaxis with ganciclovir or aciclovir will reduce the frequency and impact of these infections. Regular monitoring for evidence of CMV infection (i.e. PCR of bronchoalveolar lavage or blood specimens), and early pre-emptive treatment with ganciclovir drastically reduces the incidence and severity of subsequent CMV disease. Delaying treatment until the establishment of CMV disease has a poor prognosis.

Many patients will experience HSV reactivation if prophylactic aciclovir is not given. Some patients will experience aciclovir-resistant HSV infections, which are usually amenable to foscarnet treatment.

Many patients will experience severe viral respiratory infections (adenovirus, parainfluenzaviruses) for which no antiviral treatment is available. Viral gastroenteritis, effective with prolonged viral shedding is a problem and has similar symptoms to GVHD. Many patients develop shingles, which can be treated with famciclovir or valaciclovir.

11.6 INVASIVE INFECTIONS

Invasive infections can be subdivided into those caused by fungi (e.g. yeasts, such as *Candida albicans* and *Cryptococcus neoformans*) and those caused by moulds (e.g. *Aspergillus fumigatus* and *Rhizopus oryzae*). Overall these infections share the following features: (i) they are predisposed by being neutropenic and tend to resolve when the neutropenia recovers; (ii) they have a high mortality; (iii) they have no typical clinical picture; and (iv) they are resistant to conventional antibiotic therapy and are often the cause of a pyrexia when this therapy fails. Invasive fungal infections are difficult to diagnose with conventional culture-based techniques, but when isolated will grow on Sabouraud's agar; Sensitivity testing for fungal infections is less well developed than for bacteria, and is not routinely performed for moulds.

Fungi are almost all sensitive to amphotericin B, which is the 'gold standard' therapy. These infections will now be described in more detail.

11.6.1   Yeast infections

Yeasts are Gram-positive budding microorganisms and can be subdivided into the different species by use of the germ tube test (90% of isolates of *Candida albicans* are germ tube-positive), pattern of sugar assimilation capsule production (as seen by Indian Ink) and the urease reaction (*Cryptococcus neoformans* is positive). Virulence varies from high (*C. albicans, Candida tropicalis, Candida krusei*) to low (*Candida parapsilosis* and *Torulopsis glabrata*). Antibiotic sensitivity is also species-dependent, and isolates of *C. krusei* and *T. glabrata* are resistant to fluconazole whereas *C. tropicalis* is variable and fluconazole resistance has been reported as high as 5–10% in *C. albicans* isolates from HIV-positive patients. This is important as fluconazole is routinely used as chemoprophylaxis which has been repeatedly reported as associated with a rise in the number of infections due to these resistant species.

CLINICAL PRESENTATION

Localized infections include oral and oesophageal candidiasis where the yeast can subsequently seed down the gastrointestinal tract and disseminate.

Yeasts can **superinfect** any wound and produce a UTI. In neutropenic patients, the borderline between local and disseminated infection is blurred and clinicians tend to use aggressive chemotherapy early. An example is intravenous line colonization with *C. albicans* where, in the past, the line would have been removed and no therapy given. The high rate of candidal seeding means now that it is imperative to give systemic antifungal therapy. This is absolute with *C. albicans* but more debatable with *C. parapsilosis*. Here, removal of the line usually leads to resolution of the temperature but the yeast has been repeatedly reported as seeding to the heart, where it causes endocarditis.

Disseminated candidiasis has a non-specific clinical presentation of temperature, shock (high pulse, low blood pressure) and lack of response to broad-spectrum antibiotics. The classical findings of a typical rash ('acne'-like lesions over the abdomen and lower chest) and endophthalmitis ('white fluffy exudates') are rare. The infection may disseminate to the central nervous system and mimic a stroke, in which the clinical signs vary from hour to hour. Other suggestive features include positive urine cultures (especially in the absence of a urinary catheter) a positive swab from a chest drain, especially after upper gastrointestinal tract (oesophagogastric) surgery, a positive swab from an intravenous line and a faecal sample where yeasts are the dominant microorganisms. Blood cultures are the definitive test but are only positive in about 50% of cases subsequently proven at autopsy; hence, non-culture-based techniques for making the diagnosis have been developed. In summary, the detection of antibody is prognostic rather than diagnostic, and antigen detection can be subdivided into either **crude tests** using latex agglutination with a rabbit polyclonal for detecting the cytoplasmic antigens of *C. albicans*, or **specific tests** for candidal mannan, β-glucan, enolase (48 kDa antigen) or candidal heat shock protein 90 (47 kDa antigen). Overall these may improve the sensitivity of detection by 25%, but there is debate as to the cut-off points, the nature of the best test and a lack of standardization. Recently, tests dependent on the polymerase chain reaction (PCR) have been introduced though there is no consensus on whether or not to detect low copy number genes such as actin, lanosterol α-methylase, heat shock protein 90 or high copy number genes such as the ribosomal and mitochondial sequences. Semiquantification has been introduced by incorporating digoxigenin into the initial labelling process and binding the product to a streptavidin-coated plate. The plate is then developed in a modified enzyme immunoassay, leading to a result (expressed as an optical density) that can be used as a surrogate marker for either initiating or stopping therapy.

One specific syndrome associated with candidal infection is hepatosplenic candidiasis. Paradoxically this occurs as the neutropenia resolves, and presents as a combination of pyrexia, progressively abnormal liver function tests and multiple lesions in the liver and spleen (seen on scanning). Blood cultures are usually negative, and diagnosis by biopsy is necessary where yeasts are seen but often do not grow.

C. neoformans causes cryptococcal meningitis in HIV-infective patients, usually on high-dose steroids. Here there is a marked lymphocytosis in the cerebrospinal fluid (CSF), and yeasts can be seen in low numbers. They normally have a capsule which can be demonstrated by staining with Indian Ink. In HIV-positive patients the presentation is often with only a mild headache and no signs of meningism; additionally the CSF lacks a typical picture and yeasts can be present in large numbers. In both syndromes antigen can be detected readily by latex agglutination, which is more sensitive than microscopy.

MANAGEMENT

Management can be subdivided into prophylaxis and therapy. Prophylaxis is most often oral fluconazole, but this can be replaced by oral itraconazole – especially in units where *Aspergillus* spp. are a problem. Cross-infection on hands or on contaminated bottles, cups, toothbrushes and intravenous feeds has been reported and should be eliminated by appropriate cleaning.

In the case of candidal UTI, suggested therapies have included amphotericin B bladder washouts, oral fluconazole, oral 5-flucytosine and systemic amphotericin B. In non-neutropenic patients, efficacy has been shown with a loading dose of 400 mg fluconazole followed by 200 mg per day.

Candidal endophthalmitis is a sight-threatening ocular infection which may complicate a septicaemia in a neutropenic population. The poor penetration of amphotericin B into the eye has meant a trend to either combination therapy with 5-flucytosine or fluconazole used in doses of 800 mg per day or greater.

In disseminated candidiasis amphotericin B is the 'gold standard'. A common practice is to administer a 1-mg test dose to observe for hypersensitivity, but most practitioners have stopped doing this.

The target dosage and length of treatment is 0.6 mg kg^{-1} per day for 10–14 days, although higher dosages have been used. 5-Flucytosine can be added if there is evidence of central nervous system or renal involvement, but is visually contraindicated if the patient is neutropenic or thrombocytopenic. Amphotericin B use is hampered by the high rate of side effects, most especially nephrotoxicity, though these have recently been overcome by the production of newer lipid formulations such as Ambisome, Abelcet and Amphocil. There is consensus that these are associated with less nephrotoxicity so that they should be advocated where renal insufficiency is a problem. There is no clear consensus as to the appropriate dosage, with doses of 3–5 mg kg^{-1} per day being suggested. Their high cost is another reason which has limited their use.

11.6.2   Mould infections

There has been a great increase in the prevalence of mould infections since the advent of transplant surgery and concomitant immunosuppression. The increase is also seen in patients with prolonged neutropenia and/or bone marrow transplantation. The two main species involved are *Aspergillus* spp. and *Mucor* spp., but other less common moulds have also been implicated. Most of these moulds are primarily chest pathogens which can disseminate to other organs such as the brain. *Mucormycosis* is difficult to treat and less common than *Aspergillus*. In addition to foci in the respiratory tract, it can be initiated as a skin lesion by using non-sterile swabs for dressing wounds.

CLINICAL PRESENTATION

The clinical presentation is usually as a respiratory difficulty and a cough with concurrent pleural rub or haemoptysis. The presentation may mimic a pulmonary embolism because the mould invades bronchial arteries and can spread rapidly.

In a neutropenic patient, widespread lung diseases can be found at autopsy despite a clear chest X-ray in up to 10% of patients. The disease can be missed on bronchoscopy, and computed tomography scanning is superior at demonstrating the discrete lesions. Scanning, however, does not provide histological or morphological proof of infection. Sputum production may not occur in up to one-third of patients, and the isolation of *Aspergillus* spp. from a single sputum does not mean that it is causing the disease. However, isolation of *Aspergillus* from the normal respiratory tract is very unusual and an explanation should be sought. Repeated isolation of the same species is much more significant, especially if it is *A. fumigatus*. A mould isolated from a blood culture is usually a contaminant, with the exception of the rare patient with fungal endocarditis. A wide range of methods for serological diagnosis are available by detection of antigens and antibodies, although both are only detectable late in the disease. The detection of fungal DNA by PCR has been shown to be effective on bronchial aspirates, but there is a high rate of false-positive results. Both the performance of the tests and interpretation of the findings are specialist tasks requiring consultation with the relevant experts. Treatment is rarely delayed in order to make a substantive diagnosis.

MANAGEMENT

The main agents are available for therapy, either oral itraconazole or systemic amphotericin B. A loading dose of 200 mg of itraconazole three times daily for 3 days is recommended in patients with serious infection. This drug has been used as chemoprophylaxis in transplant units with a high incidence of invasive aspergillosis. When oral therapy fails or the patient can no longer tolerate oral therapy, amphotericin B is given at a dose of 1 mg kg^{-1} per day up to an arbitrary total dose of 1–2 g. The total dose given is limited by side effects; an alternative is to use one of the liposomal preparations of amphotericin B. Doses advocated are higher than those for systemic candidiasis at 4–5 mg kg^{-1} per day because the lower renal toxicity of these preparations allows a higher dose to be given. The success rates of treatment are low. Caspofungin is now being introduced for the treatment of fungal infections which are resistant to amphotericin B.

The development of new antifungal therapies is proceeding, rapidly fuelled by the increase in number of deaths from yeast and mould infections. These include new echinocandins and an anibody against fungi antigen hsp 90 (mycograb).

11.7   FURTHER READING

De Pauw, B.E. (1997) Practical modalities for prevention of fungal infections in cancer patients. *European Journal of Clinical Microbiology and Infectious Disease,* **16**, 32–41.

De Pauw, B.E. (2001) Treatment of documented and suspected neutropenia-associated invasive fungal infections. *Journal of Chemotherapy,* **13**, 181–192.

Edwards, J.E., Bodey, G.P., Bowden, R.A., *et al.* (1997) International conference for the development of a consensus on the management and prevention of severe candidal infections. *Clinical Infectious Disease,* **25**, 43–59.

Hughes, W.T., Armstrong, D., Bodey, G.P., *et al.* (1997) Guidelines for the use of antimicrobial agents in neutropenic patients with unexplained fever. *Clinical Infectious Disease,* **25**, 551–573.

Maki, D.G., Mermel, L.A. (1998) Infections due to Infusion Therapy. In Bennet, J.V. and Bradman, P.S. (eds) *Hospital Infections,* 4th ed. 689.

Memel, L., Fow, B., Sherertz, R., *et al.* (2001) Guidelines for the management of intravenous catheter related infections. *Clinical Infectious Disease,* **32**, 1249–1272.

Yeghen, T., Kibbler, C.C., Prentice, H.G., *et al.* (2000) Management of invasive pulmonary aspergillosis in haematology patients: a review of 87 consecutive cases in a single institution. *Clinical Infectious Disease,* **31**, 859–868.

The implant-invaded host

S.P. BARRETT

12.1 INTRODUCTION

A wide variety of procedures can be included under the general term 'invasion of the host'. Common to all is that foreign material is interposed into host tissues either temporarily or to serve some permanent purpose. Thus, a cannula introduced into a vein for a radiographic procedure, an aortic xenograft, a prosthetic joint and a lens implant can all be considered under this heading. In all cases the host suffers some degree of compromise of the normal defence functions. The use of such implanted devices is associated with a wide range of unwanted sequelae including mechanical, toxicological and immunological effects. All implanted materials share a propensity to infection which may be influenced by the nature, position and duration of the implant.

12.2 HISTORY

The use of implanted devices to serve a variety of purposes extends back at least to the seventeenth century, the early history mainly involving devices used for the drainage of body fluids such as blood, urine or cerebrospinal fluid (CSF). Metal tubes were the most popular, although alternatives such as hollowed animal bones have been recorded in the early literature. Prostheses of an essentially cosmetic nature have also been used for hundreds of years, but advances in invasive surgery during the nineteenth century led to more ambitious projects – metallic orthopaedic implants and even a wooden joint prosthesis have been recorded. The nineteenth century also witnessed the introduction of the intravenous route of infusion as a means of resuscitating cholera victims; successfully with saline in the 1830s, and less successfully with milk in the 1870s. Although the first implanted devices were used long before the discovery of microorganisms, early workers recognized that, for example, artificial drainage systems for CSF were always complicated by eventual lethal inflammation, this being indicative of the infections that it is now possible to control. Rapid advances in antisepsis, and later in antibiotics, have permitted an accelerating development of invasive procedures in the present century. Indeed, blood transfusion has become standard from around the time of the first world war, and during the past 50 years implant techniques have affected virtually every branch of surgery (Figure 12.1).

12.3 MICROBIOLOGY OF IMPLANT INFECTIONS

In comparison with the past, modern medicine permits patients to survive under much greater debility, whilst at the same time contemporary clinical practice subjects them to a far wider range of invasive procedures than before. These increasingly **varied opportunities for breaching host defences** have brought to the fore infection with microorganisms not considered important

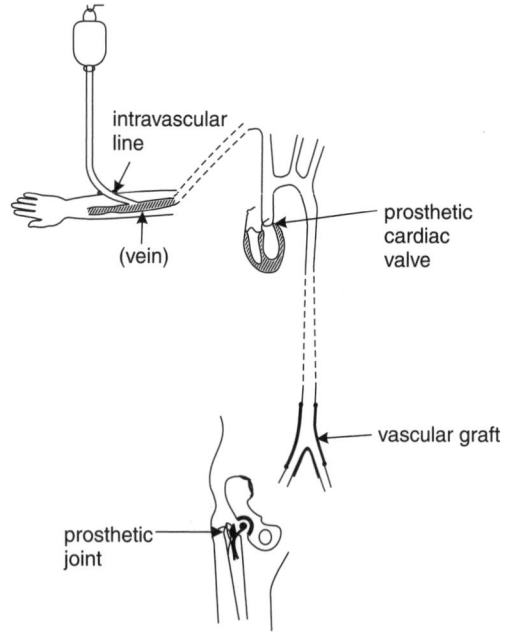

Figure 12.1 *Commonly used implants that may become infected.*

pathogens in other contexts. These 'opportunists' usually originate in the normal body flora or the everyday environment, and their prominence in the compromised host reflects not an underlying virulence but their ubiquitous nature. Because the type of patient subjected to invasive procedures has often received antibiotics, opportunists are commonly antibiotic-resistant and, depending on context, the antibiotic-resistant components of the normal flora are frequently encountered. These include coagulase-negative staphylococci, faecal streptococci and fungi such as *Candida* spp., as well as resistant environmental organisms, e.g. pseudomonads. The use of an invasive technique for infusion of potentially infected fluids, for example in enteral feeding or in blood transfusion, adds the extra dimension of possible infection with massive numbers of bacteria or with pathogenic

viruses carried asymptomatically by the donor, for example hepatitis, cytomegalovirus and HIV. With the exception of intravascular prostheses, the low virulence of most agents of implant infection means that their manifestations are rarely acute. More commonly the signs of sepsis are non-specific, sometimes with complications such as local thrombophlebitis (vascular access lines), metastatic infection, and eventual failure of the device.

12.3.1 Routes of infection

Infection can result from seeding of the device at the time of implantation or from a later bacteraemia or, in the case of invasive devices such as intravascular lines and urinary catheters, by contiguity from the insertion site on the skin (Figure 12.2). This latter route is responsible for early infections of such devices, and the intracutaneous portion of the line has been found to be the first to become colonized.

Using a correct aseptic technique, infection initiated at the time of implantation is likely to have arisen from a relatively small inoculum, for example the bacteria present on a skin squame. Unless heavy contamination or a particularly pathogenic organism is involved, a considerable amount of time may be needed for the small number of bacteria, introduced into an area where a brisk inflammatory response is occurring, to multiply sufficiently for infection to become apparent. This justifies the insertion of a peripheral vascular device, destined for short-term use, in the open ward, whilst an orthopaedic implant necessitates the environment of an operating theatre with specific aseptic precautions (see Chapter 4).

CONTAMINATED INTRAVASCULAR INFUSIONS

Manufacturing defects or faulty handling have occasionally led to the administration of contaminated intravascular

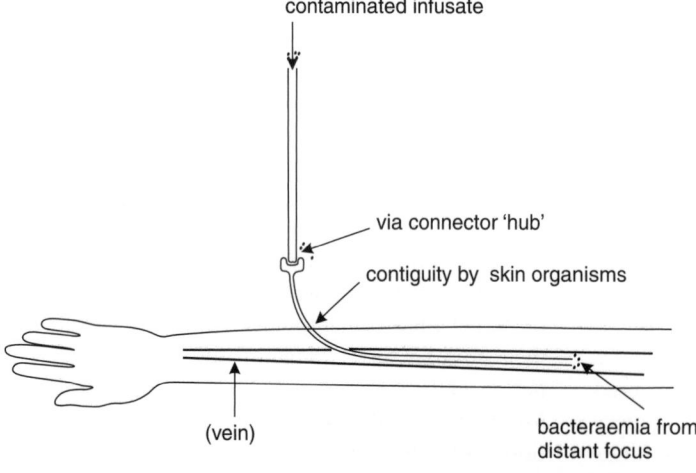

Figure 12.2 *Routes of infection of intravascular access devices.*

solutions. Since bacterial concentrations below 10^5 ml^{-1} are generally not apparent even in clear fluids, contamination will probably not be noticed before infusion. Despite the theoretical risks of a massive infusion of endotoxins, the otherwise fit patient will usually recover from the self-limiting bacteraemia; however there is a substantial risk of infection seeding onto any indwelling devices.

12.3.2 Important microorganisms

Although a vast range of bacteria and fungi has been reported from individual cases, most implant infections are due to a few major organisms:

- **Coagulase-negative staphylococci**: these are any staphylococci other than *Staphylococcus aureus*. They are sometimes referred to as *Staphylococcus epidermidis*, although strictly this term now represents one single species, and as '*Staphylococcus albus*' in older literature. Coagulase-negative staphylococci are ubiquitous commensals of the skin and upper respiratory tract and frequently resistant to most antimicrobials (Figure 12.3). These organisms account for more instances of implant infection than any other organisms.
- *Staphylococcus aureus* (the coagulase-positive staphylococcus): this is present in the normal flora of about 20% of the population and of over 30% of hospital patients. Unlike coagulase-negative staphylococci, *Staph. aureus* is carried in certain sites only (the anterior nares, axilla and perineum). It is

intrinsically more virulent, but generally less antibiotic-resistant, than the coagulase-negative staphylococci except for methicillin-resistant *Staphylococcus aureus* (MRSA). An implant infection with *Staph. aureus* results in systemic disease more often than one with coagulase-negative staphylococci.

- **Yeasts**: these are predominantly *Candida* species, most commonly *C. albicans*, and are a minor component of the normal body flora. Like all fungi, they are resistant to antibacterial antibiotics. They are a relatively rare cause of implant infection.
- **Coliforms and pseudomonads**: 'coliform' is a term used loosely to describe commensal Gram-negative rods whose presumed preferred habitat is the large bowel; it is frequently taken to include *Escherichia coli*, *Klebsiella* spp. and *Proteus* spp. etc. Pseudomonads are *Pseudomonas* spp. and related Gram-negative rods of environmental origin. Such bacteria are relatively uncommon causes of implant infection.
- **Anaerobic bacteria**: examples include *Bacteroides* spp., *Fusobacterium* spp. and the anaerobic cocci, and these seem rarely to cause implant infection. Mixed bacterial infections of implants are reported in some series.

Although coagulase-negative staphylococci are the single most commonly implicated group of microorganisms in implant infection, others predominate in certain circumstances. For example, *Staph. aureus* is the most commonly reported cause of infection in many studies of orthopaedic implants, and figures prominently in infections of vascular implants and pacemaker wires. There is insufficient information to decide whether this reflects the nature of the implants or differences between the patient groups.

12.4 PATHOPHYSIOLOGY OF IMPLANT INFECTIONS

Implants can be classified according to the type of material from which they are made. In the majority of cases these are plastics; metallic implants are largely limited to orthopaedic use and a small number of implants are of animal origin, such as porcine cardiac valve xenografts. Clearly, for an implant infection to become established there must be an initial adhesion of the infecting organism (or particle on which it is borne, e.g. a skin squame) to the surface of the implant, and this is probably governed by electrostatic interactions. Synthetic polymers used for implant manufacture show differing affinities for bacteria, and these differ between species of bacteria. Some bacteria, for example *E. coli*, show markedly low affinity for almost all implant materials, and this may explain their rarity in such infections despite being a relatively frequent cause of bacteraemia. Some implant materials with the greatest biocompatibility, for example,

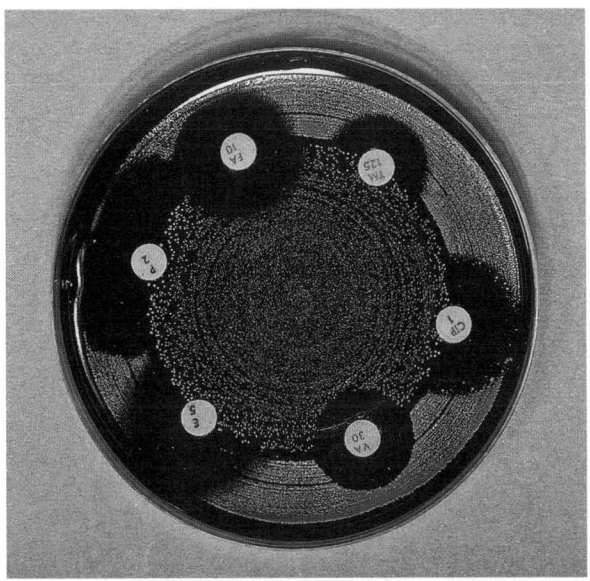

Figure 12.3 *Coagulase-negative staphylococcus (*Staphylococcus epidermidis*), demonstrating a typical multi-antibiotic-resistant pattern. In this example resistant to P (penicillin), E (erythromycin), TM (trimethoprim) and CIP (ciprofloxacin); sensitive to only FA (fusidic acid) and (VA) vancomycin.*

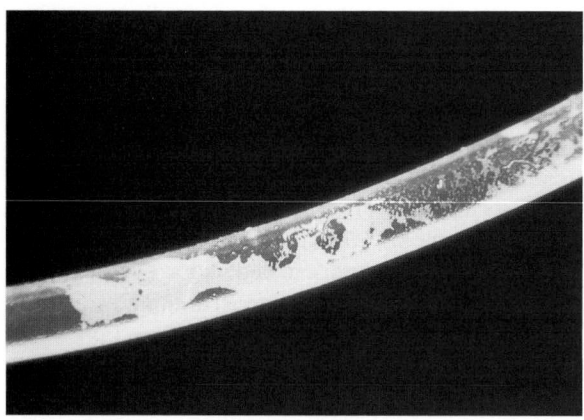

Figure 12.4 *Sheet of coagulase-negative staphylococci colonizing the lumen of a central venous infusion catheter.*

polyurethane and the silicone polymers, also demonstrate the greatest *in-vitro* affinity for bacteria and are particularly favourable to bacterial multiplication if infected pre-implantation. Those **materials most favoured by the tissues may also be most favoured by bacteria**.

Bacteria colonizing implant materials *in vitro* often multiply slowly within a complex 'biofilm'. This is an extracellular matrix produced by the organisms that protects them from host defences, impairs the access of antimicrobials, and greatly increases resistance to them. This may be of importance where, for example, bacteria colonize the lumen of infusion tubing (Figure 12.4). *In vivo*, host proteins are deposited on implants rapidly after their interposition in the tissues and before a bacterial biofilm can develop; this protein deposit masks differences in implant material surface physicochemistry and consequent affinity for microorganisms and also contributes to the difficulties of choice between different implants. The chemical nature of longer-term implants influences the type of surrounding tissue response, but it is not clear whether this influences later infection.

Microorganisms infecting an implant are in a uniquely privileged position. By colonizing a material that lacks a blood supply or any other innate means of attacking them, the microorganisms are immune from the usual means of elimination – a position akin to bacteria in necrotic tissue or in an osteomyelitic sequestrum. Furthermore, there is evidence that implant materials (particularly if metallic) exert a local immunosuppressive effect, and phagocytic cells drawn to the site of an implant show 'exhaustion'. In this privileged position the organisms excite a reaction which fails to destroy them but which involves the usual response with either an acute or a chronic inflammatory reaction. The privileged position is of course completely localized, and organisms outgrowing this limited area of protection are removed by the normal host defence mechanisms. The chronic tissue reaction both to infection and to a long-term

implant further immures the organisms and this both shields them and limits their multiplication and thus their susceptibility to antibiotics. In this situation a chronic low-grade infective process is likely to ensue, with the risk of occasional bacteraemia, and which is terminated only by failure and or removal of the device.

12.5 PREVENTION OF IMPLANT INFECTION

Infection often limits the life of an implant, and various strategies have been investigated to reduce its likelihood; their number reflects the failure of any to achieve outstanding success.

These strategies may be classed under three general headings:

1. The design and manufacture of implants with low likelihood of infection.
2. Reduction of the infection risk at the time of implantation.
3. Avoidance of infection after implantation.

12.5.1 Design of implants with reduced infection risk

Some designs of vascular access catheters have been criticised as potential infection hazards, for example, because of the proximity of connecting ports to the skin, or because manipulation causes excessive movement of the percutaneous portion. However, there is no hard evidence that design of implants *per se* has contributed to excess infection. Some have found poor positioning of a device, for example of vascular catheters in the femoral vein, to predispose to infection, but in other cases, for example chronic ambulatory peritoneal dialysis (CAPD) catheters, this has not been found an important factor.

Although much research has gone into devising implant materials that are unattractive to microorganisms, implant materials are usually chosen for their biocompatibility and mechanical properties. An affinity for microbes is a less obvious property, and the usual approach is to attempt to find methods of reducing the susceptibility to infection of materials already selected on other grounds. Two main strategies have been pursued: (i) modification of the surface of the implant so that microorganisms are less likely to adhere; and (ii) incorporation of antimicrobial compounds into the implant material in order to inhibit microbial multiplication.

Modification of the surface of implants, particularly intravascular cannulae, by **irradiation** or **coating by cationic molecules** (e.g. hydrogel, protamine, silver compounds) has been investigated as a means of reducing the implants' surface attraction for microorganisms and inhibiting the development of bacterial 'biofilm'. This approach has met with some success *in vitro*, in contrast to anionic coatings such as fluoride, which appear to attract rather than to repel bacteria. However, it remains to be shown whether this reduces implant infections, and on first principles one might expect any benefit to be limited to those infections arising at the time of implantation, i.e. before host tissue proteins have had the opportunity to adhere to the surface and alter its surface properties. More recently, pre-implantation 'sealing' of materials (e.g. Dacron) has been undertaken by bonding biological materials such as serum proteins, fibrin 'glue' and collagen; these materials provoke less tissue reaction and may thereby reduce the risk of infection.

A more obvious approach than subtle manipulation of microbe–polymer interaction is the use of implants that are 'self-sterilizing' by virtue of incorporated antimicrobials. Direct incorporation has two major constraints: (i) the incorporated antimicrobial may alter the physical properties of the implant, for example rendering it too brittle to be useful; and (ii) the antimicrobial may itself be inactivated by the manufacturing process, and particularly by the high temperatures reached during moulding. Post-manufacture bonding and impregnation have a wider scope and rely on the interaction between the implant material, the bonding agent and the antimicrobial; experimental success in reducing infection has been claimed for various antimicrobials. The choice of antimicrobials investigated in this context is limited by their physical properties and the need for activity against the most common pathogen, *Staphylococcus epidermidis*. Rifampicin has an attractive antimicrobial spectrum in this respect, and has shown promising results despite concerns about increasing thrombogenicity. However, many bacteria rapidly develop resistance to rifampicin and it may be best combined with a second antimicrobial. Other antimicrobials for which there exist reports of successful use in this way include the quinolone drugs (ciprofloxacin, ofloxacin) and aminoglycosides (e.g. gentamicin, streptomycin). The bonding or incorporation of antiseptics such as chlorhexidine and silver sulphadiazine has also provided promising results.

The incorporation of antimicrobial substances into implanted materials does not produce a permanently self-sterilizing device. Clearly, an antimicrobial molecule is not available to exert microbicidal activity if bound within the matrix of an implant material; moreover, if it is unconstrained and free to inhibit microorganisms then it is also free to diffuse out of the implant. Effective antimicrobial impregnation is therefore always limited by the time it takes for the antimicrobial to elute away. For short-term implants an antimicrobial activity time of 24h is adequate, or may even be advantageous, for example the 'depot' effect of gentamicin beads in orthopaedics. However, there is currently no means of designing an implant with permanent antimicrobial activity. There is also a theoretical drawback to the use of antimicrobials in this way, the possibility being that pro-longed low levels of the active agent may diffuse out, perhaps leading to the development of bacterial resistance.

In practice, gentamicin-impregnated bone cement has been the only antimicrobial implant to find widespread practical application, and this compound has also been incorporated into beads implanted for the local treatment of osteomyelitis. Gentamicin has a mainly Gram-negative spectrum, and is poorly effective against streptococci – which can sometimes be a critical drawback. The popularity of gentamicin as an additive owes more to the physical robustness of the molecule than to its activity against likely pathogens, and there is no reliable clinical trial data to support its use.

12.5.2   Reducing infection risks at the time of implantation

Careful study has revealed that at least a proportion of implant infections occur at the time of insertion. Large-scale clinical studies in the field of orthopaedic implantation have revealed the value of ultraclean theatre air in combination with antibiotic prophylaxis in reducing intraoperative infection of orthopaedic implants. This has been demonstrated epidemiologically where infection rates have been related to antibiotic prophylaxis and bacterial contamination of theatre air, and also by identifying bacteria isolated from infected implants to be the same as those carried either by the patient or by an operator at the time of insertion. However, ultraclean air facilities are not practicable in most hospitals and it is still not uncommon practice to implant major devices, such as orthopaedic and cardiovascular, in a standard undesignated operating theatre environment, and to insert short-term vascular lines as a ward procedure with few precautions.

SURGICALLY IMPLANTED DEVICES

Antibiotic prophylaxis is standard for orthopaedic implant surgery. It has not been found beneficial in the placement of percutaneous vascular lines, and is not generally used for the insertion of prosthetic cardiac valves. As with other branches of surgery, a wide variety of prophylactic antibiotic regimens is used, and although the predominant microorganisms in implant infection are the Gram-positive cocci, prophylactic regimens generally do not target these organisms but make use of standard broad-spectrum cephalosporins, frequently with metronidazole. Some workers favour prophylactic flucloxacillin, even though half of the *Staphylococcus epidermidis* strains are resistant. Only vancomycin and teicoplanin are active against virtually all staphylococci and, since these agents are the only remaining drugs for treating MRSA, there is reluctance to countenance their widespread use in prophylaxis. Drugs with prolonged half-lives, such as ceftriaxone and teicoplanin, could be considered for complex lengthy implant operations when infection risks are higher and their consequences devastating; the latter having the particular virtue of broad antistaphylococcal activity. As with other branches of surgery, prophylaxis is ideally given no earlier than induction, or else the patient may have acquired an antibiotic-resistant flora rendering prophylaxis futile. Implants of course lack host defences and so even the most comprehensive antimicrobial prophylaxis is at best an adjunct to scrupulous aseptic technique.

The ideal duration of antimicrobial prophylaxis for implant surgery has not been established, but there is no evidence that it should differ from that used in other forms of surgery, i.e. it should not continue more than 24 hours postoperatively. Given the potentially lethal consequences of infection of certain implants, for example in vascular surgery, some surgeons prefer to continue antibiotics until all intravascular devices have been removed in case a line-related bacteraemia results in infection of the implant. Whether this reduces the risk of implant infection, or whether it simply leads to infection with organisms resistant to the prophylactic agent, has not been determined.

INTRAVASCULAR LINES

Chlorhexidine (0.5% in 70% isopropyl alcohol) should be used to clean the skin before inserting a peripheral vascular line, the rapid evaporation of the alcohol being an advantage over other antiseptics such as iodine solutions. Disposable gloves protect the operator from blood-borne viruses as well as the patient from local infection, and the temptation to prod the insertion site to establish the position of the vein after applying the antiseptic should be resisted unless sterile gloves are used.

12.5.3 Preventing infection following device implantation

Like heart valves damaged by rheumatic fever, permanently implanted devices (e.g. cardiac valves, joint prostheses) are at continuing risk of infection from bacteraemia, and implant infections have been reported to follow procedures such as endoscopy and systemic infections such as pneumonia. Therefore, there should be a low threshold for the antibiotic treatment of any infection in patients with implants, and antibiotic prophylaxis must be considered before any invasive procedure. In the case of prosthetic cardiac valves, the British Society of Antimicrobial Chemotherapy has published guidelines for prophylaxis that take account of the type of procedure and patient history. Although prophylaxis is often not given for minor procedures to patients with other types of implant, it is prudent for those with other forms of vascular prosthesis (e.g. aortic replacement) and for more major interventions, for example when the bowel is to be transected.

Whilst a permanently enclosed implant risks infection from later bacteraemia, devices for vascular access are continually subject to the further risk of infection at the entry site from the skin flora and environmental contamination. Intravascular lines left *in situ* for prolonged periods are at increased risk of infection. The steady ingress of skin microorganisms and the slow development of infection seeded at the time of insertion is compounded by the need for the device to receive attention and by the break in the closed system each time a change of connection is made. To reduce infection, indwelling cannulae should be treated aseptically and replaced at intervals. **Short-term peripheral cannulae should remain *in situ* not more than 72 hours**, and specific measures to prevent infection have not been found generally useful. For other vascular access devices optimal practice has yet to be defined; however, it has been recommended that arterial and central venous catheters should be put in with meticulous aseptic technique and replaced every 4–6 days. In practice, the complexities of individual patients often result in much less frequent replacement, and record-keeping is often so poor that it is only the patient who can remember the date of insertion of a vascular access line. Furthermore, staff are often reluctant to replace a functioning line that appears uninfected, and consequently studies of compliance with replacement policies have given disappointing results. It is important that each unit has a system for enforcing these policies.

Numerous types of dressing have been investigated in order to minimize infection of vascular access lines. Some literature suggest that gauze dressings are associated with a lower infection rate than those of the occlusive transparent variety. However, the advantages of the latter are that: (i) continuous inspection of the insertion site is possible; (ii) the line is better anchored to the skin; and (iii) there is no need to manipulate the device for examination. The use of topical antiseptics (alcohol, chlorhexidine and iodine have been those most commonly investigated) has been reported to be of quite different value by different authors. When gauze dressings are used, the application of local antiseptics is of benefit and 5% aqueous chlorhexidine solution has been found more effective than 10% iodine in delaying line infection. Dressings should be changed at intervals of, at most, a few days. If a line has had to be inserted in an emergency without due care to hygiene then it should be replaced as soon as possible. Line insertion should not be delegated to an inexperienced operator.

The application of topical antimicrobials has been studied as a means of reducing infection rates. Antibiotic ointments have been applied, and use has been made at the skin entry site of cuffs of Dacron and other materials impregnated with antiseptics. Some success in reducing infection in CAPD catheters has been claimed, but elsewhere these methods have given marginal benefit and are not generally recommended. A few centres claim success for flushing vascular lines with heparin (sometimes adding vancomycin) after each use; however, this requires care to avoid in-use contamination of the flushing solutions and is not generally recommended. **Topical antiseptics** should always be used in preference to topical antibiotics. Antibiotic agents no longer used systemically (i.e. topically) may induce bacterial resistance to related antibiotics that are used systemically, and there is a risk of cross-sensitizing the patient to these drugs.

Often, the care of intravascular devices is not accorded the importance it deserves and much infection risk and expense could be saved by treating these implants more seriously. This has been demonstrated in some centres that have used 'IV care teams', a small group of staff whose sole remit is the insertion and care of intravascular lines. Unfortunately, the obvious expense of funding such a team, as well as the problem of finding dedicated staff, means that few institutions maintain them.

12.6   TREATMENT OF IMPLANT INFECTION

The ideal treatment of an infected implant is removal followed by replacement with a new device if required. This is necessary because, even though the sepsis is commonly due to a normally non-pathogenic organism from the patient's own skin flora, persistent infection not only undermines the patient's general health but also may lead to eventual failure of the device as well as result in serious metastatic infection, e.g. a deep-seated abscess or endocarditis.

A peripheral vascular line should always be removed if found to be infected. However, there may be well-founded reluctance to remove other devices for a whole variety of reasons, and antibiotic treatment will then have to be considered. With Gram-positive infections (staphylococci, streptococci, diphtheroids), which are the most common, these have often been controlled and even eliminated by antibiotics such as vancomycin; one study found urokinase a useful adjunct, presumably by removing (and possibly preventing) the thrombus containing the bacteria. Treatment may be need to be prolonged, often for the life of the implant. Gram-negative infections have generally proven more difficult to eradicate, although some success has been claimed using antibiotics chosen according to laboratory sensitivity tests. In an elderly or debilitated patient with, for example, an infected orthopaedic implant, long-term (months or even years) oral antimicrobials may be required. Various combinations of ciprofloxacin, co-trimoxazole and rifampicin have been used in this way, but the infecting organism has sometimes developed resistance to such therapy. If parenteral therapy is feasible, long half-life antimicrobials such as ceftriaxone and teicoplanin have clear advantages in these situations.

For hospitalized patients, antibiotic or antiseptic irrigation of an infected implant is sometimes attempted, for example of orthopaedic or vascular implants. The advantage of this type of approach is that much higher concentrations of the antimicrobial can be achieved locally and that agents, for example chlorhexidine and iodine compounds, can be used which cannot be administered systemically. The disadvantages are that antimicrobials do not penetrate as uniformly to all infected sites as would occur with systemic administration and there are risks of acute toxicity and hypersensitivity. Whilst there are case reports of patients treated successfully in this manner, irrigation as an attempt to salvage an implant should be considered only when more effective approaches have been ruled out or have failed.

Other experimental methods of treating infected implants are still under evaluation. **Micelles** ('microspheres') of lipid or other biodegradable substances can be synthesized containing various antibiotics and used to deliver high concentrations directly to an infected implant. Semi-implantable pumps have also been employed to ensure that sustained high levels of antimicrobials reach the infected device.

12.7   TYPES OF IMPLANT AND INFECTION

The anatomical position of an implant and its function have a bearing on the type of infection that can occur, and its importance. Some devices, for example urinary catheters and those involving the gut, are placed in non-sterile sites and inevitably become colonized with microorganisms but usually without serious sequelae. Strangely however, some implants that might be expected to act as a conduit for serious infections, for example orthopaedic traction pins, fortunately rarely seem to become infected. For others (e.g. vascular access lines) which serve short-term purposes and in which infection can reduce the working life of the device, their replacement is relatively straightforward. Implants in the latter group intended to serve permanent roles totally enclosed within the tissues (e.g. cardiovascular and orthopaedic prostheses) which develop an infection usually require surgical remedy (usually removal) and may have a fatal outcome.

The diagnosis of infection of an *in-situ* implant by conventional methods is often problematic; their presentation tends to be indolent with a low-grade pyrexia or loss of function, rather than as dramatic sepsis. There are often no localizing signs and imaging techniques may be unhelpful. Such non-specific manifestations are perhaps predictable, since in most cases the origin of the infecting organisms means that the patient is responding to an excessive dose of normal flora rather than infection with a virulent pathogen. **Blood cultures** should be taken and are likely to be positive for infections of vascular implants and intravascular lines. However, a high index of suspicion needs to be maintained when interpreting blood culture results, as the causative organisms are also those most frequently dismissed as 'contaminants'. The finding of an identical, normally commensal, organism in multiple or repeated sets of blood cultures is highly suggestive of implant infection. Such organisms rarely enter the bloodstream by other means, and even the worst phlebotomist is unlikely to contaminate all samples with the same organism. Interpretation may become quite complicated since it is a matter of experience that a proportion of the cultures with low-grade organisms even in cases of genuine infection can be expected to become contaminated. Moreover, depending on when collected, some blood cultures may of course be negative. Optimally, blood cultures should be taken when the patient is pyrexial. The important feature then becomes the finding of a consistent organism in a series of cultures, and this may require detailed examination of isolates. For the ubiquitous coagulase-negative staphylococci (CNS), antibiogram-typing is often the best and most reliable method in such circumstances.

Pseudobacteraemia also should be remembered, as it has led to the misdiagnosis of implant infection. This condition results from a combination of badly stored blood specimen bottles and poor blood sampling practice. Typically, the citrate in ESR bottles has become contaminated with coliforms or pseudomonads. When the same syringe is used firstly to inoculate the contaminated bottle and then secondly a blood culture, the contamination is passed on. As a consequence, the finding of unusual bacteria in the blood of a patient with minimal signs of infection raises suspicion of infection of an intravascular device. The subsequent discovery that several patients appear to have bacteraemias with an identical organism often leads to the correct diagnosis, but this may only be after inappropriate action has been undertaken.

In the case of infection of 'enclosed' implants not directly involving the main bloodstream (e.g. orthopaedic devices), blood cultures may often show nothing. In such cases radiolabelling the patient's leucocytes (indium, gallium and technetium isotopes are often used) and then reinjecting them may enable an infected implant to be demonstrated as a radiological 'hot-spot' to which the leucocytes have migrated; radiolabelled human IgG has also been used in this way.

12.7.1 Infection of intravascular lines

The peripheral intravenous access line is one of the most commonly used medical devices, and hence 'line' infections are relatively common. Peripheral lines are intended for short-term use, and it is expected that they will be replaced before infection becomes established. If left *in situ* too long, or rarely if infected with a virulent organism such as *Streptococcus pyogenes*, local infection will manifest as local erythema with pain, cellulitis and possibly thrombophlebitis. Systemic manifestations are unusual. Central access and other long-term lines may show the same local signs of infection, but since the uninfected tip is some distance from the skin entry site, infection may present without obvious local signs.

Coagulase-negative staphylococci are the commonest bacteria to infect vascular access lines and account for 30–40% of cases in most series. Enterococci, yeasts and *Staph. aureus* are also frequently encountered, whilst Gram-negative organisms (apart from *Pseudomonas* in some studies) are comparatively rare. However, bacteraemias due to line infection do not directly reflect the bacteriological findings in removed catheters; a catheter infected with a 'virulent' organism such as *Staph. aureus* is far more likely to result in bacteraemia than is one infected with coagulase-negative staphylococci. Vascular lines can be infected by various routes (see Figure 12.2). Peripheral vascular devices risk infection from adjacent skin flora and air-borne contaminants, and about one-third result from a bacteraemia caused by a distant focus. The strongest single correlation with infection of the catheter tip has been found with that of the hub (connector), which suggests that organisms migrate from the surface down the lumen.

DIAGNOSIS AND TREATMENT

There are difficulties in determining whether an *in-situ* vascular access line is infected, and one is sometimes reduced to the therapeutic test of removing it to see whether this eliminates the patient's bacteraemia or other signs of sepsis. Other methods have their advocates; for example, comparing quantitative blood cultures through the line with those from a distant vein, microscopy of material adhering to a tiny brush passed down the lumen, and quantifying colony-forming units (CFUs) of bacteria on the catheter hub and skin around the entry site. During removal, a line is inevitably exposed to contamination by any bacteria colonizing the skin entry site, and various methods have been devised to validate the diagnosis of infection after line removal. These are usually applied to the tip of the line. Among these are microscopy of impression smears stained with acridine orange to highlight bacteria, and numerous semiquantitative methods for examining the inner and outer surfaces of the line, sometimes after ultrasonic treatment to loosen adherent bacteria. The simplest laboratory method is that described by Maki, in which the catheter is rolled onto an agar surface, after which the number of CFUs developing is counted (Figure 12.5); more than 15 colonies is said to suggest infection, although some workers take a count of above 1000 CFUs in fluid flushed through the catheter lumen as significant.

In practice, the examination of removed lines often serves little purpose since the line is no longer *in situ* to

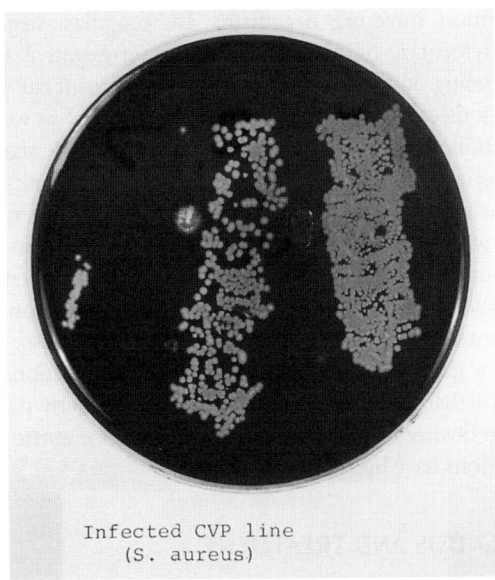

Infected CVP line
(S. aureus)

Figure 12.5 *Roll-plate technique for estimating colonization of a peripheral implanted intravascular line. An infected intravenous catheter was withdrawn from a peripheral vein, cut into sections, and three representative sections were rolled on to a blood agar plate. The increasing gradient of bacteria from the intravascular lumen to the skin entry site is clearly demonstrated. Left: intraluminal catheter tip; middle: intracutaneous portion of catheter; right: skin entry site of catheter.*

cause a problem, and most laboratories make relatively perfunctory examinations of such specimens. Clinically, a line infection is often diagnosed by the finding of 'skin' organisms such as coagulase-negative staphylococci or yeasts in several blood cultures without other localizing signs of infection, or by a spiking pyrexia (particularly when the line is flushed through) and ultimately by the disappearance of pyrexia when the line is removed (Figure 12.6).

Replacement of the infected line with a new one is the usual treatment, but it is sometimes possible to suppress an infection with antibiotics. This latter approach has been described in the salvage infected parenteral nutrition catheters when their removal might cause a problem with replacement; in this situation, high concentrations of antibiotics have been instilled into the lumen and left for prolonged periods. This should not be considered first-line therapy. Problems sometimes arise also with, for example, intensive care patients who are dependent upon multiple vascular access. Here, it is possible that infection of the tip of one line will have resulted in blood-borne infection of all others. If practicable, such patients should be given stat doses of appropriate antibiotics before removal of the infected line, and then left for as long as possible before replacement lines are inserted to allow circulating microorganisms to be cleared.

12.7.2 Prosthetic heart valve infection

Infection of a prosthetic heart valve is potentially the most lethal of implant infections, and complicates 2–4% of valve replacements with a predominance of mitral valve infection. It is clinically relevant to divide prosthetic valve endocarditis (PVE) into 'early' and 'late' onset depending upon whether it occurs more or less than 2 months postoperatively.

Although the Gram-positive cocci (staphylococci and streptococci) predominate, a wide spectrum of infecting organisms is reported in PVE, including Gram-negative rods and yeasts which are most unusual in non-implant-related ('native') valve endocarditis. *Staphylococcus epidermidis* figures prominently – unlike native valve endocarditis where it is seldom reported – and *Staph. aureus* is also common in some series. Late PVE behaves similarly to native valve endocarditis, and can be managed

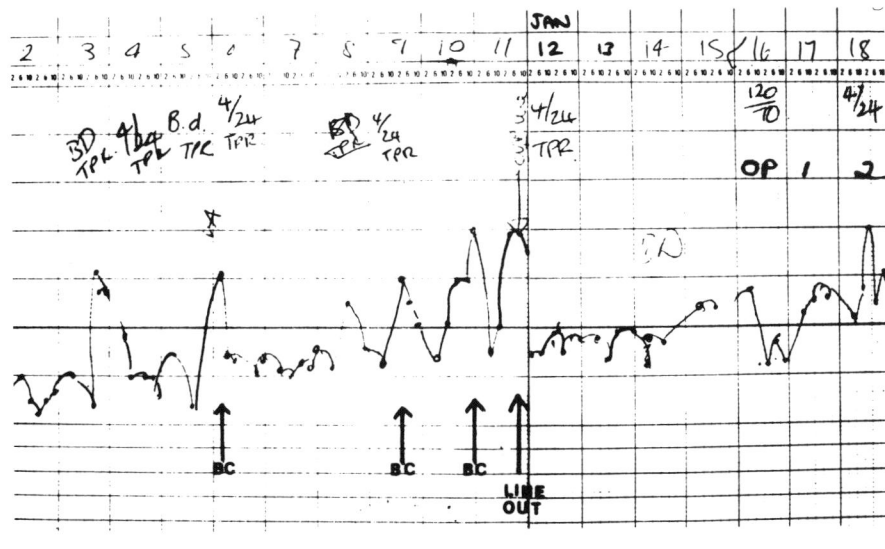

Figure 12.6 *Spiking pyrexia in a patient with a central line colonized with a coagulase-negative staphylococcus. BC = blood cultures revealed the offending staphylococcus; LINE OUT = central line removed with immediate resolution of pyrexia. The later pyrexia was due to an intraperitoneal abscess.*

medically provided that maximal and prolonged antibiotic treatment is used.

Early-onset PVE accounts for about one-third of cases and has the highest mortality; urgent replacement of the infected valve under antibiotic cover is likely to be necessary. Reflecting the situation in all recently implanted materials, *Staph. epidermidis* is the single most commonly reported organism; in some studies where early *Staph. aureus* PVE has been encountered, this has been attributed to postoperative wound infections. Late-onset PVE has an incidence of around 1% per annum and whilst lethal if untreated, more closely resembles native valve endocarditis and is more likely to be cured without surgical intervention. However, once replacement of the infected valve is deemed necessary, any delay increases the risk of mortality.

DIAGNOSIS AND TREATMENT

Examination of a **blood culture** is the mainstay of microbiological investigation and, as with native valve bacterial endocarditis, three sets collected over several hours are advisable. Interpretation of the results may be difficult because the infecting organism, often *Staph. epidermidis* or some other member of the normal flora, may at first be thought a contaminant from the skin. The finding of identical isolates of *Staph. epidermidis*, or diphtheroid bacteria, or any other component of normal skin flora in all bottles makes a strong case for PVE.

As with native valve endocarditis, combination antibiotic treatment is usually given. The multiple antibiotic resistance of the infecting bacteria and the need to maintain prolonged high levels of circulating antibiotics usually necessitate long-term intravenous therapy, and make the treatment of PVE difficult. Close liaison with the microbiology laboratory is needed to establish the best combination of antibiotics for the individual patient.

Like patients with damaged heart valves, those with a cardiac prosthesis are at risk of endocarditis if subjected to certain invasive procedures. The guidelines of the British Society for Antimicrobial Chemotherapy should be consulted for recommendations on antibiotic prophylaxis before undertaking such procedures.

12.7.3 Infection of vascular grafts

Infection of a vascular graft can be as life-threatening as infection of a prosthetic cardiac valve. Antibiotic prophylaxis is considered mandatory and cephalosporins (e.g. cefuroxime) are frequently used despite theoretical limitations of activity against coagulase-negative staphylococci. Despite this, infection still complicates up to 5% of grafts in some series. As with other implants, infection may arise around the time of surgery or later; incisions in the bacteriologically dirty groin area predispose to graft infection, as do distant infections such as those of the urinary tract.

Common infecting organisms are coagulase-negative staphylococci, *Staph. aureus* or Gram-negative rods, depending on the study. As with PVE, early and late presentations can occur. The former may manifest as wound infection, thrombosis, septic emboli and systemic signs of sepsis; later infections can present less obviously and need intensive investigation. Infection beginning around, rather than within, the graft (peri-graft infection) may begin with a wound infection or the general systemic manifestations of enclosed sepsis. In the case of aortic grafts, infection may present dramatically as massive haemorrhage associated with a graft-enteric fistula. Vascular graft infections are often lethal, perhaps in part reflecting the elderly patient group involved, and mortality rates of 70% for aortic graft infections have been reported.

DIAGNOSIS AND TREATMENT

As with prosthetic valve endocarditis, **blood cultures** are often positive. In the case of perigraph infection, aspiration around the graft under ultrasound guidance may provide fluid in which causative organisms can be identified. More complex imaging techniques such as computed tomography and radiolabelled leucocyte scans may also be needed to establish the diagnosis. Antibiotics should be given to the patient (frequently including flucloxacillin or vancomycin as a Staphylococcus will often be involved) and this may reduce the likelihood of metastatic infection. However, replacement of the graft through a non-infected field has to be undertaken as a matter of urgency. Antibiotic cover should be given before, during and after surgery, and the case for long-term antibiotic therapy is strong.

12.7.4 Infection of orthopaedic implants

Although infection of an orthopaedic implant does not generally present in the acutely life-threatening fashion of infection of cardiovascular prostheses, the eventual outcome in a patient who may be elderly and debilitated can be equally lethal.

Because load-bearing strength is of particular importance for orthopaedic implants they are made from different materials to other implanted devices, generally various alloys based on steel, nickel, aluminium, cobalt, chromium, titanium and vanadium, although synthetic polymers such as ultrahigh molecular weight polyethylene, as well as ceramic material, have also found application in this field. The metallic nature of these devices, as well as the fact that they do not encroach into major blood vessels, may explain certain differences in infection. For example in many series *Staph. aureus* has accounted for around one-third of reported infections and coagulase-negative staphylococci for only about 15% – an approximate reversal of the situation with intravenous line infections. Gram-negative rods are also more common, accounting for one-quarter of infections in some series.

The most common orthopaedic implant is the **replacement hip**, and here infection rates below 1% are expected. Analysis of large series suggests that a minority of infections occur at the time of surgery and most follow a later bacteraemia or else occur in replacements of already-infected prosthetic joints. Cephalosporin antibiotics are usually given as prophylaxis and are effective despite being weak against coagulase-negative staphylococci; 'local' prophylaxis in the form of gentamicin-impregnated bone cement is favoured by some operators. Extreme measures such as ultraclean air theatre suites, the use of exhausted (this term is used to express the use of pumped air through the sealed operation suit, and does not imply tiredness) low-porosity clothing for operators and UV light (with appropriate protection) all further reduce infection rates, but such facilities are not widely available.

DIAGNOSIS AND TREATMENT

Orthopaedic implant infections do not normally result in bacteraemia, and so blood cultures are rarely positive. Radiological investigation of loss of function may show changes that do not distinguish infection from mechanical loosening. A raised erythrocyte sedimentation rate and pyrexia provide circumstantial evidence, but direct methods such as fine-needle aspiration or a radio-labelled leucocyte scan may be needed to confirm the diagnosis. Reports of orthopaedic implant infections cured by antibiotics are rare, and replacement of the device under appropriate antibiotic cover is the usual outcome. However, since many implants are in elderly patients who may be too frail for more surgery, life-long (which may be short) suppressive antibiotic therapy is sometimes the preferred option.

12.7.5   Infection of peritoneal dialysis catheters

Peritoneal dialysis catheters are intended for long-term use and, like long-term vascular access devices, are difficult to replace if infected. Infection presents less dramatically than in cardiovascular implants and does not necessitate life-threatening surgery. However, patients with infected dialysis catheters run the risk of peritonitis which, even if successfully treated, may lead to obliteration of the peritoneal space and so compromise further peritoneal dialysis. Various factors render dialysis catheters particularly liable to infection. Because dialysis patients try to lead otherwise normal lives with their catheters sited in positions that carry a normal skin flora, they are always at risk of contamination; furthermore, the catheters must be regularly manipulated when used as the conduit for several litres of dialysis fluid. Dialysis patients may be receiving immunosuppressive drugs such as corticosteroids, and there is also the rare complication of erosion of the catheter into the bowel resulting in faecal peritonitis. Peritoneal dialysis catheters are exceptional amongst implants in being routinely managed by the patients themselves outside the hospital setting; thus, there exist the unquantifiable infection hazards of a non-standardized environment.

As with other implants, infections with coagulase-negative staphylococci predominate, although the most serious infections, entailing the greatest risk of catheter loss, are those caused by *Staph. aureus* or Gram-negative bacilli. Catheter infection with *Staph. aureus* often follows an infection at the site where the catheter penetrates the skin ('exit site infection'), and this may progress to infection along the track of the catheter ('tunnel site infection'). In some studies, nasal carriage of *Staph. aureus* has been associated with a much increased risk of catheter infection, and some authorities attempt to eliminate this before catheter implantation. Peritoneal dialysis catheters may become infected with a wider spectrum of microorganisms than other implants, including mycobacteria and even algae (*Prototheca* spp.).

Attempts to reduce infection include attention to catheter design, for example the Tenckhoff with a Dacron cuff that promotes surrounding fibrosis to prevent microorganisms migrating along the catheter's outer wall. Of particular importance is the maintenance of sterility at home, and all patients receive careful training in the aseptic care of their catheters, including instruction in the need to avoid wetting their dressings and the use of sterile water and antiseptic skin preparations.

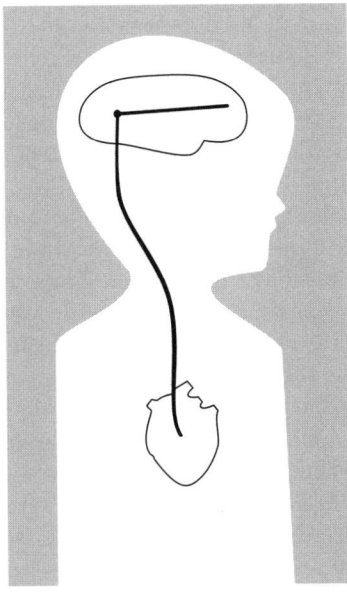

Figure 12.7 *A CSF drainage system for the relief of hydrocephalus.*

DIAGNOSIS AND TREATMENT

Local erythema and tenderness at the exit site may indicate infection, as with other implants that penetrate the skin. However, unless there is a frank discharge at the exit site, a skin swab from the site may only provide evidence of the local skin flora. The onset of peritonitis may manifest as systemic sepsis, but both immunosuppression and the indolent nature of coagulase-negative staphylococci infection may serve to mask this. If infection is suspected, dialysis fluid should be examined microscopically, when the finding of polymorphs and/or bacteria obviously points to infection. The fluid should also be cultured; some nephrologists inoculate dialysate directly into blood culture bottles for this purpose. On suspicion of infection, vancomycin may be both added to the dialysate and also given systemically on the presumption that the infecting organism is likely to be a staphylococcus; this can be modified in the light of subsequent culture results.

12.7.6 Cerebrospinal fluid drainage devices

Systems such as the 'Spitz-Holter' shunt are used to drain off excess cerebrospinal fluid (CSF) in hydrocephalus (Figure 12.7). Commonly, a cannula is inserted through a burr-hole into the cerebral ventricles and is connected to a valve implanted under the scalp with a distal drainage catheter emptying into a great vein or the peritoneal cavity. In these devices, coagulase-negative staphylococci are once again the predominant infecting organism and hence clinical manifestations are usually non-specific. Fortunately, the presence of valves in the system and the considerable length of catheter along which an ascending infection needs to migrate, usually result in therapeutic intervention occurring before the obvious complication of meningitis supervenes. Because the insertion or replacement of such devices requires general anaesthesia and neurosurgery, much of the detailed study of the mechanisms of implant infection has been made in the context of these devices. As elsewhere, it has been found that infection may be initiated either at implantation, or following a later bacteraemia. The usual attempts at bonding and encorporating antimicrobials have been tried as preventive measures, but none has found widespread application.

DIAGNOSIS AND TREATMENT

Clinicians managing patients with CSF drainage devices are usually alert to the low-grade pyrexia and malaise that may indicate infection. Occasionally, and to some extent depending on the precise positioning of the system, neglected cases have presented with pulmonary hypertension or immune-complex nephritis. Ulceration

of the subcutaneous valve through the scalp has also been reported. As with other implants, there are case reports of infections apparently cured by long-term treatment with carefully chosen antibiotics, particularly when caused by Gram-positive cocci. However, most infections necessitate eventual replacement of the drainage system.

12.7.7 Other implanted devices

A whole range of implants is used on a smaller scale in a wide range of surgical disciplines, for example grommets for chronic suppurative otitis media, artificial ocular lenses and prostheses that are often individually designed for cosmetic surgery. Infective complications of these lesser-used devices is rarely reported, although a certain amount of publicity has focused on infections of breast implants which can eventually lead to scarring and contracture. In most cases, when infections occur, removal of the implants is required, and is the mainstay of treatment. Eye infections are serious and require antibiotic treatment in addition to lens removal; enucleation is sometimes necessary. Because the eye is a microbiologically protected environment, most implant infections are iatrogenic at the time of operation.

12.8 PARENTERAL AND ENTERAL NUTRITION

Lines used for parenteral nutrition are subject to the same infectious complications as those used for other purposes; however, line infection with the yeast *Malassezia furfur* (*Pityrosporum orbiculare*) is a relatively specific complication of intravenous infusion of lipid emulsions. Most cases have been reported in neonates, and the organism is commonly found in neonatal intensive care units. Replacement of the line and amphotericin treatment may be necessary as the condition can be lethal. Rarely, *M. furfur* infection has complicated lipid administration to immunosuppressed adults.

The infections associated with enteral nutrition via a nasogastric tube are quite different. Minor contamination of an enteral feed is unlikely to be significant as the stomach commonly accepts non-sterile food. However, enteral feeds provide a ready growth medium for bacteria, and the patients receiving them often have some form of underlying immunocompromise. Common-sense steps should therefore be taken to avoid contamination that will deliver a large number of microbes, even of a commensal or generally 'harmless' variety, into the patient's gut. Although direct correlates with systemic infection are vague, an association between the degree of feed contamination and diarrhoea has been found. A further complication of the long-term presence of a nasogastric tube is an excess of lower respiratory tract infections resulting from aspirations and colonization of the upper respiratory tract with a Gram-negative flora.

12.9 FURTHER READING

Barrett, S.P. (1988) Bacterial adhesion to intravenous cannulae: influence of implantation in the rabbit and of enzyme treatments. *Epidemiol. Infect.*, **100**, 91–100.

Jansen, B. and Peters, G. (1991) Modern strategies in the prevention of polymer-associated infection. *J. Hosp. Infect.*, **19**, 83–88.

Maki, D.G., Weise, C.E. and Sarafin, H.W. (1977) A semi-quantitative culture method for identifying intravenous-catheter-related infection. *N. Engl. J. Med.*, **296**, 1305–1309.

Meers, P.D. (1983) Ventilation in operating rooms. *Br. Med. J.*, **286**, 244–245, 1215.

Pai, M.P., Pendland, S.L. and Danziger, L.H. (2001) Antimicrobial-coated/bonded and impregnated intra-vascular catheter. *Ann Pharmacother* **35**, 1255–1263.

Pratt,R.J., *et al.* (2001) The Epic project: developing national evidence-based guidelines for preventing healthcare associated infections. *J. Hosp. Infect.* Supplement 47.

Saravolatz, L.D. (1993) Infection in implantable prosthetic devices. In *Prevention and Control of Nosocomial Infections*, ed. R.P. Wenzel, Williams and Wilkins, Baltimore, 683–707.

Simmons, N.A. *et al.* (1992) Antibiotic prophylaxis and infective endocarditis. *Lancet*, **339**, 1292–1293.

Widmer, A.F. (1993) IV-related infections. In *Prevention and Control of Nosocomial Infections*, ed. R.P. Wenzel, Williams and Wilkins, Baltimore, 556–579.

Infections of skin, soft tissues and burns

R.J. SAGE

SECTION I: SKIN AND SOFT TISSUES

13.1 INTRODUCTION

The skin is the largest organ in the body, and provides one of the most significant physical barriers to infection. The normal skin is colonized by bacteria, usually considered to be of low pathogenicity. Physical damage, disease and antimicrobial chemotherapy significantly alter skin flora, often leading to colonization and/or infection with organisms of greater pathogenic potential.

As with all infectious disease, there is a delicate balance between the host immune system and potential pathogens. The range of disease is nowhere more apparent than with infection related to the skin. Minor breaches of the skin can lead to life-threatening sepsis with virulent organisms, and patients with severe immunosuppression may develop significant disease with normally benign skin flora. Substantial destruction of the skin leads to colonization and infection with a wide variety of organisms, including environmental bacteria. The seriously burned patient is a paradigm which is given separate consideration in this chapter (see Section II).

13.2 MICROBIOLOGY OF SKIN

13.2.1 Normal skin flora

The average human has approximately 1.8 m^2 of skin, colonized by vast numbers of bacteria, the quantity and type of these varying by site and by individual. In general, bacterial numbers tend to be lowest in cool, dry peripheral sites (hands and face), and highest in moist central sites (groin and axillae). Gram-positive organisms predominate, including micrococcaceae (staphylococci, micrococci) and coryneforms (diphtheroids). Gram-negative organisms, such as the enterobacteriaceae, are generally confined to skin sites adjacent to major reservoirs such as the gastro-intestinal tract; *Acinetobacter* spp. are an exception, being found on up to one-quarter of individuals, most frequently isolated from the groin, axilla and toe webs.

Most skin commensals, including acinetobacters, are organisms of low pathogenicity, causing disease only in immunocompromised patients or when inoculated into sterile sites. All, however, share a propensity to develop multiple antibiotic resistance.

On occasions, the skin and mucous membranes of normal individuals become colonized with well-recognized pathogens, thus:

- Some 10–20% of the population are colonized with *Staphylococcus aureus*. Overt infection, such as recurrent boils and carbuncles, may follow.
- Young children have a high carriage rate of traditionally recognized pathogens, often in the upper respiratory tract. The most notable example is *Streptococcus pyogenes* or β-haemolytic streptococci of Lancefield group A (βHSA), with significant implications for plastic surgery and burned patients (see page 121).
- Patients with chronic skin disease such as eczema or psoriasis are universally colonized with *Staph. aureus*, and are significant disseminators of such organisms.

13.2.2 Hospital skin flora

Hospitalization of patients leads to changes in type and antibiotic sensitivity of colonizing flora. Air-borne and environmental bacteria have an undoubted special significance for burned patients, but may be underestimated in other cases. Multiple pressures are exerted on hospital patients' microflora; some are obvious with relevance to all patients, thus:

- On average, 25% of acute ward patients receive antibiotics, although this may rise to almost 100% in certain critical care environments, significantly altering colonizing flora.
- The basic unit in which patients are cared for involves them being in close proximity; many patients are 'reservoirs' of large numbers of hospital bacteria, and are often potent disseminators of bacteria.
- Healthcare workers are frequently transiently colonized with pathogens, and often act as vectors.

As discussed later (see page 124), the physical environment and air quality are also relevant to the seriously burned patient, and may be germane to other circumstances where there is a significant skin defect. In most hospital-acquired infections (HAIs), attention has focused on either endogenous infection or transient colonization of healthcare workers. Little attention has been paid to the environment, despite increasing sophistication and complexity of equipment for investigation, monitoring and treatment. **Many cleaning policies are inadequate for complex or delicate equipment**. In the case of burned patients or those with pressure damage to the skin, highly complex low air-loss beds are frequently employed. The adequate decontamination of these beds is impossible in the normal ward setting.

Common sense suggests that other factors affect colonization and infection, but many are poorly documented or defined. Throughput, case mix and antibiotic prescribing patterns, for example, are likely to have a profound influence.

The combined effects of the multiple 'pressures' of hospitalization have a significant impact on colonizing flora of skin and mucous membranes, with subsequent implications for clinical infection:

- There is a shift from Gram-positive to Gram-negative colonizing flora. This is particularly evident in areas of damaged skin or mucous membrane colonization. Enterobacteriaceae and pseudomonads become the dominant flora.
- Highly antibiotic-resistant skin flora (primarily Gram-positive) develop. Glycopeptides (vancomycin/teicoplanin) are increasingly the only antibiotics active against many hospital strains of staphylococci and coryneforms.
- Vancomycin-resistant enterococci (VRE) are reported in the USA and recently in the UK. There is the apocalyptic prospect of vancomycin-resistant *Staphylococcus aureus* (VRSA).
- Highly resistant acinetobacters are increasingly seen in the critical care environment. In seriously burned patients subjected to prolonged critical care, totally resistant acinetobacters are now encountered.
- Replacement of bacterial flora with yeasts is well recognized in US burns units. Although rarely seen in the UK, it may be an ominous sign.

Unlike many other organs, the skin is accessible to easy visual examination. Signs and symptoms of infection are usually obvious, with pain and a classical inflammatory reaction with calor and rubor, and often also discharge. Historically, surgery has been one of the mainstays of treatment of bacterial infection of the skin. Despite many advances, surgery continues to be critical in treatment and is also increasingly important in the diagnosis of skin disease, especially infective.

13.3 MINOR SKIN INFECTIONS: SURGICAL RELEVANCE

13.3.1 Boils and carbuncles

Almost everybody has experienced a simple staphylococcal boil (Fig.13.1). These are distressing and sometimes excruciatingly painful, but are usually self-limiting and discharge spontaneously; occasionally some help may be needed from the surgeon. On occasion there is a failure to localize lesions, and regional lymph nodes become involved (lymphangitis; lymphadenitis); rarely there is evidence of systemic infection, with fever, rigor and even septic shock. In any of these circumstances, antibiotics and supportive therapy are undoubtedly indicated. Despite the emergence in many hospitals of methicillin-resistant *Staphylococcus aureus* (MRSA), flucloxacillin must still be considered the first-choice agent, as most infections are community-acquired. To increase anti-

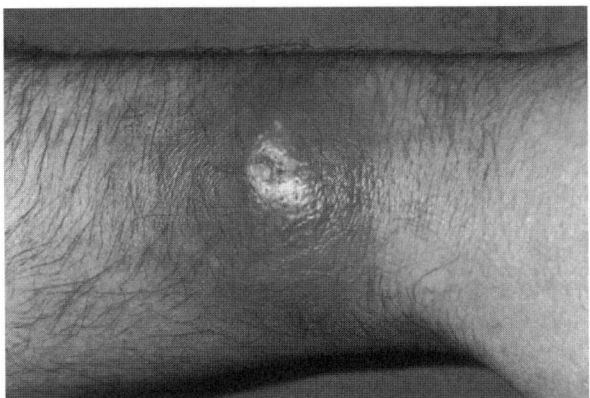

Figure 13.1 *Simple* Staphylococcus aureus *boil.*

staphylococcal activity in cases of progressive disease, sodium fusidate can reasonably be added. If the infection is not checked in the regional lymph nodes and progresses to septicaemia, then intravenous therapy is indicated. Gentamicin (2 mg kg^{-1} twice daily) and flucloxacillin is the traditional antibiotic regimen that is employed initially. If serious septic complications occur, then substantial supportive therapy will be required. Erythromycin, cephalosporins and vancomycin are alternatives, but expert advice should be sought if they are needed, as when traditional antibiotic therapy either fails or is not appropriate.

13.3.2   Scalded Skin Syndrome (Figure 13.2)

Thermal injury is not always the reason for major skin loss. Occasionally it may follow chemical burns or contact with other noxious agents. Rarely, skin loss may be a manifestation of bacterial infection, as in the case of toxic epidermal necrolysis (scalded skin syndrome). The disease is caused by toxin-producing strains of *Staphylococcus aureus* and almost invariably occurs in children. Within days of initial infection (often minor) with *Staphylococcus aureus,* large bullae appear, containing sterile clear fluid. These generally exfoliate within a few days. Within 10 days, new epidermis replaces the exuded area and recovery without scarring is usually complete.

13.3.3   Recurrent infections

Whilst conservative treatment or simple surgical drainage of abscesses is usually adequate, some patients develop multiple recurrent staphylococcal lesions. Chronic colonization with *Staph. aureus* is the predisposing cause. Carriage is eliminated in the majority of circumstances. Neither antibiotics nor surgery provide a cure, and the

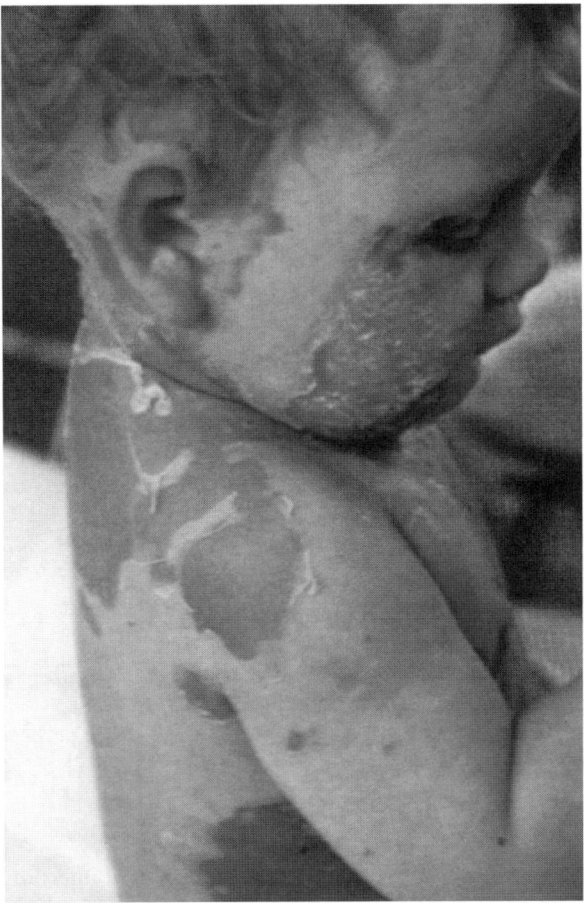

Figure 13.2 *Scalded Skin Syndrome.*

possibility of an immunodeficiency predisposing cause should be considered. A decontamination regimen is required: one programme is to use povidone-iodine surgical scrub painted all over the body prior to bathing (or preferably showering), together with mupirocin applied to the nose and other colonized sites. Triclosan or hexachlorophane are alternatives. It should be noted that concentrated disinfectants added to the bath are ineffective.

13.3.4   Folliculitis

Folliculitis is an acute infection of the hair-bearing areas of skin, leading to multiple small abscesses. It is often seen in areas subjected to shaving ('barber's rash'). Skin flora, particularly *Staph. aureus,* are the infecting agents. It is recognized that wound infections are much more common in patients shaved immediately before surgery; hence, shaving should be replaced by clipping or depilatory creams.

Whilst folliculitis is most frequently caused by *Staph. aureus,* on occasions other organisms may be involved. Recreational use of whirlpools or jacuzzis has on occasions led to an unusual form of folliculitis, with a generalized rash. *Pseudomonas aeruginosa* is the most common pathogen (Fig.13.3).

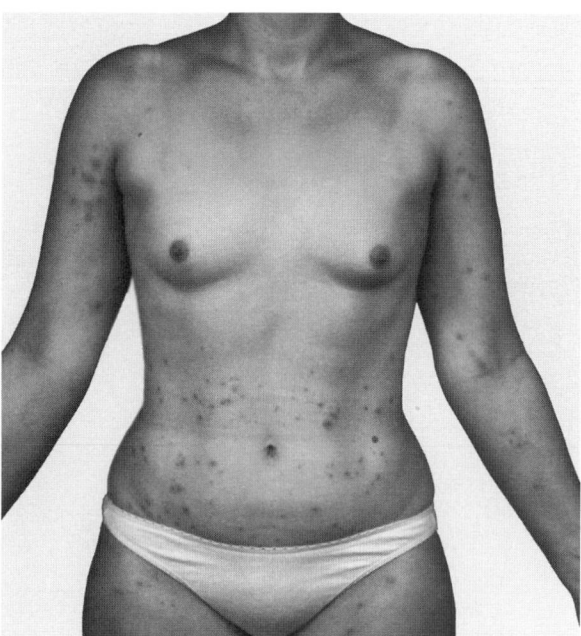

Figure 13.3 Pesudomonas aeruginosa *folliculitis. The patient had been using a Jacuzzi, note 'water line'.*

13.3.5 Hidradenitis suppurativa

Hidradenitis suppurativa is a chronic recurrent infection of the axillary or perineal sweat glands (Fig.13.4). Recurrent abscesses form in the sweat glands, initially caused by *Staph. aureus*, but *Proteus* spp. and other Gram-negative rods are frequently involved in chronic disease. Antibiotic therapy should largely be guided by culture and sensitivity testing. Courses will need to be protracted.

Initially antibiotics may help, but recurrent infections lead to sinuses, scarring and fibrosis, and excision of the apocrine areas may be required.

13.3.6 Ulceration and pressure sores

Arterial or venous generated ulceration (e.g. 'varicose ulcer') and pressure damage to the skin (e.g. 'bed sores') are common in domiciliary and hospital practice (Fig.13.5). Irrespective of aetiology, such lesions invariably become colonized with *P. aeruginosa* and faecal flora. Often, the superficial bacteriology isolates are irrelevant to the disease process. Treatment requires correction of physiological and mechanical defects, rather than antibiotic therapy. It is only when there is clinical evidence of spreading infection that antibiotics are indicated. Despite the wide range of Gram-negative isolates, anti-staphylococcal and streptococcal therapy is usually effective. Rarely, Gram-negative organisms play a role; invariably such patients have significant underlying pathology, the diabetic patient being the most obvious example.

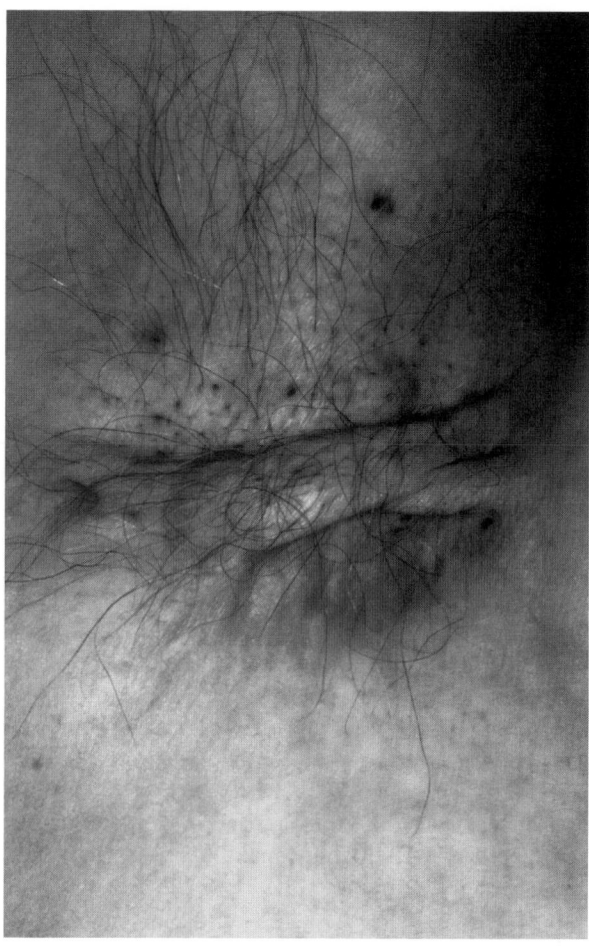

Figure 13.4 *Hydradenitis suppurativa. Surgery is considered the last resort in treatment.*

13.3.7 Mycobacterial infections

Increasingly, mycobacteria are being recognized as the cause of chronic infections of the skin and soft tissue. Often described as the 'swimming pool granuloma', *Mycobacterium marinum* has been isolated in water

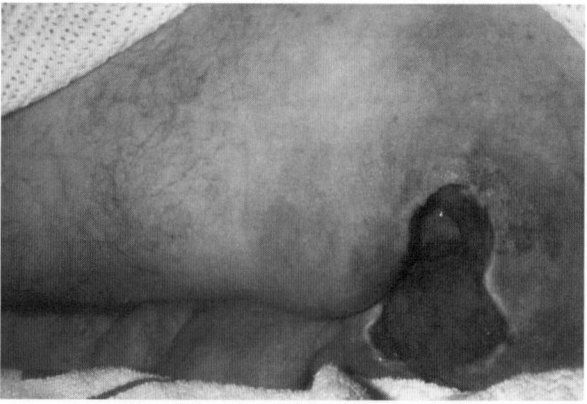

Figure 13.5 *Typical pressure sore. Antiseptics and wound care are more important than antibiotics. May require surgical debridement and possibly skin grafting.*

sports enthusiasts, but is also frequently associated with tropical fish enthusiasts. Characteristically, chronic lesions of the hands appear that fail to respond to conventional antibiotic therapy. Diagnosis often requires a skin biopsy and culture. Other superficial acid-fast bacillus (AFB) infections are increasingly recognized, such as inoculation injuries in gardeners.

Any chronic skin infection, whatever the site, should be examined for AFB infection. Short (by AFB standards) courses of rifampicin are usually effective. Normally, 6 weeks of therapy suffices.

13.3.8 Viral infections

Many viral infections have obvious cutaneous manifestations, though few have surgical relevance. Two, however, may be of note: **Herpes Simplex Virus** (HSV) and, more rarely, **Orf**.

HSV whitlows present as an acutely painful nail bed infection which may be difficult to distinguish from bacterial or fungal infection, but do not require any surgical intervention as they do not suppurate. They often occur in healthcare workers following treatment of children with HSV stomatogingivitis. If started early enough, aciclovir can limit, and sometimes abort, the infection (Fig.13.6).

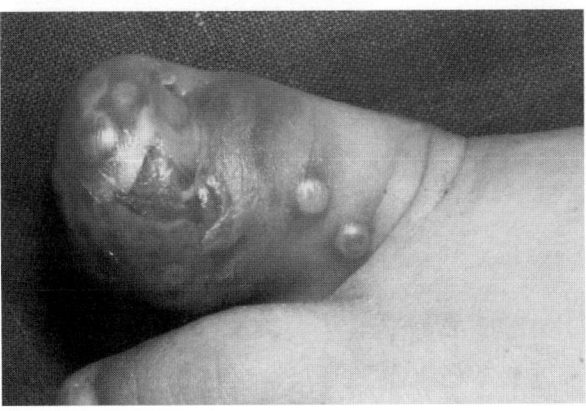

Figure 13.6 *Herpes Simplex Virus in a child. A 1-year-old boy presented to the A&E Department with an infected toe. The child was irritable and systematically unwell with a temperature of 39 °C. There was an obvious eruption with vesicles on the toe. Ulcerating lesions were also found in the mouth and satellite lesions on the upper chest. The diagnosis was primary HSV stomato-gingivitis with secondary toe lesions due to toe sucking.*

Orf is also a disease resulting from direct inoculation. Associated with farm workers, usually in the lambing season, Orf is a pox virus acquired from suckling orphan sheep. Prominent lesions develop, usually on the fingers, 1–2 cm across, these being fluid-filled and deep-seated with minor erythema (Fig.13.7). Electron microscopy reveals large viral particles that resemble smallpox virus.

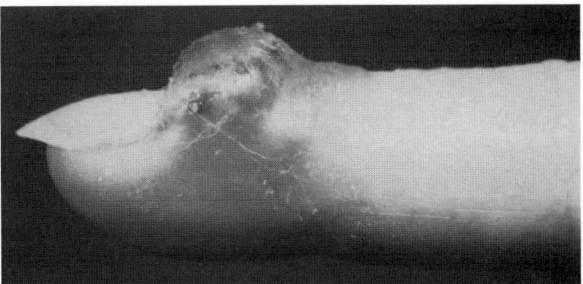

Figure 13.7 *Orf. A pox virus infection found in a farmer's wife at lambing time.*

13.4 MAJOR SKIN INFECTIONS

13.4.1 Cellulitis

Cellulitis is a serious disease, as it has the propensity to spread, initially to regional lymph nodes and subsequently the bloodstream. The most frequent and virulent organisms involved are β-haemolytic streptococci of Lancefield group A (*Streptococcus pyogenes* or βHSA); occasionally infection with Lancefield groups C and G occurs. It is frequently suggested (and believed) that *Staph. aureus* is a major cause of cellulitis, but in most cases it is a coincidental isolate from colonized skin.

In the past, Group A streptococcal disease was a frequent cause of admission to 'fever hospitals', with a diagnosis of scarlet fever, rheumatic fever or nephritis. Although such disease has been in decline for several decades, recent evidence has indicated that there has been a re-emergence of virulent strains, leading to serious skin and soft tissue disease, and longer term sequelae such as rheumatic fever.

The portal of entry of β-haemolytic streptococci is often thought to be occult, but minor cuts or abrasions, tinea pedis and minor diabetic foot lesions are frequently found if care is taken in examination. Group A streptococci rarely infect wounds in modern surgical practice, but if it occurs the sequelae are grave. It is worth noting that Group A streptococcal disease may be occupationally related (e.g. in abattoir, mortuary and farm workers). Young children also have a high carriage rate of *Streptococcus pyogenes* in their upper respiratory tract.

Initially there is rapid development of local cellulitis; within 24–48 hours lymphangitis may develop, with a characteristic red line and local lymphadenopathy. In progressive disease there is rapid generalized erythema, increasing oedema and bullous formation (Fig.13.8). Systemic symptoms become increasingly prominent with fever, rigors and confusion. Septicaemia may lead to cardiovascular collapse ('septic shock'), disseminated intravascular coagulation (DIC) and multiple organ failure; superficial skin and peripheral limb gangrene may develop.

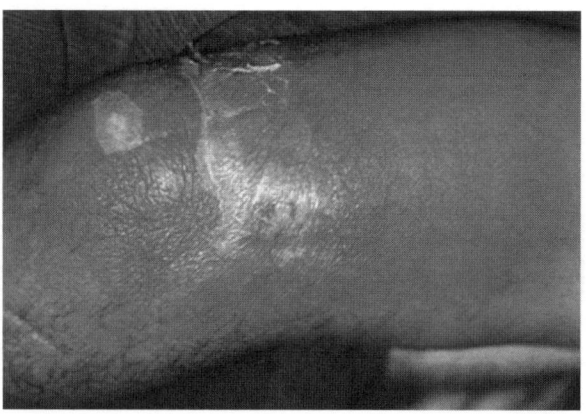

Figure 13.8 *Streptococcal cellulitis of arm. Shows remnants of bullous formation (Bouncer case history). Caused by β-haemolytic streptococci of Lancefield group A often found colonizing the oropharynx of young children.*

Early recognition is the most important element of management, and prompt early treatment with benzyl-penicillin aborts many complications. In cases of severe cellulitis with associated swelling and oedema, fasciotomy may be required to alleviate nerve entrapment syndromes. In the most extreme circumstances, critical care support is necessary, including ventilation and inotropic support.

Rarely, organisms other than haemolytic streptococci cause severe cellulitis: *Staph. aureus*, enterobacteriaceae and *Pseudomonas* spp. have been implicated. The more unusual the organism, the more likely is the patient to have significant underlying pathology.

Almost unique to children is cellulitis due to infection with *Haemophilus influenzae*. Most frequently associated with meningitis, this organism also causes cellulitis, epiglottitis and osteomyelitis. Cellulitis is usually facial and in particular peri-orbital. Initial treatment should be with a third generation cephalosporin (cefuroxime, ceftri-axone). In the UK, the use of *H. influenzae* type b vaccine (HIB) has led to haemophilus cellulitis becoming a rarity.

13.4.2 Bacterial gangrene

The majority of cases of gangrene involve anaerobic bacteria (*Clostridia* and *Bacteroides* spp.), or mixtures of anaerobes and other organisms in a 'synergistic relationship'. β-Haemolytic streptococci of Lancefield group A (βHSA) are an exception, where a single aerobic organism may lead to devastating disease, including gangrene. It is important to distinguish streptococcal gangrene from other causes as the focus of treatment differs. In most cases of infectious gangrene, surgical treatment is pre-eminent, whereas in those caused by βHSA, medicine and intensive support are required, surgical support being secondary.

STREPTOCOCCAL GANGRENE

βHSA have long been the cause of serious disease in surgical practice. In the pre-antibiotic era, βHSA were one of the most common causes of sepsis following surgical intervention, often with gangrene a major feature. In the early 1920s Meleney described cases of gangrene of the limbs caused by haemolytic streptococci, using the term 'necrotising fasciitis' (Fig.13.9). Unfortunately, he sub-sequently described other forms of bacterial gangrene referring to 'synergistic necrotising fasciitis', an entirely different disease unrelated to streptococcal gangrene.

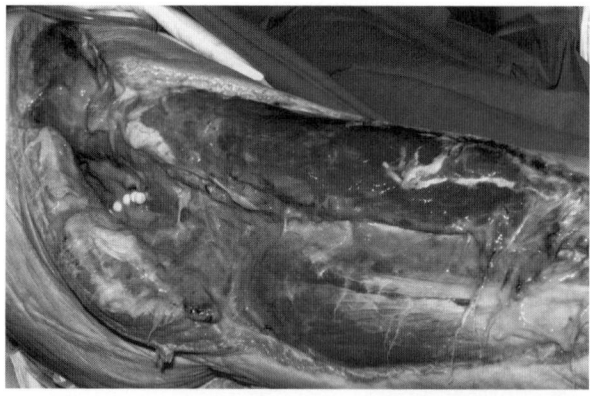

Figure 13.9 *Necrotising fasciitis. Nomenclature and microbiology confusing and academic. A mixed infection often following previous surgery, rapidly progressive painful and with a very high mortality. Gas formation found clinically (crepitus) or radiologically in the soft tissues. Requires extensive surgery, intensive support and the co-operation of surgeon, intensivist and microbiologist.*

CASE HISTORY

A 28-year-old man was admitted with massive cellulitis of his right arm with a temperature of 39°C, rigors and local lymphadenopathy (Fig.13.10). He had grazed his knuckles 48 hours previously in his job as a bouncer for a local disco, and his 3-year-old son had 'kissed Daddy better'. Group A β-haemolytic strepto-cocci were isolated from the patient's blood and from his son's throat. High-dose benzylpenicillin led to a full recovery.

CASE HISTORY

A 50-year-old acute leukaemic with neutropenia (WBC count <0.1 mm^{-3}), who was undergoing intensive chemotherapy developed fever and cellulitis of both legs. No obvious precipitating lesion was seen, despite scrupulous examination of the patient's feet. Treatment initially with an aminoglycoside and ureidopenicillin combination failed to produce any improvement. Within 24 hours, large Gram-positive rods were isolated from blood cultures. Vancomycin and metronidazole (MTE) were added to the patient's regimen, but the cellulitis progressed to involve both legs, to the groin. Death occurred 48 hours after the patient first became febrile. The Gram-positive rod was identified as *Bacillus cereus*, and was subsequently isolated in post-mortem specimens from the pericardium, pleura and blood.

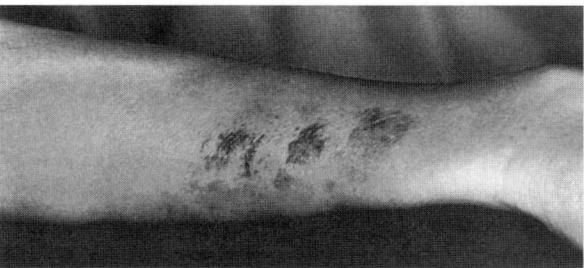

Figure 13.10 *Streptococcal cellulitis with necrosis. Necrosis is an ominous sign in steptococcal disease. Patient may require intensive support and wide debridement.*

Streptococcal gangrene is normally an extension of severe unchecked cellulitis. The diagnosis is usually obvious from the clinical presentation but is more difficult when deeper tissues are involved. βHSA may be inoculated into deeper tissues at the time of surgery or trauma. The origin of the organisms may be endogenous, from upper respiratory tract colonization of the patient, or rarely exogenous from staff carriage. Fortunately both are uncommon. Illness usually presents within a short period of inoculation (24–48 hours). Initially fever is a prominent feature, with little evidence of wound infection or cellulitis. Systemic symptoms, including rigors and mental confusion, become prominent. Haemodynamic instability ultimately occurs. Symptoms and systemic signs of deep-seated βHSA disease are generally out of proportion to those seen in the wound, especially in a previously fit patient. Discharge from the wound is likely to be thin and serosanguinous. Wound breakdown with frank infection tends to be a late feature.

Investigations should include blood and wound cultures, clotting screen and blood gases. Occasionally, a Gram stain of wound discharge reveals chains of Gram-positive cocci with relatively scanty pus cells. Early diagnosis is critical to successful treatment, and is largely dependent upon suspicion.

Antibiotic therapy should be started empirically, rather than waiting for definitive microbiology. High-dose benzylpenicillin is an essential element of any regimen. As the differential diagnosis is likely to include anaerobic forms of gangrene, metronidazole also is mandatory. Some form of anti-Gram-negative and anti-staphylococcal therapy is usually prudent, e.g. an aminoglycoside or quinolone, but expert advice from a microbiologist should be sought when initiating such complex multiple combination antibiotic therapy.

Correction of metabolic and fluid balance is often required. Inotropic and respiratory support may both be necessary, requiring the critical care team. Once stabilized, exploration of the surgical wound can be undertaken. Extensive necrosis of deeper tissues may be found, including fat, fascia and muscle, for which débridement will be essential. In advanced disease, gangrene of the peripheral limbs may occur, though this is usually caused by hypotension and vascular insufficiency rather than directly by βHSA.

GANGRENE INVOLVING ANAEROBES

Bacterial gangrene of the skin and associated soft tissues underlies a group of diseases that is not only difficult to define but also to categorize in terms of diagnosis and treatment. A confusing array of terms are used to describe process, anatomy, histology and microbiology. This is complicated by the use of eponyms, e.g. Meleney and Fournier.

The majority of cases of infectious gangrene involve anaerobic bacteria or mixtures of anaerobes and other organisms, often in a synergistic relationship. *Clostridia*, *Bacteroides* and peptostreptococci are true anaerobes and require the exclusion of oxygen to multiply. Both *in vivo* and *in vitro* they produce a variety of tissue-damaging enzymes which facilitate their invasion of skin, fat, fascia and muscle. The end product of their metabolism produces volatile fatty acids which give the characteristic foul smells associated with anaerobic infection.

Other organisms less fastidious in their atmospheric requirements survive with or without oxygen and may be involved in gangrene. The so-called 'facultative organisms' include the enterobacteriaceae (*E. coli*, *Klebsiella*, *Enterobacter* spp.) and many streptococci, and are frequently of gut origin. There is an apparently synergistic relationship between true anaerobes and facultative organisms in many infections.

Confusion is often caused by faulty description of the anatomic depth of infection. Cellulitis is the most superficial disease encountered, involving skin and subcutaneous fat. Fasciitis implies a deeper disease, involving the fascial planes and adjacent tissues. It is often a feature of gangrenous disease that there is extensive spread via fascial planes to distant sites. Myonecrosis may occur in muscle adjacent to fascial disease or, as in the case of clostridial myonecrosis ('gas gangrene'), may be a primary process.

The speed of progress of disease is also very variable, from the indolent, relentlessly progressive diseases such as Fournier's gangrene to the rapid course of clostridial cellulitis. Signs and symptoms vary enormously; with low-grade disease the patient may be afebrile with apparently minor cutaneous disease, progressing over days or even weeks; this contrasts with the acutely ill toxic patient progressing over a matter of hours. Variation in disease is in part a reflection of the virulence of the organism, but the patient's immune status is also critical. Many cases of gangrene, in modern medical practice are seen in patients with significant underlying disease.

The enormous variability of infective gangrene suggests that a spectrum of disease exists, rather than specific disease entities. Despite the enormous variability in terminology, a number of generalizations can be made:

- The first axiom of bacterial gangrene must be 'recognize the problem'. Much of the morbidity associated with gangrene results from late diagnosis. Individually, each form of gangrene is rare, but all require urgent treatment.
- Primary management is surgical, but optimal care must involve physician, intensivist and microbiologist. Surgery needs to be radical to remove all dead and infected tissue; repeated operations are often necessary, both for assessment and further débridement (Fig.13.11).

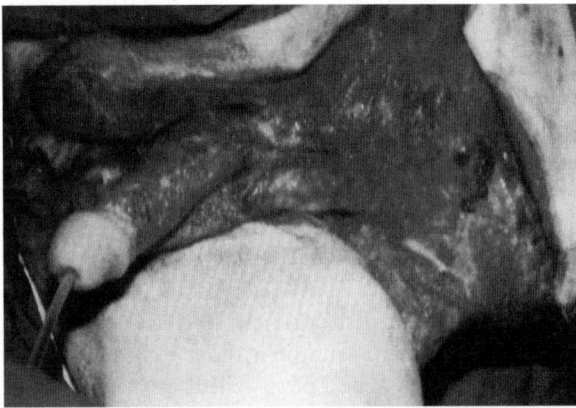

Figure 13.11 *Fournier's gangrene. Found in the perineal area of elderly debilitated patients, usually slowly progressive. Requires extensive debridement, multiple 'relook' surgery and skin grafting to cure.*

- The extent of the disease is frequently underestimated in terms of local wound disease and systemic manifestations. The more aggressive disease tends to have profound systemic effects, often resulting in DIC and multiple organ failure.
- In many circumstances, patients have significant underlying pathology. Perineal gangrene occurs in immobile oedematous patients ('Fournier's gangrene'). Synergistic necrotizing fasciitis of the abdominal wall is seen after large bowel surgery, especially in the obese.
- Although physical signs vary widely, some should alert the attendant to serious anaerobic infection. Anaerobic organisms produce gas which is clinically apparent by its foul odour and by either crepitus in tissue, or evidence of gas in the tissues on X-radiography.

It is often pointlessly academic to differentiate many of the forms of bacterial gangrene involving anaerobes; the final list is often an unsatisfactory amalgam of terminologies. A reasonable degree of differentiation into four types (Table 13.1) can be made by using pain, toxicity, appearance and speed of infection as parameters, providing it is accepted that any individual manifestation can have a spectrum of disease.

SECTION II: BURNS AND OTHER SKIN LOSSES

Substantial skin loss is a challenge to surgeon, intensivist and microbiologist. Thermal damage is by far the commonest cause, but it may also occur as a result of **electrical or chemical injury**. Infection is second only to the initial injury as the cause of mortality. Most serious septic complications follow large, full-thickness burns. A major burn is usually defined as greater than 25% full-thickness loss in adults, and 10% in children.

In the acute full-thickness burn, one of the most significant barriers to infection is removed in a matter of minutes, exposing large areas of dead tissue, with copious exudate at temperatures of 37°C or more. It is doubtful that microbiology laboratories can provide an environment more conducive to bacterial growth. The severely burned patient must also be considered acutely and seriously immunocompromised.

Most major burns are now managed in specialized centres with dedicated plastic surgeons and intensivists. Advances have led to the survival of patients with burns of ≥50%, considered almost universally fatal two decades ago. The high technology environment and specialist treatment, together with the extensive use of potent broad-spectrum antibiotics all contribute to survival, but have also created major microbiological problems. The principal adverse features of organism, patient and environment interaction are:

Table 13.1 *Differential diagnosis of gangrenous infections of subcutaneous tissues and skin*

	Bacterial synergistic gangrene	Necrotizing fasciitis	Streptococcal gangrene	Gas gangrene
Predisposing conditions	Usually follows wound infection; draining sinus	Wound infection; perineal infections	Occasionally diabetes or myxoedema, but often none; after abdominal surgery	Local trauma to deep soft tissues
Pain	Variable	Variable	Severe	Severe
Toxicity	Minimal	Marked	Marked	Very marked
Fever	Minimal or absent	Moderate	High	Moderate or high
Crepitus	Absent	Frequent	Absent	Frequent
Aetiology	Microaerophilic streptococcus plus *S. aureus* (or enterobacteria)	Usually a mixture of aerobic and anaerobic organisms	Primarily Group A streptococci	*C. perfringens* (occasionally other clostridia)
Progress	Slow	Rapid	Rapid	Rapid

- Gram-negative rods, both endogenous and exogenous, are a major cause of burn infection. *Pseudomonas aeruginosa* is pre-eminent, although other inherently antibiotic-resistant environmental bacteria (e.g. Acinetobacter) are increasingly common.
- The use of a wide variety of medical devices – endotracheal tubes, intravenous catheters, urinary catheters and others – all allow bacterial invasion of normally sterile sites.
- Usually benign skin flora become highly antibiotic-resistant and an increasing cause of bacteraemia.
- Extensive use of broad-spectrum antibiotics not only compounds bacterial resistance problems, but leads to colonization (if not infection) with *Candida* spp.
- Cross-infection commonly occurs in the unit. Despite strict infection control policies, it is difficult to control environmental factors. Colossal numbers of bacteria are found in the air at dressing times. There is also considerable difficulty in decontaminating the increasingly complex equipment.

13.5 DIAGNOSIS OF INFECTION IN BURNED PATIENTS

The clinical diagnosis of infection in the acutely burned patient is almost impossible. Every patient with a significant burn will exhibit signs and symptoms compatible with infection, i.e. be febrile, hypotensive, mentally confused and generally 'toxic'. Most initial laboratory investigations are abnormal, with neutrophilia, disturbed electrolytes, LFTs and blood gases reflecting multi-organ effects. C-reactive protein (CRP) and other acute phase proteins are massively elevated. Clinical diagnosis is difficult and microbiological diagnosis is equally problematical. Blood cultures – the normal 'gold standard' of serious infection – are prone to frequent contamination,

being often taken through burn sites, and consequently interpretation is difficult. Burn wound culture does not distinguish between colonization and invasive disease. Wound biopsy and bacterial counts is advocated in some circles, but is often academic rather than practical.

It is therefore impossible to provide a didactic approach to the diagnosis and treatment of infection in the burned patient. The suspicion of sepsis is largely dependent on the observation of trends and particularly the rates of changes in commonly monitored parameters. Examples of serious clinical import regarding presence of sepsis include:

- Increasing haemodynamic instability in a patient with apparently appropriate fluid replacement for the size of burn.
- Persistent or increasing fever above 39.5°C, especially after adequate débridement of necrotic tissue.
- Deteriorating haematological or biochemical parameters, including clotting factors, blood gases and renal function.
- A mental state at variance with sedation or analgesia.
- Clinical appearance and smell of burn wound (albeit these are highly dependent upon experience).
- Microbiological isolation of certain 'alert' organisms, βHSA providing the most obvious example.
- Any other patient or laboratory parameter that is deteriorating in the face of appropriate corrective therapy when no other cause is apparent.

It is therefore by necessity that initial antibiotic therapy in burned patients is entirely empirical, though in many cases its efficacy is impossible to assess. Nevertheless, treatment needs to have some focus. The management must, to some extent, be governed by local practice, including débridement and antibiotic cover practice. Broadly, the microbiology can be divided into early, intermediate and late septic complications. **Early infection** is likely to occur within the first few days and not later than one week; **intermediate infection** occurs in weeks 2–3; and **late infection** is seen in major burns at 3 weeks to 3 months.

13.6 EARLY COLONIZATION INFECTIONS

13.6.1 Detailed initial history

The circumstances of the burn are important. It is wrongly assumed that all burns are initially sterile. The immediate post-burn management may significantly affect the microbiology of the burn wound – well-intentioned but misguided interventions may contaminate the burn wound. Rolling patients in carpets or diving into stagnant water may lead to early contamination of the burn wound with large numbers of ubiquitous bacteria or fungi. It is therefore important to ascertain in detail the exact circumstances of the burn, and the immediate pre-hospital management.

13.6.2 Initial colonization

Initial colonization is dependent upon the site of the burn. Broadly, upper-limb and torso burns are likely to become initially colonized with Gram-positive skin organisms or upper respiratory tract flora, whereas lower-limb and perineal lesions acquire Gram-negative organisms of gut origin. Anaerobic organisms play little part in early colonization, presumably largely due to the superficial site of injury. Thus, *Staph. aureus*, enterobacteriaceae and haemolytic streptococci are the principal organisms involved early in burn infection.

The diagnosis of infection in the early management of burned patients is particularly difficult, as it is likely that all signs, symptoms and investigations will be grossly abnormal. It is difficult to ignore that much treatment in the early stages is intuitive, however unsatisfactory scientifically.

A number of initial regimens are appropriate. A quinolone plus benzylpenicillin is likely to cover most eventualities in adults, but aminoglycoside plus penicillin is perhaps more acceptable in children. Considerable care, however, needs to be taken in monitoring aminoglycosides, as much to ensure efficacy as to avoid toxicity. Aminoglycoside levels and other antibiotic levels will often be lower than expected in some individuals, as there is often massive flux of fluids in the acute phase.

13.6.3 Young children

It is a feature of young children that they carry a variety of potential pathogens in their upper respiratory tracts. *Streptococcus pneumonia*, *H. influenzae* and β-haemolytic streptococci are common examples, and may lead to rapid early colonization of burn wounds with these organisms. Group A streptococci present a particular problem, causing severe acute disease, including a toxic shock syndrome. Group A streptococci also have a marked deleterious effect on skin grafts, causing early failure.

13.6.4 Toxic shock syndrome

Toxic shock syndrome was originally associated with tampon usage, but is also well described in burned patients. Toxic shock syndrome toxin-producing strains of *Staph. aureus* have been isolated in children with the classical signs and symptoms of toxic shock. Clinically, it is impossible to differentiate staphylococcal disease from other causes of toxic shock syndrome. It should, however, be suspected in a gravely ill child with a relatively small burn wound.

13.7 MID-TERM INFECTIONS

After the first 5–7 days, the bacterial colonization of burn wounds becomes much more variable (Fig.13.12). There are multiple pressures from bacteria, both endogenous and exogenous, caused by the high technology environment in which the patient is managed. Many, however, will be influenced by the ability to remove dead tissue and achieve skin coverage of the burn wound. The faster this can be achieved, the fewer septic complications will occur.

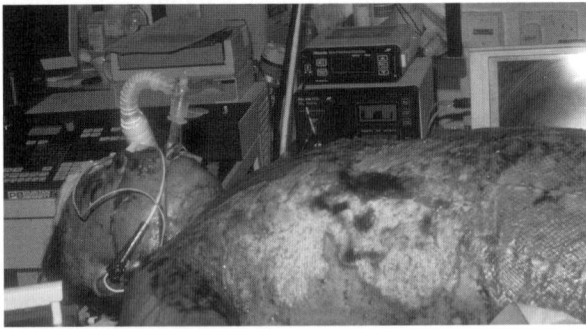

Figure 13.12 *80% burns. Second week, evidence of extensive colonization with* Pseudomonas aeruginosa. *The patient is also at risk of respiratory tract and line sepsis in the intensive care environment.*

Regular wound surveillance cultures are helpful in determining antibiotic therapy. Twice-weekly wound swabs not only identify the predominant flora of the patient and/or unit, but also the degree of antimicrobial sensitivity. Organisms are often highly resistant, partly reflecting the extensive use of early empiric therapy.

Infection does not only come from the burn wound. Endogenous and exogenous device-associated infection is thought to be common, but often difficult to prove. Extensive use of multiple venous access catheters is necessary in the management of fluid balance, endotracheal intubation is often required (especially in associated inhalation injury), and major vascular access catheters are required in patients developing renal failure.

In general, the microbiology of the second period of burns concerns Gram-negative, inherently antibiotic-resistant organisms. *Pseudomonas aeruginosa* is probably the single most significant pathogen, although others, such as *Acinetobacter* spp., may cause problems. Local unit resident problem organisms are frequently encountered.

Highly resistant Gram-positive organisms also proliferate. Methicillin-resistant *Staph. aureus* is a frequent finding, as are resistant Gram-positive skin organisms, such as *Staph. epidermidis* and coryneforms.

Anti-Gram-negative therapy needs to be tailored to local circumstances. Many of the modern, ultra broad-spectrum antibiotics will have to be deployed. Third- and fourth-generation cephalosporins, monobactams, etc., are all contenders. Local microbiology and opinions will largely dictate choice, but financial constraints may apply. Empiric therapy for suspected Gram-positive infection is much more limited; vancomycin and teicoplanin are the only practical agents. Repeated surveillance cultures should be used to guide future therapy, as a major burn will require repeated courses of antibiotics.

Provided that good wound débridement and coverage have been achieved, sepsis is increasingly likely to originate from areas other than the burn wound, particularly those related to the intensive management necessary for such patients.

13.8 LATE INFECTIONS

Surgically unresolved burns, for whatever reason, are the most likely to suffer from late infections. Disease is due to microorganisms generated by the continued effects of anti-bacterial agents and to long-term exposure to the critical care environment. Progressively resistant bacteria are encountered in the burn wound. Sites other than the burn wound become subject to infection as a consequence of the necessary invasive interventions, particularly the respiratory tract. Following the use of broad-spectrum antibiotics, **yeast** colonization invariably increases. In the USA, infection with *Candida* spp. is a well-recognized problem. In the UK, so far this is a rare problem, but is likely to increase. Surveillance cultures should monitor the

levels of bacterial and yeast colonization and help in the prediction of infection. In addition to this, regular monitoring of the burn wound, urine, stool and upper-respiratory tract cultures should be undertaken in the long term (>3–4 weeks). Anti-fungal therapy should be considered in patients isolating yeasts in three or more sites when there is clinical evidence of continuing sepsis. It should be recognized that *Candida* infection is not only a late complication, but is also seen as a slowly progressive disease in the chronically debilitated patient, rather than as a rapid acute phenomenon. Fluconazole is probably the agent of choice initially, and there may be arguments for its prophylactic use in the high-risk patient.

Some Candida spp. are inherently resistant to the imidazoles, and require amphotericin; drug interaction and toxicity are commonly encountered.

Rarely reported in the UK but frequently seen in the USA are infections of burn wounds with hyphate fungi (Aspergillus, Rhizopus, Mucor). Diagnosis is only reliably made by autopsy. Mortality is very high, as treatment involves extensive excision of infected tissue, antifungal therapy having little impact.

With all fungal disease in burned patients, there must be consultation and co-operation between surgeon, intensivist and microbiologist.

The skin is a large, uniquely observable organ. Considering the number of pathogens that may be encountered, it provides a remarkable barrier to infection. Infections present in a wide spectrum from the minor to the life threatening.

A comprehensive history and thorough examination may be a cliché, but is essential to diagnosis. Biopsy is usually relatively easy; the greatest benefit is likely to be seen if samples are sent to microbiology as well as histopathology. Best management of skin infection should involve the synergy of surgeons and microbiologists.

13.9 FURTHER READING

Hoeprich, P.D., Jordan, M.C. and Ronald, A.R. (1994) *Infectious Diseases, 5th edition*. Lippincott, Baltimore.

Kucers, A., Crowe, S., Grayson, M.L. and Hoy, J. (1997) *The use of Antibiotics: A Clinical Review of Antibacterial, Antifungal and Antiviral Drugs, 5th edition*. Butterworth–Heinemann, Oxford.

Mandell, G.L., Bennett, J.E. and Dolin, R. (2000) *Mandell, Douglas and Bennett's Principles and Practice of Infectious Diseases, 5th edition*. Churchill Livingstone, Philadelphia.

Sherris Medical Microbiology: An Introduction to Infectious Diseases, 3rd edition. Appleton and Lange, Connecticut.

Central (cardiovascular) and peripheral vascular infections of surgical importance

R. FREEMAN

SECTION I: CARDIOVASCULAR SURGERY

14.1 INTRODUCTION

With the exception of bacterial endocarditis there are few cardiovascular infections which initially present to the surgeon. Most of the infective aspects of cardiovascular surgery relate to prevention of infection after surgery and dealing with such infections when they occur. Cardiovascular surgery embraces valvular surgery, correction of congenital anomalies and coronary artery bypass grafting (CABG). Where the definition enlarges to include surgery on the thoracic aorta and other intrathoracic vascular structures, the same general principles apply. In all instances it is simplest to define five stages: **preoperative**; **intraoperative**; **immediate postoperative** (intensive care); **early convalescence**; and **long-term follow-up**. Special considerations will apply to transplantation procedures which are detailed elsewhere (see Chapter 11). This chapter centres on the performance of a typical major procedure, that is, for instance, valve replacement or CABG, whilst variations are outlined in later sections. Although some procedures are still performed without cardiopulmonary bypass (CPB), this support is so common in cardiovascular surgery that the main body of this chapter will assume its use.

14.2 PREOPERATIVE STAGE

14.2.1 Before admission

Many major cardiovascular procedures are elective, allowing some preoperative assessment. This is an opportunity in CABG candidates to assess and take action on the frequently associated chronic obstructive airways diseases in this group, the presence of which will influence postoperative chest management. This is also the stage at which many units routinely assess the patient's status in relation to blood-borne viruses, including hepatitis B and HIV. The rare possibility of large-scale spillage of blood (particularly from the heart-lung bypass machine when it may be released under pressure) can lead to uncontrolled exposure to such agents by, for instance, conjunctival contamination. Consequently it has been common practice to screen the patient for evidence of infection or carriage with hepatitis B and HIV. Consent will be needed in both instances and, in addition, counselling may be necessary for HIV screening. Nonetheless, the almost universal experience is that patients are happy to comply, given an adequate explanation for the request. The introduction of hepatitis B vaccination of staff has provided increased reassurance against one of these risks and the extensive experience of accidental exposure to HIV-positive material in recent years suggests that this risk is low and that prophylactic therapy reduces it further. However, there have been significant changes in recent years in the knowledge of blood-borne virus disease which may considerably modify the above practices.

Firstly, whereas it was the settled belief that hepatitis B surface antigen (HbsAg)-positive carriers were divisible into a minority which were of high infectivity, distinguished by the presence of the 'e' antigen, and a majority of very low infectivity, distinguished by the detection of 'e' antibody, it is now known that 'e' antigen-negative carriers can be highly infectious. This new, third group, can be identified by measuring the level of hepatitis B DNA in the blood. Such complex investigation algorithms begin to defeat the original plan to simplify procedures. It may be prudent, for the moment, to adopt 'universal precautions', such as double-gloving, visors, and so on, in all HbsAg-positive patients, whatever their 'e' status.

Secondly, a 'new' blood-borne virus disease in which an infective chronic carrier state exists (hepatitis C) can now be added to the list of agents to which the operators might be exposed but, unfortunately, not to the lists of vaccines or post-exposure prophylactic therapy. No agreed approach to this problem exists and there seems little evidence that any unit has instituted preoperative screening for hepatitis C antibody in cardiovascular surgery.

Lastly, however, it should be remembered that the incidence of abnormal results in all these screening tests is very low and that the purpose of such a screening plan is to allow the vast majority of elective patients to be managed with a minimum of extra and cumbersome precautions, to their overall benefit.

In candidates for CABG it is important carefully to examine the lower limbs when selecting vein donor sites. Indolent ulcers, both venous and arterial, must be cultured since they may be heavily colonized with *Staphylococcus aureus*, even if clinically apparently uninfected. The identification and treatment of tinea pedis is

also important for minimization of chronic erysipelas in the long term.

Although it may be obvious at this stage that some patients are likely to progress more slowly than others, it is also certain that all patients are open to the possibility of a prolonged stay in the intensive care unit (ICU) if unexpected complications develop. CPB is followed by a **variable period of colonic stasis** during which enteric organisms dramatically increase in number. This phenomenon also applies to yeasts, and it has been shown that preoperative administration of oral nystatin minimizes this effect. If the gut is adequately preloaded with nystatin tablets before admission, the incidence of postoperative *Candida* infection is greatly reduced.

14.2.2 At admission

Traditionally, patients are screened for the presence of *Staph. aureus* in the nose and throat, and a mid-stream urine (MSU) sample is taken for microscopy and culture.

The current prevalence of methicillin-resistant *Staph. aureus* (MRSA) makes such screening sensible for units serving a wide catchment area, but it must be understood that the detection of methicillin-sensitive *Staph. aureus* (MSSA) will be a common finding (i.e. the tests for its presence will be 'positive for *Staph. aureus*') and need occasion no additional action in the presence of routine prophylaxis. Detection of MRSA will require special individual precautions for the positive patient (see below).

Preoperative asymptomatic urinary tract infection is occasionally found in female patients, and may require therapy and deferment of operation, although operation may proceed under additional appropriate antibiotic cover if the clinical condition dictates it. A preoperative MSU examination is a poor predictor of postoperative urinary tract infection in both sexes, and especially so in males when estimation of preoperative urine flow rate is a much more illuminating measurement.

Immediately prior to surgery patients undergo skin preparation, topical antiseptic solutions (as discussed in Chapter 2) being applied to the operative sites, which in the case of CABG will include the vein donor sites.

14.3 INTRAOPERATIVE STAGE

Antibiotic prophylaxis has always been used in cardiac surgery, and particularly in open-heart surgery, although there is surprisingly little scientific proof of its value. Valve replacement surgery acquired a sinister association with *Staph. aureus* septicaemia and endocarditis in its early days but this may have been, in retrospect, one facet of the *Staph. aureus* pandemic of the time and not a specific association. Nonetheless, the extremely **serious consequences of infection of the intracardiac operative site**, especially when a prosthesis is involved, have continued to sustain the argument for routine prophylaxis, and the practice is universal. More recently, attention has focused on the prevention of infection after CABG. In the first instance prophylaxis is directed against the organisms causing early prosthetic valve endocarditis (EPVE), and in the second against the organisms causing sternotomy wound infection and mediastinitis. In practice the overwhelming burden of the organisms concerned in each instance are staphylococci (*Staph. aureus* and the coagulase-negative staphylococci), so that a similar regimen suffices for both. Some authorities have advised a narrow-spectrum agent such as an isoaloxozyl penicillin (flucloxacillin, nafcillin), whereas others prefer a cephalosporin (cefuroxime, cefamandole): both are acceptable. Broader- spectrum agents (gentamicin, extended spectrum cephalosporins) have been used or added, but the side effects encountered (toxicity, superinfections) outweigh any (theoretical) advantages. In cases of penicillin allergy the narrow-spectrum approach can be maintained by the substitution of clindamycin. If MRSA is detected it may be necessary to offer prophylaxis with vancomycin or teicoplanin B. Choice between one of several simple regimes is less important than ensuring the correct usage of the drug chosen. The regimen used, which must not commence until immediately prior to surgery, should ensure:

- An immediate high concentration of the agent in the blood when first incision is made. Large doses (where the agent is relatively non-toxic) should be used, for instance, 2 g of flucloxacillin or nafcillin.
- A duration of effect throughout the procedure. Cardiac surgical procedures are often long. In addition, the cessation of CPB (well before the end of the whole operation) can cause a sudden fall in the concentration of the prophylactic drug. For both these reasons, a 'top-up' dose is often given after 2–3 hours or at the end of CPB.
- Adherence to the 'three-dose regimen'. As with other surgical procedures, the formation of the wound coagulum in the hours after surgery dictates that further prophylaxis is unnecessary. The possibility that the operative site remains prey to postoperative bacteraemias (see below) requires action in its own right rather than extension of the perioperative prophylaxis.

One peculiarity of open-heart surgery deserves mention. In most open-heart operations using CPB, cardioplegia is used, whereby the tissues of the operative field are purged of blood and filled with a balanced salt solution which contains antibiotics. Thus, the site of operation may also be purged of antibiotic. This factor requires further study.

Great care and attention to detail is required of those assistants inserting the many intravenous and intraarterial lines used, since they may overlie the intraoperative site and be connected to liquid-bearing transducers. Rarely, **contamination of the CPB machine** can occur and result in bloodstream contamination. Clusters of EPVE with the same organism should raise this suspicion.

14.4 IMMEDIATE POSTOPERATIVE STAGE (INTENSIVE CARE)

Most cardiothoracic surgical patients spend only a short time on the ICU. During this time microbiological concern is directed towards several aspects.

14.4.1 The respiratory tract

With good humidification, physiotherapy and bronchial toilet using sterile suction tubes, chest infection can be minimized. Cultures of sputum/tracheal secretion are often prepared routinely, and nearly 50% will grow *Haemophilus influenzae*. Treatment of this finding in the absence of radiological abnormalities does not have a beneficial effect in most patients and is unnecessary. If broad-spectrum antibiotics have been used for prophylaxis, *Escherichia coli* and similar organisms will be found instead.

The development of **radiological abnormalities** on the chest X-ray is highly correlated with preoperative left ventricular failure and pulmonary oedema. Although tracheal cultures are occasionally positive, the lesions are non-infective in most instances.

14.4.2 Lines

Cardiothoracic patients have several common lines inserted. These are a left atrial (LA) line which measures pressures, a right atrial (RA) line which is preferentially used to administer inotropes, and a venous line (VL) which allows access to the great veins. An arterial line (AL) is also common. All of these invasive lines are potential portals of entry for bacteria, commonly those from the skin (coagulase-negative staphylococci, diphtheroids and, occasionally, streptococci). Coliforms are unusual line-based invaders as are yeasts and both only occur after prolonged antibiotic therapy.

The major preventive measure is the earliest possible removal of the lines, although the addition of sodium metabisulphite to the flush system used on the venous, LA and RA lines is an effective adjunct. Pulmonary artery catheterization (Swan–Ganz) is occasionally necessary, but those catheters must be removed within 24 hours of their introduction since they are extremely likely to cause right-sided endocardial trauma, complicated by right-sided infective endocarditis after this time.

14.4.3 Early fever

The majority (75–80%) of patients undergoing CPB manifest a high fever 2–6 hours after discontinuation of the CPB, marked as the time of aortic cross-clamp removal. This is an endotoxin-mediated event and is almost always self-limited. Although blood cultures may be taken they are usually negative and the patient responds well to antipyretics. CPB leads to temporary underperfusion of the gut, and this is why the endotoxin release occurs, the delay in the fever being due to the subsequent generation of endogenous pyrogens, principally tumour necrosis factor alpha (TNFα). Nonetheless, this insult may occasionally be much more serious leading to a prolonged paralytic ileus, small bowel infarction or acute pancreatic necrosis, all of which should be borne in mind if the early fever does not remit as expected.

14.4.4 Urinary tract infection

Typically, urinary tract infection presents in early convalescence (see below) but it can present in the immediate postoperative stage when it is often accompanied by septicaemia.

14.4.5 Antibiotic management

From the foregoing it can be seen that the majority of patients can be managed expectantly. Clear lung fields, an expected remission of the predictable early fever and rapid removal of the various lines will allow safe withholding of antibiotics additional to the relatively narrow spectrum prophylaxis, confidence being enhanced by examination of urine, tracheal secretions and blood cultures where necessary.

Microbiological concerns multiply whenever patients develop non-infective complications dictating a prolonged ICU stay. Long-stay patients frequently become colonized with Gram-negative bacilli, but the significance of these findings is often doubtful. If **tracheostomy** is performed the necessary *humidification* greatly promotes colonization with *Pseudomonas aeruginosa*. As before, treatment should be directed against the patient's condition and not the laboratory report, though the development in ill patients of an acute respiratory distress syndrome (ARDS) lung picture may make it impossible to distinguish the appearances from Gram-negative pneumonitis. Rapid massive deterioration in respiratory function with ready isolation of Gram-negative bacilli from tracheal secretion and the blood should prompt

consideration of contamination of the humidification equipment.

In view of the above it might be argued that cardiothoracic patients should receive selective decontamination of the digestive tract (SDD). The benefits of this procedure are anyway disputed, but such benefits as may result are generally only apparent after 2 or more weeks. All but a few percentage of cardiothoracic patients will be off the ICU and even out of hospital by that time. SDD is not, therefore, recommended as a routine measure and those who might have benefited are beyond its institution by the time their unpredictable need is clear.

14.5 EARLY CONVALESCENCE

The move from ICU is usually accompanied by the removal of most of the intravascular lines and the urinary catheter. Microbiological (or putative microbiological) problems may be encountered in several areas.

14.5.1 Chest infections

The pain associated with median sternotomy inhibits coughing and expectoration. It is to be expected that sputum culture will produce a range of organisms not normally found in the site. These will include *H. influenzae*, *E. coli*, *Proteus*, *Klebsiella* and *Ps. aeruginosa*. Their significance must be judged against the patient's general condition, and that of the respiratory tract in particular. Patients should normally be afebrile at this stage. If no significant lung field abnormality (clinical or radiological) is present, these organisms are likely to represent no more than an altered 'normal flora'.

14.5.2 Urinary tract infections (UTIs)

Typically, UTIs occur in the early convalescent stage after catheter removal, and at this stage it is a predominantly male problem. The incidence is approximately 10%, and 10% of those affected progress to Gram-negative septicaemia.

The development of postoperative UTI in males after open-heart surgery is correlated with abnormal peak urine flow rates preoperatively (but not with positive preoperative MSU cultures). It may represent a complication of incomplete voiding which is clinically silent in normal ambulatory life. Treatment is directed against the isolated organism (it should be assumed to be a Gram-negative bacillus if urgent blind therapy is necessary). Affected male patients should have their bladder function assessed after recovery. Such episodes of Gram-negative septicaemia are highly unlikely to result in intracardiac

General experience is that it is difficult if not impossible to eradicate the infection without removing the box or, at least, re-siting it. Infection of only the superficial wound, (most commonly due to *Staph. aureus*) however, may respond entirely to antibiotic therapy.

De-novo insertions of pacemakers boxes should be accompanied by antibiotic prophylaxis against the common skin flora. A suitable choice would include flucloxacillin, nafcillin or clindamycin. Where MRSA is a problem such drugs as vancomycin and teicoplanin will be preferred. Re-siting of an already infected box should be preceded by a short period of chemotherapy against the infecting organism(s), guided by results of blood cultures or aspiration cultures from around the box, followed by re-implantation under cover of an *additional* drug to which the organisms are sensitive but which is not part of the treatment regimen. In all instances the prophylactic drug should be given according to the principles of 'three dose' prophylaxis. Good local antisepsis and skin preparation is also important in all pacemaker insertions, a suitable topical preparation being providone-iodine.

The second situation in which cardiac surgeons encounter pacemakers problems is in assisting cardiologists to deal with infected transvenous pacemakers. In the common scenario the patient presents with fever, rigors and positive blood cultures. In some cases the organism is *Staph. aureus*, when a severe septicaemic picture occurs, but in most cases the organism is a coagulase-negative staphylococcus when a less violent illness is the rule. In either case initial medical treatment, including appropriate antibiotics, will have served to stabilize the condition. The predominant short-term consideration is eradicating the infection from the electrode implantation site in the right ventricle. The right ventricular implantation site usually comprises an area of granulation tissue or granulomata which has become infected. Although analogous to right-sided bacterial endocarditis (including, occasionally, embolization to the lungs), the presence of the foreign body precludes eradication of the infection by antibiotic therapy alone, even if prolonged for up to 6 weeks and carefully managed as for endocarditis. Attempts may be made to remove the electrode transvenously, but the tissue reaction around the ventricular endocardial implantation site is often too strong and this fails, or the lead snaps to leave a proximal remnant.

The microbiological experience is that this infection will not resolve until the foreign body is removed at ventriculotomy. The patient should continue to receive appropriate antibiotics directed against the known organism throughout the operation, and for up to 2 weeks thereafter. If an alternative pacemaker is to be inserted at the same time (possibly an epicardial device) an *additional* antibiotic likely to be active against the skin flora of a patient receiving the existing treatment should be given for prophylaxis (three doses) and discontinued immediately afterwards. In patients already being treated with flucloxacillin or clindamycin a common choice is either teicoplanin or vancomycin, but in these cases, microbiological advice should be sought. Where the patient is to be sustained without a pacemaker for a short period after removal, subsequent elective re-implantation should follow the scheme outlined earlier.

14.9 ENDOCARDITIS

14.9.1 Native valve endocarditis (NVE)

Endocarditis can present to cardiac surgeons in two settings. First, surgery may be necessary in the treatment of NVE and, second, prosthetic valve endocarditis (PVE) is one of the major complications of cardiac surgery itself. Prosthetic valve endocarditis is described in section 14.9.2.

SURGERY IN NVE

The treatment of NVE is a highly skilled and often complex matter, involving a **close partnership between cardiologist and microbiologist**. It is, therefore, highly likely that microbiological advice will be already available if the need for surgery arises. This account assumes, therefore, that the antibiotic therapy in place at the time of surgical consultation will be appropriate, and is concerned only with those microbiological aspects which centre on the surgery. In the modern era, NVE is recognized to be either acute (in which case the organism is almost certain to be *Staph. aureus*) or subacute (usually streptococcal).

ACUTE ENDOCARDITIS

In acute endocarditis the clinical picture is that of a septicaemia with additional acute ulcerative damage to the heart which may be structurally normal before the onset. Osler's term 'endocarditis maligna' is very descriptive. Acute ulcerative damage to the heart probably occurs in 30% of *Staph. aureus* septicaemias, and progression to abscess formation can occur within hours or days. Presentations include valve destruction, annular abscesses with associated conduction defects, intracardiac fistulae, septic pericarditis, and many more. The operative indications in these circumstances are evident and pressing. Softer indications include increasing heart failure, recurrent emboli and apparent inability to eradicate the infection. There is also a belief in some circles that surgery is mandatory in acute *Staph. aureus* endocarditis. Finally, the modern ability to image the vegetations and intracardiac structures has led some to advise that the detection of large vegetations alone is an indication for intervention.

Optimal antibiotic therapy, rapidly and aggressively given within 2–3 days at most of the onset of *Staph.*

aureus endocarditis will frequently achieve medical cure without surgery. This presumably is because it prevents the progress to abscess formation (so characteristic of this organism) and, therefore, reduces the resultant intracardiac sequelae which are the common indications for surgery. Patients beginning therapy, however adequate, more than 7 days after the onset of the disease will almost always require surgery. There is no good evidence that in an otherwise uncomplicated case removing vegetations solely because they are visualized or large confers any benefits, and it is wise before accepting that infection has not been controlled by (or has apparently recurred during) expectedly adequate therapy, to ensure that extracardiac abscesses (especially splenic) are not the cause of the problem.

Whilst surgery (when indicated) must usually be performed immediately, it is occasionally possible to delay it. This may be advantageous, all else being equal, since prosthetic valves inserted into a septic annulus frequently become incompetent as the infection heals, requiring replacement later. Antibiotic prophylaxis must be given and must be *additional* to the therapy which the patient will be receiving. The drug chosen should be known to act against the infecting organism but must also be likely to work against skin bacteria resistant to the ongoing therapy. In the case of MRSA infections a logical choice for the prophylaxis will be teicoplanin or vancomycin. Only three doses should be given, the patient throughout this time also receiving the endocarditis treatment drugs. These latter should continue after the prophylaxis stops if necessary. Thereafter management is as for standard valve replacement (see above). It is re-emphasized that the exclusion of, or, when present, drainage and treatment of, extracardiac abscesses is an important step prior to surgery, since such lesions will pose an obvious threat to the newly implanted valve. If three or more days of adequate antibiotic therapy has been given to the patient prior to operation it is unusual for the infecting strain to be isolated from excised operative tissues. Positive cultures from an operation several days after the start of therapy should lead to a re-appraisal of the regime being used.

SUBACUTE BACTERIAL ENDOCARDITIS (SBE)

Patients with SBE have usually been infected with the culprit organism for at least 3 months before presentation. Fortunately, the organisms involved (streptococci from the oral, respiratory or upper alimentary tract – 'Streptococcus viridans' – or from the lower alimentary or genitourinary tract – 'Strep. faecalis') are of low-grade pathogenicity and the infection smoulders rather than ignites, causing weight loss, anaemia and other non-specific abnormalities as a background to physical signs which are dominated by those in the heart. Again, the Oslerian term, 'endocarditis lente', is much more descriptive than its modern equivalent. (The organism

names are given in parentheses because modern bacterial taxonomy no longer recognizes these names and has supplanted them with many specific streptococcal species. The terms, however, remain familiar to clinicians and, small nuances apart, the sense and associations of the traditional names will suffice for this account.)

Typically, the patient with SBE will have pre-existing, non-infective cardiac pathology, either acquired (rheumatic) or congenital. The low-virulence organisms of SBE can still, in their privileged site, cause intracardiac suppuration, and annular abscesses (with conduction defects), fistulae and valve destruction can still occur. The pace of the progression is, however, much slower, although the already compromised cardiac performance in many patients may hasten this. Indications for surgery are, therefore, much the same as in acute endocarditis and prophylaxis for the operation should follow the same principles. Since infected emboli in SBE usually result in sterile infarcts rather than metastatic abscesses the possibility of peripheral lesions is not as threatening.

A common concern in all patients receiving surgical intervention during the course of infective endocarditis is the need for extra therapy postoperatively. There is little evidence on this matter, and it is thought that the total course of treatment should be given as dictated by the nature of the disease and that no specific alterations should be occasioned by the surgery, it being regarded as an event within the planned treatment.

14.9.2 Prosthetic valve endocarditis (PVE)

PVE is traditionally divided into **early prosthetic valve endocarditis** (EPVE), which manifests itself within 60 days of operation, and **late prosthetic valve endocarditis** (LPVE), which presents at any time thereafter. The watershed of 60 days is not universally accepted and the interval has ranged from 60 to 90 days; however, all authorities have agreed that PVE presenting more than 3 months after surgery is unrelated to the operative procedure. The assumed division between EPVE and LPVE is reflected in the microbiology of the two conditions. Staphylococci (*Staph. aureus* and coagulase-negative staphylococci) and other skin organisms such as diphtheroids predominate in EPVE, whereas the organisms found in LPVE are much more those of native valve endocarditis (see section 14.9.1), such as streptococci. However, coagulase-negative staphylococci account for a significantly greater proportion of cases of LPVE than would be expected if the parallel with NVE was exact.

Recently, large actuarial studies of risk factors for PVE have shown that the hazard of PVE is highest at 3–6 weeks after operation, but remains elevated for 12 months after operation. These studies, which were statistically powerful and notable for the completeness of the data, strongly suggest that the watershed should now be placed at 12 months and that PVE presenting up to 1 year after operation often has its genesis in events occurring at operation or in the immediate postoperative period. Interestingly, this change in the definition of EPVE removes most (but not all) of the CNS component in LPVE, a finding which complements the risk analysis.

The large actuarial studies also found several specific risk factors for PVE. These included:

- The use of mechanical (rather than biological) prosthetic valves.
- The duration of operation. This might reflect the 'fall-off' in prophylactic antibiotic concentrations in prolonged CPB referred to earlier, and reinforces the practice of 'top-up' doses.
- Multiple valve replacement. It might be argued that this merely makes it likely that the operation will be long, but multiple valve replacement remains an independent risk factor after appropriate correction for duration of operation.
- Pre-existing NVE or PVE. This is a very potent risk factor, and remains so even when correction is made in those instances when the new PVE is due to a different organism to that found in the antecedent episode. This suggests that some patients may be unduly susceptible to PVE. One approach to this is to prefer allografts to mechanical prostheses in patients with previous NVE or PVE.

Several other risk factors (age, diabetes, etc.) showed weak and unsurprising associations.

Early PVE

EPVE can present early and within the original admission. It rapidly becomes clear in these early presentations that the valve is malfunctioning and dehiscence (leading to intractable heart failure) is common. Reoperation is inevitable and will reveal that the infection is on the suture line. Although EPVE is the correct designation for this situation, it is actually an interoperative wound-site. Later presentations of EPVE (after first discharge) may involve dehiscence, but are also likely to have some of the non-cardiac features of endocarditis (emboli, renal impairment, etc.). The possibility of PVE should never be far from the mind for any patient with a prosthetic valve. Blood cultures are usually positive, and confirmation of the diagnosis (once suspected) is usually straightforward. Very rarely fungi may be involved. In the case of yeast (*Candida*) infection the patient behaves very similarly to a bacterial PVE and the organism can usually be found in blood cultures. The much rarer EPVE with dimorphic fungi such as *Aspergillus* is very difficult to diagnose. Blood cultures are inevitably negative, and the quickest way to diagnose the condition is histology and culture of material removed at embolectomy surgery following one of the major emboli with which the disease

characteristically presents. Examination of the serum for *Aspergillus* antibodies may also help.

Prevention of EPVE

Prevention of EPVE centres around operative prophylaxis and prevention of postoperative bacteraemias. The former has been dealt with earlier and is the principal defence against intraoperative infection occurring at implantation. Although it has been suggested that prolonged exposure of the operative site and the introduction of a prosthesis might necessitate the complicated and expensive clean air systems used in hip replacement surgery, there is no evidence in open-heart surgery that such methods will be of benefit. However, a high level of asepsis and theatre discipline are essential in the crowded modern cardiac theatre. A dedicated theatre is considered essential, to which restricted access is desirable.

Postoperative bacteraemias

Theatre implantation of microorganisms apart, suspicion has focused on postoperative bacteraemia (not necessarily clinically detectable) as the major route whereby suitable organisms of the kind which are recovered from EPVE (staphylococci and diphtheroids) gain access to the valve. In a prospective, multicentre study 171 patients with prosthetic heart valves who had developed bacteraemia during their postoperative stay were followed for 12 months. Overall, 43% developed (E)PVE, which was diagnosed at the same time as the bacteraemia in 75%. In the other 25% there was a significant, sometimes very long, interval between bacteraemia and PVE. Some of these latter patients presented well beyond the previous watershed of 60 days, and in the past would presumably have been dubbed LPVE. Most of the bacteraemia/PVE episodes were with staphylococci or diphtheroids, and portals of entry were predominantly intravascular catheters, skin sepsis and wounds. Occasional examples of PVE were associated with bacteraemia due to Gram-negative bacilli and fungi, but always when the portal of entry was other than the urinary tract. No instance of PVE was related to infections (all Gram-negative bacilli) arising from the urine. In those instances in which no portal of entry could be found the PVE and bacteraemia were coincident, suggesting that some at least of these were examples of EPVE resulting from theatre-based infection. A very important finding was that prolonged, endocarditis-like treatment of the bacteraemia as an insurance against PVE had no significant protective effect. In other words, prevention of postoperative bacteraemia is the all-important measure. Once bacteraemia has occurred (and has been diagnosed) antibiotic therapy is unlikely to rescue the situation and is not certain to prevent PVE.

All the above argues for the meticulous approach to line care, the earliest possible removal of intravascular lines, the avoidance wherever possible of Swan–Ganz catheterization, and the early diagnosis and prompt treatment of skin and wound infection advocated earlier.

Late PVE

Once the risk period of EPVE is past, patients with prosthetic valves remain at risk of LPVE. As indicated earlier, the organisms involved are predominantly those of NVE. It is thought that this change in microbiology reflects the endothelialization of the prosthesis, presenting a surface onto which streptococci have a facility to adhere in contrast to the unendothelialized surface of the early postoperative phase. Risk factors are, therefore, exactly those which apply to the acquisition of NVE and include dental surgery, genitourinary surgery, gut surgery, etc. Prophylaxis for these occasions should be on precisely the same lines as for NVE.

Established streptococcal LPVE has a much less sinister course than EPVE, and many such patients will be successfully treated without surgery. Dehiscence is much less common – possibly because the infection and resultant vegetations are on the valve cusps rather than within the annulus. Complications similar to those of NVE, including annular abscesses, can occur and surgery may be required under similar indications as for NVE.

Staph. aureus infection follows the same, if not worse, course as in NVE and requires particularly aggressive management.

SECTION II: PERIPHERAL VASCULAR SURGERY

The term peripheral vascular disease is used here to distinguish the subject from cardiovascular disease. It is clear that the two areas will overlap in some instances, but the following account deals with those aspects which relate distinctly to the peripheral system. Arterial disease dominates the picture, but some mention of the infective aspects of venous problems is included.

In contrast to cardiac surgery, primary infections of the peripheral vascular system often present to the surgeon for initial diagnosis and management, although one particularly common condition – the management of the infective complications of peripheral vascular disease in diabetes – is usually in concert with a physician. A second, major area of microbiological interest in vascular surgery is the prevention, diagnosis and treatment of infections associated with vascular (arterial) prosthetic surgery.

14.10 PRIMARY (SPONTANEOUS) ARTERIAL INFECTIONS

Many 'spontaneous' arterial infections are associated with a discernible predisposing or underlying condition (Table 14.1), and the term is one of traditional or historical, rather than scientific, value. The condition is often misdiagnosed, or at least not recognized preoperatively, in many cases. The presentation will depend upon the aetiology and the location of the lesion. Diagnosis is more likely to be accurate in those patients with bacterial endocarditis in which the suspicion of mycotic aneurysms is (or should be) high and the patient is often already in hospital. Modern imaging techniques can offer much in all categories of spontaneous arterial infection.

Table 14.1 allows some prediction of the likely organisms to be encountered. It is generally agreed that the antibiotics used should be bactericidal wherever possible, and that drugs of a low toxicity and which can be given in very high dosages should be preferred. The precarious renal state of many arteriopathic patients is another important factor. Hence, beta-lactam antibiotics (penicillins and cephalosporins) figure largely among the agents chosen.

Table 14.1 *Spontaneous arterial infections*

	Mycotic aneurysm	Infected aneurysm	Microbial arteritis	Traumatic infected pseudoaneurysm
Aetiology	Endocarditis	Bacteraemia	Bacteraemia	Vessel trauma, narcotic addiction
Age (years)	30–50	Over 50	Over 50	Under 30
Incidence	Rare	Unusual	Common	Common
Site	Visceral, intracranial, aorta and peripheral arteries	Distal aorta	Aortoiliac, superficial femoral arteries; congenital or traumatic vascular defects	Femoral, carotid or sites of injection
Bacteriology	*Staph. aureus Streptococcus*	*Staphylococcus, Escherichia coli*	*Salmonella* species	Polymicrobial flora

Adapted from Wilson, S.E., Van Wagenen, P. and Passaro, E. Jr (1978): *Curr. Probl. Surg.*, **15**:1.

In **mycotic aneurysms** complicating bacterial endocarditis therapy may well be in progress, but if not, a combination of a penicillin (penicillin itself or amoxycillin) and an aminoglycoside (usually gentamicin) is appropriate for undiagnosed cases of streptococcal endocarditis (subacute endocarditis) which will have a history of weeks or even months. In patients presenting with a short history of hours or days and a septicaemic picture in addition to intracardiac signs, *Staph. aureus* must be suspected and large doses of an isoaloxozyl penicillin (flucloxacillin, nafcillin) should be given, if necessary in addition to amoxycillin and gentamicin. Suspicion of MRSA will dictate vancomycin or teicoplanin. Since vancomycin is also anti-streptococcal, its use for anti-staphylococcal purposes will permit the omission of amoxycillin and a combination of vancomycin and gentamicin will cover all the possibilities. However, the use of two nephrotoxic and ototoxic drugs will require expert microbiological support and frequent assays.

Blind therapy for infected aneuryms of the distal aorta (see Table 14.1) should encompass anti-staphylococcal drugs and an agent active against coliform organisms such as *E. coli, Klebsiella, Proteus*, etc. Pseudomonads are unlikely unless the causative bacteraemia was probably acquired in hospital. An appropriate regime is commonly achieved by the addition of a broad-spectrum penicillin (e.g. azlocillin, piperacillin,) or a later-generation cephalosporin (e.g. cefuroxime, cefamandole, ceftazidime) to the anti-staphylococcal therapy outlined earlier. Other drugs meriting consideration might be quinolones (ciprofloxacin) and penems (imipenem, meropenem). Choices will also be governed by local factors, particularly the prevalence of resistance to common antibiotics in Gram-negative bacilli. Potential regimens are many in number, some even combining the two elements into one preparation (co-amoxyclav, imipenem, tazobactam). The early administration and high dosage of the regimen is more relevant than the specific content (assuming a sensible choice), together with the realization that infection of distal aortic aneurysms has a very high mortality rate and medical treatment alone is rarely successful.

Microbial arteritis due to *Salmonella* also has a high mortality. It can take several clinical forms: **focal arteritis** with aneurysm formation and rupture, a diffuse **suppurative endarteritis** and, occasionally, **local infection** centred on a pre-existing degenerative lesion. Recent advances in anti-salmonella chemotherapy (particularly the introduction of fluoroquinolones) have improved matters, although treatment often needs to continue for many months after apparent cure, in addition to any necessary surgery.

Arterial infection after, (and often long after) vascular trauma commonly has a complex microbial flora. The description 'trauma' in this instance is not referring to major trauma but to iatrogenic procedures such as arterial puncture for cardiac catheterization or, more important-

antly and commonly, as an accidental complication of parenteral drug abuse. In this latter group an enormous range of organisms occurs. The infection is usually centred on a previously unsuspected pseudoaneurysm.

Finally, all clinicians should remain vigilant for the remote possibility that infected aneurysmal lesions can occur as a complication of a contiguous tuberculosus lesion, particularly of lymph nodes.

Management of all these patients must be by a combination of appropriate antibiotic therapy and surgery. Antibiotic therapy should be in large doses (preferably bactericidal), and will often need to be continued for several weeks after surgery. The surgical principle is to isolate the infected area from the arterial circulation. Clearly, the site and situation of the individual lesion will determine whether this is by simple ligation, diversion or prosthetic bypass. If it is impossible to do other than maintain arterial continuity through the infected area itself, it is recommended that tissue grafts be used rather than prosthetic material.

14.11 VASCULAR TRAUMA AND INFECTION

Infection closely following non-endogenous and non-iatrogenic vascular trauma (usually road traffic accidents) requires thoughtful management. A variety of organisms can be involved, all of which may be derived from the flora of viscera (particularly the gut) if the trauma is penetrative, and may alternatively be a collection of organisms derived from the environment. Antibiotic prophylaxis and therapy needs to cover a very wide range, including anaerobic, organisms (both *Clostridium* and the gut-derived *Bacteroides* species). Therefore, metronidazole must be given in addition to whatever other antibiotics are selected. The presence of dead tissue, especially muscle, makes post-traumatic arterial infection a distinct category in this very important regard. Such patients are normally given β-lactam antibiotics (penicillins or cephalosporins) and metronidazole at admission to prevent gangrene. However, in cases in which environmental material has been driven into the tissues, and in particular in instances of close-range gunshot wounds to the lower limbs ('knee-capping'), organisms of the *Bacillus* species may be introduced. The common species involved is *B. cereus* which is a potent source of proteolytic enzymes and other toxins. Characteristically *B. cereus* infection develops after 2–3 days and results in a severe necrotizing cellulitis which can progress to septicaemia and death. *B. cereus* strains are almost always resistant to all β-lactam antibiotics, including even the most recent varieties. Treatment must be with a non-β-lactam drug, and ciprofloxacin or teicoplanin are suitable. Whether or not such drugs should be added to the β-lactam plus metronidazole prophylaxis given at admission is debatable, and it would be an expensive addition to benefit a minority of patients. Nonetheless, patients in these categories should be closely observed, specimens should be obtained, and this possibility should be borne in mind.

14.12 GANGRENE

The infective aspects of gangrene can be divided into: (i) ischaemic gangrene (the moist gangrene which follows arterial occlusion or trauma); and (ii) gangrene primarily due to infection.

14.12.1 Moist gangrene

Infection is inevitably present and a complex bacterial flora is the rule, most commonly comprising faecal organisms (coliforms, enterococci, etc.). The important organisms are the anaerobes, whether of the *Bacteroides* species or the clostridia. All anerobic organisms will flourish in dead tissue or in any area in which the blood supply is failing. Whereas the *Bacteroides* species will cause local infection and abscess formation, it is the ability of clostridial infection to affect organs and systems well beyond the local area which makes them so important. It is important to note that these organisms are endogenous. Gangrene (and gas gangrene) is not a communicable infection and does not require barrier nursing with the important exception of streptococcal gangrene or necrotizing fasciitis (see below).

Many clostridia are saccharolytic, and this is especially true of the commonest species implicated in moist ischaemic gangrene; *Clostridium perfringens* (*Cl. welchii*). Sugars in the muscle and glycogen are metabolized to produce vast quantities of gas, leading to the well-known emphysematous appearances, detected clinically as **crepitus** and easily seen on X-radiography. *Cl. perfringens* does not do this in healthy (well-vascularized) tissue; indeed, it can, if looked for, commonly be recovered from healthily healing abdominal wounds after gut surgery. Hence, gas in the tissues is an ominous sign. Furthermore, *Cl. perfringens* produces several potent exotoxins, notably a lecithinase known as alpha toxin, an oxygen-labile haemolysin. When released into the circulation, this causes intravascular haemolysis with consequent anaemia, jaundice and, when free haemoglobin is produced, renal failure. No amount of antibiotic, however appropriate, will influence this condition. Alpha toxin can be rendered ineffective in the blood by very high arterial pO_2 levels under hyperbaric oxygen therapy, allowing correction of anaemia and lessening of haemolysis, but this simply gains a respite and presents the surgeon with a fitter patient on which to carry out the definitive therapy, such as amputation. Antibiotic therapy, which is essential to defend the

Table 14.2 *Common diabetic foot infections*

Acute infections	Chronic infections
Localized cellulitis	Osteomyelitis
Infective arthritis	
Necrotizing cellulitis or fasciitis	
Deep space infections	
Gangrene, non-clostridial and clostridial	

Adapted from Bridges, R.M. and Deitch, E.A. (1994) *Surg. Clin. North Am.*, **74**, 524.

viable and borderline ischaemic tissues, must include a potent anti-anaerobe drug. Metronidazole and clindamycin cover both *Bacteroides* and clostridia; penicillins cover only the latter.

14.12.2 Primary infective gangrene

Infection with a mixture of organisms, one of which is an anaerobe, the other being of a non-clostridial or non-*Bacteroides* species, can give rise to synergistic gangrene in which the non-anaerobic organism is thought to create the anaerobic conditions for the anaerobe to flourish. The tissue planes affected are either the fascia or subcutaneous fat, and trauma or operation allowing faecal and other organisms access to these tissues is a common antecedent. Sadly, the condition is no respector of surgeons or patients, and can follow minor procedures in good-risk patients. Depending on its location the condition is variously called Meleney's or Fournier's gangrene, and it also corresponds to the non-streptococcal variety of necrotizing fasciitis. As with all gangrenous infections, antibiotic therapy must include anti-anaerobic drugs (see above), but surgical excision of the affected area (which must be extensive and include a generous rim of viable tissue) is the curative procedure.

The other variety of necrotizing fasciitis is caused by *Strep. pyogenes*, the dramatic tissue destruction being due to the many enzymes and toxins produced by this organism. This condition is discussed elsewhere (see p. 122)

14.13 DIABETES

Diabetes is so common that it merits specific mention, although many of the infective problems will have been dealt with earlier. Common diabetic foot infections are listed in Table 14.2. In general, it can be assumed that the organisms involved will be those causing similar but less extensive infections in non-diabetics. However, three factors must be borne in mind in diabetes. First, all infections spread more quickly, are more extensive and are more likely to suppurate than resolve. Second, although anaerobic organisms do cause infections in diabetes, the use of crepitus as the hallmark of clostridial infection is misleading. Common aerobic organisms such as *E. coli* can produce gas when growing in diabetic tissues. Third, in diabetic patients fungal infection, especially due to *Candida* species, is common.

14.14 VENOUS INFECTIONS

Surgeons are occasionally summoned to assist when intravenous catheters, central venous catheters, umbilical catheters and other such devices have become detached and embolize. This is the only common circumstance in which veins become infected in an analogous way to arteries. The organisms involved will be *Staph. aureus*, coagulase-negative staphylococci, diphtheroids and other members of the skin flora, which may include coliforms and yeasts in immunocompromised patients, diabetes and those receiving many antibiotics. Removal is essential and antibiotic cover will be necessary, usually against both aerobes and anaerobes.

Venous ulcers are a common accompaniment of diabetes and of peripheral vascular disease in general, as well as presenting along with varicose veins requiring surgical attention. These ulcers will always contain organisms since they contain granulation tissue and are moist. Coliform organisms, including *Pseudomonas aeruginosa*, are commonly isolated. Compression therapy to remove the oedema together with appropriate local antiseptics form the basis of management, and are especially important prior to surgery. Systemic antibiotic therapy is nihilistic (and may lead to colonization with even more resistant organisms) unless: (i) the ulcer is surrounded by a cellulitic flare; (ii) frank pus is present; or (iii) *Staph. aureus*, *Strep. pyogenes* or *Bacteroides fragilis* are isolated, in which case flucloxacillin, penicillin or metronidazole, respectively, should be prescribed. It will be particularly important to remove these bacteria before surgery in an adjacent area.

SECTION III: ARTERIAL PROSTHETIC SURGERY

The reported incidence of infection after prosthetic graft implantation ranges from 0 to 3.5% and depends on the site of implantation. Acknowledged risk factors include: (i) operation under emergency conditions; (ii) a groin incision; (iii) subcutaneous routing of the prosthesis; (iv) early reoperation (usually for bleeding); and (v) wound-related early complications such as lymphocoele, haematoma or cellulitis. Many of these are unavoidable and can only lead to careful observation and anticipation.

Much more debatable is the claim that up to 40% of apparently innocent aneurysmal contents removed at elective operation will grow organisms on culture. These results were obtained using enrichment techniques designed to recover very small numbers of organisms in the original material. Most microbiologists will be sceptical of such claims. Similar claims have been made in many other fields and often found to be spurious, especially so when the organisms concerned are coagulase-negative staphylococci which are such common contaminants. Nonetheless, in some series a clear relationship appears to have been demonstrated between such positive cultures and subsequent graft infection. The topic merits further study. Modern molecular biological methods might clarify matters, not relying on culture to demonstrate *in situ* the presence of small numbers of microorganisms.

14.15 GRAFT INFECTIONS

In an analogous manner to prosthetic endocarditis, graft infections are conventionally classified as early or late, the dividing point taken to be (about) 4 months. **Early infection** is taken to be related to events surrounding the implantation or immediate perioperative period. Infections occurring within 30 days of surgery are thought to relate almost certainly to operative factors, and a 30-day incidence of infection greater than 1.5% is taken by many to require immediate review of operative conditions and of antibiotic prophylaxis.

14.15.1 Early graft infection

This is predominantly due to *Staph. aureus* (80%) with Gram-negative bacilli (*E. coli*, *Proteus*, *Klebsiella*, etc.) accounting for much of the remainder. Early graft infection is closely associated with the fate of the operative wounds, and in particular, the groin wound. Wound haematomas, lymphatic leaks and, clearly, wound infections, are all complications which threaten the prosthesis. Gram-negative infections have become proportionately more common with the use of antibiotic prophylaxis, but may also occasionally be linked with urinary tract-based and catheter-related bacteraemias. They also increase proportionately with duration of hospital stay and preoperative debility. A particularly devastating infection is caused by *Ps. aeruginosa*, possibly because of the potent enzyme production by this organism. Haemorrhage from the graft is a sign associated with Gram-negative infection.

Early infection is characterized by fever, leukocytosis and, when severe, the associated phenomena of the sepsis syndrome. When related to the wound it is an important early step rigorously to assess the nature of the wound infection and its depth in relation to the prosthesis. **Cellulitis** of the skin or infection extending only to the subcutaneous tissues may be treated as a wound infection and is often apparently successful, the graft being spared. However, it is likely that the incidence of late graft infection is higher in patients with these apparently resolved early infections. When wound infection extends to the graft, or to tissue planes adjacent to the graft, surgery will be necessary under appropriate and vigorous antibiotic therapy. The detection of organisms in the peripheral blood in grafted patients with a known wound infection is also a pointer to graft involvement, even if this is not apparent at the time.

Perioperative prophylaxis is largely directed towards preventing early infection and, therefore, is chosen to cover *Staph. aureus* and coliforms. Typically, this is achieved by using a cephalosporin (e.g. cefuroxime, cefamandole), the use following the three-dose format. Since many coagulase-negative staphylococci will be resistant to this regime the undoubted general success in its use tends to lend weight to the argument that some of the claims related to preoperative presence of coagulase-negative staphylococci may be spurious.

A recent innovative approach is to incorporate appropriate antibiotics into the prosthesis itself, and various drugs have been evaluated for their effect when bonded into the prosthetic material. This interesting approach will no doubt progress further in years to come.

14.15.2   Late graft infection

At least 50% of graft infections present in an indolent manner, not often associated with systemic signs and symptoms, and even without laboratory evidence of a marked inflammatory process, many months or even years after operation. Signs and symptoms often relate to the site of the graft and include pain, swelling, fistula formation and dysfunction of adjacent organs. Again, modern imaging techniques are invaluable in diagnosis. The microbiology is often obscure (up to 60% remain of unproven origin). It is thought that a very low-grade infection of a biofilm occurs, and coagulase-negative staphylococci have emerged as the most frequently isolated organism, albeit after enhanced enrichment methods. Whether or not these organisms are indeed the culprits and whether or not they gain access during the perioperative period (perhaps from line-based bacteraemias) is unknown. Peripheral vascular surgery may

be able to draw useful lessons from the cardiac surgical experience outlined elsewhere. Treatment involves surgery (see above) together with judicious use of bactericidal antibiotics, pre-, peri- and postoperatively. When cultures are available, choice will be dictated by tests on these but in their absence coagulase-negative staphylococci are assumed and some resistance is also assumed. Combinations of rifampicin with other anti-staphylococcal drugs (clindamycin, fusidic acid or vancomycin) form the basis of many regimes.

A final area of uncertainty is whether or not long-term survivors of graft implantation should undergo episodic prophylaxis for dental and other bacteraemia-prone procedures in the same way as is done for those with prosthetic heart valves. Opinion is divided, but many favour this approach, believing that the consequences of infection are so disastrous that the costs of many unnecessary episodes of prophylaxis are more than outweighed by the savings (financial and human) accompanying one successfully prevented case.

14.16   FURTHER READING

Cardiovascular surgery

Calderwood, S.B., Swinski, L.A., Waternaux, C.M. *et al.* (1985) Risk factors for the development of prosthetic value endocarditis. *Circulation*, **72**, 31–37.

Daebbeling, B.N., Pfaller, M.A., Kuhns, K.R. *et al.* (1990) Cardiovascular surgery prophylaxis. *J. Thorac. Cardi. Vasc. Surg.*, **99**, 981–989.

Freeman, R. and Hall, R.J.C. (1996) Infective Endocarditis. In *Diseases of the Heart*, eds D.G. Julian, *et al.* W.B. Saunders Company Ltd, London, 889–910.

Ivert, T.A., Dismukes, W.E., Cobbs, C.G. *et al.* (1984) Prosthetic value endocarditis. *Circulation*, **69**, 223–232.

Peripheral vascular surgery

Bandyk, D.F. (1990) Graft infection: a dreadful challenge. *Serv. Vasc. Surg.*, **3**, 77–80.

Buckels, J.A.C. and Welson, S.E. (1987) The prevention and management of prosthetic graft infection. In *Vascular Surgery, Principles and Practice*, ed. S.E. Wilson, McGraw-Hill, New York, 889–897.

Strachan, C.J.L., Newson, S.W.B. and Ashton, T.R. (1991) The clinical use of an antibiotic bonded graft. *Eur. J. Vasc. Surg.*, **5**, 627–632.

15

Infections in trauma

P.J. SANDERSON

15.1 MICROBIOLOGY OF TRAUMA

15.1.1 Sources of organisms

Trauma wounds will almost always be contaminated by bacteria. In civil injuries, the organisms will originate from the skin and clothing as well as from the environment of the road or farm, whereas in warfare, bullets or shrapnel will most likely be sterile, but they will carry fragments of clothing and skin into the wound. In bomb blast injuries the internal organs and serous cavities may be contaminated by the normal flora of the gut and respiratory tract.

15.1.2 Types of organisms

Staphylococcus aureus carried on the skin and clothing is the most common cause of trauma wound sepsis. This organism is responsible for the majority of soft tissue, bone and joint infection in trauma, although haemolytic streptococci, anaerobes and coliforms may also be involved on occasion. In abdominal injury, rupture of the gut releases anaerobes (e.g. *Bacteroides*, anaerobic streptococci), enterococci and coliforms (e.g. *Escherichia coli*, *Proteus*, *Enterobacter*) into the peritoneal cavity, and peritonitis may result after some hours. In head and neck injuries, infections may arise from organisms of the upper respiratory tract, for example anaerobes, streptococci and *Staph. aureus*, whilst in urinary tract injury, it is coliforms that predominate (Table 15.1).

The spores of *Clostridium perfringens* and *Clostridium tetani* survive in the environment, particularly in soil and manure, and when seeded into a wound on impact may germinate under anaerobic conditions to cause gas gangrene and tetanus.

Trauma in **certain environments** may result in infection with particular organisms, for example in salt water with vibrios, and in fresh water with aeromonads. Animal bites often become infected with *Pasteurella multocida*, and human bites with bacteria of the mouth (see p. 148). There is a tendency in trauma wounds of diabetics for infection with mixed organisms, but it is debatable whether the frequency of infection in these patients is actually increased.

15.1.3 Later infection

Later infection in trauma arises either from contamination of wounds by the patient's own organisms originating from neighbouring sources (e.g. skin, faeces, etc.), or from exogenous organisms originating by poor aseptic technique or cross-infection. Antibiotics may influence both the type of organism and its sensitivities, and resistant coliforms, pseudomonads and *Candida* spp. may act as secondary invaders under their influence.

Table 15.1 *Organisms causing infection in trauma patients*

Site	Common organisms	Occasional organisms and secondary invaders
Soft tissues Bones and joints Hand	*Staph. aureus* Group A streptococci	Coliforms Anaerobes *Pseudomonas*
Peritoneal cavity	Coliforms Anaerobes	*Pseudomonas* *Staph. aureus* *Strep. faecalis*
Thoracic cavity Head and neck	*Strep. pneumoniae* Anaerobes *Staph. aureus*	Coliforms Group A streptococci *Haemophilus* spp.
Bites – human	*Staph. aureus* Group A streptococci Anaerobes *Eikenella*	Coliforms
– animal	*Pasteurella multocida*	*Staph. aureus* Coliforms Anaerobes

15.2 SPECIMENS AND LABORATORY REPORTS

15.2.1 Obtaining samples

In severe trauma, samples of tissue obtained by debridement, or swabs, can (and should) be cultured early **before signs of infection develop**, for example in penetrating wounds of road or farm accidents. These may reveal the presence of clostridia or *Staph. aureus*. Samples of faecal spillage in the peritoneal cavity and of urine in urinary tract injury should also be sent to the laboratory routinely at surgery. Otherwise it is doubtful if routine early sampling is justified in trauma in the absence of signs of infection.

If infection is suspected, samples should be obtained before starting antibiotics. Specimens of tissue or pus are much more efficient than swabs, and anaerobes are more likely to survive the journey to the laboratory if retained in such media. Swabs should be sent in a transport medium. Samples should reach the laboratory as soon as reasonably practicable, and if likely to be delayed should be held at 4°C in a refrigerator.

15.2.2 Interpretation of reports

A microbiology report of a wound swab or tissue should be strictly interpreted in relation to the clinical findings. Contaminated wounds may yield irrelevant organisms, and clean wounds may be colonized (but not infected) by potentially pathogenic organisms. Culture of coliforms and anaerobes, as well as of *Staph. aureus*, does not necessitate systemic antibiotic treatment unless accompanied by observed signs of infection. The detection of haemolytic streptococci of group A, on the other hand, does indicate the need for treatment, whether signs of infection are present or not, since these organisms are regarded as always potentially (inevitably) pathogenic. The culture of clostridia will suggest gas gangrene, and in the absence of typical signs the patient requires careful observation. The recovery of *C. tetani* in a wound demands the use of penicillin.

A Gram-stained film will detect the presence of polymorphs and thus support the clinical diagnosis of infection (but this is not a substitute for clinical inspection). The detection of bacteria in the film indicates the presence and morphology of bacteria in the wound. This finding may confirm the relevance of the culture result and provide an indication of the numbers of bacteria present. Many laboratories report an approximate quantitation of the culture, but this is a variable finding and is an unreliable indication of the presence of infection.

15.3 ANTIBIOTIC PROPHYLAXIS OF INFECTION IN TRAUMA

15.3.1 Indications for prophylaxis

Prophylaxis is required in trauma when vulnerable tissues or organs are exposed to contamination. The following types of trauma justify single dose, or short-term prophylaxis. In **compound fractures**, infection may arise in the exposed and damaged bone, and prophylaxis is mandatory. **Penetrating wounds** may allow growth of both anaerobes and aerobes in deep tissues. In head injuries, access to the **meninges** may result in meningitis, and similarly

CASE HISTORY

A shot in the neck

A bullet entered the right thorax and lodged against T2 in a Post Office raider. There was extensive damage to the right lung (Figure 15.1). A drain was inserted and flucloxacillin and amoxycillin given as prophylaxis. Healing was rapid, and at 1 week the drain was removed. Antibiotics were stopped at 10 days, after which the wounds resolved without infection.

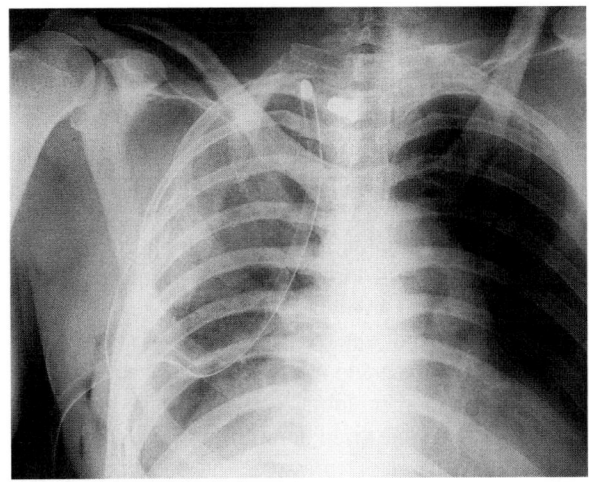

Figure 15.1

injuries resulting in the exposure of lung tissue, the peritoneal cavity and urinary tract to exogenous or endogenous organisms may result in infection. Complicated injuries to the hand may justify prophylaxis.

However, unless such injuries are present prophylaxis is contraindicated, the disadvantages being the damage to the normal flora brought about by systemic antibiotics, with consequent invasion by opportunist or secondary pathogens, as well as the selection of resistant strains and additional cost.

15.3.2 Timing and duration of prophylaxis

If prophylaxis is indicated, the antibiotic should be given as soon as possible after injury. An intramuscular injection can be administered by paramedical staff, at the scene of accident or on reception in the A&E department. It is not appropriate to delay administration until the patient reaches the operating theatre.

15.3.3 Appropriate antibiotics (Table 15.2)

It is essential to treat against *Staph. aureus* in all trauma wounds requiring prophylaxis. In limb injuries, flucloxacillin alone will be sufficient, but in abdominal injury with ruptured viscera, then cover against coliforms and anaerobes will also be required, and this is adequately provided by a second-generation cephalosporin and metronidazole. In head, neck and thoracic trauma, the respiratory flora and anaerobes require treatment with amoxycillin and metronidazole as well as with co-amoxyclav alone. Broader-spectrum or newer agents are not required because prophylaxis is aimed at the environmental or patient's flora, which are not likely to be resistant to antibiotics if he/she has not been in hospital or treated with antibiotics. Alternative regimens are listed in Table 15.2.

In types I and II compound fractures and in head and neck injuries, a single dose (or at most a 24-hour period of cover) will be sufficient. In type III compound fractures and in thoracic and abdominal injuries, up to 3 days'

CASE HISTORY

Prophylaxis for a compound fracture

A rider fell from his horse and suffered a compound fracture of the ankle; the wound was contaminated by manure. In hospital, cefuroxime prophylaxis was given and the fractures fixed by screws. Four days later infection developed in the wound, and a swab yielded *Bacteroides* organisms. Metronidazole was begun at 1 week after the trauma, but osteomyelitis due to *Bacteroides* resulted. The infection probably occurred by *Bacteroides* inoculation into the wound at the point of injury, and was not preventable by cefuroxime.

In trauma, the history is relevant; for example, in heavy contamination, farmyard or war injuries, prophylaxis with metronidazole in addition to cefuroxime may be justified to prevent anaerobic infections.

CASE HISTORY

Infection in a broken arm

A man fell against a pavement kerb and grazed and fractured his forearm. A plaster was applied, but after 3 days severe pain and swelling of the hand led to its removal. Some days later cellulitis and lymphangitis of the forearm was diagnosed. Oral penicillin was given, but the cellulitis spread to the shoulder and trunk (Figure 15.2). A haemolytic streptococcus group A was reported by the laboratory. Thereafter, intravenous penicillin and flucloxacillin were given and incisions made into the forearm to relieve pressure. The patient made a complete recovery.

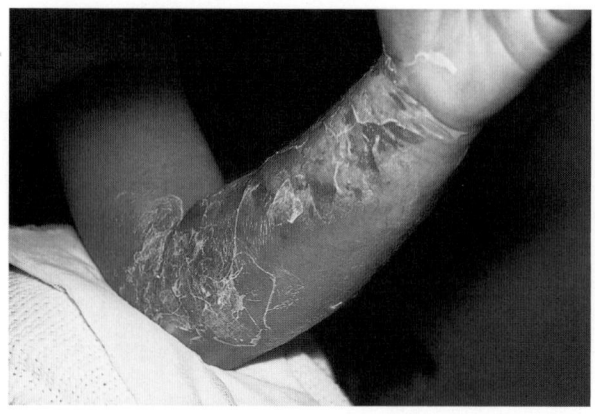

Figure 15.2

---

prophylaxis is appropriate, depending on the clinical findings and progress of the patient.

15.3.4 Surgical treatment

Surgical techniques are as (or more) important as antibiotics in reducing infection in trauma. Debridement of dead tissue and elimination of dead space and haematomas help to exclude a nidus for infection; indeed, debridement is crucial and may need to be repeated. Adequate vascularity must be established and any fractures stabilized to aid the response to infection. If wounds are closed by primary suture or too early, then infection may be encouraged or its presence disguised. Minor infection in the pin tracts of external fixation devices does not prevent fur-

Table 15.2 *Appropriate antibiotics for prophylaxis and treating infection resulting from trauma*

Site	Prophylaxis	Treatment
Soft tissues Bones and joints Hand	Flucloxacillin	Flucloxacillin Benzylpenicillin Metronidazole
Peritoneal cavity	Cefuroxime and metronidazole	Cephalosporin/ ciprofloxacin/ gentamicin Thienamycin Metronidazole
Thoracic cavity Head and neck	Amoxycillin and metronidazole Co-amoxyclav	Amoxycillin Metronidazole
Bites – human	Flucloxacillin and metronidazole	As for prophylaxis
– animal	Cephalosporin and metronidazole	As for prophylaxis

ther surgery, but if the infection extends to the bone it will need to be treated first.

15.4 TREATMENT OF INFECTION IN TRAUMA

15.4.1 Diagnosis

The initial two steps in dealing with infection in trauma are: (i) to suspect it; and (ii) to obtain good samples for culture. Repeated clinical examination, good communication with nursing staff and adequate specimens will help in delivering timely and focused care. Specimens should be taken from deep in the wound where the infection is most active, and include tissue and bone or the intramedullary canal if infection complicates intramedullary nailing. A series of three specimens enhances the reliability of the bacteriology; if the same bacteria are repeatedly isolated it is supporting evidence that they are playing a pathogenic role. Samples contaminated by skin or extraneous bacteria are less likely to yield consistent results. Swabs from sinuses can be particularly misleading, as they are often contaminated by organisms of the skin. Swabs should be driven deep into a wound or sinus tract and skin contact avoided; preferably, tissue samples should be obtained as in all deep and inaccessible wounds.

15.4.2 Management and antibiotics (Table 15.2)

Infection after trauma to the soft tissues, the hand and bones and joints, is likely to result from *Staph. aureus* (see Table 15.1), and flucloxacillin is therefore the appropriate first choice for treatment, being the most potent anti-staphylococcal agent available. Flucloxacillin is safe and rapidly excreted via the kidneys, and can be given at 500 mg and 1 g at 6-hourly intervals in adults. In penicillin-allergic patients, erythromycin or clindamycin can be used as a substitute. Most *Staph. aureus* strains are sensitive to erythromycin, which is also given at 500 mg or 1 g 6-hourly, though prolonged use should be avoided in order to prevent liver and ototoxicity. Clindamycin is an effective anti-staphylococcal and anti-anaerobe agent, but its reputation for inducing *Clostridium difficile* diarrhoea has detracted from its use. If group A streptococcal infection is clinically suspected, or confirmed by the laboratory, penicillin should be added, being more potent than flucloxacillin for this rapidly infective organism.

Abdominal sepsis resulting from trauma will be due to the patient's own gut flora (with possible *Staph. aureus* in penetrating injury) and resistant strains and pseudomonas are less likely pathogens. Broader cover including for coliforms and anaerobes is required from the beginning, and a cephalosporin plus metronidazole is satisfactory. Cephalosporins provide safe cover against Gram-negative organisms, and in this context those which are also active against *Staph. aureus* (e.g. cefuroxime) are particularly relevant. Ciprofloxacin and gentamicin are also appropriate for coliforms. Third-generation cephalosporins are not indicated unless there is evidence of resistant strains or poor clinical response which may be due to more resistant secondary invaders.

In head and neck trauma infection, penicillin, amoxycillin with metronidazole, or augmentin alone, are appropriate since the endogenous organisms of the upper respiratory tract will respond to these first-line agents.

Initially the intravenous route should be used; when a clinical response has been obtained antibiotics can be given orally. Prolonged courses of treatment, for example beyond 10 days or 2 weeks should be avoided. Doses need to be adjusted in line with renal function, but penicillins and cephalosporins are well excreted unless creatinine clearance is reduced to less than half. Gentamicin treatment requires serum assays to be carried out and is best avoided if the patient is in shock. In limb injuries where there is bone damage, treatment of infection should be early and active enough to prevent osteomyelitis. In types I and II compound fractures the oral route is acceptable, but if there is pyrexia or signs of systemic infection, and in type III fractures, the intravenous route is mandatory.

Laboratory reports, particularly when resistant or unusual strains, for example *Pseudomonas aeruginosa* or methicillin-resistant *Staphylococcus aureus* are reported, require careful assessment. The relevance of the sample (e.g. was it a cleanly taken deep tissue or bone specimen, or was it a superficial swab taken close to the skin surface?) must be considered, as must be the clinical appearance of the wound. The need for treatment is determined by the clinical findings, and not by the laboratory report. Hence, the advice of a microbiologist will be helpful in deciding on the relevance of isolates, especially in complicated or prolonged convalescence where more resistant secondary invaders may be encountered.

Gentamicin beads provide local concentrations of gentamicin in a convenient form. Gentamicin is active against Gram-negative organisms and also *Staph. aureus*, but not streptococci or anaerobes. The beads may be useful for abscesses, or evacuated haematomas, and in local infections where the blood supply may be restricted, such as Brodie's abscess. They are probably best used in conjunction with systemic antibiotics.

Table 15.3 *Organisms causing infection after intramedullary fixation of fractures*

Organism	No. isolated
Staphylococcus aureus	11
Staphylococcus epidermidis	5
Enterococcus spp.	3
Gram-positive	3
Pseudomonas spp.	5
Enterobacter spp.	4
Gram-negative	8
Total	39

15.5 BITES, GAS GANGRENE AND TETANUS

15.5.1 Bites

Bites, both animal and human, often result in infection. The mouth contains large numbers of organisms and so a bite may introduce them into deep and susceptible tissues. The range of organisms in the human mouth includes *Staph. aureus*, group A streptococci, anaerobes and *Eikenella* spp. in dogs and cats *Pasteurella multocida* is also frequent.

If infection develops it is often polymicrobial, and any treatment before bacteriological guidance needs to be broad spectrum. In human bites, augmentin or flucloxacillin with metronidazole will be appropriate; in animal bites, augmentin or a cephalosporin with metronidazole is required. In secondary infection or late infection, coliforms and anaerobes can also be involved. Bone, joint, deep compartment and tendon infection should be looked for actively. In contaminated deep or complicated wounds of the hand prophylaxis at the time of injury is justified.

15.5.2 Gas gangrene

Although most cases of gas gangrene follow trauma, some follow surgery (including clean surgery) and very occasionally occur without antecedent trauma or surgery. The usual dominant organism is *Clostridium perfringens*, and sometimes *C. septicum*, *C. histolyticum* or other less frequent species. Spores enter tissues from the soil, bowel or patient's skin. Clostridia produce exotoxins; alpha lysin destroys lecithin, leading to local tissue destruction and red cell lysis; theta haemolysin leads to haemolysis and cardiotoxicity, while hyaluronidase, collagenase and proteinase aid spread of the organism through the tissues. Other non-clostridial organisms can produce gas in tissues; examples are *Escherichia coli* and anaerobes, but these infections progress more slowly and have less systemic effects than gas gangrene and may occur in tissues already gangrenous as a result of poor blood supply.

The skin becomes bruised, then blackens and is tense and painful; crepitus may be detected on palpation. Soft tissue X-radiography may detect gas in tissues, sometimes without crepitus or before it develops. The infection spreads rapidly, and the patient appears ill. Debridement and release of tension by opening the wound and tissue planes must be considered early, not only to ensure the vascular supply but also to destroy the anaerobic conditions on which the organism depends. Usually, muscle tissue is affected leading to myonecrosis, but gas gangrene can be limited to the subcutaneous tissues with the same consequences.

Serous wound discharge or tissue samples should be sent to the laboratory for a Gram film and culture. If Gram-positive bacilli are seen the diagnosis should be assumed, but a negative film does not exclude the disease.

Initial treatment is with high doses of benzylpenicillin, together with surgery to the wound. If the condition progresses, then hyperbaric oxygen should be considered. Careful monitoring of the pulse rate, blood pressure, haemoglobin and renal function is required, since the systemic effects of the toxins may soon appear. Red cell lysis leads to a falling haemoglobin and renal dysfunction, whilst the pulse is raised disproportionately to the temperature. Pericardial effusion and diarrhoea may also develop, and eventually circulatory collapse supervenes.

The diagnosis of gas gangrene depends on clinical awareness, and a successful outcome is more likely the earlier treatment begins. The help of physicians in managing a developing case should be sought.

15.5.3 Tetanus

In tetanus, *Clostridium tetani* spores are implanted in a wound and germinate in anaerobic conditions to produce a toxin, tetanospasmin (Figure 15.3). Spores usually originate from soil or manure, but may enter tissues

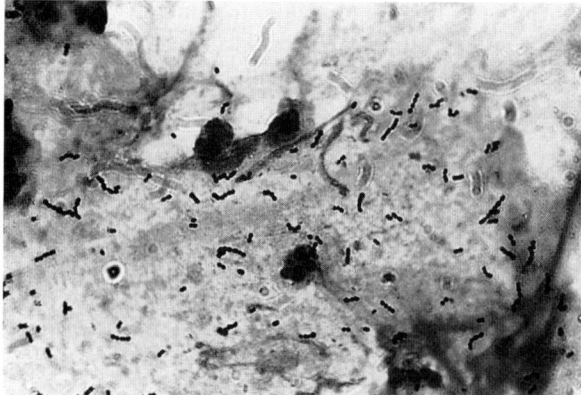

Figure 15.3 *A Gram stain of* Clostridium tetani, *showing terminal spores.*

from the gut and tetanus can occur after bowel and other types of surgery. The toxin enters the bloodstream and is alone responsible for the disease; it invades myoneural junctions and travels in nerve axons towards the central nervous system, where inhibitory impulses acting on motor neurones are blocked by selectively depressing neurotransmitter release.

Diagnosis is clinical; swabs and tissue samples may confirm the diagnosis if the organism is cultured. Muscle spasm usually begins in the jaw and face, since the facial nerve roots are shorter. Local tetanus can also occur.

Treatment includes penicillin to prevent further production of toxin, and human anti-toxin to neutralize any circulating tetanospasmin, but the evident effects of the toxin on the central nervous system cannot be reversed and, indeed, may progress after diagnosis. Patients require specialist care with sedation, muscle relaxants and artificial ventilation; full recovery is possible after some weeks.

TETANUS PREVENTION

Protection is brought about by large-scale immunization with tetanus toxoid. The purified toxin is treated with formaldehyde, converting it to an immunogenic, but innocuous toxoid. Immunogenicity is enhanced by absorption to an aluminium adjuvant.

Wounds at particular risk are those with significant devitalized tissue: puncture wounds; contact with soil or manure; and any wound sustained more than 6 hours before treatment. The anti-tetanus prophylaxis required, for both clean and 'at-risk' wounds, depends on the patient's immunization status, and is indicated in Table 15.4. For wounds at risk, except in patients with a documented completed course of immunization within the past 10 years, a dose of human anti-tetanus immunoglobulin is recommended. This material is prepared from pooled plasma from blood donors. While anaphylactic reactions are rare with either vaccine or human antiserum, practitioners should be familiar with their management.

Table 15.4 *Protection against tetanus*

Immunization status	Clean wound	Tetanus risk wound*
Course completed or booster within 10 years	Nil	Nil
Course completed or booster more than 10 years ago	Booster dose	Booster plus dose of antiglobulin
Not immunized, unknown status or incomplete course	3-dose course of immunization	3-dose course plus antiglobulin

*Wounds with significant devitalized tissue; contact with soil or manure; evident sepsis; puncture wounds; wounds sustained more than 6 hours before treatment.

CASE HISTORY

Fatal gas gangrene

A reserve soldier on military exercises suffered a severe crush injury to the leg which resulted in the limb being amputated. At the first wound dressing some slight bruising in the stump was noted. Two days later the patient became ill, with raised pulse and falling blood pressure. The stump was discoloured blue/black and discharging foul smelling serous exudate. *Clostridium welchii* was grown from tissue samples. Debridement, antibiotics, support therapies and later hyperbaric oxygen failed to save the soldier's life.

Amputation requires prophylaxis. The early signs of gas gangrene can be minimal, but suspicion of the diagnosis requires action.

15.6 PREVENTION OF OTHER COMMUNICABLE DISEASES

15.6.1 Rabies

In animal bites sustained abroad, the degree of risk for rabies is assessed according to country. In deciding whether prophylaxis is required, the advice given in *Immunisation against Infectious Disease* published by the Department of Health (1996) and available to all doctors, should be followed.

15.6.2 Blood-borne viruses

Possible exposure to hepatitis B may occur in trauma wounds exposed to blood or secretions of other people, particularly human bites. Vaccine or immunoglobulin are not given unless the 'donor' is known to be hepatitis B-positive or in a risk group, because the incidence of infectivity for hepatitis B in the UK population is low, i.e. about 0.1% or less. If exposure could have occurred, then 'donor' blood should be tested for hepatitis B markers if possible. The use of vaccine or immunoglobulin will depend on the nature of the exposure and the immune status of the patient: advice should be sought from the local control of infection doctor.

It is probable that the hepatitis C virus can be transmitted in a similar way to hepatitis B. At present, there is no vaccine or immunoglobulin for prevention.

HIV

Although infectivity of HIV in blood is less than for hepatitis B, transmission by blood contaminating human bite and other wounds has been described. Patients should be carefully assessed for risk, counselled and offered appropriate prophylaxis if the 'donor' is known positive or high risk, but not otherwise. This should be carried out as soon as possible after wounding, and advice sought from the local control of infection doctor. Testing the 'donor' for HIV status may help in deciding whether to continue the course of prophylaxis, but this requires permission and is not necessary in making the decision of whether to give an initial dose, which is based on an assessment of the 'donor' (see Chapter 6).

15.7 FURTHER READING

Bozorgzadah, A., Pizzi, W.F., Barie, P.S. *et al.* (1999) The duration of antibiotic administration in penetrating abdominal trauma. *American Journal of Surgery,* **177**, 125–131.

Medeiros, I. and Saconato, H. (2001) *Antibiotic prophylaxis for mammalian bites.* Cochrane database systematic review (2), CD 001 1738.

Stevens, D.L. and Bryant, A.E. (2002) The role of clostridial toxins in the pathogenesis of gas gangrene. *Clinical Infectious Diseases*, **35** (Supplement 1), S93–100.

Velmahos, G.C., Jindal, A., Chan, L. *et al.* (2001) Prophylactic antibiotics after severe trauma: more is not better. *International Surgery*, **86**, 176–183.

Velmahos, G.C., Konstantinos, G.T., Sarkisian, G. *et al.* (2002) Severe trauma is not an excuse for prolonged antibiotic prophylaxis. *Archives of Surgery*, **137**, 537–542.

Infections in orthopaedic surgery

P.J. SANDERSON AND G.R. SERJEANT

16.1 ORGANISMS AND PATHOGENESIS

16.1.1 Organisms in bone and joint infection

The predominant organism of haematogenous bone and joint infection in children and adults is *Staphylococcus aureus*. In neonates, a wider range of organisms, predominantly group B streptococci and coliforms, occur. In children, group A streptococci and *Haemophilus influenzae* are found in addition. Salmonellas occur in sickle cell disease, whilst *Neisseria gonorrhoreae* and *Streptococcus pneumoniae* may cause joint infection in younger and older adults respectively (Table 16.1).

At present in the UK, reported cases of osteomyelitis caused by methicillin-resistant *Staph. aureus* (MRSA) are rare. Similarly, there are few cases of resistant strains of *Staphylococcus epidermidis* (MRSE) causing implant infections. However, the incidence of these strains is rising elsewhere (e.g. in the USA), and such infections need to be monitored and reported.

Table 16.1 *Organisms causing haematogenous osteomyelitis in different age groups*

	Common organisms	**Less common organisms**
Neonates	Group B streptococci Coliforms	*Staph. aureus* Group A streptococci Anaerobes
Children	*Staph. aureus*	Group A streptococci *Haemophilus influenzae*[a] *Strep. pneumoniae*
Young adults	*Staph. aureus*	*Salmonella*[b] *Brucella*[c]
Older patients	*Staph. aureus*	Coliforms[d] *Pseudomonas*[d] Anaerobes

[a] Incidence probably declining with Hib vaccination.
[b] Specially in sickle cell disease.
[c] Relevant occupational and geographical history.
[d] Often secondary invaders in chronic disease, maybe primary pathogens in the foot.

Other organisms are involved in bone infection according to clinical circumstances; *Staph. epidermidis* is the most common cause of implant infection, while coliforms and *Pseudomonas spp.* are associated with vertebral osteomyelitis. Coliforms and anaerobes are found in osteomyelitis of the feet associated with diabetes or arterial insufficiency.

16.1.2 Pathogenesis

There are various sources of organisms causing bone infection. In haematogenous osteomyelitis the source will usually be unrecognized, but rarely metastatic spread from a local infection may occur. In most implant infections the organisms have entered the wound at the time of surgery on skin scales released from surgical staff, or in some cases from the patient's own skin and contaminated instruments. In trauma, the organisms are carried into the wound from the environment, skin and clothing of the patient.

To initiate infection, bacteria must first adhere to a surface, and this has led to the concept of the 'race for the surface' in implant infection. Biomaterial or allograft surfaces present free energy sites which are available for occupation by protein (fibronectin), thus forming a biofilm, or bacteria. Protein paves the way for colonization by tissue cells, which if successful prevents adhesion by bacteria competing for the same sites. The production of slime by some strains of *Staph. epidermidis* reduces antibiotic penetration and may aid their colonization of such surfaces. However, if antibiotic is already present in the milieu of these sites before the arrival of bacteria, prevention of colonization and bacterial growth is much more likely than if bacterial adhesion and slime production have occurred.

What determines the site of haematogenous osteomyelitis is unknown. Sometimes there is a history of previous minor trauma to the affected site, but it is uncertain how this could affect pathogenesis. Turbulent blood flow and lack of polymorphs in the metaphyseal sinusoids might be relevant in the metaphyses of long bones, the classic site of osteomyelitis. In sickle cell disease both local occlusion of small blood vessels and overburdened polymorphonucleocytes may allow bacterial adhesion to endothelium and subsequent bacterial growth. In the feet of diabetics and arteriopaths, local soft tissue infection may invade adjacent bone, and bone elsewhere is subject to contiguous infection.

16.2 SPECIMENS AND LABORATORY REPORTS

16.2.1 Specimens

In general, 'Antibiotics without bacteriology is guesswork'. The recovery of a pathogen allows antibiotic treatment to be specific against that organism, for without it treatment must encompass a broader spectrum of organisms with the disadvantages of increased side effects, costs and a less certain outcome. This is particularly relevant in orthopaedic infection where deep-sited infection may require longer duration of therapy than usual. Every effort should be made to obtain relevant material for culture; if a histological examination is in progress, then part of the sample also should be cultured. It should be noted that: tissue, bone or pus are more efficient than swabs; the specimens should be taken by experienced staff, taking care to avoid contamination from skin organisms; transport should not be delayed; and both direct and enrichment cultures should be performed. A **Gram stain** may reveal the presence of polymorphs and organisms in the wound (if in sufficient numbers to be seen), and this should support (or not) the clinical diagnosis of infection. Treatment should begin if possible after samples have been obtained, even if this involves surgery. In deep infection it is useful to obtain three samples of tissue or bone; consistency of isolates supports their pathogenic role.

16.2.2 Laboratory reports

The clinical relevance of a microbiology report depends largely on the quality of the specimen, and reports should be interpreted strictly according to the clinical findings in the patient. The frequent isolation of *Staph. epidermidis* from implant infections demonstrates the problems of whether the organism is truly infective in the deep tissues, or whether the swab has been contaminated from the skin. The question also remains whether the organism is simply contaminating the tissue surfaces in the absence of a true infection. The finding of polymorphs and bacteria on a Gram film confirms their presence in the wound, and if the bacterial morphology correlates with the culture result it supports the relevance of the cultured organisms. It is always good practice to discuss the implication of reports with a microbiologist, however.

16.3 OSTEOMYELITIS

16.3.1 Acute haematogenous osteomyelitis

DIAGNOSIS

In any form of osteomyelitis there are difficulties both in the clinical diagnosis and in obtaining a pathogen. A delay in diagnosis often occurs because bone infection is not suspected, and a source is seldom apparent. Bone pain and fever, sometimes with a history of trauma, are the classic but limited symptoms. As the focus of infection enlarges, pus collects beneath the periosteum, dead bone forms a sequestrum, and eventually pus penetrates to the surface through a sinus. Frequently patients will have received antibiotics intermittently, and these may have altered the clinical course and reduced the chance of isolating an organism.

It is worthwhile undertaking aspiration or biopsy for bacteriological culture, and blood cultures are very important. The white blood cell (WBC) count, erythrocyte sedimentation rate (ESR) and C-reactive protein level (CRP) may be raised and should be monitored during illness as they are useful markers of response to treatment. An X-ray examination is usually not helpful in diagnosis, since some 30–50% of bone loss is required to detect bone destruction, which needs at least 14 days. Soft tissue swelling with displacement of muscle planes may accompany underlying bone infection, and this can be detected earlier.

^{99m}Technetium scanning will detect areas of increased vascularity in sepsis, new bone formation or prosthesis loosening, but will not distinguish between them. ^{111}Indium white cell labelling will detect areas of white cell accumulation, of whatever cause, and is useful if the results of X-radiography and ^{99m}Technetium scanning are negative. At present, the patient's granulocytes are purified, labelled and re-injected but, in future, labelled monoclonal antibodies against granulocytes might be available; this would be simpler as it involves only a single injection. Magnetic resonance imaging (MRI) is also relevant, particularly for spinal infection and examination of joints, as it may reveal changes earlier than X-radiography.

TREATMENT

The organisms associated with acute osteomyelitis of long bones are predominantly *Staph. aureus*, with group A streptococci, *Strep. pneumoniae*, anaerobes and coliforms occurring much less frequently (Table 16.1). Once a diagnosis has been made, the patient is committed to a course of intravenous and follow-up oral antibiotics for at least some weeks (Table 16.2). The actual length of treatment is debatable, from not less than 3 weeks to as long as 6 months. As stated, such treatment should begin intravenously but can be continued by mouth once a good initial response has been obtained, as judged clinically by symptoms and function.

It is important to detect and remove dead or sequestered bone and any foreign bodies (including metal) which will prevent antibiotic cure and lead to chronic infection. Good antibiotic penetration is ensured by using high doses intravenously, and this route should be used for 2 weeks; oral therapy can then be continued for around 2 months. At this stage it is useful to monitor the antibiotic activity in the patient's blood by 'back titration' to check that the oral dose is sufficient. At 2 hours after ingestion the serum should kill the pathogen or a

Table 16.2 *Treatment of osteomyelitis*

1. Guided by sensitivities of organism if available – particularly important with advent of flucloxacillin (methicillin)-resistant strains of *Staphylococcus aureus*.

2. Standard therapy:
   Flucloxacillin 1–2 g q.d.s., i.v. daily for 14 days
   Fucidin 500 mg t.d.s orally daily for 14 days
   Then orally, flucloxacillin 1 g t.d.s and fucidin 500 mg t.d.s for 2–6 months, depending on clinical response.

3. In true penicillin allergy:
   Clindamycin 600 mg q.d.s daily, i.v. for 2 weeks, followed by 450 mg orally, **or** erythromycin (clarithromycin) 1 g daily (500 mg b.d.), i.v. for 2 weeks, followed by 500 mg once or twice daily orally.

laboratory control strain of *Staph. aureus* at a dilution of at least 1:8; this will be the 'peak' level.

Appropriate antibiotics for treatment are determined by the organism recovered, and by the predominance of *Staph. aureus* as the usual pathogen. If this organism is cultured from the patient it may be assumed to be the pathogen, but if another type of organism is recovered in a clinical picture of acute osteomyelitis, it is carefully to assess its role. For example, *Staph. epidermidis* is an unlikely cause of acute haematogenous infection; coliforms may be secondary invaders and may have a source of infection elsewhere, for example in the urinary tract. Anaerobes can be pathogenic alone, but often occur with other organisms, as does *Pseudomonas*, and both may also be secondary invaders. The results of good quality specimens (e.g. bone or affected tissue) can be relied upon, especially if several samples have been obtained and have yielded the same organism.

Nevertheless, whatever type of organism is recovered, it is appropriate to include potent anti-staphylococcal activity when selecting the antibiotics for treatment. This is not only because the prime role of *Staph. aureus* in acute and chronic haematogenous osteomyelitis may be obscured by secondary invaders, but also because of its ability to persist in bone infection despite return of function.

Flucloxacillin is thus the antibiotic of choice, a dose of 4–6 g per day being required in adults. In view of the acute and destructive nature of the infection a second antibiotic is given in order to improve the rapidity of response by a synergistic or additive action. A combination also helps to provide a total kill of organisms by utilizing different modes of action of antibiotics. The usual second agent is fusidic acid, given by mouth at 500 mg three times daily.

Flucloxacillin is a safe, penicillin-type antibiotic which is excreted via the kidneys; hence, large doses can be given provided that renal function is normal. It is the most potent agent available against *Staph. aureus*. Fucidin has good activity against Gram-positive and Gram-negative cocci, penetrates bone and joint fluid well, and is well tolerated by mouth; however, when given intravenously, reversible liver function changes may occur.

If the patient gives a history of allergy to penicillin it is important to check this carefully, since the potency of flucloxacillin against *Staph. aureus* makes it the drug of choice in osteomyelitis. A clear history of a rash, or of breathing difficulties, or loss of consciousness possibly indicating an anaphylactoid reaction, confirms probable allergy. Erythromycin should then be used, again intravenously (at 2–4 g per day) in combination with fucidin. Erythromycin tends to thrombose peripheral veins and may require a central line; it is associated with liver function changes and, at these doses and duration, with inner-ear toxicity. Alternatively, clindamycin with fucidin is an effective combination in view of the good bone penetration by these agents.

Clindamycin is associated with *Clostridium difficile* diarrhoea, but most individual patients avoid this and it is otherwise well tolerated. Its reputation for this complication is unfortunate in this context, since it is highly effective in osteomyelitis and it has been used successfully as the first-line antibiotic of choice for osteomyelitis. It can be given either by mouth or intravenously. Gentamicin as a second agent to flucloxacillin has the disadvantage of requiring repeated serum assays and dose adjustment, although the single daily dosing regimen is easier to manage and equally effective and safe. It provides cover against coliforms and *Pseudomonas*, as does ciprofloxacin; both agents also have some activity against *Staph. aureus*, which is valuable in this context.

In neonates the incidence of group B streptococci and coliforms makes an exception to the use of flucloxacillin; here, a cephalosporin with anti-staphylococcal activity (e.g. cefuroxime), is appropriate until a bacteriological diagnosis is available. The incidence of *Haemophilus influenzae* osteomyelitis in younger children suggests that the second agent to flucloxacillin in the age group 2 to 5 years should be gentamicin or a cephalosporin; there is a 5 to 30% resistance rate to amoxycillin. *Haemophilus influenzae* bacterium (Hib) vaccination seems to be successful in reducing bone and joint infection as well as meningitis, caused by this organism.

In osteomyelitis due to MRSA the antibiotic of choice is either vancomycin or teicoplanin. These glycopeptides continue (at present) to be the only reliably active agents against this dangerous organism. They act against all Gram-positive cocci, and may also be useful in rare, resistant infections with *Strep. faecalis* (enterococci) and other unusual Gram-positive strains. One problem is that vancomycin is toxic to kidneys and requires serum assay; teicoplanin is used in lower doses and does not require monitoring.

Although some strains of MRSA may show 'in-vitro' sensitivity to clindamycin and gentamicin, it is uncertain whether they should be used in combination with vancomycin and teicoplanin. A better choice is rifampicin; this broad-spectrum bacteriocide is normally reserved for treating tuberculosis, but it is a valid choice here and in other non-responding, serious bacterial bone or joint infections. Side effects include the staining of body secretions and liver toxicity, and advice from a microbiologist and/or a chest physician should be obtained if its use is to be considered. New antibiotics active against Gram-positive bacteria continue to appear. The main problem organism is MRSA. This organism is able to develop resistance to rifampicin fairly rapidly and it should be used in combination with other agents to which the organism is susceptible. Similarly, staphylococci readily become resistant to quinolones in most infected sites. The number of bacteria present in chronic osteomyelitis is small; for this reason some surgeons/microbiologists do use ciprofloxacin in long-term suppressive therapy for osteomyelitis. Published evidence on the efficacy of new fluoroquinolones is awaited. Quinapristin/dalfopristin is a parental antibiotic which may be of value in penicillin-hypersensitive persons. Linezolid is a further compound with a different chemical structure and mode of action to other antibiotic classes. It can be given by mouth or parenterally and is active against almost all staphylococci. It may well have a role in combination with parental agents as initial therapy or as maintenance therapy in ambulent patients. Further results with all these new agents are awaited.

After initiating treatment in hospital, intravenous therapy can be continued at home in suitable patients by the use of syringe pumps. This approach would allow a longer period of intravenous therapy, and so reduce the overall length of treatment by avoiding the oral route.

In summary, well-controlled antibiotic therapy is necessary for cure. Every case of chronic haematogenous osteomyelitis is a case of failed treatment of acute osteomyelitis. Other complications of failure to treat adequately include the general effects of any longstanding infection, i.e. metastatic infection, recurrence and possibly amyloid. Brodie's abscess most likely results from an episode of acute bone infection (see also p. 156).

16.3.2 Vertebral osteomyelitis

Diagnosis of this condition is again difficult; osteomyelitis at this site occurs typically in elderly patients with persistent, localized back pain. Sometimes there is a history of urinary infections or instrumentation. A plexus of veins (Batson's veins) draining both the bladder and the lumbar vertebrae may account for this association, and for the increased incidence of coliforms and *Pseudomonas* as pathogens. Infection is most frequent in the lumbar or thoracic spine; in the cervical spine osteomyelitis may arise by direct spread from local infection in the neck.

Infection usually begins in the metaphyseal area of the vertebral body close to the anterior longitudinal ligament, and may then spread across the adjacent intervertebral disc to the same site of the next vertebrae. This leads to characteristically sited X-ray changes in the vertebral bodies. The disc soon becomes involved, leading to early narrowing of the disc space; this contrasts with tuberculosis, where disc narrowing occurs later. Progress may result in vertebral collapse and paravertebral abscess.

Blood cultures and percutaneous aspiration or formal biopsy should be carried out for bacteriological culture. Attempts to isolate any organism are particularly relevant in view of the wider range of organisms that may be involved. Radiolabelling techniques may also be helpful in diagnosis and localization.

In the absence of a bacterial isolate, broad-spectrum antibiotics (in addition to anti-staphylococcal cover by flucloxacillin) are required and include quinolones or gentamicin to provide cover for coliforms. A history of urinary tract infections should be sought, and the sensitivities of any urinary pathogens taken into account. If *Pseudomonas* has been isolated it is appropriate to initiate treatment with two anti-pseudomonal agents; selection from ceftazidime, ciprofloxacin and gentamicin is appropriate, all of them being active against *Pseudomonas* and each having some (but incomplete) activity against *Staph. aureus.*

Where the patient's history is relevant, or the clinical response slow, mycobacterial infection, brucellosis or fungal infection should be investigated. Specific culture should be requested, and there are serological tests for *Brucella* infection.

16.3.3   Osteomyelitis in the foot

Deep soft tissue infection of the feet in diabetics, and less often in arteriopaths, may lead to osteomyelitis by contiguous spread. It may not be suspected unless X-radiography is performed, but it may account for a slow response to antibiotics. Again, at this site a wider range of organisms including anaerobes may be involved. A suitable choice of antibiotics is clindamycin, which provides good cover against *Staph. aureus* and anaerobes, with a cephalosporin or quinolone for Gram-negative, i.e. coliform, cover. There is a slight advantage to ciprofloxacin in also providing cover for *Pseudomonas.* Both clindamycin and ciprofloxacin can be given by mouth, and this route may be justified since the infection is not usually extensive but may need prolonged treatment. An active approach with broad-spectrum, more prolonged treatment, may prevent or reduce loss of useful tissue by amputation (Table 16.3).

Puncture wounds of the soles of the feet may penetrate deep tissue structures, joints or bone. Organisms from soil and from the heavily colonized soles of shoes and trainers, which may include *Clostridium* spp. and *Pseudomonas* spp., can lead to infection. If the bone or joint has been penetrated, then single-dose prophylaxis should be considered, usually and best given intravenously.

Table 16.3 *Treatment of infection in diabetic feet*

1. Often involves *Staphylococcus aureus* together with coliforms and anaerobes, superficial swabs may be misleading.

2.
1st choice	**2nd choice**	**Also**
Flucloxacillin	Clindamycin	Trimethoprim
Ciprofloxacillin	Ciprofloxacin	Erythromycin
Metronidazole		

3. Initially intravenously, then by mouth for 2–4 weeks.

4. If osteomyelitis present, increase dose and duration of intravenous flucloxacillin.

5. Re-assess surgical approach after appropriate course of antibiotics.

16.3.4   Chronic osteomyelitis

This may follow acute haematogenous osteomyelitis, or it may result from trauma or implant infection. In each of these situations the original infecting organism is likely still to be involved, and even if not recovered bacteriologically should be assumed still to be present when deciding on antibiotics. However, a persisting site of infection, poor blood supply or fracture instability allow other organisms to invade, and mixed cultures are often found. Coliforms, *Pseudomonas* spp. and anaerobes are associated with chronic bone infection and may occur as true pathogens, apparently alone or in mixed infections. Neighbouring soft tissue infection or contamination, especially of open lesions or sinuses which are often found concomitantly, may lead to spurious culture results. Initially intravenous treatment is advantageous and should last between 2 to 4 weeks depending on the severity of the lesion and clinical progress. Progress may be slow and dependent on the removal of dead bone, haematoma, dead space and metal work. Good blood supply and stability of ununited fractures is also needed.

The antibiotic regimen chosen should be active against *Staph. aureus.* Additional antibiotics should be selected according to culture results from reliable tissue or bone samples. If no bacteriology is available, then coliforms and anaerobes should be covered.

Appropriate antibiotics include combinations of flucloxacillin with ciprofloxacin, or a cephalosporin with anti-staphylococcal activity; metronidazole may be added to both if necessary. If *Pseudomonas* is suspected to have a pathogenic role, the use of two agents with anti-pseudomonal activity, (e.g. ceftazidime, gentamicin or ciprofloxacin) is efficient. Thienamycins are relevant, but are not required if the strain is sensitive to the agents mentioned. In view of the lack of oral agents active against *Pseudomonas,* there is a role for domiciliary intravenous therapy for chronic pseudomonal osteomyelitis. Ciprofloxacin can be used by mouth, but subsequent resistance by the organisms can develop.

CASE HISTORY

A 'sportsman knee'

A man aged 22 years experienced a painful knee when running. A lateral release operation was performed, but 6 days later the knee became exquisitely painful and tender, with some swelling and reddening of the skin. He attended an A&E department where a haematoma was diagnosed; 14 hours later he re-attended and an aspirate of the joint was obtained. This yielded *Staphylococcus aureus* 2 days later. The man was then admitted and treated with intravenous flucloxacillin. A slow recovery ensued, although further aspiration was not performed. Unfortunately, the patient lost a season of sporting activity and the chance of a place on a National team.

Irrigation systems to deliver local antibiotics are difficult to set up, and are of doubtful value. Moreover, they may be vulnerable to contamination from handling and improperly prepared fluids, leading to secondary infection. It is more reliable to ensure that there are adequate serum concentrations of antibiotics, and a good blood supply.

Gentamicin beads provide good local concentrations of the antibiotic, with activity against staphylococci and coliforms. They are particularly useful in cavities and in treating pseudomonal infection, but should be used in conjunction with adequate systemic therapy.

In infected fracture, non-union, radical débridement to remove sequestra and loose metal ensuring stability and vascular supply are required. Repeated debridement, with plating, bone grafting and skin flaps may be necessary as healing progresses. The use of external stabilizing devices allows improved management of infected fracture sites by avoiding foreign bodies in the wound area, and facilitating good access for debridement and dressings.

16.3.5 Brodie's abscess

This is a chronic abscess in bone without antecedent evidence of infection. Typically, a young adult complains of local pain on use. X-radiography shows a lucent defect bordered by sclerotic reaction, usually in a long bone. Biopsy is required for confirmation by histology and culture, since osteoid osteoma or malignancy may present in a similar way. Occasionally *Staph. aureus* will be recovered.

16.3.6 Discitis

Infection of the intervertebral (usually lumbar) discs can occur primarily in children, and also after spinal operations or unusually as a primary infection in adults. Diagnosis is difficult; children and adults present with chronic back pain without increased WBC count, but may have a raised ESR. X-radiography shows narrowing of the disc space, with or without irregular erosion of the adjacent vertebral end plates. Biopsy or aspiration may

yield *Staph. aureus*. Prolonged antibiotic therapy, possibly for as long as 6 months, with agents active against this organism is required, with progress monitored by X-radiography and ESR. Postoperative cases may follow initial recovery, with increased symptoms, WBC count and X-ray changes after some weeks. Clinical suspicion should be aroused in postoperative cases where recovery is slow and new symptoms develop.

16.4 INFECTIVE ARTHRITIS

Haematogenous bacterial joint infection occurs predominantly in the knee followed by the hip, shoulder and ankle, with other joints involved less frequently (Table 16.4). The causative organisms are similar to those in osteomyelitis. In neonates, group B streptococci and coliforms, and in children group A streptococci and *Haemophilus* (where Hib vaccination is not carried out) are important minority pathogens in addition to *Staph. aureus*. In young adults, *Neisseria gonorrhoeae* infection may result in systemic symptoms with polyarthritis. Characteristic erythematous papules (which may become vesicular) often appear on the skin and help in the diagnosis, since the joint fluid usually fails to yield the

Table 16.4 *Percentage frequency of joint involvement in infective arthritis*

	Children	Adults
Knee	41	48
Hip	23	24
Ankle	14	7
Elbow	12	11
Wrist	4	7
Shoulder	4	15
Interphalangeal and metacarpal	1.4	1
Sternoclavicular	0.4	8
Sacroiliac	0.4	2

Adapted from Mandell, G.L., Douglas, R.G. and Bennett, J.E. (eds), *Principles and Practice of Infectious Disease*, 3rd edition. John Wiley & Sons, New York.

organism. This organism can also present as a mono-articular suppurative joint infection with recovery of the organism from joint fluid. Blood cultures are helpful in both forms, as indeed they are in any bacterial arthritis. *Streptococcus pneumoniae* joint infection may occur in any age group. Precipitating events for infective arthritis include intra-articular steroid injection, recent knee operation and trauma, in each of which *Staph. aureus* is usual. In septicaemia, metastatic infection may develop in a joint. Rheumatoid arthritis and perhaps diabetes and other concomitant illness may predispose to joint infection.

Diagnosis requires blood cultures and joint aspiration. Acute mononuclear arthritis should always arouse suspicion of bacterial infection, although gout, chondrocalcinosis and rheumatoid arthritis may present in a similar way. Similarly, in a warm, painful and swollen joint after surgery or trauma, a haematoma needs to be carefully distinguished from infection by the level of pyrexia, WBC count and culture of aspirate.

Treatment needs to be prompt; an initial choice of flucloxacillin intravenously with fucidin by mouth is appropriate, with alternative antibiotics as for osteomyelitis (Table 16.5). Depending on the patient's response, a total of 2–4 weeks' treatment is usual with the first one or two weeks' treatment given intravenously. Intra-articular injections of antibiotics are not necessary since adequate systemic doses will enter inflamed joints.

Other causes of infective arthritis include *Candida* spp., as a secondary invader or opportunist in immunocompromised patients. Mycobacteria and *Brucella* spp. may cause monoarticular arthritis. Viruses, including hepatitis B and rubella, and mycoplasmas are associated with arthritis occurring as part of a systemic infection with these organisms.

Infectious diarrhoea with *Shigella*, *Salmonella*, *Campylobacter* and *Yersinia* is occasionally followed by postinfectious or 'reactive' arthritis, usually 2–3 weeks after the acute illness. The organisms cannot be recovered from joint fluid, and the arthritis – which occurs more often in patients with HLA B27 – is abscribed to the immune response. In Lyme disease due to injection of *Borrelia burgdorferi* (a spirochaete) by ticks, arthritis is often a presenting symptom, but organisms are not obtained and the typical skin rash and exposure history should be sought.

Osteomyelitis in sickle cell disease

Sickle cell disease represents a group of syndromes consequent on the inheritance of the haemoglobin S (HbS) gene from one parent, and an abnormal haemoglobin gene from the other parent. The most common form of sickle cell disease at birth is **homozygous sickle cell (SS) disease** in which the HbS gene is inherited from both parents, but other conditions include the double heterozygote sickle cell-haemoglobin C (SC) disease, sickle cell-β^+ thalassaemia and sickle cell-β° thalassaemia. The relative frequencies of these conditions at birth in Jamaica is 1 in 300 for SS disease, 1 in 500 for SC disease, 1 in 3000 for S-β^+ thalassaemia, and 1 in 7000 for S-β° thalassaemia. The **sickle cell trait** (AS) genotype in which the HbS gene is inherited from one parent and a normal gene for HbA from the other parent is a harmless carrier state, and should not be included within the term sickle cell disease.

Sickle cell disease is characterized by a tendency for the HbS molecules in red cells to polymerize on deoxygenation causing the cell to sickle. Sickled cells lack the pliability of normal erythrocytes and are rapidly destroyed in the circulation (haemolysis). They also block the flow in blood vessels (vaso-occlusion), causing ischaemia and death of the tissue supplied. These processes are most common in the relatively severe SS disease and S-β° thalassaemia, but less common in the mild SC disease and S-β^+ thalassaemia. Ischaemic damage is common in the bone marrow because of its high metabolic demands, the result being bone marrow necrosis. The clinical pattern of such necrosis is determined by the age of the patient; the condition affects the small bones of the hands and feet (dactylitis) in young children, the shafts of the long bones (avascular necrosis of bone) in older children, and the juxta-articular areas of the long bones (painful crisis) in older children and young adults. A special form of the latter process may also affect the femoral head which, with continued weight-bearing, may collapse resulting in characteristic avascular necrosis of the femoral head and (somewhat less importantly) of the humeral head.

Necrotic bone marrow is prone to infection by organisms gaining access to the blood, and such bacteraemias are more common in SS disease, probably because of the early loss of splenic function. The resulting osteomyelitis is most commonly caused by *Salmonella* species and may result in extensive bone damage, drainage of pus through chronic sinuses, and death of parts of the bone which then remain as a sequestrum. Clinically, there is a spectrum of involvement with pain and swelling of the affected area of bone and systemic symptoms such as fever, but the clinical distinction of sterile avascular

Table 16.5 *Treatment of infective arthritis*

1. Guided by sensitivities of organism – particularly important with advent of flucloxacillin (methicillin)-resistant strains of *Staphylococcus aureus* and role of other organisms.

2. Initial standard therapy if no isolate available:
   Flucloxacillin 1–2 g q.d.s., i.v. daily
   Fucidin 500 mg t.d.s orally daily for 1 week,
   thereafter continue i.v. or orally, depending on clinical response.

3. In penicillin allergy:
   Clindamyin **or** erythromycin for 1 week i.v. and then orally
   as above in doses as for osteomyelitis

necrosis from osteomyelitis is not easy, even with modern scintigraphic and nuclear medicine techniques. A diagnosis of osteomyelitis is more likely with more extensive swelling and systemic symptoms, more dramatic radiological change, and the presence of a sinus. The frequency with which organisms are isolated depends upon the aggressiveness of investigation and is higher with aspiration of bone marrow, trephine biopsy, or grinding up and culture of removed sequestra. Although blood cultures may be negative even in the presence of confirmed osteomyelitis, it is wise to treat with anti-*Salmonella* therapy such as chloramphenicol or third-generation cephalosporins. **Surgery** may be indicated to improve drainage, evacuate dead or infected bone, or removal of sequestra. Osteomyelitis complicating avascular necrosis of the femoral head presents a special challenge because of its position. This complication is underdiagnosed, and should be suspected in cases with particularly rapid destruction of the femoral head. Surgery may require removal of the infected femoral head, but total hip replacement cannot be contemplated until local infection has been eradicated.

(Contributed by G.R. Serjeant)

16.5 IMPLANT INFECTIONS

Most infections of prostheses whether immediately postoperative, early (i.e. up to 3 months after operation) or late, arise from organisms seeded into the operation site at the time of surgery. Although antibiotic prophylaxis is now universal, occasional failures of prophylaxis are to be expected for a number of reasons: resistant organisms; a large input of organisms; sequestration of bacteria in haematomas or other areas with poor blood supply; 'resting' organisms; or a lag phase extending to a time when serum levels are declining. More than one predisposing cause is possible in an individual case, especially with poor technique or a contaminated environment.

Infection occurring within 10 days of surgery should be rare and is nearly always due to *Staph. aureus*. A swollen, warm joint within a few days of surgery is usually due to haematoma, but infection is always to be considered. If infection is found soon after surgery, the theatre procedures should be reviewed, since it is probably infected with *Staph. aureus* and originated during surgery and may indicate a lapse in procedure or an unrecognized source of infection.

Infection which appears weeks to several months after surgery is commonly due to *Staph. epidermidis*, with coliforms, anaerobes and *Staph. aureus* as less common causes. Symptoms are difficult to distinguish from those of loosening. The WBC count is seldom raised, but if the ESR or CRP are raised this suggests infection; [111]indium labelling and [99]technetium scanning are positive in both. In most cases there is little opportunity to culture the organism, but aspiration of the joint is worthwhile because the joint space communicates with the interface between metal and bone. This procedure should be performed more often, repeated if necessary and may be diagnostic. Previous intermittent antibiotics will reduce positive cultures.

The frequency of late haematogenous infection is difficult to decide upon; reports in which the proposed source organism and pathogen are well correlated are few in number.

Treatment is also difficult, and is often started on a 'trial' basis because of uncertain diagnosis and lack of an isolate. Nevertheless, a formal period of broad-spectrum, anti-staphyloccocal, intravenous antibiotic is worthwhile, followed by oral administration for some weeks if a clinical or ESR response appears. Appropriate antibiotics are similar to those described for osteomyelitis, with a broad-spectrum approach. Thus, an anti-staphylococcal cephalosporin with metronidazole, flucloxacillin with gentamicin, and clindamycin are all appropriate. If there is a past history of colonization or infection with MRSA or MRSE, consideration will have to be given to using teicoplanin or vancomycin; however, these glycopeptides are active only against Gram-positive organisms, and additional cover for coliforms and anaerobes might be required (Table 16.6).

In very frail elderly patients who are unfit for revision arthroplasty, in patients who refuse operation, or where revision would be difficult because of loss of bone stock, a long-term, (perhaps permanent) course of suppressive antibiotics can be considered. Patients have been maintained in some circumstances on long-term oral cephalosporins and ciprofloxacin, the aim being to suppress clinical symptoms and prevent further deterioration. Unfortunately, failure and side effects often occur.

16.6 HAND INFECTIONS

Hand infections are common, dangerous and taxing. Their importance, especially in association with trauma needs to be recognized. Loss of useful hand and finger

Table 16.6 *Treatment of joint implant infection*

1. Infection will be almost impossible to eliminate without removal of the implant.

2. Joint aspiration in order to obtain organisms (may be diagnostic).

3. Two-stage replacement procedure probably preferable. After removal, intravenous flucloxacillin and fucidin, clindamycin or rifampicin for 1–2 weeks, then continue 2 weeks after replacement.

4. In frail, elderly patients, or poor bone stock, where further operation would be problematical or refused by patient, long-term suppressive therapy can be worthwhile.

tissues (e.g. pulp), or even parts of a digit, can have a devastating impact on employment.

In acute purulent infection there should be a low threshold for exploration and debridement. Antibiotics alone are unlikely to cure deep compartmentalized infections, for example, in the palmar spaces, tendon sheaths or joints of the hand.

The organisms most often initiating infection are *Staph. aureus* and group A streptococci. Anaerobes are not infrequent. *Eikenella* spp. and *Pasteurella multocida* may follow human and animal bites respectively, while coliforms are usually secondary invaders. In deep trauma and bite wounds prophylaxis is appropriate (see Chapter 15; Table 15.2).

In deep infection, antibiotics should be given intravenously, then orally after 2–7 days, depending on the response – which should be rapid in uncomplicated cases. Flucloxacillin and metronidazole are appropriate first-choice agents (in animal bites, cephalosporin and metronidazole). Frequent re-evaluation of progress is called for, especially if antibiotics alone are used. In the latter case early response should be forthcoming; if not, exploration and investigation should be made for deep space infection, spreading infection along fascial planes, and infection of tendon sheaths, bone and joints. In trauma a search should be made for foreign bodies, and in bites for deeper unsuspected infection or damage, e.g. in punch injuries of the metacarpophalangeal joint.

Herpes simplex causes a **whitlow**, a non-purulent painful swelling of the fingers or thumb. Often there is a history of contact and there may be surface vesicles. The lesion should not be incised. Acyclovir may or may not influence the self-limiting course of infection, but if prescribed, it should be given early-on.

The hand can be the site of unusual infection, e.g. **erysipelothrix** if there is contact with fish or farm animals, especially pigs; anthrax after contact with raw hides; and *Mycobacterium marinum* after abrasions acquired from aquaria or swimming pools. Other mycobacteria, including *M. tuberculosis,* are a cause of tenosynovitis.

16.7 UNUSUAL INFECTIONS

Tuberculosis should always be considered in unusual or non-responding musculoskeletal lesions, particularly in Asians. Definitive diagnosis rests upon histology and culture, the former being more sensitive and faster. X-radiography may reveal underlying bony lysis, and a chest X-ray is usually positive. Bone infection most commonly presents in the spine followed by the limb joints, but may occur in any part of the skeleton.

The history is insidious, the lesion persisting in some cases despite usual antibiotic treatment. Chemotherapy is by rifampicin and isoniazid, with pyrazinamide, streptomycin or ethambutol as a third agent. Triple therapy is for an initial 2 to 3-month period, followed by 1–2 years' therapy in total. The advice of a chest physician should be sought.

Less common mycobacterial infections are *Mycobacterium marinum*, which may cause a granulomatous soft tissue lesion and *M. avium intracellulare*, which may cause a metastatic bone infection from a pulmonary focus in immunocompromised patients.

Brucellosis may also present as a chronic granulomatous lesion, often in the spine. Suspicion should be raised by a history of relevant occupation, exposure or geographical origin, particularly the Middle East. Diagnosis rests upon culture (the laboratory should be informed of the suspected diagnosis as culture is not routine) and serology, which is usually reliable. Treatment is dual therapy with doyxcycline, co-trimoxazole or rifampicin, for 6 weeks, with the advice of an infectious disease expert.

Fungal infections, apart from candidiasis, are rare and occur predominantly in immunocompromised patients as opportunist pathogens. A longstanding, granulomatous lesion not responding to treatment, where mycobacteria have been excluded, requires histological examination for these organisms. In the Americas, blastomycosis, coccidioidomycosis and histoplasmosis occur as true pathogens, but the absence of a travel history will exclude these. These and the following infections require specialist advice in diagnosis and treatment:

CASE HISTORY

Recurrent spinal tuberculosis

A middle-aged Asian lady who did not speak English presented with backache. X-ray revealed a lytic lesion at T6, and softening of the psoas shadow. As blood cultures and chest X-radiography were negative, she was started on antituberculosis therapy and sent home. Two months later she presented at another hospital with more severe symptoms and a psoas abscess, from which *Mycobacterium tuberculosis* was cultured. Therapy was restarted and the care of the patient shared with the chest clinic. She made a good recovery. The case had not been notified initially and she did not attend outpatient clinics. She had stopped taking therapy on discharge from hospital.

- **Candida** occurs more often in joints than bone. It is easily cultured, and care must be taken to exclude contamination. Demonstration of mycelial infiltration of tissue by wet potassium hydroxide preparation or histology confirms pathogenicity. Treatment is with fluconazole or amphotericin for more serious lesions.
- **Aspergillus** may extend from the lungs to ribs or the spine, and from the paranasal sinuses to the orbital bones. Again, demonstration of actual tissue invasion is required for diagnosis, as the organism is easy to culture and specimens may be contaminated. Treatment is difficult, amphotericin is partially effective, and surgery may well be required.
- **Cryptococcosis** is a ubiquitous yeast-like fungus which infects the lungs primarily, but may metastasize to the meninges, soft tissues and bone. Histology and culture will make the diagnosis and distinguish the lesion from sarcoma and other tumours. A serological test for the antigen may be helpful in disseminated disease. Treatment involves amphotericin, flucytosone and surgery.
- **Mycetoma** of which 'Madura foot' is one form, is caused by a number of fungi, mainly in India, Africa and Central America. The tissues become 'woody', sinuses and later bone infection may develop. Histological demonstration of fungal invasion and positive culture confirm the clinical diagnosis. Treatment involves sulphones, streptomycin or other agents depending on the species found, together with surgery.
- **Miscellaneous fungi**, e.g. *Pseudoallescheria boydi* and *Mucor* occur, and require expert help in diagnosis in treatment.

16.8 ANTIBIOTIC PROPHYLAXIS

16.8.1 Rationale

The presence of antibiotic in the tissues and blood during the insertion of prostheses has been shown to reduce subsequent infection seven-fold; infection seriously threatens the viability of the implant. Prophylaxis is routine for prosthetic surgery and has become conventional for surgery involving most metal implants, e.g. pin and plating. Antibiotic prophylaxis has an additive effect to that of ultraclean air laminar flow theatre systems. The timing, duration and type of antibiotic required for prophylaxis has become established over the past two decades, but many surgeons still use inefficient regimens, often only given in small doses, and continued after 24 hours when no added benefit accrues.

Prophylactic antibiotics should be given intravenously at the start of the operation; that is, after anaesthesia is established and before the first incision. The aim of prophylaxis is to kill organisms being deposited within the field of operation while the tissues are exposed; once the incision is closed this route of infection ceases (see Section 16.1). Thus, provided that the operation does not extend beyond 3 hours, a single dose is sufficient. Replenishment at 3 hours is necessary, since the half-life of many penicillin-type antibiotics is about 90 minutes.

16.8.2 Antibiotics regimens

The organisms found in implant infections determine the choice of drug. The predominance of staphylococci and the lesser incidence of anaerobes and coliforms make those cephalosporins which have potent anti-staphylococcal activity appropriate. Flucloxacillin and gentamicin are also appropriate, and in both regimens metronidazole is given. Resistance among staphylococci increasingly threatens the efficacy of these antibiotics, and substantial numbers of *Staph. epidermidis* (MRSE) and *Staph. aureus* (MRSA) show resistance to flucloxacillin and cephalosporins. Isolates from infected prostheses should be monitored for their antibiotic susceptibilities to help decide on policies for prophylactic regimens. Patients previously infected or colonized with resistant staphylococci should probably receive teicoplanin or vancomycin for prophylaxis. Any intercurrent infection in a patient due for a planned procedure should be eliminated before surgery.

CASE HISTORY

A non-responding spinal abscess

A middle-aged man presented with a spinal abscess. Tissue removed at operation failed to culture organisms (including *Mycobacterium tuberculosis*), and he was treated with anti-staphylococcal antibiotics. One month later, neither symptoms nor signs had improved; compliance was checked and serological tests for fungi considered. A re-examination of the patient's history revealed that he had worked in the Middle East. Serological tests for brucellosis were positive, and a cure was achieved with appropriate therapy.

CASE HISTORY

A successful hip replacement?

A 60-year-old woman underwent a hip replacement for arthritis. About 6 months later, progressive intermittent pain occurred in the hip, particularly when walking. There was no pyrexia, raised WBC count or X-ray changes, but the ESR was slightly raised. At 10 months after the surgery antibiotics were given because of continuing symptoms, but without much benefit. However, a serological test available at the time indicated raised antibodies to *Staphylococcus epidermidis*. Further antibiotic treatment was without effect. A two-stage replacement operation was performed, and *Staphylococcus epidermidis* was recovered from tissue samples. Intravenous antibiotics were given for 2 weeks before the second stage, and continued for 2 weeks postoperatively; this led to a cure.

16.8.3   Procedures requiring antibiotic prophylaxis

Prophylaxis should be given for operations requiring the implantation of prostheses and metal work. Operations involving bone without insertion of metal and arthroscopic procedures, especially short-time procedures, do not justify prophylaxis, in view of the low incidence of infection. However, prophylaxis is required in limb amputation, primarily to prevent gas gangrene since clostridial spores resist skin disinfection. Compound fractures also require antibiotic prophylaxis or therapy (see Chapter 15).

In patients undergoing prosthetic replacement for loosening or infection, multiple tissue samples should be cultured on removal of the old prosthesis. In a two-stage procedure the antibiotics for treatment or prophylaxis can be orientated to the isolates found.

Irrigation of wounds with antibiotic solutions for prophylaxis during or after surgery is unnecessary (if adequate systemic antibiotics are given), as this may introduce contamination.

16.8.4   Preventing infection in prosthetic joints

Infections in prosthetic joints can occur months or years after insertion, and although most are probably due to hitherto 'quiescent' organisms which were seeded at the time of surgery, some are due to haematogenous spread from a remote source. This is the reason for protecting prostheses in conditions where bacteraemias may occur, e.g. in dirty or clean/contaminated surgery, bladder catheterization, soft tissue and other infections, and periodontal disease treatment. However, there is scanty evidence for the efficacy of such prophylaxis. Perhaps in rheumatoid patients, who are more susceptible to prosthetic infection, there is more justification,

otherwise individual experience will dictate practice. Appropriate antibiotics are those with a broad spectrum and good anti-staphylococcal activity which can be given orally, e.g. co-amoxyclav, cephalosporin or clindamycin.

16.8.5   Antibiotic-containing cement

Various antibiotics (usually gentamicin) can be incorporated into cement and will leak into surrounding tissues after insertion, giving protection from infection. Even without systemic antibiotics gentamicin cement is effective, but it is advisable and common practice also to use systemic antibiotic prophylaxis. Impregnated cement is commonly used for revision arthroplasty, which has a greater risk of infection than primary. Gentamicin cannot be detected in serum or urine beyond a few days, but probably continues to be present at the implant–bone interface for many months. The possibility of generating bacterial resistance and allergic reactions seems remote.

16.8.6   Prophylaxis and tourniquets

Extruding blood from a limb and applying a tourniquet will prevent diffusion of antibiotics from the blood stream to the operation site. However, it has been shown that adequate levels of antibiotics will reach joint fluid 20 minutes after intravenous injection, and such a time interval should be allowed between injection and the application of a tourniquet.

Recently, it has been shown that injection of antibiotic into veins in the foot after applying a tourniquet results in effective antibiotic concentrations in the knee, the penetration being thought to occur via the lymphatic system. Indeed, this would lead to a simpler approach to prophylaxis for knee replacement.

16.9 FURTHER READING

Adams, J.C. and Hamblen, D.L. (1995) *Outline of Orthopaedics*, 12th edition., Churchill Livingstone, Edinburgh.

Coombs, R. and Fitzgerald, R.H. (1989) *Infection in the Orthopaedic Patient*. Butterworths, London.

Gustilo, R.B., Gruninger, R.P. and Tsukayama, D.T. (1989) *Orthopaedic Infection: Diagnosis and Treatment*. W.B. Saunders, Philadelphia.

Howard, R.J. and Simmons, R.L. (1995) *Surgical Infectious Diseases*, 3rd edition. Appleton and Lange, East Norwalk, Connecticut, USA.

Infections in neurosurgery

E.M. BROWN AND R. BAYSTON

17.1 INTRODUCTION

In recent years the prognoses of patients with a broad range of neurological diseases have been improved and the status of contemporary medicine in general has been enhanced by remarkable developments in neurosurgery. These include the introduction of sophisticated and highly sensitive diagnostic techniques, such as computerized tomography (CT) and magnetic resonance imaging (MRI), novel and imaginative operative procedures and innovative, non-operative therapeutic modalities. It is disappointing therefore that developments in the prevention and treatment of infection in neurosurgical patients have not kept pace with progress in virtually all other aspects of the specialty. Indeed, current practice and guidelines for prophylaxis and therapy in neurosurgery owe almost nothing to evidence-based medicine. This is largely because contemporary practice has been, and continues to be, heavily influenced by tradition, personal experience, innate conservatism and, in particular, a literature that is replete with poorly designed and executed clinical trials. It is against this background that the prevention and treatment of patients with those infections most commonly encountered in neurosurgical practice are addressed.

17.2 CHEMOPROPHYLAXIS

Although the incidence of infection following neurosurgery is relatively low, this complication is an important cause of patient morbidity. Apparently trivial or superficial sepsis at the operative site may progress to osteomyelitis, meningitis, cerebritis, abscess formation or even death. It may delay the patient's discharge from hospital, lead to further surgery and ultimately increase the overall cost of hospital care. Antibiotics have been used extensively for many years to prevent post-operative infections, although unequivocal support for their efficacies does not exist. This is not because there have been too few attempts to resolve this issue, but rather because virtually all of the many clinical trials have suffered from major flaws in design and/or execution. The following recommendations relating to chemoprophylaxis in neurosurgery draw heavily on guidelines issued by the Infection in Neurosurgery Working Party of the British Society for Antimicrobial Chemotherapy.

17.2.1 Clean non-implant procedures

In the absence of prophylaxis the incidence of infection following clean, non-implant neurosurgical procedures has varied widely from less than 1% to 18%, with 3–4% being the average. Most early studies demonstrated that antibiotics reduce the incidence of post-operative infection; however, all but three of these were retrospective. The more recent trials, most of which were prospective, have also shown that prophylaxis in clean neurosurgical procedures is significantly better than either a placebo or no treatment. Although these studies enrolled far fewer patients than would be necessary to demonstrate statistical significance, the likelihood that they all independently reached the wrong conclusion is remote. This led four reviewers and the authors of a working party report on infections in neurosurgery to recommend that prophylaxis should be administered to patients undergoing clean, non-implant surgical procedures. However, in none of these cases was a distinction made between craniotomy and spinal surgery, and a closer inspection of the data yields a different impression, at least insofar as the benefits of prophylaxis to spinal surgery patients are concerned.

In four prospective controlled studies which were published in neurosurgical journals the investigators evaluated the efficacy of prophylaxis in clean non-implant neurosurgical procedures and calculated the post-operative wound infection rates for patients undergoing craniotomy separately from those undergoing spinal surgery. Despite clearly differentiating between the procedures, they then combined the data for the two categories of patients and concluded, on the basis of the overall results, that the use of prophylaxis was associated with a statistically significant benefit in terms of reducing the incidence of post-operative wound infections. In doing so, the investigators allowed the much larger craniotomy data to exaggerate the effects of prophylaxis on patients undergoing spinal surgery. When the wound infection rates for patients undergoing craniotomy and spinal surgery are analyzed separately, they confirm the efficacy of prophylaxis in craniotomy patients, but suggest that it is not of benefit to spinal surgery patients. It must be acknowledged that all four trials were underpowered, thereby raising the possibility of a Type II error.

The only study in the orthopaedic literature which investigated the efficacy of antibiotic prophylaxis in patients undergoing lumbar spinal surgery (laminectomy or discectomy) also failed to show that prophylaxis was significantly better than placebo in terms of reducing the incidence of post-operative wound infection. This study, in common with those described above, was underpowered and the results must be interpreted with caution. For the time being, the role of antibiotic prophylaxis in spinal surgery must be regarded as undetermined and each surgeon will therefore need to reach a decision independently whether or not to adopt this practice. A special case might be made for patients undergoing discectomy, for whom discitis is an infrequent but serious post-operative complication. To date, no prospective, randomized clinical trials in which adequate numbers of patients were enrolled have evaluated the efficacy of antibiotic prophylaxis in this clinical setting. However, based on the limited results of animal studies and two flawed clinical trials, and because of the severe morbidity associated with discitis and the marginal benefits of antibiotics on the course and outcome of this infection once it develops, it is widely perceived that the benefits of prophylaxis outweigh the risks in patients undergoing discectomy.

Many different antimicrobials have been used as prophylaxis in clean non-implant neurosurgery. While all of these agents have been reported to be effective, very few comparative studies have been undertaken to establish whether any single antibiotic, or combination of agents, has clear superiority over the other regimens.

A suitable prophylactic agent should achieve therapeutic concentrations in the tissues of the operative field; the ability to penetrate into cerebrospinal fluid (CSF) is not a prerequisite. The choice must also take account of the nature and susceptibility patterns of the principal pathogens, these being *Staphylococcus aureus*, aerobic Gram-negative bacilli (AGNB) and streptococci. Flucloxacillin, which has been a popular choice in the past, is suboptimal because it does not provide cover against AGNB. In a number of studies, cephalosporins were found to be active *in vitro* against more than 80% of the bacteria isolated from operative site infections. Although experience with these agents in neurosurgery has been limited to a few non-comparative clinical trials, albeit with excellent results, either a first- or second-generation cephalosporin, e.g., cefradine, cefazolin, cefuroxime and cefamandole, fulfils the above criteria. Patients who are allergic to cephalosporins and those who are known to be either colonized or infected with strains of methicillin-resistant *S. aureus* (MRSA) should receive a combination of a glycopeptide (vancomycin or teicoplanin) and gentamicin. Single doses, given by the intravenous route at induction of anaesthesia, are adequate unless the procedure extends beyond 4 hours (8 hours if prophylaxis comprised a glycopeptide and gentamicin), in which case intra-operative doses (50% of the initial dosage) should be administered every 4 hours (8 hours if prophylaxis comprised a glycopeptide and gentamicin) for the duration of the surgery; vancomycin and gentamicin must be used with caution in patients with impaired renal function or who might be at risk of developing toxicity following treatment with these drugs. Additional doses in the post-operative period are not indicated and extending the duration of prophylaxis to 'cover' lines, drains or catheters is unwarranted. The dosing regimens are summarized in Table 17.1.

17.2.2 Clean-contaminated procedures

Clean-contaminated neurosurgical operations are those procedures during which, deliberately or otherwise, one or more cranial air sinuses are crossed in the absence of

Table 17.1 *Dosages and routes of administration of antibiotics recommended for prophylaxis in patients undergoing neurosurgical procedures*[a]

Antibiotic	Dosage of first dose	Dosage of subsequent doses[b]	Route of administration
Cefradine	1 g (25 mg/kg)[c]	500 mg (12.5 mg/kg)	intravenous
Cefazolin	1 g (25 mg/kg)	500 mg (12.5 mg/kg)	intravenous
Cefuroxime	1.5 g (25 mg/kg)	750 mg (12.5 mg/kg)	intravenous
Cefamandole	1 g (25 mg/kg)	500 mg (12.5 mg/kg)	intravenous
Co-amoxiclav	1.2 g (30 mg/kg)	600 mg (15 mg/kg)	intravenous
Metronidazole	500 mg (7.5 mg/kg)	250 mg (4 mg/kg)	intravenous
Vancomycin[d]	1 g (15 mg/kg)	500 mg (7.5 mg/kg)	intravenous
Teicoplanin	800 mg (10 mg/kg)	400 mg (5 mg/kg)	intravenous
Gentamicin[d]	3 mg/kg (3 mg/kg)	1.5 mg/kg (1.5 mg/kg)	intravenous
Vancomycin	10 mg[e]	NA[f]	intraventricular
Gentamicin	3 mg	NA	intraventricular

[a]Adapted from: Infection in Neurosurgery Working Party of the British Society for Antimicrobial Chemotherapy, *Lancet* 1994; **344**: 1547–51.
[b]Administered at 4-hourly intervals (8-hourly for glycopeptides and gentamicin) for operative procedures of ≥ 4 hours duration (≥ 8 hours if patient is receiving a glycopeptide/aminoglycoside regimen).
[c]Dosage for children.
[d]Must be used with caution in patients who have impaired renal function or who are at risk of toxicity from these drugs.
[e]Adminstered in 1 mL of water for injection.
[f]Not applicable (additional doses not required).

pre-existing infection; operations which gain access via the naso- or oropharynx also fall into this category. Transphenoidal and transoral surgical procedures differ from those that cross the air sinuses by virtue of the fact that the surgical wound remains within the contaminated field. In the case of transphenoidal surgery there is only a limited degree of wound closure and the local anatomy facilitates natural drainage away from the wound site. Whether the incidence of wound infection following transoral/transphenoidal surgery is higher or lower because of these factors is not known.

There are virtually no useful data on the incidences of infection associated with such procedures, reports from the 1960s and 1970s being discounted because of the significant changes in surgical technique that have since been introduced. It is reasonable to assume, however, that the incidence of post-operative infection following clean-contaminated operations is not less than that following clean operations and, for this reason, prophylaxis is deemed appropriate for procedures falling into the former category.

The choice of antibiotics to be used as prophylaxis against wound infection following clean-contaminated procedures should take account of the local mucosal flora which normally comprise a mixture of both aerobic and anaerobic bacteria. Because of the latter organisms, co-amoxiclav would be a suitable choice; a combination of a first- or second-generation cephalosporin and metronidazole should be given to penicillin-allergic patients. (See Table 17.1 for the dosages of these agents.)

A single dose of either regimen should be administered with induction of anaesthesia. For prolonged operations, further doses should be given at 4-hourly intervals until the end of the procedure.

17.2.3 Cerebrospinal fluid shunt surgery

Infection remains one of the most frequent and potentially serious complications of CSF shunt surgery. Although infrequently fatal, each episode of ventriculitis increases the degree of neurological damage, especially if it is accompanied by shunt obstruction. Considerable morbidity may also result from secondary complications such as septicaemia, adhesive peritonitis and shunt nephritis. Reported rates of infection have varied from 0–39%. While most fall within the range of 10–15%, more recently, rates of 2–5% have become more common. Approximately 70% of infections are diagnosed within the 2 months immediately following implantation, the incidence declining thereafter. This suggests that the pathogens are probably introduced at the time of the operation.

A large number of studies have attempted to determine whether prophylactic antibiotics minimize the risks of infection in patients undergoing shunt surgery. However, many of the published clinical trials have been either uncontrolled or have used historical control groups and have included so few patients that the data are unsuitable for statistical analysis. These criticisms aside, the contradictory results of the studies make it impossible to conclude whether antibiotics have an impact on the incidence of infection. Two recent meta-analyses have attempted to resolve this issue. Each showed that only one or two of the trials included in the analyses achieved statistical significance favouring prophylaxis (although the others demonstrated a trend in the same direction), but when all of the studies were analyzed together, the administration of antibiotics was associated with a statistically significant reduction in the incidence of shunt infection. More detailed analysis of the data by one of the groups of investigators revealed that a protective effect was limited to those studies in which the rates of infection for the control groups were in excess of 15%. There are two major flaws in these analyses. Firstly, the selection criteria used by both groups of investigators were poorly discriminating, the 'quality scores' allocated to some studies being so low that it is questionable whether they should have been included. Secondly, even if the authors' conclusions are valid, there were so many different prophylactic agents and routes of administration that the meta-analyses provide no guidance for neurosurgeons regarding the optimal regimen. For these reasons, the conclusions of the meta-analyses are not considered to be sufficiently robust to resolve the controversy surrounding the role of antimicrobial prophylaxis in shunt operations. It is not possible therefore to make recommendations either for or against the use of prophylaxis in shunt surgery on the basis of the existing evidence.

For those neurosurgeons who elect to use prophylactic antibiotics, there is no consensus of opinion regarding the optimal regimen, nor is there agreement on the most appropriate method of administration. In most instances, antibiotics have been given parenterally. However, some surgeons have instilled these drugs directly into the ventricles. Others have given them by both the intravenous and intraventricular routes, while still others either soaked the shunts in antibiotics or irrigated the shunt system just before implantation. The results associated with these diverse techniques of administering prophylaxis have been so variable that they cannot usefully be evaluated.

The majority of infections following shunt surgery are internal and are secondary to colonization of the shunt lumen. Skin commensals are the predominant pathogens, up to 90% of infective episodes being caused by coagulase-negative staphylococci (CoNS), more than 60% of which are resistant to multiple antibiotics, including methicillin. Other common pathogens include *S. aureus* (13–27%) and AGNB (10–20%), with streptococci, *Propionibacterium acnes, Corynebacterium* spp. and a wide range of other organisms accounting for the remainder. While a combination of vancomycin and gentamicin provides the most effective cover against this spectrum, neither of these antibiotics achieves therapeutic concentrations in the CSF when given by the intravenous route to patients with non-inflamed meninges. In order to ensure that CSF concentrations are adequate, both vancomycin and gentamicin should therefore be instilled into the ventricles during the operation (see Table 17.1 for dosages); the method of introducing these agents will depend on the type of shunt used. It must be emphasized, however, that the basis for choosing this regimen is entirely empirical; its efficacy has not been evaluated in controlled clinical trials. Furthermore, the product licence for vancomycin does not currently cover intraventricular administration, although widespread experience has demonstrated that delivery of the drug by this route is safe.

External infections, which involve the tissues adjacent to the shunt tubing, as distinct from internal infections, are rare following shunt surgery. In the event that antibiotic prophylaxis is considered necessary to prevent such infections, it would be appropriate to give a single dose of a first- or second-generation cephalosporin (cefradine, cefazolin, cefuroxime or cefamandole), administered at induction of anaesthesia by the intravenous route, as for other clean neurosurgical procedures (see Table 17.1 for dosages).

An alternative and potentially more effective means of preventing infection involves the use of shunts impregnated with antibiotics. Preliminary investigations indicate that a device which has been developed along these lines is resistant to colonization by the organisms commonly associated with shunt infection. If clinical trials confirm these favourable results, the incidence of shunt infection could be reduced dramatically.

Irrespective of whether or not antibiotic prophylaxis is administered, scrupulous hygiene and surgical technique at the time of shunt implantation are essential. A sample protocol for shunt insertion is shown in Table 17.2.

17.2.4 Skull fracture and CSF fistula

Meningitis is a serious complication of head injury. Approximately 11–25% of individuals with CSF leaks become infected, although the incidence has been as high as 38%. The delay from the time of injury until the onset of meningitis is also very variable. In a retrospective study of 16 cases of meningitis for which the intervals between trauma and infection were known, six presented in the first week, two in the first month and three in the first year; four occurred after an interval of more than one year (range 2–31 years). The cumulative risk of meningitis increases with persistence of the leak and may exceed 85% after 10 years.

The bacterium which is most commonly associated with post-traumatic meningitis is *Streptococcus pneumoniae*; other organisms which are part of the flora of the upper respiratory tract have been implicated less frequently. Episodes of meningitis caused by *S. aureus* and AGNB occur in patients who have been hospitalized for prolonged periods, who have recently received antibiotics or who have penetrating or open wounds.

Table 17.2 *Perioperative protocol for shunt insertion*

Pre-operative period

- Selection of patients

  Look for any focus of infection at proposed wound sites

  Defer surgery if unexplained pyrexia

  Avoid placing valve in recently opened incision or drain site

  Consider intraventricular vancomycin for 2 days before shunt insertion if EVD is *in situ* (see 'Ventriculitis in patients with EVDs')

- Apply betadine shampoo on the night before operation and on the morning of surgery
- Schedule surgery early on list if possible

Operative period

- Generous shaving of scalp (in anaesthetic room only), except babies
- Surgeon selects shunt equipment carefully
- All equipment ready to be opened in theatre
- Minimum number of personnel in operating theatre
- All personnel to wear masks and keep movements and talking to a minimum
- Theatre doors must be kept closed during shunt implantation (unless absolute emergency). Place 'NO ENTRY' sign on outside of theatre door
- Surgical instruments must be covered until the start of the operation
- Careful skin preparation with betadine and/or chlorhexidine for at least 2 min
- Change gloves after draping. While gowned up and wearing clean gloves, assemble shunt equipment and immediately submerge in irrigation solution (small bowl of saline containing gentamicin at a concentration of 20 mg/L)
- Meticulous haemostasis throughout, avoiding haematomas
- Gloves must be changed again before handling shunt tubing
- Avoid contact of shunt tubing with skin edge
- Cover tubing and valve with chlorhexidine-soaked swabs when exposed to air
- Flush through the valve system (no need to test opening pressure)
- Consider instilling vancomycin 10 mg and gentamicin 3 mg into the ventricles as prophylaxis prior to closure

Early publications emphasized the importance of antibiotics as a means of reducing the high risk of meningitis in patients with fractures of the skull complicated by CSF leaks. This recommendation, which appears to have been based wholly on the perceived or theoretical risks of infection and the experiences of the authors, has been reproduced in successive generations of both neurosurgical and general surgical textbooks. This has ensured that prophylaxis continues to be standard practice in many centres in the UK, although there is a great diversity of opinion regarding the optimal antibiotic regimen and for how long it should be administered. Moreover, there is little experimental or clinical evidence to suggest that this strategy is actually of benefit to patients.

A number of studies have assessed the efficacy of prophylaxis in patients with dural fistulae. With one exception, all of the studies were retrospective and involved small numbers of patients. Only one concluded that the routine administration of antibiotics prevented meningitis but, in this case, it is difficult to discern the relative contributions of prophylaxis and early operative intervention.

Two recent reviews of the literature, evaluating 347 patients and 848 patients respectively, also attempted to determine whether antibiotics were of benefit to patients with basal skull fractures; both demonstrated that prophylaxis does not reduce the incidence of meningitis in these patients.

The controversy surrounding the role of prophylaxis in this clinical setting will be resolved only by a prospective, randomized trial comparing a placebo with an appropriate antibiotic, or combination of antibiotics, prescribed in adequate dosage(s). Since skull fractures with CSF leaks account for a small percentage of head injuries requiring hospital admission, it would be difficult to recruit the very considerable number of patients required for such a study without involving several centres. The existing evidence does not support the use of prophylactic antibiotics in patients with CSF fistulae. Furthermore, the rationale quoted for such prophylaxis is theoretically flawed and there is a stronger theoretical argument against this line of management. Instead, the early diagnosis of meningitis should be encouraged by adequately counselling patients and their relatives regarding the signs and symptoms of infection and by informing general practitioners of the risks. Appropriate empirical therapy can then be instituted with minimal delay should this complication develop. In a large neurosurgical centre in the USA, patients with CSF fistulae are routinely immunized against *S. pneumoniae*. No cases of pneumococcal meningitis in 850 patients were reported following implementation of this intervention.

17.2.5   Penetrating craniocerebral injuries

Penetrating craniocerebral injuries (PCCI), in the military or civilian context, include gunshot wounds (from high- and low-velocity weapons) and penetration by sharp instruments such as knives, screwdrivers or arrows and pencils and other wooden objects. The most common infections following such injuries are osteomyelitis of the skull, meningitis and brain abscess.

Injuries caused by low-velocity bullets are principally due to the crushing effect exerted by the bullet as it passes through the tissues. The passage of high-velocity bullets, on the other hand, sets up secondary shock waves and cavitation that lead to rapid pressure pulses which cause devastating tissue destruction remote from the missile tract. High-velocity bullet wounds to the brain are therefore associated with much more severe, and more often fatal, injuries and the predominance of patients with intracranial injuries caused by low-velocity bullets surviving to be treated in military hospitals is related to this.

Gunshot wounds following failed suicide attempts, where there is a greater likelihood of involvement of the sinuses or oropharynx, are associated with an increased risk of bacterial contamination. In low-velocity bullet wounds, skin, hair, bone fragments and clothing may be driven into the brain along the bullet track, carrying bacteria with them. PCCI caused by penetration by sharp instruments such as knives and screwdrivers may produce small entry sites which give the impression that the injury is purely superficial. In these cases, bone fragments are often displaced and may be driven into the brain, piercing the dura and allowing bacteria to gain entry.

Accurate information about the agents causing infections associated with PCCI is incomplete for several reasons. Most studies were conducted before modern microbiological techniques were available and the results are therefore unreliable. In some cases, swabs were obtained after antibiotics had been administered. In others, swabs and/or tissue or bone samples were not cultured directly, but were placed into broth and cultured after a period of incubation. It is therefore impossible to determine the weight of bacterial growth in these specimens. Investigators often failed to speciate staphylococci, thereby precluding differentiation between *S. aureus* and CoNS which are common skin contaminants. Finally, the isolation of bacteria from removed bone, tissue and metal fragments from patients with PCCI is not the same as isolating pathogens from infected sites such as pus and CSF. Notwithstanding these confounding factors, the causes of infection in this setting are likely to be predominantly Gram-positive bacteria (*S. aureus*, possibly CoNS and streptococci), followed by AGNB and a miscellany of anaerobes, including *Clostridium* spp.

The principles of managing military and civilian gunshot and shrapnel wounds are as follows: debridement of both entrance and exit wounds; removal of necrotic tissue, haematoma, and bone fragments; removal of intracranial bone and metal fragments, where these are accessible, and foreign material including hair and clothing; and closure of the dura, with reconstruction if necessary. Although the presence of indriven fragments may be perceived as creating an obvious risk of infection, this does not appear to apply to bone and metal fragments, and healthy brain should not be compromised in the course of retrieving these.

Assessment of the published literature does not permit accurate conclusions about the efficacy of antibiotic prophylaxis in patients with PCCI, there having been no controlled trials. Moreover, it is unlikely that prospective studies of the role of antibiotics in the prevention of infection will ever be undertaken. Bacteriological data from published studies are also insufficiently reliable to facilitate recommendations. None the less, it is widely perceived that antibiotics play an essential role in the prevention of infection following PCCI. Although the administration of short courses, or even single doses, of prophylaxis are currently recommended in other surgical settings, there are sufficient data to suggest that, if there is any likelihood of retained fragments of organic material, however small in size, a 5-day course is more appropriate. For military craniocerebral injuries, civilian intracranial gunshot wounds and civilian penetrating intracranial injuries from other causes, antimicrobial prophylaxis should comprise the following: intravenous co-amoxiclav 1.2 g every 8 hours or intravenous cefuroxime 1.5 g, then 750 mg every 8 hours, with intravenous metronidazole 500 mg every 8 hours (or 1 g every 12 hours per rectum or 400 mg every 8 hours by mouth). The corresponding regimens for children are: intravenous co-amoxiclav 30 mg/kg every 8 hours or intravenous cefuroxime 25 mg/kg every 8 hours with metronidazole given orally, intravenously or per rectum, 7.5 mg/kg in each case. The dosages of these agents are summarized in Table 17.1. Administration of one of the above regimens should begin as soon as possible following injury and continue for 5 days post-operatively. Human anti-tetanus immunoglobulin 250–500 IU intramuscularly should also be administered to all patients and their vaccination status brought up to date in line with current guidelines.

17.3 HYDROCEPHALUS SHUNT INFECTIONS

17.3.1 Epidemiology

Shunting as a means of controlling hydrocephalus was adopted after the introduction of the silicone shunt. Originally, CSF was drained from the lateral cerebral ventricle to the right atrium via the superior vena cava (ventriculoatrial or VA shunt). Drainage to the peritoneal cavity (ventriculoperitoneal or VP shunt) was subsequently introduced; other routes are used occasionally.

Soon after the introduction of shunting for hydrocephalus in the late 1950s, infection became a recognized complication of the procedure. Although the rates of infection have generally fallen over the years, in adults, rates of 3–5% are not unusual, while higher rates are seen in children, particularly in the first few months of life when incidences of 15–20% have been reported. There is no difference between VA and VP shunts in terms of the infection rate.

Shunt infections can be divided into three groups. Internal infections are the commonest type, infection beginning as colonization of the inner surfaces of the shunt. Less common are external infections, involving the outer surface and surrounding tissues. Rarely, infection may arise following perforation of the bowel or bladder by the distal end of a VP shunt. After an interval, the first two types of infection often spread and become indistinguishable, although important differences in aetiology and treatment remain.

17.3.2 Pathogenesis and aetiology

Both research and experience have shown that virtually all cases of internal infection arise at the time of insertion or revision of a shunt. The causative bacteria, most commonly *Staphylococcus epidermidis*, originate in most cases from the patient's skin and are found in the incisions during shunt placement despite rigorous skin preparation and other measures. These organisms are capable of adhering to the shunt tubing and of persisting for very long periods in a quiescent state. External shunt infections also tend to develop at operation and are an example of surgical wound infections exacerbated by the presence of biomaterial. They are usually caused by *S. aureus*, which is less capable of adhering to the shunt but which is able to resist phagocytosis on the outer surfaces of the shunt and to cause inflammation, suppuration and necrosis. Occasionally this is not directly related to surgery but is secondary to erosion of the skin overlying the shunt, often in babies or in patients who are malnourished. Polymicrobial shunt infections are seen in patients with VP shunts following bowel perforation by the distal end of the catheter which may protrude from the anus. In these cases, infections are caused by intestinal organisms such as AGNB and anaerobes.

17.3.3 Diagnosis

VA and VP shunt infections and the three types of infection described above differ in terms of clinical features.

Internal infections involving VA shunts probably represent the greatest diagnostic challenge. Symptoms, sufficiently serious to warrant medical attention, often do not appear for months or even years after surgery, although vague aches, pains and sporadic fevers occurring during this time may be elicited. Patients may present with fevers, sometimes with rigors as well, or, if the infection is longstanding, the presenting features may be those of immune complex disease, i.e., rash, arthropathy and nephritis. Blood cultures should be taken as a matter of course, but these may show either contamination with *S. epidermidis* or be consistently sterile. The shunt reservoir should also be tapped (lumbar puncture is not indicated), although, here again, a negative result should not, in the presence of symptoms, exclude shunt infection. It is important that both a Gram's stain and culture of aspirated CSF be carried out, irrespective of the cell count. A reliable test for VA shunt infection, which depends on detecting high titres of antibody to *S. epidermidis*, is currently available.

Patients with internal infections of VP shunts present very differently, although there is still considerable variation in symptoms. Generally, patients present within approximately 6 months of operation and, in most cases, the inflammatory response in the peritoneal cavity eventually causes shunt obstruction. However, distal shunt obstruction may be unrelated to infection and these cases must be distinguished. While patients with VP shunt infections may present with headache and vomiting as the only features, most complain of abdominal pain, bloating or tenderness; fever is noted in about 50% of cases. Later, reflux of infected CSF up the outside of the distal catheter gives rise to erythema over the shunt track. Blood cultures obtained from patients with VP shunt infections are almost always sterile and shunt aspiration again can yield negative culture results if the infection is confined to the distal catheter. Even samples of CSF taken from the abdomen at revision can be sterile, owing to rapid phagocytosis. Unfortunately, there is currently no serological test available for patients with VP shunt infections, although estimation of the serum C-reactive protein (CRP) concentration can be helpful. However, any patient presenting with shunt-related symptoms, even if it is only obstruction, within 6 months of surgery should be suspected of having an infected shunt.

External infections in all shunt types present with erythema, serous or purulent discharge or wound dehiscence.

VP shunt infections secondary to visceral perforation are often surprisingly mild and the reason for referral may be the appearance of the catheter tip at the anus or in the vagina. However, shunt aspiration usually reveals enteric organisms in large numbers. Though rare, this complication can occur at any time.

17.3.4 Management

When shunt infections were first recognized 40 years ago, patients were treated with large intravenous doses of methicillin or cloxacillin, in common with patients with serious staphylococcal infections at other sites. This treatment was invariably unsuccessful and, eventually, two main explanations were identified. The first was pharmacological. In order to eradicate the pathogen within the shunt, it is necessary for antibiotics to which it is susceptible to be present in the ventricular CSF. Furthermore, the meninges usually exhibit only a minimal inflammatory response to *S. epidermidis* and the blood-CSF barrier is not patent. Consequently, intravenously-administered drugs (with some exceptions) do not achieve therapeutic concentrations in the CSF. The second is related to the biological state of the bacteria inside the shunt. These organisms are present within biofilms, a state which increases the concentration of antibiotic needed to exert a bactericidal effect by at least 1000-fold.

Clinical trials have confirmed that the highest cure rates in patients with shunt infections are associated with removal of the shunt and the Infection in Neurosurgery Working Party of the British Society for Antimicrobial Chemotherapy concluded that this is an essential step in the management of patients with shunt infections. However, the availability of novel drug regimens may cause this situation to change.

The choice of antibiotics should not be guided solely by the results of susceptibility testing. Aminoglycosides (e.g. gentamicin), β-lactams (e.g. penicillin and cephalosporins) and glycopeptides (e.g. vancomycin and teicoplanin) all fail to penetrate into the CSF in sufficient concentrations when given by the intravenous route and only rifampicin, chloramphenicol and trimethoprim will do so, regardless of the inflammatory response. Of the latter drugs, only rifampicin and trimethoprim are active against staphylococci, there being no place for chloramphenicol in this clinical setting. For intraventricular use, vancomycin and/or gentamicin are the drugs of choice.

The recommended treatment of patients with shunt infections caused by *S. epidermidis* or *S. aureus* is shunt removal, insertion of an external ventricular drain (EVD) and the administration of rifampicin (600 mg bd, initially by the intravenous route, then orally, or, in children 20 mg/kg/day in two divided doses) and vancomycin (10–20 mg once daily intraventricularly via

the EVD or a separate Ommaya reservoir). Vancomycin is safe when given intraventricularly and high CSF concentrations can be expected. The dosage is determined on the basis of the estimated CSF volume and not the age or body weight. Clinical and microbiological responses should be evident by the fourth day and treatment should be continued for 7–10 days, the last dose of each drug being given on the day on which a new shunt is implanted; there is no case for continuing treatment post-operatively. Rifampicin should never be given alone as resistance develops rapidly under these circumstances. In a few cases, it may be necessary to administer vancomycin or teicoplanin by the intravenous route. The above regimen is also appropriate for coryneforms, and patients with infections caused by enterococci can be treated with a combination of inventricular vancomycin and gentamicin (2–3 mg once daily). While it is currently recommended that the shunt be removed, in the case of infections caused by *S. epidermidis* (but not *S. aureus*), a 2-week course of intraventricular vancomycin and oral rifampicin, without shunt removal, may be successful as long as the shunt is not obstructed (E.M. Brown, unpublished data).

External shunt infections can rarely be treated successfully without shunt removal, although, if the diagnosis is made early, an attempt might be made. In this case, intraventricular antibiotics should be avoided because of the risk of introducing infection into the ventricular system, and intravenous flucloxacillin, cefuroxime or a glycopeptide, depending on the pathogen and its susceptibility, should be given. The relapse rate is high. If a decision is made to remove the shunt, treatment with the above regimen should be instituted, with the inclusion of intraventricular therapy, preferably given through an Ommaya reservoir placed on the contralateral side.

Shunt infections caused by AGNB should be treated by shunt removal and the administration of intravenous antibiotics, chosen according to the susceptibility of the isolate. The usual regimen comprises a third-generation cephalosporin, with or without an aminoglycoside.

Patients with polymicrobial infections secondary to visceral perforation should be treated in the same way as patients with meningitis, i.e., with antibiotics active against enterococci, AGNB and anaerobes. Appropriate options are ampicillin, gentamicin and metronidazole or a combination that includes a cephalosporin or co-amoxiclav; the therapy should be reviewed in the light of culture and susceptibility test results. The shunt must be removed promptly. Laparotomy is contraindicated and the perforation usually seals spontaneously.

Shunt infections caused by *Candida* spp., although uncommon, are challenging owing to difficulties associated with eradicating the yeast. The shunt should routinely be removed as *Candida* spp. colonize the tubing and will eventually occlude it. Amphotericin B, together with flucytosine or fluconazole, should be given by the intravenous route. There is no benefit, and some risk, associated with the intraventricular administration of amphotericin B. Occasionally, cure has been reported following treatment with fluconazole alone.

Community-acquired meningitis caused by the meningococcus, pneumococcus or *Haemophilus influenzae* is observed occasionally in shunted patients, but with a higher incidence than in the general population. In such cases, it is unnecessary to remove the shunt. Indeed, shunted patients with meningitis often have a milder course and respond more rapidly to treatment than patients without shunts. This is thought to be due to relief of intracranial pressure by the shunt. Antibiotic therapy should be the same as that recommended for patients with community-acquired bacterial meningitis who do not have shunts.

17.4 BRAIN ABSCESS

17.4.1 Epidemiology

Brain abscess is a focal (or, less frequently, multifocal) process that develops within the brain parenchyma. It is a relatively rare disease, with a reported incidence that varies from 0.32 hospital admissions per 100 000 population per year in the UK to 1.1 per 100 000 population per year in the USA; therefore, between four and ten cases will present annually to a neurosurgical department. The incidence of brain abscess is higher in immunocompromised patients, and those hospitals to which large numbers of patients with the Acquired Immunodeficiency Syndrome (AIDS) are admitted can expect to see particularly large numbers. The mean age of patients is 35–40 years, with a peak incidence in the second and third decades; approximately 25% of all brain abscesses occur in children (peak incidence 4–7 years of age). There is a male preponderance, with a male:female ratio of 2–3:1.

17.4.2 Pathogenesis

Brain abscesses develop as a consequence of implantation in the brain substance of bacteria or bacterial emboli from either local or distant septic foci. In the majority of cases, organisms gain access by direct spread from contiguous infected foci, e.g. acute or chronic otitis media (with or without mastoiditis), sinusitis, dental infections and meningitis (albeit rarely). Middle ear and sinugenic infections together account for 40–70% of brain abscesses, although aggressive antibiotic therapy of otitis media has led to a decrease in the incidence attributable to the former in most developed countries. The incidence of odontogenic abscess is approximately 10%. Metastatic or haematogenous spread from a distant focus accounts for 20–25% of brain abscesses. The most common sources are chronic pyogenic lung diseases, such as empyema, bronchiectasis and lung abscesses, which are now uncommon in the UK. Others include osteomyelitis, intraabdominal infections, pelvic infections, skin and soft tissue infections, septicaemias and infective endocarditis. Cyanotic congenital cardiac disease in patients with right-to-left shunts, particularly Fallot's tetralogy, is associated with 5–10% of cases overall, but with up to 25% of all brain abscesses in children. Brain abscesses complicate cavernous sinus thrombosis secondary to septic thrombophlebitis of the anterior facial vein or malignant tumours involving the cranial bones. Organisms may also gain access to the brain following implantation through a penetrating wound of the head which may be traumatic or iatrogenic, i.e., following neurosurgery or in association with an intracranial pressure monitor; this route accounts for 5–10% of brain abscesses. Finally, 10–30% of cases are cryptogenic.

Most abscesses (75–90%) are solitary, occurring, in descending order of frequency, in the frontal, temporal, frontoparietal, parietal, cerebellar and occipital lobes; the locations in the brain reflect the site of predisposing, and usually adjacent, foci of infection. For example, frontal lobe abscesses are characteristically secondary to frontal or ethmoidal sinusitis or dental sepsis, while temporal lobe and cerebellar abscesses are secondary to infections in the middle ear/mastoid cavity or sphenoidal sinuses. Brain stem and thalamic abscesses are characteristically the result of haematogenous spread from a distant focus. Multiple lesions, on the other hand, account for 5–25% of abscess. They are almost always metastatic, spreading via the bloodstream from distant foci of infection, and are most frequently located in the area of the brain supplied by the middle cerebral artery (parietal, anterior temporal and posterior frontal lobes).

17.4.3 Pathology

Regardless of the origin of the infection, brain abscesses are thought to develop in areas of pre-existing necrosis, this being a principal requirement for their initiation. The first stage in the development of an abscess is an acute cerebritis which normally lasts about 3 days. This is followed by a late cerebritis of 4–9 days' duration, culminating in a necrotic central focus. The formation of a collagen capsule around the developing abscess starts after 10 days and is usually complete by 14 days. The capsule, which limits the spread of infection within the brain, tends to be thinner on the medial aspect, thereby accounting for the tendency of abscesses, on rare occasions, to rupture into the ventricles. Metastatic abscesses are characteristically less well encapsulated and this may account for their tendency to spread. The oedema surrounding an abscess often occupies a greater volume than the abscess itself and therefore makes an important contribution to raised intracranial pressure.

17.4.4   Aetiology

As many as 50% of brain abscesses are monomicrobial and a similar percentage are polymicrobial. Between 20% and 25% are culture-negative, either because the patient has already received antibiotic treatment or because laboratory diagnostic techniques have been less than optimal. Aerobic bacteria have been isolated from between 50% and 75% of lesions and anaerobes from 25–50%. Streptococci, predominantly microaerophilic and anaerobic species, are the most commonly recovered organisms (40–70%), regardless of the source. Abscesses that are secondary to penetrating trauma have, in the past, been caused by *S. aureus*, but Enterobacteriaceae are increasing in frequency. AGNB, particularly *Proteus* spp. and *Pseudomonas aeruginosa*, are also common pathogens in patients with otogenic brain abscesses. A very broad range of other bacterial species have been occasionally isolated. In those parts of the world where protozoa and helminths are endemic, brain abscesses can develop secondary to amoebiasis, schistosomiasis, echinococcosis, trichinosis or *Taenia solium* (cysticercosis). Finally, in immunocompromised patients, a wide variety of uncommon bacteria, fungi and parasites are being identified with increasing frequency; these include mycobacteria, *Aspergillus* spp., *Candida* spp., *Cryptococcus neoformans*, *Listeria monocytogenes*, *Actinomyces* spp., *Nocardia* spp., *Toxoplasma gondii* (the most common cause of brain abscesses in AIDS patients) and *Acanthamoeba* spp.

17.4.5   Clinical manifestations

The clinical spectrum of patients with brain abscesses ranges from fulminating to indolent and can vary in duration from hours to weeks. Headache is the most common symptom (occurring in $\geq$ 75% of patients). If it is the only complaint, there is a high likelihood of misdiagnosis and if accompanied by a discharging ear, there is a risk that it will be attributed to otitis media. Nausea and vomiting, presumably secondary to raised intracranial pressure, are common (affecting approximately 50% of patients). Other prominent features are fever (40–60%), dizziness, impaired consciousness and papilloedema (40–60%). Focal neurological signs (in 50% of patients) vary according to the location of the abscess, but may include hemiparesis, focal seizures and visual and speech disturbances. Diffuse neurological dysfunction is usually associated with abscesses in the occipital or temporal lobe and is characterized by coma, generalized seizures, behavioural disturbances and confusion. Meningism, which is a feature in approximately 25% of cases, is also characteristic of abscesses in the occipital or

temporal lobe and may be secondary to concomitant meningitis or rupture of the abscess into a ventricle or the subarachnoid space. Other clinical features may reflect the extracranial underlying disease, e.g. ear or nasal discharge.

The differential diagnosis in patients with brain abscesses includes a myriad of other diseases, the most common being herpes simplex encephalitis, subdural empyema, cerebral metastasis, bacterial meningitis, primary brain tumour, vascular lesions, tuberculosis and toxoplasmosis.

17.4.6   Diagnosis

The principal diagnostic procedures are radiological. A plain skull x-ray is often normal in patients with brain abscesses, but may show a mid-line shift (in $>$ 50% of patients), gas in the abscess cavity (rare) or evidence of sinusitis or mastoiditis. A contrast-enhanced CT scan is the single most useful investigation and is more sensitive than isotope brain scans once the abscess has progressed beyond the cerebritis stage. It usually shows a ring-enhancing lesion surrounded by oedema or, less commonly, either nodular enhancement or areas of low attenuation without enhancement. Displacement of the ventricles by the adjacent abscess is often evident and signs of sinusitis or middle ear disease/mastoiditis should also be sought. The CT scan lacks specificity, however, and it may be difficult to distinguish a brain abscess from other mass lesions, especially neoplasms. MRI is at least as specific and sensitive as CT and may be superior, especially in the early (cerebritis) stage of the disease and in terms of detecting multiple small abscesses. However, in common with the CT scan, it suffers from not being able to reliably differentiate between an abscess and a neoplasm. Demonstration of an hypo-intense rim on T_2-weighted MRI images, which is unusual in this lesion, but occasionally seen, can be very helpful in facilitating the diagnosis. Radionuclide scanning is sometimes helpful, particularly when used in conjunction with ^{99m}Tc-HMPAO. It is very rarely needed when MRI is available and is most likely to be of value following surgery. Finally, a white cell or a ^{99m}Tc-HMPAO scan may help to differentiate a brain abscess from a neoplasm.

Lumbar puncture is generally unhelpful, the findings on microscopy tending to be highly variable and non-specific; organisms are isolated from $<$ 10% of CSF samples. It may also be a dangerous procedure, leading to coning in up to one-third of patients. It should be performed, therefore, only if meningitis is suspected and when a CT scan confirms that it is safe to do so. An EEG is usually abnormal in patients with brain abscesses, but the findings are non-specific. For this reason, it is considered a non-essential investigation. The peripheral white blood cell (WBC) count is raised in 30–60% of patients and the CRP will be significantly elevated in most cases. Blood cultures are positive in 10–20% of patients and are essential investigations if a systemic focus is suspected; they may be particularly helpful in patients who are not managed surgically. When present, samples of sputum or nasal or ear discharge should also be cultured.

17.4.7 Surgical management

Most patients with brain abscesses undergo surgery as part of their management. Surgery is associated with a number of advantages, including confirmation of the diagnosis, removal of infected and necrotic material, relief of raised intracranial pressure, accurate identification of the aetiological agent(s) (thereby facilitating optimal antimicrobial therapy) and enhancement of the activities of the antibiotics.

Removal of pus is achieved by craniotomy and drainage or excision of the abscess or by aspiration through a burr hole, preferably with CT- or MRI-guided stereotaxy. The type of procedure is dictated by the depth, size and location of the abscess, the number of abscesses, the stage of development, the clinical status of the patient and the risk of post-operative complications. The superiority of one or the other of these techniques remains controversial. Some neurosurgeons claim that there are more frequent sequelae (mainly epilepsy), greater morbidity from trauma and a higher incidence of mortality with excision. Others have suggested that excision is associated with a lower incidence of mortality and offers immediate decompression, a lower recurrence rate, a shorter period of hospitalization and a shorter course of antibiotics. The overall consensus is that there is probably no difference between the two options, but that aspiration is appropriate for patients who are too ill to undergo a more extensive surgical procedure, who have multiple abscesses or whose abscesses are poorly encapsulated or in deep, critical or less accessible areas of the brain, while excision should be undertaken in the presence of foreign material, in patients with superficial, solitary or multiloculated abscesses and for abscesses that fail to resolve following aspiration. If patients have shown favourable clinical responses to antibiotic treatment, further aspirations of the abscess cavity are unnecessary.

Non-surgical management should be restricted to highly selected groups of patients who are neurologically intact and who fulfil the following criteria: small abscesses (< 3 cm in diameter); poor medical condition which precludes surgery; high density lesion (cerebritis); no predisposing factor; multiple abscesses; and inaccessible abscesses or those in deep or eloquent brain locations. The best results are obtained when bacteria are identified in blood cultures. A number of reports have confirmed that patients can be managed successfully without surgery, but the strategy relies on CT monitoring in order to detect exacerbations as early as possible.

17.4.8 Antimicrobial chemotherapy

Several antibiotics, including benzylpenicillin, ampicillin, cefuroxime, chloramphenicol, co-trimoxazole, ceftazidime and metronidazole, have been detected in brain abscess pus in therapeutic concentrations, but this is not necessarily predictive of their therapeutic efficacy; there is little information currently available regarding the penetration of newer agents.

The complexity of the physiological, surgical, pharmacological and bacteriological parameters that influence the outcome of treatment of patients with brain abscesses, together with a lack of data from prospective, randomized clinical trials, have undermined efforts to make recommendations for optimal empirical therapy. For many years, a combination of penicillin and chloramphenicol was the most widely used regimen and, indeed, most patients responded favourably to it. More recently, however, extended-spectrum β-lactams, particularly third-generation cephalosporins, in combination with metronidazole, have been administered with increasing frequency.

The initial choice of empirical antibiotic therapy can be facilitated by a number of considerations, including the location of the abscess, the precipitating source of infection (e.g. middle ear infection, a history of sinusitis or trauma etc.), the odour of the pus (which may suggest the presence of anaerobes) and a Gram's stain of the pus. Treatment should be initiated as soon as the diagnosis is confirmed. The recommendations summarized in Table 17.3 constitute appropriate first-line empirical therapy. Treatment should be modified, if necessary, in the light of the results obtained from culturing aspirated pus. Initially, all antibiotics should be administered by the intravenous route. The efficacy of instilling antibiotics directly into the abscess cavity is unconfirmed. Moreover, antibiotics administered by this route may diffuse rapidly into the surrounding tissues and precipitate seizures. Current evidence does not support the routine instillation of antimicrobial agents into brain abscess cavities.

The optimal duration of treatment of patients with brain abscesses remains a controversial issue, current practice owing more to tradition than to scientific evidence. Recommendations have ranged from 4–8 weeks of parenteral therapy, followed by prolonged courses of oral therapy (assuming suitable agents are available), if the abscess has been excised or aspirated, and even longer (up to 12 weeks of parenteral therapy) when management has been conservative. The lack of uniformity of opinion regarding an optimal duration is due both to a failure to attempt to resolve this question by prospective clinical trials and to the absence of reliable criteria for monitoring patients' responses to therapy.

Table 17.3 *Initial empirical antibiotic therapy of patients with brain abscesses[a]*

Source	Location	Antimicrobial regimens[b]
Paranasal sinuses	frontal lobe	Cefuroxime 1.5 g tds, cefotaxime 2 g qds or ceftriaxone 3–4 g od and metronidazole 500 mg tds
Teeth	frontal lobe	Cefuroxime 1.5 g tds and metronidazole 500 mg tds
Middle ear (less often, sphenoidal sinuses)	temporal lobe	Ampicillin 2–3 g tds and metronidazole 500 mg tds plus either ceftazidime 2 g tds or gentamicin 5 mg/kg od[c]
Middle ear (less often, sphenoidal sinuses)	cerebellum	Ampicillin 2–3 g tds and metronidazole 500 mg tds plus either ceftazidime 2 g tds or gentamicin 5 mg/kg od[c]
Penetrating trauma	depends on site of wound	Flucloxacillin 2–3 g qds or cefuroxime 1.5 g tds, cefotaxime 2 g qds or ceftriaxone 3–4 g od
Metastatic and cryptogenic	multiple lesions (usually in area supplied by middle cerebral artery)	Depends on source: benzylpenicillin 1.8–2.4 g 6-hourly if infective endocarditis or cyanotic congenital heart disease; alternatively, cefuroxime 1.5 g tds or cefotaxime 2 g qds or ceftriaxone 3–4 g od with or without metronidazole 500 mg tds

[a]Reproduced from: Infection in Neurosurgery Working Party of the British Society of Antimicrobial Chemotherapy, *British Journal of Neurosurgery* 2000; **14**: 525–30.
[b]Adult dosages.
[c]Gentamicin serum concentrations must be monitored.

Serial CT and MRI scans cannot be used to provide an objective endpoint for discontinuing antibiotics as scan appearances may suggest ongoing infection for up to 10 weeks after the successful completion of therapy; in one published report, complete resolution of CT signs on discharge was observed in respect of only three of 18 patients. There is preliminary evidence from two studies that antibiotics can be discontinued once the serum CRP concentration falls to within the normal range, provided that patients have undergone either drainage or excision of their abscesses, that the abscesses are solitary, that there is improvement in the clinical condition and that the fever has resolved. In most cases, this will be within 2 weeks of starting appropriate therapy. In a minority of patients the CRP concentrations will be within the normal range, or only slightly elevated, at the time of presentation. The most likely explanation for this observation is that the abscess has been completely walled off and the infection no longer exposed to the physiological processes that drive the inflammatory response – analogous to sequestra in patients with chronic osteomyelitis. Although, in these patients, the CRP cannot be used to monitor response to therapy, it may still not be necessary to administer antibiotics for more than 2 weeks, so long as the abscess

has been excised or drained. A further complication is that, while the CRP is a very sensitive criterion for monitoring response to therapy, it is not specific. Therefore, if there is an intercurrent infection or other inflammatory process, such as a deep vein thrombosis or pulmonary embolism, the CRP concentration may remain elevated. Finally, there is preliminary evidence to support a switch from parenteral to oral therapy when the CRP concentration has fallen below 50 mg/L, so long as there is an absence of systemic signs of infection, the patient is able to tolerate antibiotics by mouth and appropriate agents are available.

17.4.9 Adjunctive therapy

Steroids are commonly used to reduce oedema, but are of no proven benefit in terms of reducing morbidity, the incidence of neurological sequelae or the duration of hospitalization. The consensus is that they should be avoided unless there is significant oedema with raised intracranial pressure and rapid neurological deterioration; even then, they should be used for short periods only. Anticonvulsants may be appropriate in patients with seizures and are often started empirically as prophylaxis.

17.4.10 Prognosis and complications

In the past, the incidence of mortality has ranged from 20–50%. More recently, however, incidences of 5–20% have been reported. This improved outcome has been attributed to more sensitive and specific radiological techniques (which allow earlier diagnosis and better localization), superior surgical techniques (in particular, the introduction of stereotactic brain biopsy and aspiration), more reliable microbiological methods and more effective antibiotic therapy. Outcome does not appear to be influenced by the location of the abscess, the number of abscesses, predisposing factors, the nature of the pathogen(s) or the type of surgery. A poor prognosis is, however, related to the initial clinical status of the patient, particularly the level of consciousness (which is indirectly related to a delay in diagnosis), and is associated with rapidly progressing neurological impairment, multiple, deep or multiloculated abscesses and rupture of the abscess into a ventricle.

Complications include cortical thrombophlebitis (leading to focal epilepsy or hemiparesis), rupture into a ventricle or subarachnoid space (leading to meningitis and/or ventriculitis, coma and death), tension pneumocephalus and non-communicating hydrocephalus. Neurological sequelae (25–50%) include hemiparesis, cranial nerve palsies, epilepsy, memory deficits, behavioural disorders, ataxia, blindness and hemianopia.

Intraventricular rupture is a particularly serious complication and is associated with a mortality rate exceeding 80%. As well as the administration of appropriate antibiotics systemically, management should comprise open craniotomy with aggressive debridement of the abscess cavity and lavage of the ventricular system with normal saline containing one or more appropriate antibiotics suitable for intraventricular instillation, i.e. vancomycin and gentamicin, each at a concentration of 10 mg/L.

17.5 SUBDURAL EMPYEMA

Subdural empyema is a collection of pus in the space between the dura and the arachnoid, the outermost layers of the meninges. It occurs less commonly than brain abscess, but still accounts for approximately 20% of all intracranial infections; a typical neurosurgical department will therefore see between two and three cases per year. While all ages are affected, 76% of cases occur in the second and third decades. There is a male preponderance, the male:female ratio being 4:1.

17.5.1 Pathogenesis

In 50–70% of patients, infection spreads to the dura, either directly or, more often, indirectly via venous drainage, from the paranasal sinuses (particularly the frontal and ethmoid sinuses). A further 10–20% originate in the middle ear or mastoid cavity and, in 5%, spread is from a distant focus, usually the lungs, via the bloodstream. Subdural empyema may also occur secondary to trauma, surgery, dental infection, brain abscess, cranial osteomyelitis or an infected subdural haematoma; in 15% of cases the source is unknown.

17.5.2 Pathology

Infection may involve one or both cerebral hemispheres and develops over the convexities of the hemispheres, at the base of the brain or along the falx cerebri; the posterior fossa is rarely involved and less than 10% of subdural empyemas are infratentorial. The empyema may be loculated. Focal osteomyelitis and/or extradural abscess co-exist in up to 50% of patients. Oedema of the brain parenchyma develops rapidly and contributes to the mass effect.

17.5.3 Aetiology

The organisms associated with subdural empyema closely resemble those causing brain abscesses although, unlike brain abscess, most infections are monomicrobial. Streptococci (aerobic, anaerobic and microaerophilic) are the predominant pathogens, being isolated from 50–75% of patients. Anaerobes account for 5–10% of infections and S. aureus and AGNB (causing 15–25% and 5–10% of infections, respectively) are usually associated with trauma or surgery. Finally, a miscellany of other organisms, including H. influenzae, S. pneumoniae, Neisseria meningitidis and Group B β-haemolytic streptococci, has also been isolated.

17.5.4 Clinical features

The signs and symptoms of subdural empyema are related to raised intracranial pressure, focal pressure, meningitis, systemic effects and the underlying infection. Acute subdural empyema has been described as the most imperative surgical emergency. Patients present with a history of short duration and the course of the disease is rapid and fulminating. The most common clinical features include headache, pyrexia, meningismus, nausea and/or vomiting, impaired consciousness, focal neurological deficits (including hemiparesis, hemiplegia and dysphasia), focal or generalized seizures and papilloedema. Concurrent sinusitis or otitis media have been reported in 60–90% of cases.

In patients with subacute subdural empyemas, the history is longer (usually weeks) and infection is most commonly secondary to trauma or surgery. Patients complain of chronic localized headache, and tenderness and erythema are present over the craniotomy incision or the site of the trauma.

In infancy, subdural empyema is usually secondary to meningitis. The clinical features are similar to those in adults, i.e. high fever, seizures, vomiting, lethargy, irritability, a bulging fontanelle, neck stiffness and coma.

The clinical features of subdural empyema are non-specific and the following conditions must be included in the differential diagnosis: brain abscess; extradural abscess; cortical thrombophlebitis; meningitis; thrombosis of the cavernous or lateral sinus; sphenoid sinus empyema; tuberculous meningitis; encephalitis; septic infarct secondary to endocarditis; and exacerbation of otitis media or sinusitis.

17.5.5   Diagnosis

Plain skull films are rarely helpful, although they may demonstrate concurrent sinusitis or otitis media. An unenhanced CT is often normal. Contrast, which is mandatory, frequently demonstrates very subtle changes with only slight displacement of the enhancing capsule away from the vault. However, because of its greater sensitivity and specificity, MRI with gadolinium enhancement has become the diagnostic procedure of choice.

Peripheral WBC counts are usually high ($20–30 \times 10^9$/L). An EEG often reveals non-specific abnormalities and is therefore not particularly helpful. Similarly, the findings in the CSF are non-specific; the WBC count is not invariably elevated and the differential cell count is highly variable. On the grounds that a lumbar puncture rarely provides valuable diagnostic information and is potentially dangerous, this procedure is justified in only the most exceptional circumstances.

17.5.6   Surgical management

In most cases, the rapid progression of a subdural empyema necessitates early surgical intervention, although small numbers of patients have been treated conservatively. Surgical drainage relieves intracranial pressure and facilitates both the choice of optimal antibiotic therapy and the activities of the antibiotics administered. Drainage can be achieved either by multiple burr holes with irrigation of the subdural space or by craniotomy, but neurosurgeons are at variance regarding the superior approach. Advocates of craniotomy claim that it is associated with a higher incidence of survivors, better decompression and lower rates of complications and reaccumulation. It is the surgery of choice for patients with posterior fossa empyema if the pus is too tenacious to be removed through a burr hole or if there is reaccumulation of pus. On the other hand, if infection of the cranial bone flap complicates craniotomy, replacement of the flap may not be possible until the infection has resolved, thereby leaving a defect. Recurrences, which may be multiple, are common, necessitating further surgery in up to 50% of patients. Serial serum CRP concentrations should be used to monitor patients' responses. Failure of the CRP concentration to fall or a rise following an initial decline in a patient who is receiving appropriate antibiotics in adequate dosages is probably the earliest indication of reaccumulation.

17.5.7   Antibiotic therapy

Although treatment is almost invariably empirical, the choice of agents can be guided by knowledge of the predominant pathogens, the presumed source and the odour and a Gram's stain of the pus. A second- or third-generation cephalosporin, such as cefuroxime 1.5 g qds, cefotaxime 2–3 g qds or ceftriaxone 3–4 g od or 2 g bd, in combination with metronidazole 500 mg tds, would be appropriate empirical therapy for most patients with subdural empyema. Neonates, in whom subdural empyemas are often secondary to meningitis, can be given the same regimen, but without the metronidazole. Patients who develop subdural empyemas following neurosurgery should receive a combination of flucloxacillin 2–3 g qds and ceftazidime 2 g tds. Therapy should be modified, if necessary, in the light of culture and susceptibility test results. Initially, all antibiotics should be administered by the intravenous route. Instillation of antibiotics into the subdural space is a common practice, but there is no evidence that it is beneficial and β-lactam antibiotics may be epileptogenic. There is no consensus regarding the optimal duration of therapy and no clinical trials have been conducted with the aim of resolving this issue. Most patients have been treated for between 3 and 4 weeks, although in common with patients with brain abscesses, antibiotics can be discontinued once the serum CRP concentration returns to normal. This will usually be 2 weeks after starting appropriate therapy.

Other therapeutic adjuncts include prophylactic anticonvulsants and mannitol and steroids to reduce intracranial pressure.

17.5.8   Prognosis and complications

Without prompt diagnosis and the initiation of effective treatment, subdural empyema is rapidly fatal. In the past, mortality rates have ranged from 25–40% but, more recently, with the introduction of better diagnostic and therapeutic measures, rates have fallen to between 10% and 20%; if the patient is alert at the time of presentation, mortality rates are usually less than 10%, but are up to 75% if the patient is comatose.

When therapeutic intervention is prompt, there is a high likelihood of complete recovery in survivors. Complications include reaccumulation of pus, focal or generalized seizures, hemiparesis, aphasia and corticothrombophlebitis.

17.6 NON-TUBERCULOUS SPINAL EXTRADURAL (EPIDURAL) ABSCESS

A spinal extradural abscess is a localized suppurative infection of the space between the outermost layer of the meninges, the dura mater, and the vertebral column. It is an uncommon condition and even large neurosurgical centres can expect no more than 3–4 cases per year. While all ages are affected, the mean age is between 50 and 60 years; the disease is rare in infants and young children. The male:female ratio has been reported as varying from 1–2:1.

17.6.1 Pathogenesis

Spinal extradural abscesses almost always originate from foci of infection elsewhere in the body, with spread to the extradural space either via the bloodstream or the lymphatic system, or directly from a contiguous focus of infection. Skin and soft tissue infections are the most common sources of bacteraemias leading to extradural infections, but other foci include infective endocarditis, pharyngitis, mastoiditis, pneumonia, urinary tract infections, periodontal infections, intraabdominal infections and infected vascular catheters. Abscesses may also occur following direct spread from vertebral osteomyelitis (present in more than 50% of chronic abscesses, but in only 15% of acute abscesses), perinephric, retropharyngeal or psoas abscesses, decubitus ulcers or persistent/congenital dermal sinus tracts. Infections have been reported, albeit rarely, following penetrating injuries, lumbar punctures, spinal surgery, epidural anaesthesia and CT-guided needle biopsy and in association with the use of temporary epidural catheters. A history of prior back trauma has been noted in 10–35% of patients, leading to suggestions that haematomas or damaged tissues may predispose to haematogenous seeding. Other predisposing conditions include diabetes, intravenous drug abuse, degenerative joint disease, renal failure and cirrhosis.

17.6.2 Pathology

Owing to the lack of resistance to the longitudinal spread of infection through the extradural space, several (on average, between three and six) vertebral segments are affected, although there have been reports of the entire length of the spinal cord being involved. Involvement of the thoracic spine occurs in 50–80% of cases, the lumbar spine in 17–38% and the cervical spine in 10–25%; in children, infection usually affects the cervical and lumbar regions. Abscesses are located posterior to the cord in more than 70% of patients, but may also be anterior or circumferential. Acute abscesses consist of granulation tissue containing loculated pus, while chronic abscesses consist of both granulation and fibrous tissues. As the abscess enlarges, it may compress the spinal cord, cause myelomalacia or cord necrosis or extend into the subdural or subarachnoid space.

17.6.3 Aetiology

Pathogens are isolated either from blood cultures or intraoperative specimens or both. *S. aureus* is the predominant aetiological agent, accounting for 60–90% of infections. Other common organisms include streptococci (approximately 20%), AGNB (approximately 15%), particularly *Escherichia coli* and *P. aeruginosa*, and anaerobes (up to 7%); a very broad range of bacterial and fungal species have been reported less frequently and multiple organisms have been isolated from 5–10% of patients.

17.6.4 Clinical features

Spinal extradural abscesses may develop acutely or chronically. Acute cases are more likely to exhibit the classical features of infection, i.e. high fevers, rigors and raised peripheral WBC counts, consistent with spread by the haematogenous route, while chronic cases are more likely to be secondary to slowly developing contiguous foci of infection, particularly vertebral osteomyelitis. Classically, the disease progresses through four phases: phase I, focal vertebral pain at the affected level of the spine, with localized tenderness and fever; phase II, nerve root pain, with radiculopathy and/or paraesthesiae; phase III, weakness, with motor and sensory deficits and/or bladder or bowel dysfunction; and phase IV, paralysis. The first three phases progress at rates varying from days in acute cases to weeks or months in chronic cases. However, the weakness phase (III) can progress to the paralysis phase (IV) within hours, irrespective of whether the course of the disease is acute or chronic.

Back pain, with or without neurological deficits, may be attributed to an enormous range of disease processes. This, and the relative rarity of spinal extradural abscess, have led to a high percentage of patients with this disease being initially misdiagnosed, although the presence of systemic signs of infection may help to narrow the spectrum. Included in the differential diagnosis of spinal extradural abscess are the following: musculoskeletal pain secondary to strain or trauma; vertebral or intervertebral disc space disease (degenerative or inflammatory); vertebral osteomyelitis; tuberculous osteomyelitis; transverse myelitis (associated with bacterial, viral or parasitic infection, vaccination or autoimmune disease); meningitis; intradural or extradural neoplasms (primary or metastatic); Guillain-Barré syndrome; vascular lesions; spinal subdural abscess; epidural lipomatosis; epidural sarcoidosis; intraspinal infection; and spinal cord haematoma.

17.6.5   Diagnosis

Spinal extradural abscess should be considered in any patient with back pain and radicular symptoms, especially in the presence of the signs of infection. Prompt diagnosis is essential if permanent neurological sequelae are to be avoided.

Plain X-ray films of the spine are normal in many patients, but may show signs of vertebral osteomyelitis or other findings suggestive of infection in the spinal canal. CT, with contrast enhancement, is useful in diagnosing vertebral osteomyelitis and distinguishing between extradural and subdural infections. However, as it is a relatively insensitive technique for diagnosing extradural abscesses and may fail to define the longitudinal extent of the infection, it is rarely used. Gadolinium-enhanced MRI is superior to CT and is currently the diagnostic procedure of choice in the initial evaluation of patients with suspected extradural abscesses. It usually shows an heterogeneously enhancing extradural mass with compression of the adjacent neural structures. MRI accurately identifies both extradural abscess and osteomyelitis, differentiates between extradural abscess and other spinal cord lesions with which it can be confused and precisely delineates the longitudinal extent of the infection and loculations of inflammatory tissue.

A raised peripheral WBC count and ESR are common findings, especially in patients with acute disease, but are non-specific and therefore unreliable. Samples of blood for culture should always be taken and yield a pathogen in up to 70% of cases. A lumbar puncture should not be performed routinely because of the risk of spreading infection to the subdural or subarachnoid space. Examination of CSF typically shows ranges characteristic of a parameningeal focus of inflammation, with a raised WBC count of usually no more than 150/cmm (much less if the abscess is chronic) and comprising a mixture of polymorphonuclear leucocytes and lymphocytes or predominantly polymorphonuclear leucocytes; the protein concentration is raised (markedly so in the presence of a complete block) and the glucose concentration normal, unless there is coincidental meningitis. A Gram's stain is usually negative and the CSF is sterile in up to 80% of cases. Material obtained from the abscess should always be submitted for Gram's stain and culture.

17.6.6   Surgical management

Surgical drainage with decompression laminectomy, as soon as the diagnosis is made in order to optimize neurological recovery and to reduce the potential for rapid progression to complete and permanent paralysis, is considered to be the cornerstone of surgical management. The extent of the procedure will depend on the extent of the abscess, as demonstrated by radiological imaging. In children, a limited laminectomy may be undertaken to minimize the risk of subsequent spinal deformity. Occasionally, anterior spinal decompression is necessary, particularly when the cervical spine is involved and pus is present in the ventral extradural space. Immediate stabilization with graft, and even plates and screws, have recently been used successfully in the acute stage. It has been recommended that a wound drain be inserted at the time of primary drainage as a means of preventing recurrence of the extradural collection. Primary closure of the wound reduces both the amount of discomfort experienced by the patient and the duration of hospital stay. CT-guided percutaneous needle aspiration has been used as an alternative to laminectomy in selected patients, but this approach has not been validated by clinical studies and it should not normally be used in place of surgery. Antibiotic therapy alone may be considered if a patient's general condition precludes surgery or if the patient has no or only minimal neurological deficit on presentation. The latter group should be monitored closely with regular neurological examinations and MRI studies, and surgical intervention instituted immediately in the event of sudden neurological deterioration.

17.6.7   Antibiotic therapy (Table 17.4)

The initial empirical regimen, the choice of which can be facilitated by a Gram's stain of any pus that is obtained at surgery, should provide cover against the predominant pathogen, *S. aureus*. Flucloxacillin 2–3 g qds is therefore the drug of choice, with a first-generation cephalosporin, such as cefradine 2–3 g qds, for patients who are allergic to penicillins. If there is any reason to suspect AGNB, a second- or third-generation cephalosporin (cefuroxime 1.5 g tds, cefotaxime 2–3 g qds or ceftriaxone 3–4 g od or 2 g bd) or a fluoroquinolone (ciprofloxacin 400–600 mg bd) would be appropriate, unless *P. aeruginosa* is likely, in which case, ceftazidime 2 g tds (together with flucloxacillin) should be administered. An anti-anaerobic agent, such as metronidazole 500 mg tds, should be added to the empirical regimen if anaerobes are suspected on the basis of the original focus of infection and/or foul-smelling pus. Treatment should be modified, if necessary, in the light of the results of culture and susceptibility testing. Initially, all antibiotics should be administered by the intravenous route. While the optimal

Table 17.4 *Empirical antibiotic therapy of patients with pyogenic vertebral osteomyelitis*

Clinical setting/suspected pathogen	Regimen[a]
First-line	flucloxacillin 2–3 g qds (+ fusidic acid 500 mg bd po)[b]
First-line (penicillin allergy)	cefradine 2–3 g qds (+ fusidic acid 500 mg bd po)[b]
Elderly patient and/or suspicion of aerobic Gram-negative bacillus	cefuroxime 1.5 g tds, cefotaxime 2–3 g qds or ceftriaxone 3–4 g od or 2 g bd
P. aeruginosa[c]	ceftazidime 2 g tds + flucloxacillin 2–3 g qds[d]

[a]Adult dosages.
[b]For the first 10–14 days if and when *S. aureus* is confirmed as the causative organism.
[c]Suspected in intravenous drug abusers and patients with long-term indwelling urinary catheters.
[d]To provide cover against *S. aureus* (cefradine 2–3 g qds in case of penicillin allergy).

duration of therapy has not been determined, most patients have received antibiotics for 3–4 weeks, although shorter courses may be equally effective. The response to treatment should be monitored by serial measurements of the serum CRP concentration. If there is concurrent osteomyelitis, the drugs should be given for a total of 6 weeks. The role of steroids in the management of patients with spinal extradural abscess is controversial. They have not been shown convincingly to improve outcome and, with prompt diagnosis, early surgical decompression and effective antibiotic therapy, are probably unnecessary.

17.6.8 Prognosis

The prospect of a complete recovery is high if intervention is begun before or during the second (root pain) phase of the disease, i.e. before there is significant neurological deficit. The prognosis worsens rapidly when there is a delay in making the diagnosis and once weakness develops. There is little likelihood of full recovery if surgery is delayed by more than 24 hours after the onset of paralysis and no chance if the delay is more than 48 hours. The overall incidence of mortality is reported to be 13%, but 5% in patients treated surgically.

17.7 TUBERCULOUS SPINAL EXTRADURAL ABSCESS

The incidences of subacute and chronic tuberculous spinal extradural abscesses in the UK and USA have fallen dramatically in the past 30 years, although, with the recent resurgence of tuberculosis in general and the increase in the incidence of HIV infection, it is likely that patients with this disease, perhaps in greater numbers, will continue to present to neurosurgical units. In one series from New York, seven of 27 (25%) cases admitted during the 10-year period, 1968–1978, were caused by *Mycobacterium tuberculosis*.

Tuberculous spinal extradural abscess usually develops following spread from contiguous tuberculous vertebral osteomyelitis or spondylitis. Rarely, disease may arise in the absence of spinal or pulmonary infection and is presumably secondary to haematogenous spread from a distant focus. In common with tuberculous vertebral osteomyelitis, abscesses may occur at any level of the spine, but are most common in the mid- and lower thoracic and lumbar spine, followed by the sacroiliac and cervical spine. The intervertebral disc may be the first tissue affected, with subsequent tracking of pus along the longitudinal ligaments or via adjacent marrow spaces, thereby producing infection in multiple vertebrae.

The clinical features of tuberculous spinal extradural abscess closely resemble those of chronic non-tuberculous spinal extradural abscess, although the symptoms of the former may be present for even longer periods (mean, 3 months; range, 2 weeks–7 years). None the less, the disease may progress at a rapid pace. Back pain is the most common symptom and may be accompanied by weight loss, other non-specific constitutional symptoms, anaemia and a raised serum alkaline phosphatase concentration. Fever and leucocytosis are usually absent, but the tuberculin test is positive in more than 70% of cases. Less than 50% of patients have radiological evidence of active pulmonary tuberculosis. X-rays of the spine are usually abnormal and often show bone destruction. The CT scan can be helpful in defining the extent of the disease and detecting calcification within the abscess which provides a clue to a tuberculous aetiology. In contrast to non-tuberculous abscesses, the advantages of MRI over CT in the diagnosis of tuberculous spinal extradural abscess have not been demonstrated. If myelography is contemplated, it should be preceded by MRI. Material obtained at surgery should always be stained and cultured (positive in more than 70% of cases).

The role of surgery in the management of patients with spinal extradural abscesses is controversial. Many patients will respond to medical therapy alone, with surgical decompression being reserved for patients with profound neurological deficits secondary to involvement of the cervical or upper thoracic spinal regions, when paraplegia is present or for those who experience rapid loss of neurological function or further deterioration of spinal cord function despite appropriate antimicrobial chemotherapy. Others advocate that surgery be performed on any patient with neurological impairment. Drainage of the abscess is not normally required unless it encroaches on the spinal cord. All patients should receive a course of antituberculous therapy (advice regarding appropriate treatment should be obtained from a specialist in respiratory medicine) for between 6 and 9 months, depending on the regimen. Those with co-existing osteomyelitis are usually treated for 12 months.

17.8   VERTEBRAL OSTEOMYELITIS

Vertebral osteomyelitis can be subgrouped into pyogenic and granulomatous types.

17.8.1   Pyogenic vertebral osteomyelitis

Until recently, vertebral osteomyelitis was an uncommon disease. However, the incidence has been increasing as the result of both the growing number of injecting drug users and the increasing use of intravenous access devices with resultant nosocomial bacteraemia. Vertebral infection accounts for 2–4% of all cases of pyogenic osteomyelitis. Affected patients are usually in the fifth to seventh decades, with an average age of 50 years; indeed, the vertebrae are the most common sites of haematogenous osteomyelitis in patients more than 50 years of age. Once found principally in children, the disease is now rare in younger populations. The male:female ratio is as high as 2:1.

Pyogenic vertebral osteomyelitis is usually caused by haematogenous spread of microorganisms from a distant site to the richly vascularized bone adjacent to the disc cartilage. Less often, it follows direct contamination, such as at a surgical procedure, direct extension from a contiguous focus, as in a pharyngeal abscess, or oesophageal instrumentation or perforation. The pathogen and the inflammatory reaction destroy the cartilage end-plate and extend into and destroy the intervertebral disc. Spread to adjacent vertebrae via the ascending and descending branches of the posterior spinal artery is common. The lumbar region is affected in at least 45% of cases where spread is haematogenous, followed by the thoracic spine (35%) and the cervical spine (20%). If the inflammatory process transcends the periosteum, pus accumulates in the surrounding soft tissue, such as the extradural space, where it causes an abscess in approximately 17% of patients. The most common factors predisposing patients to vertebral

osteomyelitis, but identified in only a minority of cases, are diabetes mellitus, immunosuppressive therapy (including oral steroids), intravenous drug abuse, intravenous cannulation, alcoholism, old age, haemodialysis, genitourinary tract instrumentation, previous spinal surgery and blunt trauma to the back. Important sources of infection are the genitourinary and respiratory tracts, skin and soft tissues and teeth. In approximately 37% of cases, a source of infection is not identified.

S. aureus is the most common infecting organism, although, in intravenous drug users, *P. aeruginosa* is the predominant pathogen. AGNB (usually originating in the genitourinary tract) account for up to 30% of aetiological agents, and a miscellany of other organisms, including *H. influenzae*, *Streptococcus pyogenes*, *Salmonella* spp. (in patients with sickle cell disease), anaerobes (in patients with infections involving the neural arch, as opposed to the vertebral body or disc), *Nocardia* spp., *Candida* spp. and *Brucella* spp., accounts for the remainder. As many as 5% of infections are polymicrobial.

Most patients present with subacute manifestations. Back pain of at least 2–3 weeks' duration is the most common symptom (reported by up to 100% of patients). Localized tenderness is also present in at least 90% of cases, but fever is observed in only 20–50%. Motor and sensory neurological deficits, including paralysis, are found in 6–15% of patients. Other clinical features include malaise, weight loss, limitation of back movement and chest wall and abdominal pain. The relative rarity of the disease and the low specificity of the signs and symptoms have resulted in the diagnosis being delayed or missed altogether. A high index of suspicion in a patient with severe back pain and tenderness and malaise is therefore the key to diagnosing pyogenic vertebral osteomyelitis.

Radiological evidence of vertebral osteomyelitis usually lags behind the clinical findings by weeks or even months. Early changes detected by plain X-ray films (which are non-specific) are narrowing of the intervertebral disc space, subchondral lucency, soft tissue swelling and bone destruction and formation of reactive bone. A bone scan can detect spinal abnormalities in more than 90% of patients in the early stages of infection, often within 24 hours of the onset of the process, but the specificity of this technique is lower (about 80%). Both CT and MRI scans are highly sensitive and specific, demonstrate evidence of osteomyelitis (paravertebral soft tissue swelling and bone destruction) before radiological changes occur and are helpful in delineating the full extent of the disease.

The peripheral WBC count is normal in more than 50% of patients, but the ESR and serum CRP concentration are almost invariably elevated. The definitive diagnostic procedure is a bone biopsy or aspiration of disc space tissue; the importance of establishing the aetiology cannot be overemphasized. An open biopsy may be necessary when culture of material obtained at closed aspiration fails to yield a pathogen. Although blood cultures are sterile in more than 50% of patients, it is reasonable to assume that a significant blood culture isolate is the cause of the infection.

Surgical debridement and drainage of bone and associated soft tissue abscesses are unnecessary to achieve cure, except when the infection extends, e.g. when there is a paravertebral or extradural abscess or progressive paraplegia. Similarly, bed rest and immobilization with a brace are no longer regarded as important components of management and are rarely recommended.

Antimicrobial therapy should be guided by the results of a biopsy and/or blood cultures. The initial empirical regimen should provide cover against the predominant pathogen, *S. aureus*, i.e. a combination of flucloxacillin 2–3 g qds and fusidic acid 500 mg bd; a first-generation cephalosporin, such as cefradine 2–3 g qds, can be used in place of flucloxacillin in patients who are allergic to penicillins. In elderly patients and in those in whom there is reason to suspect that the infection is caused by an AGNB, the treatment of choice is a second- or third-generation cephalosporin (cefuroxime 1.5 g tds, cefotaxime 2–3 g qds or ceftriaxone 3–4 g od or 2 g bd). If *P. aeruginosa* is the likely pathogen (e.g. in intravenous drug abusers and patients with long-term indwelling urinary catheters) the initial therapy should be ceftazidime 2 g tds; it should be combined with flucloxacillin 2–3 g qds because of the inadequate cover provided by ceftazidime against *S. aureus*. Treatment should be modified, if necessary, in the light of the results of culture and susceptibility testing. All antibiotics should be administered by the intravenous route (with the exception of fusidic acid which can be given by mouth) for a minimum of 2 weeks, followed by oral therapy if a suitable agent is available. The optimal duration of therapy has not been determined and recommendations in the literature have varied widely. Many authorities advocate treatment for 6 weeks, a period that is recommended for patients with osteomyelitis at other sites, and this seems appropriate. However, there are reports of relapse in patients who have been given what was considered optimal therapy for an adequate duration, and it may be prudent, therefore, to treat patients with symptoms of ≥ 1 month's duration at the time of presentation, or whose diagnoses have been markedly delayed, for 3 months in total. A falling serum CRP concentration is a reliable indication that the patient is responding to treatment.

The outcome of uncomplicated vertebral osteomyelitis is usually good, with most patients recovering fully. Paraplegia complicates the disease in 4.5–13% of cases and 3–40% of patients experience relapses. Other complications include spinal deformities, extradural, subdural, paravertebral, retropharyngeal, mediastinal, subphrenic or retroperitoneal abscesses, meningitis, lesions of the aorta (mycotic aneurysms, infected aneurysms and pseudoaneurysms) and, in patients with haematogenous vertebral osteomyelitis, metastasis to other sites.

17.8.2 Granulomatous vertebral osteomyelitis

Of the granulomatous types of vertebral osteomyelitis, tuberculosis is the most prevalent worldwide. Spinal tuberculosis was once common, but its incidence declined dramatically during the latter half of this century. However, with the increasing incidence of tuberculosis in general, neurosurgeons can expect to see an increase in the number of patients with this disease. Currently, spinal involvement accounts for approximately 50% of cases of tuberculosis of the skeletal system in adults.

It is believed that tuberculous vertebral osteomyelitis is caused by haematogenous spread of the organism early in the course of the initial infection, although, in some cases, spread is via the lymphatics. Infection of the pleura or kidneys can also spread through the paraaortic lymph nodes, with erosion of one or more vertebrae. The first lumbar vertebra is the most frequently affected, followed by the thoracic and then cervical vertebrae. While solitary lesions are observed, multiple lesions are typical. The vertebral body is affected more commonly than the posterior elements, but, in some patients, the latter are predominantly affected. The disease process typically begins with destruction of the anterior portion of the vertebral body adjacent to the subchondral plate. As the lesion enlarges, the infection may spread beneath the anterior or posterior longitudinal ligaments to the adjacent intervertebral disc, subsequently involving the peripheral disc tissue, or to an adjacent vertebra, producing a similar lesion in that bone. Tuberculosis frequently extends to the adjacent ligaments and soft tissues where a paravertebral abscess may develop. After it becomes established in the peripheral tissues it may remain localized or extend for a considerable distance, e.g. to the psoas muscle as a 'cold' abscess. Less commonly, sufficient granulomatous material and pus may accumulate in the extradural space to produce neurological changes (Pott's paraplegia).

The clinical features of tuberculous vertebral osteomyelitis closely resemble those of the chronic form of pyogenic vertebral osteomyelitis; in common with pulmonary tuberculosis, the disease may smoulder for years before it is recognized. Fever and leucocytosis are uncommon, but the tuberculin test is positive in the majority of patients. The appearances on plain X-ray films of the spine are usually abnormal and differ from those of pyogenic infection; in the former, radiological changes are usually observed in the anterior-inferior part of a vertebral body and typically produce a large anterior soft tissue mass. The MRI findings in tuberculous vertebral osteomyelitis include sparing of the disc space. The definitive diagnostic procedure is a fine needle aspiration.

Once the diagnosis is confirmed, anti-tuberculous therapy should be initiated (advice regarding a suitable regimen should be obtained from a specialist in respiratory medicine) and administered for 12 months. Internal fixation in the acute stage is being used with increasing frequency. Otherwise, surgery is not normally indicated unless Pott's paraplegia develops, in which case early decompression and drainage are necessary to avoid permanent damage to the spinal cord, cauda equina and nerve roots.

Most patients respond to treatment and recover fully. With the introduction of modern anti-tuberculous therapy, complications that were commonly observed in the past, including severe spinal deformities, Pott's disease and Pott's paraplegia, have been virtually eliminated.

17.9   DISCITIS

Discitis, inflammation of the intervertebral disc, is an uncommon but severe and debilitating infection. Most cases are iatrogenic, resulting from direct inoculation of bacteria into the disc during spinal surgery. Injury to the end-plates, operative trauma to small vessels, haematomas in the intervertebral space and necrotic tissue caused by the surgery provide suitable conditions for bacterial growth. Discitis may complicate other procedures during which the intervertebral disc is violated, such as discography, chemonucleolysis, discometry, intradiscal steroid injections and percutaneous nucleotomy. It can also result from direct spread from other contiguous foci of infection, although haematogenous spread to avascular discs from a remote source of infection is uncommon; when this does occur, it is usually seen in patients with urinary tract infections or in intravenous drug abusers. In children, discitis may present as a primary infection, this being rare in adults.

The incidence of discitis has increased in recent years, both because of the increasing numbers of invasive procedures undertaken to diagnose and treat disease in human discs and because of the availability of modern, more sensitive and specific diagnostic techniques. The incidence following discectomy is between 1% and 5%, depending on the extent of the procedure, and that following other interventions involving disc violation is approximately 2% (range 1–3.4%). The lumbar vertebral level is most frequently affected (> 80% of cases), followed by the cervical and thoracic levels.

Discitis following intradiscal injection was previously thought to be a chemical or aseptic reaction, but it is now widely believed that all cases are initiated by bacterial infection. The most common pathogens are *S. aureus* (causing up to 100% of post-operative infections) and

CoNS. AGNB, including *P. aeruginosa*, account for up to 30% of pathogens and a miscellany of other organisms, including anaerobes, causes the remainder.

The pathological features of discitis include destruction of the cartilage end-plates, herniation of nuclear material from the intervertebral disc into the adjacent vertebral bodies and extensive replacement of the nucleus pulposus by granulation tissue.

Patients with post-operative discitis present with back pain, usually within 2 weeks of surgery (although the onset can range from days to months), following an initial period of relief from the pre-operative symptoms. Indeed, severe back and/or leg pain may be the only symptoms. The most common physical findings include paravertebral muscle spasm, a strongly positive straight leg-raising test, a limited range of spinal movements and spasticity. The incidences of neurological signs and symptoms are highly variable. Patients may complain of constitutional disturbances, particularly malaise. Fever has been reported in between 4% and 50% of patients, depending on the series. Pain or neurological deficits in post-discectomy patients may be regarded as a consequence of failed surgery or recurrent disc herniation or may be dismissed in a 'neurotic' patient. This, together with the absence of fever, leucocytosis and haematological, biochemical and radiological criteria that are sufficiently sensitive and specific ensure that diagnosis is difficult and often delayed.

Laboratory findings tend to be non-specific. WBC counts are often within normal limits. The ESR is raised in 80–90% percent of cases, but is non-specific and remains elevated for up to 3 months following surgery, even in non-infected patients, thereby precluding its use as a diagnostic criterion. An elevated serum CRP concentration is a common finding. However, it too is non-specific, although superior to the ESR in terms of diagnosing infection. Blood cultures are rarely positive and a percutaneous disc biopsy, with CT guidance, is positive in between 17% and 90% of cases. This is the definitive diagnostic procedure, but is associated with a high false-negative rate. Plain X-rays are unhelpful in the early stages of the disease and may be normal or show only non-specific changes. Narrowing of the disc space with end-plate erosion, bone destruction and formation, demineralization and sclerosis, with or without fusion, appear several weeks after the initial symptoms. CT and MRI scans are more sensitive and specific (up to 97% sensitivity and specificity) than other imaging techniques and increase the likelihood of an early diagnosis. However, these investigations tend not to be undertaken at early stages of the disease. Moreover, an abnormal bone scan is not conclusive evidence of discitis and can persist in patients without infection for up to 1 year following discectomy. Diagnosis therefore requires a high-index of suspicion in a patient with increasing back pain ≥ 2 weeks into the post-operative period and following an initial pain-free interval.

Management of patients with discitis is usually conservative. Most authors have favoured some form of immobilization, ranging from a plaster jacket to bed rest, although there is no evidence that immobilization of any duration has an effect on outcome. Rigid immobilization is widely regarded as unnecessary. The role of antibiotics remains controversial. Clinical observations and evidence from animal studies suggest that the disease is self-limiting. Indeed, the clinical course and outcome have been reported to be similar in treated and untreated patients. Other investigators have questioned the efficacy of antibiotics on the grounds that many of these agents, particularly the β-lactams, which have been the most commonly used therapeutic agents, are undetectable in discs following intravenous administration. However, the studies on which these observations were based were performed in animal models or in patients with diseased, non-infected discs. Penetration of antibiotics is less limited in cases of disc space infection in adults as local tissues are hyperaemic and because invasive granulation tissue is usually present as a response to infection. There is no agreement about the absolute necessity of giving antibiotics to patients with discitis, including children with primary discitis, but some authors have suggested that appropriate antibiotics may hasten recovery, although this has not been proven. None the less, most patients have received courses of these drugs following attempts to identify the aetiological agents. Empirical therapy should be directed against the predominant pathogen, S. aureus. The drug of choice is therefore flucloxacillin 2 g qds or a first-generation cephalosporin, such as cefradine 2 g qds, in patients who are allergic to penicillins. A glycopeptide (vancomycin or teicoplanin) should be administered if there are good reasons to suspect that the pathogen is MRSA. Treatment should be modified, if necessary, in the light of culture and susceptibility test results. The optimal duration of therapy has not been determined, but most patients have received antibiotics for 6 weeks, 2 weeks by the intravenous route followed by 4 weeks of oral therapy if a suitable agent is available. The CRP is a useful criterion for monitoring the response to treatment. Surgical management should be tailored to the individual patient. Some authors have advocated surgery for all patients, while others have recommended surgery only if conservative management has failed or if an abscess or extradural mass is detected.

A favourable outcome depends on early diagnosis, identification of the causal agent and initiation of specific therapy. Delays in diagnosis are associated with difficulties in subsequent management and a poor outcome. With appropriate treatment, relapses are uncommon. None the less, fewer than 50% of patients return to work and normal daily activities. Complications are uncommon. In a minority of cases, discitis progresses to vertebral osteomyelitis.

17.10 POST-OPERATIVE MENINGITIS

17.10.1 Bacterial meningitis

The incidence of bacterial meningitis complicating neurosurgical procedures is low, varying from 0.5% in patients who have undergone clean procedures with antibiotic prophylaxis to 6% in those who have undergone clean-contaminated procedures without prophylactic cover. Craniotomy following trauma or for the resection of tumour is the procedure most frequently associated with post-operative meningitis. Close proximity to the heavily colonized scalp, or the need to enter the frontal, sphenoidal or mastoid air sinuses allows direct contamination of the operative field and secondary CSF leakage facilitates the entry of potential pathogens into the subarachnoid space.

AGNB, including E. coli, Klebsiella pneumoniae, P. aeruginosa and Acinetobacter spp., which together account for 60–70% of cases, followed by S. aureus, are the most common aetiological agents. The clinical features of meningitis, which usually presents within the first 7–10 days following surgery, include headache, fever, neck stiffness, nausea and vomiting and, occasionally, an altered level of consciousness. The onset is sometimes insidious and it may be difficult to distinguish meningitis from the neurological symptoms and signs that are associated with the underlying disease or that are common in the early post-operative period. Examination of the CSF is the definitive diagnostic procedure, although a CT scan is frequently performed first in order to determine that a lumbar puncture is safe. When a lumbar puncture is unsafe, it may be necessary to carry out a ventricular puncture (although ventricular and lumbar CSF samples in patients with obstructive hydrocephalus may differ markedly in terms of the cell counts and biochemical profiles) or to treat empirically. The CSF protein concentration and leucocyte count are almost always elevated, but, if the sample has been obtained within 12 hours of the onset of symptoms, the white cell count may be low or even within the normal range; a repeat CSF examination (where practical) 24 hours later usually demonstrates a marked increase in the number of cells. The glucose concentration is normally depressed in the presence of infection, but a Gram's stain may be negative in up to 70% of patients with culture-positive infections. In common with the clinical presentation, CSF parameters (both cellular and biochemical) may be altered in the post-operative period as a result of the surgery itself, and especially in the presence of subarachnoid haemorrhage, thereby confounding efforts to confirm the diagnosis.

A third-generation cephalosporin, such as cefotaxime 2–3 g qds or ceftriaxone 3–4 g od or 2 g bd, should be administered as initial empirical therapy, unless the patient has already received broad-spectrum antibiotics,

Table 17.5 *Systemic^a antibiotic therapy of neurosurgical patients with post-operative bacterial meningitis^b*

Clinical setting/pathogen	Regimen
First-line empirical therapy	Cefotaxime 2–3 g qds or ceftriaxone 3–4 g od or 2 g bd
Patient has recently received a broad-spectrum antibiotic or confirmed *P. aeruginosa*	Ceftazidime 2 g tds
Suspected or confirmed ESBL-producing Enterobacteriaceae or *Acinetobacter* sp.	Meropenem 2 g tds
Methicillin-susceptible *S. aureus*	Flucloxacillin 2–3 g qds
Methicillin-resistant *S. aureus*	Vancomycin 1 g bd^c or teicoplanin 12 mg/kg body weight od (after three loading doses) plus rifampicin 600 mg bd

^{a}See text for intraventricular regimens.
^{b}Reproduced from: Infection in Neurosurgery Working Party of the British Society for Antimicrobial Chemotherapy, *British Journal of Neurosurgery* 2000; **14**: 7–12.
^{c}Trough and peak serum concentrations must be monitored.

in which case ceftazidime 2 g tds should be prescribed in order to provide cover against *P. aeruginosa*. Meropenem 2 g tds is the drug of choice for patients with infections caused by *Acinetobacter* spp. which are increasing in frequency and which tend to be resistant to multiple antibiotics. Those with infections caused by methicillin-susceptible strains of *S. aureus* should be treated with flucloxacillin 2–3 g qds. Either vancomycin 1 g bd or teicoplanin 12 mg/kg body weight od after three loading doses is the drug of choice for the treatment of patients with meningitis caused by strains of MRSA and should be administered in combination with rifampicin 600 mg bd po. However, glycopeptides penetrate poorly into CSF and, if the patient has failed to respond to systemic therapy, it may be necessary to implant an Ommaya reservoir and to instil vancomycin (10 mg every third day) directly into the ventricles. Treatment should be modified, if necessary, once the results of culture and susceptibility testing are available. Because AGNB can develop resistance to β-lactams during the course of therapy, ideally, CSF should be obtained for culture at regular intervals (every 4–5 days) in order to ensure that it has been sterilized. If a patient with infection caused by an AGNB is severely ill, the response to therapy is delayed or the pathogen is not eradicated by systemic therapy alone, gentamicin (3–4 mg, assuming a normal ventricular volume) should be given intraventricularly every third day; the threshold for doing so should be low. The total duration of therapy should be 2 weeks if the infecting organism is *S. aureus* and up to 3 weeks if it is an AGNB. The various regimens are summarized in Table 17.5.

17.10.2 Aseptic meningitis

Patients may develop so-called aseptic or chemical meningitis up to several days after intradural neurosurgical procedures. This complication, which occurs more frequently than bacterial meningitis, has been reported in as many as 70% of children undergoing posterior fossa surgery but, despite the association of aseptic meningitis with posterior fossa procedures, the syndrome has been observed in 50% of patients following operations in other sites. The condition is thought to be the result of chemical irritation, caused either by blood or blood degradation products which are introduced into the subarachnoid space during surgery or by factors released by dural substitutes. Aseptic meningitis normally responds favourably to high dosages of steroids which reduce meningeal inflammation and the likelihood of serious long-term complications.

The course and symptoms in patients with aseptic meningitis are indistinguishable from those in patients with bacterial meningitis. A patient with either disease may have a stiff neck, spiking fever, headache and nausea. When CSF analysis is performed, it demonstrates a low glucose concentration, an elevated protein concentration and a pleiocytosis with a predominance of polymorphonuclear leucocytes – as in bacterial meningitis. Indeed, the ranges of values of CSF parameters found in infected patients overlap significantly with those found in non-infected post-operative patients; even a Gram's stain of the CSF may be negative in up to 70% of patients with culture-positive meningitis. The desirability of avoiding the unnecessary administration of antimicrobial chemotherapy to patients with aseptic meningitis and the potentially adverse effects associated with giving steroids to patients with bacterial meningitis have prompted a search for diagnostic tests that can reliably and rapidly distinguish between the two disease processes. Many such tests have been evaluated, although, with two exceptions (see below), not in post-operative neurosurgical patients. They have included measurements of CSF concentrations of lactate, ferritin, total amino acids, CRP, endotoxin, various cytokines [interleukin (IL)-1, IL-2, IL-6 and IL-10 and tumour necrosis factor (TNF)-α], β_2-microglobulin, adenosine deaminase and nitric oxide, as well as plasma procalcitonin and amyloid A concentrations and the blood/CSF glucose ratio. However, results have varied widely from study to study, with some groups of investigators reporting that the concentrations of certain variables increase in patients with bacterial meningitis and others finding that the levels of the same variables are low or even undetectable. The observation that the concentrations of some variables are elevated only in the early stages of bacterial meningitis and decline rapidly thereafter are a further source of confusion. Finally, surgery-related changes in the composition of the CSF that occur in the early post-operative period may compromise the value of many of these diagnostic criteria.

Two groups of investigators have attempted to distinguish between aseptic and bacterial meningitis specifically in post-operative neurosurgical patients. In a retrospective study, one group reported that CSF lactate concentrations ≥ 4 mmol/L have high sensitivity, specificity and positive and negative predictive values in terms of identifying patients who develop bacterial meningitis following craniotomy. A second group evaluated the utilities of four pro-inflammatory cytokines (TNF-α, IL-1β, IL-6 and IL-8) in differentiating between post-neurosurgical aseptic and bacterial meningitis. Although the CSF concentrations of TNF-α, IL-1β and IL-6 were significantly higher in patients with bacterial meningitis than in those with aseptic meningitis, only IL-1β was sufficiently reliable to be used as a diagnostic criterion for discriminating between aseptic and bacterial meningitis. These investigators also observed that, within 24 hours of initiating antibacterial therapy, the CSF concentrations of IL-1β declined by > 50% and returned to normal over the following few days, the implication being that the CSF concentrations of this cytokine must be measured before antibiotic treatment is commenced. Although the results of both studies are promising, the potentially devastating consequences of failing to administer antibiotics to patients who have incorrectly been diagnosed as having aseptic meningitis make it essential that the efficacies of both the CSF lactate concentration and the CSF IL-1β are validated by additional prospective investigations. Measurement of the serum procalcitonin concentration also shows considerable potential as a means of identifying patients with bacterial meningitis. However, this variable has, to date, been assessed principally for its ability to differentiate between bacterial and viral meningitis. Currently, therefore, it must be concluded that no single laboratory test or combination of tests has emerged as being sufficiently specific and sensitive to enable it to be used to discriminate, with the 100% accuracy that is required, between bacterial and aseptic meningitis at the time of presentation. For the time being, isolation of a pathogen from the CSF of post-operative neurosurgical patients must remain the definitive diagnostic test, although this means that the diagnosis can be made only retrospectively.

Owing to the difficulties of accurately identifying patients with bacterial meningitis prospectively and the morbidity and mortality resulting from delays in initiating treatment, all patients who present with the clinical and laboratory features of post-operative meningitis should receive empirical therapy with a broad-spectrum antibiotic such as cefotaxime 2–3 g qds or ceftriaxone 3–4 g od or 2 g bd. If the CSF is subsequently found to be sterile (usually after 2–3 days), antibiotic treatment can be discontinued, providing that such drugs had not been given during the 24–48 hours before the lumbar puncture was performed.

17.11 VENTRICULITIS IN PATIENTS WITH EXTERNAL VENTRICULAR DRAINS

Patients with EVDs are at risk of developing ventriculitis, the risk being lowest during the first 4 days that the drain is *in situ*, rising over the first 10 days and falling off markedly thereafter; the risk is also related to the degree of aseptic technique employed to insert and maintain the drain. The incidence has been reported to be as high as 40%, but, more commonly, between 10% and 17%. It has previously been proposed that the infection rate could be lowered by prophylactically exchanging EVDs at 5-day intervals. However, it was subsequently demonstrated that the infection rate in patients in whom EVDs were replaced after < 5 days was not lower than that in patients in whom the drains were exchanged at intervals of > 5 days. The investigators therefore recommended that drains should be removed from non-infected patients as early as is practicable, but that they should not be exchanged routinely.

In common with intravascular line-related infections, the predominant aetiological agents are CoNS. Because the pathogens are low-grade, the signs and symptoms of infection are often subtle and may even be inapparent. Pyrexia is an almost invariable finding and, indeed, may be the only sign in patients who are unresponsive. On the other hand, it is a common feature of neurosurgical patients and not exclusively related to the presence of infection. Headache, nausea and/or vomiting and, less frequently, altered mental status are other recognized features in responsive patients. As the infecting agents often fail to elicit brisk inflammatory responses, neck stiffness is uncommon. For the same reason, there may be very few, or even no, white blood cells on microscopic examination of a sample of CSF. The diagnosis is therefore based on the isolation of a presumptive pathogen from the CSF. However, the incidence of contamination is high in this setting and the diagnosis should be confirmed by identifying the same bacterium in a second specimen; samples should be collected from the EVD itself or, if present, from an Ommaya reservoir, but not from the drainage bag. If the causative organism is a CoNS, the patient should be treated by instilling vancomycin (5–20 mg, depending on the ventricular volume, i.e. 5 mg for patients with 'slit' ventricles, 10 mg for those with ventricles of normal volume and 15–20 mg for those with greater than normal volumes) directly into the ventricles and clamping the drain for approximately 15 min. If CSF is draining freely (i.e. ≥ 100 mL/day), a daily dose should be administered, but, if there is no, or negligible, CSF drainage (< 50 mL/day), the dose need be repeated only every third day; patients from whom intermediate volumes of CSF (50–100 mL /day) are draining should be given doses on alternate days and those from whom very large volumes (> 200 mL/day) are draining may require higher dosages or twice-daily instillation. The frequency of dosing must be reviewed daily and should be based on the amount of fluid drained since the previous dose. Treatment for 5–7 days is usually adequate. If the drain is no longer required, it should be removed immediately after administration of the last dose in order to avoid relapse or reinfection; otherwise it should be replaced for the same reason. In the event that a bacterium other than a CoNS is isolated, treatment should be guided by the results of suscepti-bility testing.

A patient with an EVD *in situ* may undergo implanta-tion of a CSF shunt, although, unbeknown to the sur-geon, the CSF may not be sterile at the time that the procedure is performed. This can arise either because the culture results for a sample of CSF collected 2–3 days before surgery are not available until during or after implantation or, alternatively, because the CSF became infected in the interval between obtaining a pre-opera-tive sample for microbiological investigation and the procedure itself. In order to minimize the risk of this happening, a sample of CSF should be obtained for cul-ture from all patients 2–3 days before the surgery, irre-spective of whether or not ventriculitis is suspected, and vancomycin (10 mg) instilled into the ventricles imme-diately thereafter. The dose of vancomycin should be repeated once daily until the time of surgery if there is

free drainage of CSF (≥ 100 mL/day), but only one dose in total is necessary if there is no or minimal drainage. If the surgery is postponed for up to 2 days, vancomycin prophylaxis should be continued until the procedure has been carried out, but, if it is delayed for longer periods or, indeed, indefinitely, prophylaxis should be disconti-nued. Should culture of the sample obtained 2 days before surgery confirm that the CSF was sterile, no further post-operative doses are required. However, if a susceptible Gram-positive bacterium is isolated, treatment with vancomycin (10 mg instilled once daily into the ventricle through a separate reservoir) should be continued until the fourth post-operative day.

17.12   FURTHER READING

Infection in Neurosurgery Working Party of the British Society for Antimicrobial Chemotherapy (1994) Antimicrobial prophylaxis in neurosurgery and after head injury. *Lancet*, **344**, 1547–51.

Working Party on the Use of Antibiotics in Neurosurgery of the British Society for Antimicrobial Chemotherapy. (1995) Treatment of infections associated with shunting for hydrocephalus. *Br. J. Hosp. Med.*, **53**, 368–73.

Infection in Neurosurgery Working Party of the British Society for Antimicrobial Chemotherapy (2000) The management of neurosurgical patients with postoperative bacterial or aseptic meningitis or external ventricular drain-associated ventriculitis. *Br. J. Neurosurg.*, **14**, 7–12.

Infection in Neurosurgery Working Party of the British Society for Antimicrobial Chemotherapy (2000) The rational use of antibiotics in the treatment of brain abscess. *Br. J. Neurosurg.*, **14**, 525–30.

Bayston, R., de Louvois, J., Brown, E.M., Johnston, R.A., Lees, P. and Pople, I.K. (2000) 'Infection in Neurosurgery' Working Party of British Society for Antimicrobial Chemotherapy. Use of antibiotics in penetrating craniocerebral injuries. *Lancet*, **355**, 1813–17.

Infections of the face

M.A.O. LEWIS

18.1 INFECTIONS OF CONGENITAL ABNORMALITIES

18.1.1 Cleft lip and palate

Bacterial colonization of the mouth begins shortly after birth, and within the first week of life a commensal microflora comprising of viridans streptococci (predominantly *Streptococcus salivarius*), *Staphylococcus albus* and anaerobic streptococci has developed. Other bacteria which appear during early weeks include, *Neisseria* spp., *Lactobacillus* spp., *Fusobacterium* spp. and *Actinomyces* spp. In addition to being present in the mouth, these microorganisms also colonize the nasal and facial clefts of patients with cleft lip and palate.

The initial management of a neonate with a cleft is likely to involve the provision of a specialized acrylic denture, referred to as a feeding plate. The initial series of feeding plates is worn constantly for between 3 and 9 months depending on the nature of the cleft and timing of surgical repair. The acrylic plate provides a site for proliferation of members of the oral microflora, and therefore the appliance should be cleaned in 0.2% solution of chlorhexidine gluconate for 30 minutes each day. Candidal colonization, acquired from vaginal carriage in the mother, occurs in the mouths of 1 in 20 neonates, and therefore oral candidosis can be a recurrent problem due to fungal infection of the feeding plate. A microbiological swab should be taken from the palatal surface of the plate in addition to the oral mucosa to confirm the presence of candida. In addition to thorough cleaning of the plate in

0.2% chlorhexidine gluconate, it may be necessary to provide antifungal therapy. It is becoming increasingly accepted that the efficacy of topical antifungal agents is poor, and therefore if therapy is required then this should be given systemically. Suggested regimens for antifungal therapy are as follows:

- Fluconazole by mouth or intravenous infusion, 3–6 mg kg^{-1} on the first day, and there after 3 mg kg^{-1} daily (every 72 hours in neonates up to 2 weeks old, every 48 hours in neonates aged 2–4 weeks).
- Itraconazole, but this is not recommended in children.

18.2 INFECTIONS OF THE LIPS

18.2.1 Macrocheilia

Recurrent or persistent swelling of the lips is a frequent feature in Crohn's disease, orofacial granulomatosis and Melkersson–Rosenthal syndrome. Opportunistic infections involving skin and oral commensal bacteria subsequently occur, both at the angles of the mouth and in the vertical fissures that often develop in the midline of the lips (Figure 18.1).

A separate microbiological swab should be taken from each affected site and sent for bacteriological and mycological culture. Coagulase-negative staphylococci are usually encountered, although *Candida* spp. are also occasionally isolated, particularly if the patient wears dentures.

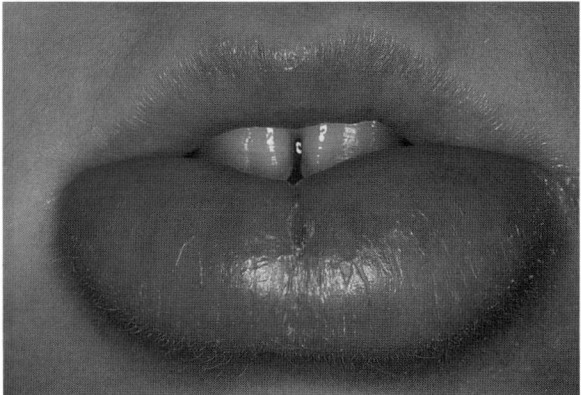

Figure 18.1 *This 10-year-old boy who has Crohn's disease has complained of lip swelling, a recognized feature of the condition, for 2 years. The painful midline fissure had mistakenly been diagnosed as herpes labialis (cold sore), and the patient had been prescribed several courses of topical aciclovir cream. Herpes labialis heals within 10 days regardless of treatment, and therefore the protracted nature of this lesion should have prompted an alternative diagnosis. A microbiological swab of the lip yielded a heavy growth of* Staph. aureus*. The topical application of mupirocin led to resolution of the infection within 7 days.*

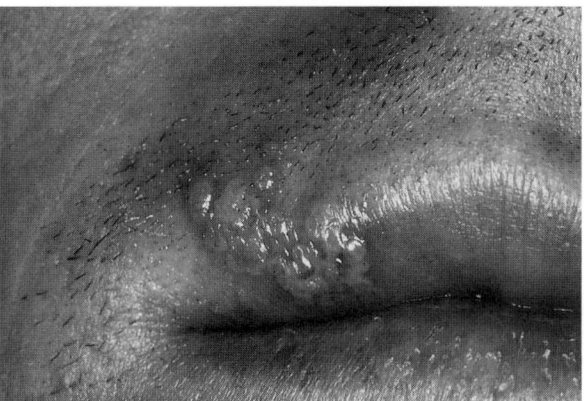

Figure 18.2 *Vesicular lesions of recurrent herpes labialis.*

Treatment is by application of a topical antimicrobial, dependent upon whether only staphylococci are isolated. If this is the case, then mupirocin 2% ointment should be applied up to three times daily for up to 10 days. Alternatively, fusidic acid 2% cream may be applied two or three times daily.

If staphylococci **and** *candida* spp. are isolated, then miconazole nitrate 2% cream should be applied twice daily.

18.2.2 Recurrent herpes labialis

The signs and symptoms of recurrent herpes labialis represent reactivation of latent herpes simplex virus (HSV) in the orofacial tissues, in particular the sensory nerves. HSV type 1 is almost exclusively involved, although HSV type 2 is occasionally isolated from herpes labialis. A number of factors, such as exposure to ultraviolet light, emotional stress or immunosuppression, have been implicated as 'triggers' of viral reactivation. Although the mechanism by which these factors initiate viral replication are not fully understood, it has been suggested it involves a detrimental effect on local lymphokine production by lymphocytes, prostaglandin synthesis and other actions of the immune defence system.

An episode of herpes labialis progresses through a number of distinct clinical phases, including blister formation (Figure 18.2). The initial localized tingle (prodrome) is followed by stages of papule, blister, ulcer and

crust prior to complete healing of the skin within 10–14 days. The sequence of events involved in recurrent herpes labialis is sufficiently characteristic that it is rarely necessary to confirm the diagnosis by virological investigation. However, if there is doubt then a swab should be taken for viral culture. Serology demonstrating the presence of antibody to HSV can be used to determine if the patient has previously had an episode of primary HSV infection, but is not helpful in diagnosis of herpes labialis since a detectable increase in HSV antibody levels does not occur during an attack.

Topical treatment based on chemicals such as phenol, ammonia, tannic acid, povidone-iodine, urea, extract of melissa, tea tree oil or zinc sulphate are helpful in some patients. The use of these non-specific agents is based on the fact that they may either dry the ulcer or moisturize any crusting to prevent painful cracking of the tissues, rather than have any specific effect on the virus. Idoxuridine, which closely resembles thymidine in structure, was one of the first specific antiviral agents used in the treatment of HSV infection. The drug can be applied topically onto lesions as a 5% solution in dimethyl sulphoxide (a vehicle that facilitates penetration of the skin). Idoxuridine can speed the time to healing of the cold sore and reduce severity of pain, although patients may complain of a stinging sensation on application and an unpleasant taste. In recent years, the use of idoxuridine has reduced considerably due to the development of two new topical antiviral agents:

- **Aciclovir:** this is applied as a 5% cream, every 4 hours (five times daily) for 5 days, starting at the first sign of attack. Aciclovir has been promoted extensively in many parts of the world as an effective form of treatment for herpes labialis, although it is stressed that early application is required to produce most benefit. There is evidence that topical aciclovir has an effect on recurrent herpes labialis but this format of the drug has not been licensed for general use in some countries including Canada and the USA.

- **Penciclovir** is the first antiviral agent to be developed specifically for the topical treatment of herpes labialis. Penciclovir 1% cream should be applied every 2 hours during waking hours for 4 days. At present, it is not recommended in children aged under 16 years. Penciclovir convincingly impacts the course of a cold sore by reducing the time to healing, the severity of pain and the period of shedding of HSV from the lesion.

Apart from considering the provision of topical antiviral therapy, patients who suffer recurrent herpes labialis should be given simple advice to reduce the incidence of attacks. Known trigger factors should be avoided if possible, and the application of total sun block on and around the lips can prevent lesions in those sufferers who develop herpes labialis after exposure to ultraviolet light. The fluid exudate from the blister is extremely infectious, containing approximately 10^6 HSV per millilitre, and sufferers should appreciate the risk of spread of virus to other body sites. This is particularly important if the patient wears contact lenses, since infection may spread to the eye via the fingers.

Some patients suffer frequent repeated attacks of herpes labialis in the absence of any recognized trigger factor, and in these circumstances consideration may be given to the provision of prophylactic systemic antiviral therapy. The use of oral aciclovir 200 mg two or three times daily over a period of 6 months in an attempt to suppress herpes labialis has been suggested, but there are obvious financial implications of this type of prophylactic approach.

18.2.3   Syphilis

Syphilis characteristically affects the genitalia and is caused by a motile spirochaete, *Treponema pallidum*. However, primary infection with *T. pallidum* may occur on the mucous membranes of the mouth or lip and present as painless ulcer (chancre) with enlargement of regional lymph nodes.

T. pallidum cannot be routinely cultured *in vitro* (although the organism can be grown in the testes of rabbit), and therefore diagnosis must be made by examination of the exudate collected from the ulcer in a fine capillary tube. Dark-field microscopy or silver staining should be used to detect the presence of motile spirochaetes. Routine investigation also involves serology. The Veneral Diseases Reference Laboratory (VDRL) test may be negative in early primary infection, whilst the fluorescent *Treponema* antibody absorbed test FTA(abs) should be positive. Procaine penicillin for 10–21 days is the treatment of choice. If the patient has a hypersensitivity to penicillins then tetracycline, doxycycline or erythromycin can be used for 14–21 days.

18.2.4   Staphylococcal lip lesions

Erythematous, painful lesions on the lip may develop due to staphylococcal infection, particularly in hospitalized or medically immunocompromised patients. If such symptoms develop then a swab should be taken from the affected mucosa and sent for culture. An appropriate topical antimicrobial should be provided and includes mupirocin 2% ointment applied up to three times daily up to 10 days, or fusidic acid 2% cream applied two or three times daily.

18.3   INFECTIONS OF MAXILLOFACIAL INJURIES

Trauma to the facial tissues due to a road traffic accident, sports injury or assault occurs frequently. Such trauma to the facial skeleton invariably results in the introduction of bacteria from the skin and/or the oral flora into the facial wound (Figure 18.3). Fortunately, most patients with facial injuries seek professional help relatively quickly, and therefore the potential for infection is reduced by the provision of appropriate treatment. However, patients may occasionally delay hospital attendance for many days and in these circumstances clinical infection which complicates management can develop. Although antibiotics are prescribed routinely in the presence of obvious infection, there is a wide difference of opinion on the need for prophylactic

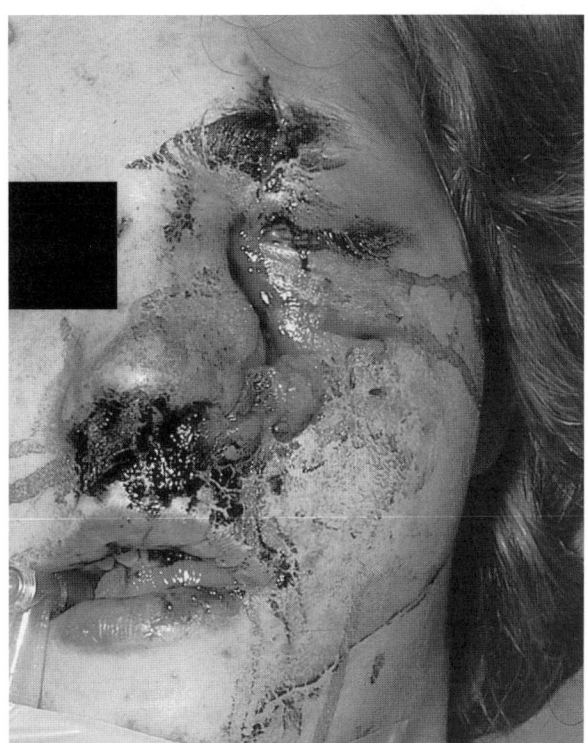

Figure 18.3 *Severe maxillofacial facial injury.*

antibiotic therapy in the management of facial injuries. Clean facial injuries in healthy patients have a surprising capacity to heal without infectious complications, so that prophylaxis in this group is probably unnecessary.

18.3.1 Facial lacerations

Superficial lacerations involving the face, neck and scalp have the potential to become infected with members of the commensal skin microflora, such as *Staphylococcus epidermidis* and *Propionibacterium acnes*. Soft tissue wounds should be treated within 24 hours by thorough cleaning prior to suturing. Infection in lacerations is rare and there is seldom a need to prescribe antibiotic therapy. Repaired wounds may be covered by dry gauze or a commercial wound dressing, although the benefit and effect on scar formation of this aspect of management are uncertain. If infection develops in a wound, a swab should be taken and sent for culture. In these circumstances an antibiotic with known activity against staphylococci, such as flucloxacillin, can be provided empirically prior to the availability of the results of any microbiological investigation. Wounds that cannot be closed by sutures or adhesive strips, and/or which may become infected, benefit from applications of topical agents. For example, mupirocin 2% ointment may be applied up to three times daily up to 10 days, or fusidic acid 2% cream may be applied two or three times daily.

18.3.2 Fractured maxilla

Fractures involving the middle third of the facial skeleton are likely to produce a bleed into the maxillary sinuses, and therefore there is an opportunity for infection. In addition, high-level or severe maxillary injuries can result in a leak of cerebrospinal fluid and a potential for intracranial infection. Antimicrobial treatment in such cases must therefore involve **an antibiotic that will cross the blood-brain barrier**. In the past, sulphonamides were used routinely for such patients, but the 'second-generation' cephalosporin, **cefuroxime** (1.5 g given intravenously every 6–8 hours) is now the drug of choice. Antimicrobial therapy should be provided until the time that the injury is treated surgically. There is rarely any need for medication after fixation of the fracture.

18.3.3 Fractured zygomatic arch

Although fractures of the zygomatic complex often produce bleeding into the maxillary sinus, infection at this site is rare. Patients with zygomatic fractures do not routinely require prophylactic antibiotics particularly if it is only the zygomatic arch that is involved. However, in severe cases where the fracture is compound, or an intra-oral approach is used for reduction and fixation, there is a potential for either maxillary sinusitis or periorbital cellulitis. In these circumstances, amoxicillin (250 mg every 8 hours) or, if the patient has a hypersensitivity to penicillins, erythromycin (250–500 mg every 6 hours) should be provided and continued for at least 7 days.

18.3.4 Fractured mandible

Antibiotic therapy is unnecessary for a fracture of the mandible occurring in an edentulous patient where there is no communication of the injury into the oral cavity or overlying skin. However, there is benefit in providing prophylactic antibiotics in cases involving teeth or tearing of the oral mucosa. Amoxicillin or benzylpenicillin can be provided intravenously until the time of reduction and fixation of the fracture. Alternatively, some surgeons prefer to use either co-amoxiclav or a combination of amoxicillin and metronidazole. There is no requirement for antimicrobial therapy once the fracture has been stabilized.

18.3.5 Other fractures

A patient may occasionally delay presentation with a fracture for many days, particularly in parts of the world where medical assistance is not readily available. In such cases suppurative infection may develop, and pus at the site of fractures will inevitably delay healing and complicate management. Alternatively, postoperative infection sometimes delays healing of fractures where there is poor fixation and mobility of the bone segments. In either of these situations, a pus sample (preferably obtained by aspiration rather than on a swab) should be sent for culture. The infection is invariably mixed in nature and involves three or four bacterial species, often the 'Streptococcus milleri' group (*Strep. anginosus*, *Strep. constellatus* and *Strep. intermedius*), *Actinomyces* spp., *Prevotella* spp. and *Eubacterium* spp. Susceptibility testing should be undertaken, since in recent years there has been an increase in the frequency of isolation of penicillin-resistant strains of *Prevotella* spp. Resistance in these isolates is due to production of β-lactamases. Empirical treatment should involve the intravenous provision of either co-amoxiclav (375 mg every 8 hours) or a combination of amoxicillin and metronidazole (250 mg amoxicillin every 8 hours combined with metronidazole 200 mg every 8 hours). Antibiotics should be discontinued when signs of resolution develop.

If the patient is allergic to penicillins, then erythromycin (250–500 mg) should be given every 6 hours, combined with metronidazole 200 mg every 8 hours.

18.4 SUBCUTANEOUS ABSCESS OF DENTAL ORIGIN

Chronic infection at the apex of a necrotic tooth or unerupted tooth may spread through the tissues to produce a chronic discharging sinus on the skin of the face (Figure 18.4). Such a lesion is occasionally mistaken for an infected sebaceous cyst, or even a squamous cell or basal cell carcinoma. Radiographs of the mandible will reveal the source of infection at the apex of a tooth. A pus sample, preferably obtained by aspiration of the skin lesion, should be sent for culture. The isolation of staphylococci is likely to reflect contamination of the sample from the skin flora rather than being representative of the underlying dental infection, which characteristically involves a mixture of strict anaerobes. Treatment should involve the removal of the dental cause of infection, either by extraction or root canal therapy of the affected tooth; antibiotics are not usually required.

18.5 SALIVARY GLAND INFECTIONS

The main excretory duct of the parotid gland has been found to have a microflora in health, composed predominantly of α-haemolytic streptococci, in particular

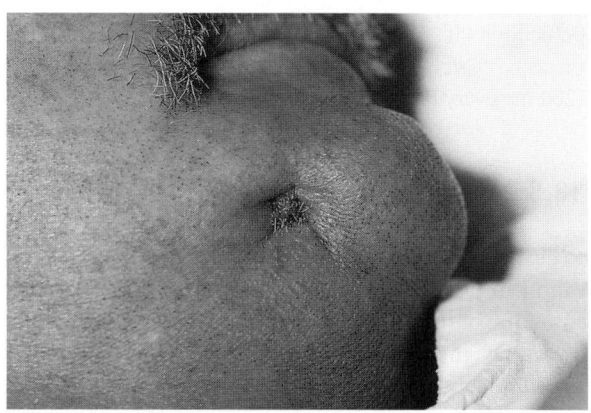

Figure 18.4 *This patient, who had had full dentures for many years, was referred for an opinion on the cause of a chronic discharging sinus in the right mental region that had been present for 10 months. The patient's medical practitioner had examined the mouth and found no evidence of oral pathology. A biopsy of the skin lesion reported inflammatory changes only with no evidence of malignancy. It was only at this stage that a dental opinion was sought. An orthopantomograph revealed an unerupted premolar lying in the body of the mandible. Surgical removal of the buried tooth led to resolution of the discharging sinus. This case illustrates the importance of undertaking radiographic examination of the jaws to exclude the presence of intra-bony pathology. Clinical examination of the mouth alone is not sufficient. (Photograph courtesy of Prof J.G. Cowpe, Bristol Dental School.)*

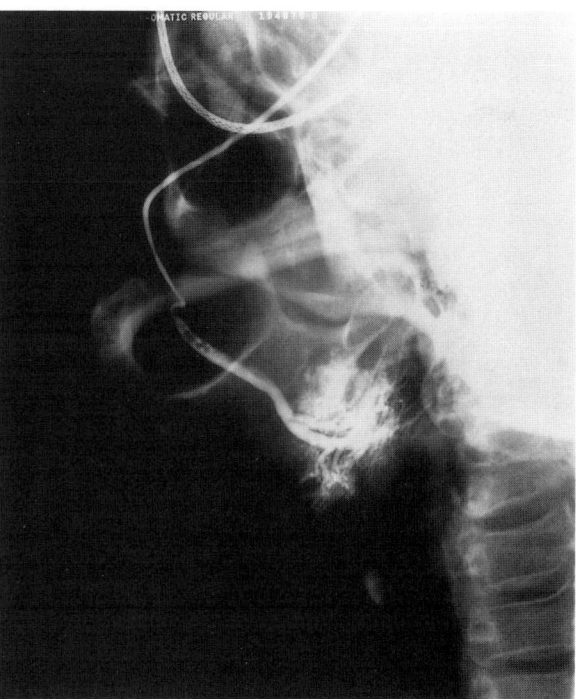

Figure 18.5 *Sialogram of parotid salivary gland showing duct dilation and gross loss of normal gland architecture.*

Strep. sanguis and *Strep. mitis*. Bacterial colonization is low at 10^3 cfu ml^{-1} during health, but the level and complexity of the flora increases with reduced saliva flow. Although it has not been investigated in such detail, it is likely that a similar commensal flora exists in the main duct of the submandibular gland.

Sialography is a structural investigation of the major salivary glands involving the infusion of contrast medium into the main excretory duct (Figure 18.5). The procedure has been shown to produce a bacteraemia involving organisms from within the duct, and this has led to suggestions that antibiotic prophylaxis should be considered when the procedure is performed on patients at risk of developing infective endocarditis. However, at the present time sialography is not included in the list of procedures routinely requiring antibiotic prophylaxis, probably due to the low level of the associated bacteraemia.

18.5.1 Acute suppurative sialadenitis

Acute bacterial infection may develop in any one of the major salivary glands, but is particularly common in the parotid gland. Patients present with a painful swelling of the affected gland and a discharge of pus at the orifice of the main excretory duct (Figure 18.6). The aetiology of suppurative sialadenitis usually represents an ascending infection of the duct involving members of the oral flora. The most common predisposing factors are either reduced salivary flow due to Sjögren's syndrome or

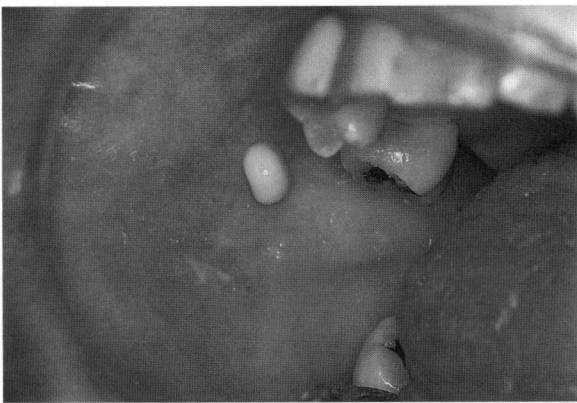

Figure 18.6 *This 55-year-old female presented with swelling of the left parotid salivary gland and a discharge of pus at the duct orifice. Episodes of acute infection occurred approximately every 6 months. The patient has rheumatoid arthritis, and clinical examination revealed xerostomia and xerophthalmia. A diagnosis of Sjögren's syndrome with suppurative parotitis was made. The acute infection resolved following a 5-day course of amoxicillin 250 mg capsule three times daily for 5 days. Culture of the discharge yielded a mixed growth of* Strep. milleri *group and* Fusobacterium nucleatum, *both of which were sensitive to amoxicillin. It is preferable to treat each episode of infection as it occurs rather than providing long-term antibiotic therapy in such patients.*

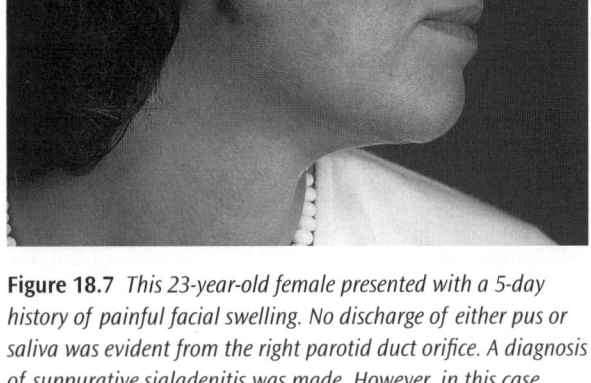

Figure 18.7 *This 23-year-old female presented with a 5-day history of painful facial swelling. No discharge of either pus or saliva was evident from the right parotid duct orifice. A diagnosis of suppurative sialadenitis was made. However, in this case pus had uncharacteristically tracked externally rather than intra-orally. The patient responded well to a 5-day course of metronidazole tablet 400 mg three times daily. Culture of an aspirate yielded a growth of* Fusobacterium nucleatum *and anaerobic Gram-positive cocci. A sialogram undertaken following resolution of the symptoms demonstrated multiple sialectasis within the gland.*

blockage of the duct by a salivary stone. Historically, parotitis involving *Staph. aureus* was a particular problem in hospitalized surgical patients, but this postoperative complication is now rare due to a better understanding of maintaining fluid balance and reduced likelihood of *Staph. aureus* colonization of the mouth which is further diminished by regular oral hygiene measures. More recently, pus from suppurative sialadenitis has been found to yield a mixture of two or three bacterial species, such as α-haemolytic streptococci, *Haemophilus* spp., *Eikenella corrodens*, *Prevotella* spp. and strictly anaerobic Gram-positive cocci. Quantitative microbiological studies of suppurative parotitis have revealed a viable flora of 10^6 cfu ml^{-1}.

Knowledge of the microbiology of suppurative sialadenitis has become clearer due to the use of improved sampling techniques. Ideally, pus should be collected by aspiration of the duct orifice in order to minimize the risk of sample contamination from the oral flora. If a swab technique is used, then great care should be taken to avoid sample contamination from the adjacent oral mucosa. Rarely, in recurrent infection, pus may also spread extra-orally (Figure 18.7) and an aspirate can be obtained externally. Specimens must be cultured using methods capable of isolating strict anaerobes. Susceptibility testing should be routine, since although penicillin-resistant species are relatively rare in this condition they have been encountered more frequently in recent years. Antimicrobial therapy should be prescribed and amoxicillin (250 mg every 8 hours) remains the antibi-

otic of choice with erythromycin (250–500 mg every 6 hours) reserved for patients with hypersensitivity to the penicillins. If microbiological investigation reveals the presence of strict anaerobes, then the use of metronidazole (200 mg every 8 hours) should be considered.

18.5.2 Recurrent parotitis of childhood

Recurrent parotitis of childhood is a relatively rare condition in which sufferers develop a purulent discharge from one of the parotid glands about two or three times a year. Diagnosis can be confirmed by the characteristic appearance (sialectasis) on a sialogram of the affected gland (Figure 18.8). Sialography should not be performed until the acute episode of infection has resolved. The microbiology of the infection is similar to that encountered in other forms of suppurative sialadenitis. It has been suggested that patients would benefit from long-term antibiotic therapy, although most patients are managed adequately with the provision of amoxicillin or erythromycin as and when acute symptoms develop.

18.5.3 Rare bacterial infections of the salivary glands

Infection of the salivary glands with *Mycobacteriun tuberculosis* has been reported, either as a result of ascending

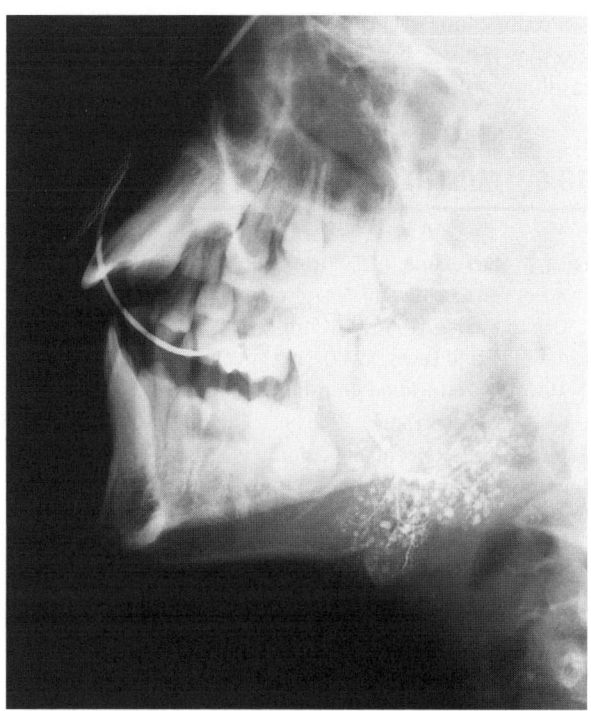

Figure 18.8 *Sialogram showing characteristic sialectasis in the parotid gland of a patient with chronic parotitis of childhood.*

infection from the mouth or due to spread from adjacent tissues. In particular, tuberculosis may develop in the salivary glands due to reactivation of tubercle bacilli in region lymph nodes. Antituberculous therapy is required.

18.5.4   Mumps (endemic parotitis)

Mumps, which is characteristically associated with painful swelling of the major salivary glands, is caused by an RNA paramyxovirus. Differentiation from suppurative sialadenitis can be made by the absence of a purulent discharge from the salivary duct orifice. Diagnosis can usually be made on the basis of clinical symptoms, especially if bilateral signs are present. However, if there is doubt then serological investigation to demonstrate the presence of specific IgM antibody can be used. In addition, a sample of saliva, collected by cannulation of the parotid duct, can be examined by electron microscopy or tissue culture to demonstrate the presence of virus. Antibiotics are not required for treatment.

18.5.5   Rare viral infections of the salivary glands

Cytomegalovirus, a member of the herpes group, can cause symptomatic infection in salivary glands referred to as **cytomegalic inclusion disease**. The name is derived from the large inclusion bodies seen within the nucleus of salivary duct cells. Other viruses rarely implicated in salivary gland disease include parainfluenza virus type 2 and type 3, echo viruses and Coxsackie viruses.

18.6   NASAL INFECTIONS

Approximately 40% of adults harbour staphylococci in the anterior nares. Whilst this is usually asymptomatic, clinical infection can develop, particularly in children. A swab should be taken and the patient provided with a topical antibacterial agent. Topical therapy is normally mupirocin 2% ointment applied up to three times daily up to 10 days, or fusidic acid 2% cream applied two or three times daily. If an outbreak of hospital infection with staphylococci is traced to a nasal carrier, similar management is indicated.

18.7   AURAL INFECTIONS

18.7.1   External infections

Skin commensals, particularly *Staph. epidermidis*, *Staph. aureus* and *Micrococcus* spp., are associated with the development of localized suppurative lesions referred to as **boils** or **furuncles**. Larger lesions are also sometimes called **carbuncles**. Treatment is with appropriate antibiotic in cases of exceptional severity, but in most cases the lesion can be treated in the expectation of rapid resolution, usually by discharge of pus. Lesions in sensitive situations (e.g., in the auditory canal) may benefit from antibiotic treatment, for example flucloxacillin 250 mg every 6 hours for 3–5 days.

18.7.2   Otitis media

Acute otitis media arises due to infection spreading from the nasopharynx into the middle ear via the Eustachian tube. Episodes of otitis media are often recurrent, and characteristically develop after the common cold. The bacteriology of this infection often involves *Haemophilus inflenzae*, *Strep. pneumoniae* or *Strep. pyogenes*. Because of the possibility of complications (which may be serious, e.g. rupture of the tympanic membrane, mastoiditis, meningitis), antibiotics (amoxicillin 250 mg every 8 hours or erythromycin 250 mg every 6 hours) should be given for at least 72 hours.

Otitis media may become chronic, resulting in pathological changes in the tissues ('glue ear') and discharge of pus. The microbiology of the chronic infection is similar to the acute form, although it is usually a mixed flora often containing Gram-negative bacilli, in particular *Pseuodomonas* spp. *Staphy. aureus*, enterobacteria and *Prevotella* spp. have also been isolated from chronic otitis media, although the role of these bacteria remains unclear. Treatment should be cleaning of the ear followed by the application of a topical broad-spectrum antimicrobial in the hospital clinic. The results of culture and susceptibility tests are occasionally helpful.

18.7.3 Ramsay–Hunt syndrome

Ramsay–Hunt syndrome is a relatively rare infection of the geniculate ganglion involving varicella-zoster virus (VZV). The syndrome consists of facial nerve palsy, vesicular eruptions on the external auditory meatus, and ulceration of the mucosa in the oropharynx. Hearing loss, which is sometimes irreversible, may occur. Diagnosis is made on clinical presentation although it may be helpful to demonstrate a four-fold rise in antibody titre to VZV by serology. Treatment should involve provision of a systemic antiviral agent at an early stage, for example famciclovir 250 mg every 8 hours or 750 mg once daily, or valaciclovir 1 g every 8 hours.

Prednisolone at a dose of 40 mg daily should also be given to reduce inflammatory oedema and encourage resolution of the facial nerve palsy.

18.8 FURTHER READING

Bagg, J., MacFarlane, T.W., Poxton, I.R., Miller, C.H. and Smith, A.J. (1999) *Essentials of Microbiology for Dental Students.* Oxford University Press, Oxford.

Lamey, P.-J. and Lewis, M.A.O. (1997) *A Clinical Guide to Oral Medicine*, 2nd edition. British Dental Association, London.

Lewis, M.A.O. and Lamey, P.-J. (1993) *Clinical Oral Medicine.* Butterworth-Heinemann, Oxford.

Lewis, M.A.O., MacFarlane, T.W., Lamey, P.-J., Leishman, R.E. and Howie, N.M. (1993) Quantitative bacteriology of the parotid salivary gland in health and disease. *Microbiol Ecology in Health and Disease*, **6**, 29–34.

Marsh, P. and Martin, M. (1999) *Oral Microbiology*, 4th edition. Wright, London.

Samaranayake, L.P. (1996) *Essential Microbiology for Dentistry.* Churchill Livingstone, London.

Schuster, G.S. (1990) *Oral Microbiology and Infectious Disease.* B.C. Decker, Inc., Philadelphia.

19

Infections in ophthalmic surgery

D.V. SEAL AND L.A. FICKER

19.1 INTRODUCTION

The eye embraces both a **sterile compartment** (the anterior chamber, iris, lens, vitreous, retina and choroid) and a **dirty compartment** (the lid margin, palpebral and bulbar conjunctiva and nasolacrimal system, which is heavily colonized by aerobic and anaerobic microbial flora). A careful distinction must be made between the two compartments, particularly during surgery when the dirty compartment communicates with the sterile one. This results in hospital-acquired infection, often from the patient's own flora, which at the worst causes a devastating endophthalmitis that, more often than not, results in a blind eye. To avoid this unhappy situation requires an understanding of the risk factors involved and how best to avoid them. In order to meet this requirement, this chapter considers the eye under the following headings: (i) the dirty compartment; (ii) the sterile compartment; (iii) prophylaxis of surgical (ophthalmological) infection; and (iv) management of postoperative infections to prevent blindness.

19.2 THE DIRTY COMPARTMENT

Bacteria indigenous to the eyelids and conjunctival sac are important for providing a normal flora. This will limit the presence of pathogenic organisms, but if this normal flora enters the sterile anterior chamber it can become pathogenic, as discussed below. It is important to understand this complex flora. The lid margins exhibit both a perma-nent flora (staphylococci, diphtheroids and *Propioni-bacterium acnes*) and transient pathogens (streptococci and coliforms), which have arisen from the throat flora or the hands. Environmental factors are also important; thus, conjunctival cultures can be positive for fungi (most frequently with *Aspergillus* spp. and *Penicillium* spp.) in 25% of farmers, but in only 9% of city residents. *Candida* spp. can be expected on 1% of lid margins in the UK.

The lid margins may also be colonized with *Staphylococcus aureus*, especially in atopes. Although similar cultures may be obtained from the two eyes, cultural findings from normal lids vary over a 48-hour period. For this reason, it is no longer customary to perform pre-operative cultures. It is advisable, however, to assume that there is lid colonization with *Staph. aureus* in atopes, especially in those with active eczema, albeit at a different site, before ocular surgery.

To reduce the number of bacteria present on the conjunctiva, topical antibiotic drops given one day before surgery can be effective in reducing the bacterial flora of the eye, but are not proven to prevent endophthalmitis. Various preparations are commercially available; fusidic acid as Fucithalmic 1% gel is effective against staphylococci, whilst gentamicin sulphate (0.3%) decreases both lid and conjunctival staphylococcal cultures but is ineffective for streptococci and *P. acnes*. Broad-spectrum cover such as that given by chloramphenicol is useful, but should be used with caution because of its idiosyncratic toxicity for bone marrow; its advantage is penetration of the surface epithelium.

The nasolacrimal system provides a microaerophilic environment which supports the growth of non-fastidious anaerobic bacteria, such as *P. acnes* and *Actinomyces* spp., and becomes infected with endogenous flora. Recurrent unilateral conjunctivitis due to an antibiotic-sensitive bacterium such as *Haemophilus influenzae*, can be the presenting symptom of a canaliculitis due to *Actinomyces* spp. (formally *Streptothrix* or *Leptothrix*), or *Arachnia propionica*. The organism does not usually invade the canaliculus wall, but instead forms a 'fungal' ball which obstructs the lumen.

19.3 THE STERILE COMPARTMENT

In contrast to the dirty compartment, the intra-ocular compartment is sterile and possesses mechanisms which maintain this situation. Anterior chamber-associated immune deviation (ACAID) exists to protect the single cell-layered corneal endothelium (which is of prime importance in the corneal 'pump' mechanism and unable to regenerate) from immune-mediated damage by cell-mediated immunity (CMI) or delayed hypersensitivity (DH) to microbial antigens within the sterile anterior chamber (AC). This is achieved by avoidance of CD8 cytotoxic T-lymphocyte (CTL)-mediated cytolysis and inhibition of CD4Th1 lymphocyte response. These aims are achieved, firstly, by an absence of class I MHC expression on endothelial cells so avoiding lysis by class I restricted CTLs (similarly to the brain). The problem with this mechanism, however, is the inability to prevent persistent viral infection in the cornea. Second, by prevention of a CMI reaction which is achieved through the camerosplenic axis; thus microbial antigen in the AC is discharged in the aqueous to the venous blood flow, and so to the spleen instead of the lymphatics. This results in the production of T suppressor (T_s) lymphocytes that migrate back to the AC to inhibit Th1 lymphocytes. These T_s cells also suppress a DH response systemically to the specific antigen. This systemic protection is lost if the spleen (which is the source of the T_s cells) is removed, so that a functioning spleen is essential for developing and maintaining ACAID. Similar splenic production of T_s cells can be observed with intravenous injection of antigens, reflecting the release of antigen from the AC to the venous flow.

The AC also contains TGF (tumour growth factor)-β which renders local antigen processing cells 'tolerogenic' and is another necessary part of ACAID – particularly if the host has systemically enhanced DH to the specific antigen. Within the AC, there is also the need for TNF-α, interleukin (IL)-4 and IL-10 to induce an ACAID response to an antigen. Not all antigens, however, induce ACAID, notable exceptions being purified protein derivative of *Mycobacterium tuberculosis* and some experimental tumour allografts. The reasons and mechanisms for such antigen selection remain unclear. The principle of immune deviation extends to the posterior segment.

There is a clearance mechanism for dealing with microorganisms that contaminate the anterior chamber during surgery or perforating trauma. This is demonstrated by the fact that approximately 25% of patients having cataract surgery will have some bacteria (at around 20 cfu ml^{-1}) in the anterior chamber at the end of surgery, but only 0.3% are expected to develop endophthalmitis. These bacteria are removed with the aqueous by the aqueous drainage mechanism. Those bacteria that cause infection have usually adhered to the plastic intra-ocular lens, formed a biofilm around themselves and are resistant to phagocytosis by polymorphonuclear cells.

19.4 PROPHYLAXIS OF SURGICAL INFECTION

A number of general points should be considered in the prophylaxis of surgical infection:

- **Site preparation**: there should be preparation of the lids with a plastic 'steri-drape' to cover the lid margins, followed by the application for 5 minutes of 5% povidone-iodine in balanced salt solution to the conjunctiva and cornea. Instruments must be sterile and a 'no-touch' technique used.
- **Radial keratotomy**: sight-threatening bilateral microbial keratitis has been reported following radial keratotomy. This operation can be followed by difficult-to-treat, fastidious bacterial infection with organisms such as *Nocardia* spp. and *Mycobacterium chelonae* that are resistant to first-line antibiotic regimens. It is considered safer to avoid bilateral surgery.
- **Corneal graft surgery** (penetrating keratoplasty): for safe collection of donor material, see Section 19.4.4 'Eye banking'.

19.4.1 Cataract surgery

The expected rate of endophthalmitis following modern cataract surgery with intraocular lens implantation varies approximately from 0.1 to 0.5%. While these rates are relatively low, endophthalmitis and the subsequent risk of blindness in the affected eye cause much distress to the patient with resulting monocular vision and lack of stereoscopy, and this in turn results in immobility and the need for social care. This presents the surgeon with a challenge, namely to reduce the infection rate further, without expensive measures.

Surgical technique reflects the skill of the operator, with those less experienced having more complications. Surgical time is proportionate to infection rate. In cataract surgery, bacteria (predominantly coagulase-negative staphylococci or *P. acnes* and occasionally *Staph. aureus* and streptococci) may gain access to the anterior chamber during irrigation, with the irrigation fluid being contaminated in up to 30% of operations. This level of contamination may be less with uncomplicated phacoemulsification technology, due to reduced volumes of irrigation, but endophthalmitis has been reported. Sutureless wound closure may be another risk factor. To combat bacterial contamination of irrigation fluid, some surgeons add an antibiotic, such as gentamicin, to the irrigation fluid at 5 mg l^{-1}. This may be efficacious against coagulase-negative staphylococci, but *P. acnes* and streptococci are resistant. This mode of prophylaxis is not yet proven, and endophthalmitis may still occur despite such measures. The addition of vancomycin to the irrigation fluid is discouraged as this antibiotic is essential for treatment of potentially resistant staphylococcal endopthalmitis, and should be reserved for this purpose.

Air-borne contamination with coagulase-negative staphylococci of the opened, sterile intra-ocular lens occurs on up to 47% of occasions prior to placement in the eye. This could be reduced by carrying out surgery in ultraclean air conditions. In addition, if the intra-ocular lens touches the conjunctival surface, then up to 80% can become contaminated with coagulase-negative staphylococci, 12% with *Staph. aureus* and 18% with *P. acnes*. Injectable intra-ocular lenses may reduce this risk by isolating the intraocular lens from the ocular surface flora. This happens because the conjunctival surface is not sterile, even after the use of prophylactic antibiotics and antiseptics. Repeated entry of the anterior chamber by instruments carries the same risk. A recent study of DNA-typing by restriction fragment length polymorphism between postoperative coagulase-negative staphylococci cultures from lids and those causing endophthalmitis has shown similarity in 85% of cases, demonstrating that the majority of, but not all, infection is due to the patient's own flora.

Careful closure of the wound is important. Loose sutures carry bacteria and may cause a stitch abscess directly or on suture removal. This is often due to *Staph. aureus*, arising from contamination with lid flora, particularly in atopes. This can be a particular problem in diabetics or those with rheumatoid arthritis, both of whom are particularly susceptible to *Staph. aureus* infection due to the inability of their polymorphonuclear cells to phagocytose this organism adequately. The infection can progress from a stitch abscess to a sclerokeratitis, which may be refractory to the usual combination of topical gentamicin forte and cefuroxime and require debridement by a lamellar keratectomy.

In the UK and USA, fungi (*Candida* spp., *Aspergillus* spp.) are known occasionally to cause endophthalmitis following cataract surgery, the source being the lid or contamination of irrigation fluids and rarely aerial contamination with spores. Studies in the UK have shown that 4% of blepharitic lids are contaminated with *Aspergillus* spores, possibly because the inflamed surface

is 'sticky'. In comparison, in the Indian subcontinent, *Aspergillus* spp. are recorded more frequently as causing postoperative cataract surgery infection.

Subconjunctival antibiotics are routinely given by some surgeons as prophylaxis for cataract surgery. There is debate whether to give them immediately prior to surgery, at the onset of anaesthesia, (as currently practised in other surgical disciplines), during surgery or immediately after surgery. The most established practice is to give one subconjunctival injection of cefuroxime (125 mg) at the end of surgery, and this practice is to be encouraged (though it is not proven) for prevention of endophthalmitis. Cefuroxime penetrates the anterior chamber and is intended to provide prophylaxis against *Staph. aureus*, *Strep. pyogenes*, coagulase-negative staphylococci and *P. acnes* infection. Gentamicin, as an alternative, is bactericidal for staphylococci, but has no effect on streptococci and *P. acnes*, making it less useful. The addition of gentamicin to the irrigation fluid is controversial and unproven. It is thought that antibiotic irrigation fluids have only a small effect on bacterial numbers in the limited period of exposure. An alternative approach is to instill an antibiotic, such as cefuroxime 1 mg, into the anterior chamber after the lens has been removed.

Some surgeons favour giving topical antibiotic drops for 2–6 weeks after cataract surgery to prevent postoperative infection, although this regimen will not prevent endophthalmitis, as the antibiotic will not penetrate into the anterior chamber in sufficient concentration, and may only prevent a stitch abscess. Chloramphenicol is often used in the UK but is not encouraged, and other preparations such as Polytrim are a good alternative. There is probably little point in giving postoperative antibiotic drops for longer than 24 hours after the epithelium has healed over the wound and/or the sutures.

Attempts should always be made to isolate the infecting bacterium or fungus by an intravitreal tap. This is especially important when several cases of endophthalmitis occur together or within a few days of each other. It is more usual to isolate unrelated bacteria, such as *Staph. aureus* of different phage types, coagulase-negative staphylococci of different biotypes, streptococci of different biotypes, and *P. acnes*, than the same organism. If the same organism is isolated, especially if it is *Strep. pyogenes* or *Staph. aureus*, the advice of professional microbiologists should be sought, as it indicates that a staff member is carrying the organism. Occasionally, there may be an epidemic of post-surgical *Candida* endophthalmitis. The unit should be temporarily closed to surgery and staff investigated to identify the carrier or the contaminated irrigation fluid, etc. With staphylococcal or streptococcal infection, staff are usually the source, mainly from sore throats or exacerbations of eczema or other dermatoses.

When the organisms are different, there should be a review of the surgical techniques used and a consideration of ways to reduce the chances of infection happening in any one patient. Past (pseudo) outbreaks have occurred in summer when operating theatre fans have broken or conditions have been excessively hot. When these problems have been corrected, the outbreak has stopped; it relates to excessive staphylococcal shedding by staff.

SIMULTANEOUS BILATERAL CATARACT SURGERY

Some surgeons have maintained that simultaneous bilateral cataract surgery is valuable in elderly, frail patients in order to restore binocular vision. There is no doubt that this is correct from the viewpoint of restoring visual acuity, but the risk must be borne of possible bilateral endophthalmitis rendering the patient totally blind. Although rare, this does occur. The problem at the time of writing is that a large clinical trial has not yet been conducted to establish whether antibiotics are effective for prophylaxis of acute post-surgery endophthalmitis and, if they are found effective, by which route they are best given. This essential information will probably be available within 5 years, but until it is known, it is probably wiser to restrict cataract surgery to one eye at a time.

19.4.2 Trauma to the eye: retention of an intra-ocular foreign body

Intra-ocular penetration of a projectile into the posterior segment of the eye is a medical emergency, especially metal splinters arising from hammering farmyard equipment, dirty or soil-contaminated items and machinery. A recent 20-year review found that 8% of patients with an intra-ocular foreign body (IOFB) developed endophthalmitis, and half of these lost all light perception. While antibiotic prophylaxis for IOFB removal has been advocated, this is not universally practised. Some ophthalmologists guess which fragments are contaminated with bacteria and give antibiotics to only these patients. However, this is no longer justifiable, and **all patients with an IOFB require antibiotic prophylaxis**.

Bacillus spp. are the most virulent pathogens carried by an IOFB, and are responsible for 50% of cases of endophthalmitis, most of which result in severe visual loss. *Staph. aureus*, coliforms, streptococci and occasionally *Clostridium perfringens* can also cause sight-threatening endophthalmitis. If trauma takes place in a rural area, there is more likely to be a polymicrobial infection. Because magnet removal is crude, a track of necrotic tissue is left behind which is seeded with bacteria. It is for this reason that we advocate, in common with others, that antibiotic prophylaxis be used for all IOFB removals.

The following regimen is suggested. Cephalosporins are excluded because *Bacillus* spp. produce β-lactamases that inactivate them:

- **intravitreal** gentamicin 200 μg (or amikacin 400 μg) + vancomycin 1000 μg (or clindamycin 1000 μg) or, if not possible or inappropriate, subconjunctival gentamicin 40 mg + clindamycin 34 mg. (It is recommended to use only 125 μg gentamicin intravitreally if a full vitrectomy has been performed and a reduced dose of vancomycin or clindamycin at 500 μg.)
- **topical** gentamicin (forte) 15 mg ml^{-1} + clindamycin 20 mg ml^{-1}.
- for severe injuries, give intravenous therapy (with the same drugs as given intravitreally) for 3 days; give adequate dosage for weight, but assay to avoid systemic toxicity, especially for renal and VIII nerve function.

If the patient presents early with good vision and the IOFB is recognized and treated as above, then the chances of endophthalmitis are reduced; without an X-ray being taken the IOFB can be missed or dismissed as non-penetrating or the cause of a possible corneal abrasion. If the IOFB is missed, and the patient returns after 24 hours with loss of vision and pain, then it is a medical emergency. To save vision, the IOFB needs prompt removal with the instillation of intravitreal antibiotics – any delay or dependence on intravenous antibiotics alone will contribute to a blind eye.

19.4.3 Management of atopic patients

The atopic individual has a symbiotic relationship with *Staph. aureus*, which colonizes the skin, including that of the eyelids and nasal mucosa to a high degree. *Staph. aureus* also colonizes, and may infect, eczematous skin. Care is therefore needed when planning surgery particularly if the patient has an associated blepharitis. The following regimen is suggested:

- Whole-body bathing, including shampooing hair, with chlorhexidine (4%)-impregnated soap (Hibiscrub) 72 hours prior to surgery.
- Topical anti-staphylococcal prophylaxis for 72 hours prior to surgery with fusidic acid gel (Fucithalmic).
- Apply 5% povidone-iodine in balanced salt solution to the conjunctivae for 8 minutes before operating.
- Postoperative oral fusidic acid 750 mgs (enteric-coated capsules) three times daily or trimethoprim 200 mg twice daily for 5 days (together with subconjunctival cefuroxime 125 mg immediately postoperatively).

19.4.4   Eye banking

The rate of bacterial endophthalmitis complicating penetrating keratoplasty in the USA and Europe is 0.1 to 0.8%, with 45 cases of bacterial endophthalmitis being reported in the literature up to 1993. A higher incidence of endophthalmitis has been shown in patients receiving corneas from a Sri Lankan eye bank (1.3%) than in those receiving eye bank tissue from Western sources (0.14%). This reflects methods of collection and the storage of whole eyes for transplantation, as well as the health of the donor.

The donor should meet the following criteria:

- They must have been in previously good health with no history of hepatitis, multiple blood transfusions or chronic infectious disease.
- There must be no history of neurological or dementing diseases; in addition, 'auto-immune'-type diseases should also be excluded.
- The donor's blood or tissue must be tested and be negative for the presence of hepatitis viruses B and C and the human immunodeficiency virus (HIV).

At present it is not possible to test for exposure to prions, particularly for those associated with Creutzfeld–Jakob or bovine spongiform encephalopathy (BSE) disease, but when this becomes possible, it should be done. There is one recorded case of Creutzfeld–Jakob disease being transferred from a donor to a recipient with corneal grafting. As with experimental transfer of prion-infected tissue within the same species, the development of disease is more rapid than the 'natural' occurrence and the patient died within 18 months of corneal graft surgery. Graft material should **not** be accepted from suicide victims or prison deaths under virtually any circumstances, but especially so when the material is purchased for money rather than being donated.

Aminoglycosides (gentamicin and streptomycin) have long been favoured for bank storage, but these antibiotics do not inhibit the growth of either streptococci or fungi. A newer medium, viz. Optisol GS contains gentamicin ($100 \, \mu g \, ml^{-1}$) and streptomycin ($200 \, \mu g \, ml^{-1}$). Stored corneal material can be contaminated with bacteria, resulting in microbial keratitis and endophthalmitis.

Rather than import whole donor eyes or corneas, each country should set up its own National Eye Bank. It is not surprising that the practice of importation of tissues is associated with an increase in the rate of bacterial endophthalmitis, as well as encouraging the transfer of tissue-associated viruses. The export of human donor material from one country to another is hazardous and contravenes World Health Organization regulations. Such practice, especially when carried out on a commercial scale, also encourages the acquisition of human donor material in the most dubious of circumstances. This practice must be resisted by ophthalmologists worldwide.

19.5   MANAGEMENT OF POSTOPERATIVE INFECTIONS

19.5.1   Peri-ocular infection

ORBITAL (POST-SEPTAL) CELLULITIS

Orbital cellulitis is a retroseptal infection of the extra-ocular orbital contents presenting with pain, lid oedema, proptosis and diplopia due to impaired extra-ocular muscle function. A few cases follow penetrating injury, surgery or are secondary to panophthalmitis, but the majority occur in association with sinusitis. The condition commonly affects children, where spread to the orbit across the thin orbital plate of the ethmoid bone occurs. Retroseptal infection requires multidisciplinary management because of the risk of extension to the eye or cranial cavity. Subperiosteal abscess with displacement of the globe, or cavernous sinus thrombosis with headache and neck stiffness can develop. Loculated pus must be drained. Delayed or inadequate treatment may lead to blindness or death.

Pathogens from the sinuses include *Strep. pyogenes*, *Staph. aureus, H. influenzae* and anaerobic bacteria if there is chronic sinusitis. Phycomycetes may be involved in diabetic patients. Post-traumatic orbital cellulitis is often polymicrobial when *Clostridia* spp. can cause gas gangrene; distinction from necrotizing fasciitis and other types of microbial gangrene needs to be made. Systemic antibiotic therapy is required with large doses, for which purpose co-amoxyclav or cephalosporins with metronidazole are suitable. If extension of infection is thought to be occurring into the meninges, then antibiotics are additionally required that penetrate into the central nervous sytem such as chloramphenicol, co-trimoxazole (Septrin) or rifampicin.

PRESEPTAL CELLULITIS

Preseptal cellulitis may resemble orbital cellulitis when intense lid swelling is present, but the presence of normal ocular movements and absence of globe inflammation in preseptal disease helps to distinguish the two. Eye movement can usually be detected despite a tense swelling of the lids. The infection is limited anteriorly to the orbital septum, but delay in therapy can result in extension to the orbit (periorbital cellulitis). The differential diagnosis can be resolved by magnetic resonance imaging. In a study of 35 children, preseptal cellulitis was associated with sinusitis in 17, with ocular infection in 11 (seven conjunctivitis and four dacryocystitis), and with an infected wound in six. Some 73% of those with ocular infection were aged less than 2 years.

Parenteral therapy is designed to cover the common causative organisms: *H. influenzae, Staph. aureus, Strep. pneumoniae* and *Strep. pyogenes. H. influenzae* is the commonest cause of orbital cellulitis in young children, and in this age group co-amoxyclav or cefuroxime are the drugs of choice. In view of the emergence of multiple-resistant strains of *H. influenzae*, consideration should be given to the use of a 'third-generation' cephalosporin such as cefotaxime, particularly when the clinical response is poor or resistant organisms are isolated from nasal swabs. In adults, therapy is directed against streptococci and *Staph. aureus* with high-dose intravenous benzylpenicillin alternating with fluclo-xacillin or, in advanced cases, clindamycin or vancomycin. Anaerobic cellulitis occurs following trauma, particularly with human or animal bites, and the latter can include infection by *Pasteurella* spp. or group G β-haemolytic streptococci for which co-amoxyclav is the antibiotic of choice.

NECROTIZING FASCIITIS

This is a potentially lethal infection of the deep subcutaneous tissue of the eyelid above the fascial layer, initially appearing as a preseptal cellulitis. It is caused by β-haemolytic streptococci of Lancefield group A (*Strep. pyogenes*) or groups C and G, together with *Staph. aureus* in 25% of cases. It usually arises as a community-acquired infection, often associated with minor trauma, but can follow contamination of a surgical wound.

Streptococci penetrate the skin in small numbers to cause a necrotizing cellulitic lesion, with septic thrombo-phlebitis of dermal vessels, that spreads upwards over the forehead or downwards over the cheek. Initially, there is ulcerative necrosis at the site of invasion, that later extends over and undermines erratically, other subcutaneous tissues, depending on the vessels thrombosed. The first 48 hours are the most vital for the patient, particularly if the pathogenesis of the infection is missed. Patients usually suffer from profound toxaemia, may rapidly develop the 'toxic shock syndrome' and die from septicaemia. This is a medical emergency and patients must be treated with large doses of benzylpenicillin (adults, 3 megaunits, 4-hourly) in order to obtain adequate tissue perfusion in the presence of the thrombosing infection, together with flucloxacillin or another anti-staphylococcal antibiotic. Gram-negative bacteria and anaerobes do not normally initiate this infection at this site.

The spreading edge of the necrotizing infection should be marked with a pen – it can advance by as much as 2.5 cm per hour. If the spreading edge of the lesion has not stopped advancing after 24 hours, then surgical debridement is indicated to remove the infected subcutaneous tissue; otherwise the lesion spreads further because of the failure of antibiotics to penetrate into the thrombosed tissue. If the infection responds within 48 hours, then the edge regresses considerably, and ulcerative necrosis is confined to the lid. After a further 5 days, the characteristic eschar has formed and all the subcutaneous swelling resolved. The eschar will slough off eventually,

often leaving a damaged lid for reconstructive surgery. Early debridement of the lids has been advocated by some, but others (including the present authors) recommend conservative therapy as described above. The patient should be investigated for latent diabetes or immunocompromisation early during convalescence.

19.5.2 Conjunctival infection

A stitch infection requires suture removal, which should be sent to the laboratory for culture. A topical antibiotic should be used for 3 days. A glaucoma drainage bleb infection requires intravenous and topical antibiotics to prevent intra-ocular contamination.

19.5.3 Corneal infection

Postoperative microbial keratitis should be managed as for presentation of the infection from other causes, e.g. trauma. A scraping should be performed for microscopy and culture and antibiotic treatment started empirically with either ciprofloxacin or ofloxacin 0.3% topically, or the combination of a cephalosporin at 5% and gentamicin forte at 1.5%. Drop therapy should be given every 15 minutes for the first hour, and then hourly day and night for 3 days. An organism is usually identified without difficulty in postoperative infection within 24 hours, and the antibiotic sensitivity within another 24 hours; this allows retargeting of the antibiotics if there is no clinical response.

19.5.4 Vitreous and retina infection

ENDOPHTHALMITIS

Endophthalmitis generally follows cataract, squint or other surgery on the globe, and implies infection of the vitreous compartment together with the retinal and uveal coats of the eye. It is most commonly encountered as an exogenous infection involving either intra-ocular surgery (such as cataract, glaucoma or occasionally squint surgery, when pathogens harboured on the lids and conjunctival sac may determine the infecting organism(s)), or following penetrating injury to the eye. The formation of thin-walled drainage blebs after glaucoma surgery using mitomycin C may predispose to late infection. Bacterial and fungal endophthalmitis may also follow penetrating keratoplasty, with over 45 cases reported in the literature.

Bacteria causing acute endophthalmitis include *Strep. pyogenes*, *Strep. pneumoniae*, *Staph. aureus* and entero-bacteriaceae; enterococci occasionally cause endophthalmitis and have so far remained sensitive to vancomycin. Causes of chronic endophthalmitis include coagulase-negative staphylococci, *P. acnes*, *P. arachnia*, *P. granulosum*, *Corynebacteria* spp., *Candida parapsilosis* and *Aspergillus* spp. including *A. terreus*. Surgeons should be wary of operating on atopic or allergic patients until they are sure that the lids are not heavily colonized by *Staph. aureus*, or that appropriate prophylaxis is used.

Following cataract surgery, patients can present:

- acutely, with fulminant endophthalmitis often due to *Staph. aureus*, *Strep. pyogenes* or *Strep. pneumoniae* within 5 days of surgery during which vision is often lost;
- sub-acutely, with infection at up to 6 weeks after surgery, often due to coagulase-negative staphylococci, and with vision reduced but retained; it is these patients who were mainly investigated in the Endophthalmitis Vitrectomy Study Group (1995) when full vitrectomy was shown to be of benefit only if vision was reduced to light perception; or
- with chronic low-grade infection, often due to *P. acnes* and occasionally coagulase-negative staphylococci.

They present initially as 'hypopyon uveitis' within 6 weeks of surgery, that fails to respond to corticosteroids and needs eventual vitrectomy with intravitreal antibiotics and often intra-ocular lens exchange. There is granulomatous inflammation and characteristic white capsular plaque.

Following trauma, it is *Bacillus* spp. that are commonly isolated, while other bacteria responsible for the remaining 50% of cases include *Staph. aureus*, streptococci and coliforms and occasionally *Clostridium perfringens* or *Cl. bifermentans*, the latter being associated with soil contamination of a foreign body injury.

Whatever the basis of the infection, endophthalmitis is a potentially blinding disease, with irreversible tissue damage occurring within 24–48 hours. Therefore, early diagnosis and prompt treatment are essential. Symptoms of acute infection include pain, loss of vision, and lid and conjunctival swelling. If the patient is a young child, it is essential to examine the eye fully under general anaesthesia, especially if there has been recent squint surgery.

Signs of acute endophthalmitis include: (i) reduced visual acuity (VA) down to perception of light; (ii) conjunctival and corneal oedema; (iii) a cloudy AC with cells, hypopyon or fibrin clot; or (iv) vitreous clouding precluding a view of the retinal vessels (often, no view of the posterior segment is possible). However, it is worth stressing that loss of the red reflex when the vitreous is viewed through the pupil may be a poor guide to the state of the vitreous – which may be most opaque anteriorly where the inflammatory process has begun. If the pupil is observed while transilluminating the sclera, the red reflex may become apparent and can then form a better guide to control of the disease. Ocular echography is a useful

adjunct for the clinical evaluation of infectious endophthalmitis, especially in eyes with opaque media.

The patient requires immediate investigation with AC tap and vitrectomy. Gram stain and semi-quantitative culture of aqueous and vitreous should be performed. Isolation of any bacterial colonies on direct inoculation of agar plates cultured aerobically, micro-aerophilically or anaerobically should be deemed indicative of culture-positive endophthalmitis. A two prong combination of intravitreal antibiotics should be instilled selected from either vancomycin (1 mg) or cephazolin (or ceftazidime) (2 mg) plus either gentamicin (0.2 mg) or amikacin (0.4 mg); 0.1 ml of each of the two chosen antibiotics should be injected intravitreally after the tap has been performed.

Patients may present within 6 weeks of cataract surgery with reduced VA, and signs of inflammation in the AC that have been managed with corticosteroids. They should be managed as for acute endophthalmitis (see above). If vitrectomy is not indicated, an AC tap and a vitreous tap will be required to confirm infection and to identify the microbe responsible; antibiotics (as above) should be instilled simultaneously into the vitreous.

Patients presenting late with 'hypopyon uveitis', that has failed to respond to corticosteroids, should be investigated for chronic infection and the possibility that the inflammation is due to infection within the capsular sac with *P. acnes*, other propionibacterium species or coagulase-negative staphylococci. This can be established, even at a late stage after one year or more, by an AC and vitreous tap followed by Gram stain and culture; both samples should be collected as only one or other may be culture-positive. There may be insufficient numbers of organisms present in the sample to yield a positive Gram stain in the presence of a positive culture; laboratories should be aware that *P. acnes* can appear as a Gram-variable cocco-bacillus when stained from the AC or vitreous. To isolate *P. acnes*, there must be strict anaerobic growth conditions with incubation for at least 14 days. The polymerase chain reaction (PCR) technique has been found more sensitive to identify bacteria within these specimens than culture. There may be viable *P. acnes* organisms sequestered within lens capsular remnants which may require surgical removal and intra-ocular lens exchange to prevent recurrent or persistent endophthalmitis. Initial management, however, should involve the instillation of intravitreal vancomycin when the tap is performed.

Bacterial endophthalmitis is treated by a combination of intravitreal and systemic antibiotic therapy. Subconjunctival therapy is a less satisfactory alternative to the intravitreal route. An antibiotic combination is injected intravitreally and repeated, as required according to the clinical response, at intervals of 48–72 hours depending on the persistence of the drugs selected within the eye. Intravitreal antibiotic doses are scaled down to avoid retinal toxicity, but the margin for error between effective chemotherapy and undesirable toxicity is narrow for the aminoglycosides (for gentamicin, 200 µg is effective but 400 µg is toxic, causing macular infarction); thus, the total dose injected needs to be highly accurate, which can be difficult to achieve. For this reason, a combination of intravitreal vancomycin (for Gram-positive bacteria) and ceftazidime (for Gram-negative bacteria) is now favoured. In addition, it is now advised that if a full vitrectomy is performed, the dose of intravitreal antibiotic given should be reduced by 50%.

DILUTION SCHEDULES

It is well recognized that pharmacists are trained to produce the required meticulous dilutions more accurately than doctors, and hence the intravitreal antibiotic should always be made up in pharmacy departments whenever possible as part of their emergency service. In cases of emergency only, a method for diluting the drugs in the operating theatre is given below. The procedure must use sterile equipment and be undertaken on a sterile surface; ideally, the hospital makes up sterile packs with bottles in advance for this purpose. All drugs should be mixed by inverting the bottle 25 times, avoiding frothing. Some important 'do's' and 'don'ts' are:

- **Never** return diluted drugs to the same vial or syringe for further dilution.
- Do **not** use syringes more than once.
- **Never** dilute at greater than 1 in 20.
- Do **not** re-use bottles for further dilution until they have been washed, rinsed and sterilized.

Acute purulent endophthalmitis should be treated with additional systemic antibiotic therapy, with the same drugs as used for intravitreal therapy. This regimen will maintain effective intravitreal levels of the drug for a longer period by reducing the diffusion gradient out of the eye. High doses are required, and there is a need to be aware of the risks of systemic toxicity. Systemic antibiotic therapy alone, except for chloramphenicol, is **not** effective for treatment of endophthalmitis when all vision will be lost unless high levels of antibiotics are achieved in the tissues at once and most effectively by intravitreal administration.

The use of oral probenecid (dose 500 mg every 12 hours) retards the outward transport of penicillins, cephalosporins and ciprofloxacin across the retinal capillary endothelial cells, thus extending the half-life of the drug within the vitreous. Probenecid also raises the plasma level by blocking secretion of these drugs by the proximal renal tubule.

After 24 hours, if there is a clear clinical response, prednisolone can be added to the systemic regimen to reduce the vitreous inflammatory response and subsequent vitreous organization (oral prednisolone 60 mg daily on a reducing scale). For the same reason, dexamethasone is often added to the intravitreal injection (dose = 400 µg

in 0.1 ml; use the commercial preparation containing 4 mg ml^{-1}) but is contraindicated in the case of fungal infection. Antibiotic therapy is modified after 24–48 hours according to the clinical response and the antibiotic sensitivity profile of the cultured organism.

If intravitreal instillation of antibiotics is not possible medically, although it can be performed under local anaesthesia in a clean examination room, then systemic therapy with chloramphenicol can be given. Chloramphenicol penetrates the ocular tissues well, and was used in the past effectively to treat bacterial endophthalmitis. Although reversible bone marrow hypoplasia may occur (albeit unlikely with short-course therapy), the chance of idiosyncratic irreversible marrow aplasia cannot be excluded. Again, this is unlikely in that it occurs 13 times more commonly with daily dosages in excess of 4 g, at an approximate occurrence rate of 1 in 50 000 doses.

FUNGAL ENDOPHTHALMITIS

Exogenous fungal endophthalmitis is invariably sight-threatening unless managed aggressively by surgery combined with anti-fungal chemotherapy. Although it is rare in the UK, usually being associated with trauma, it can follow cataract and other surgery in rural settings in tropical and hot countries. The filamentous fungus, *Fusarium*, and to a lesser extent *Aspergillus*, cause infection following trauma with soil contamination.

The fungi responsible for endogenous endophthalmitis in Europe and northern America include *Candida* spp. (the commonest isolate and the one associated with drug addiction or intravenous cannulae), followed by *Aspergillus* spp. which are frequently bilateral and secondary to systemic infection involving endocarditis or immune-suppresssion and transplantation. *Fusarium* spp. can present similarly with bilateral infection in the immunosuppressed patient.

Because of the toxicity of the most effective antifungal agents, the relatively narrow activity spectrum of some agents, and the difficulties of clinical diagnosis, treatment is rarely instituted in the absence of direct evidence of a fungal aetiology, based at least on the results of smears. Effective therapy requires mycological identification and, preferably, information about drug sensitivity. The number of drugs available for ocular use is limited, not only by problems of local and systemic toxicity, but by poor solubility or ocular penetration characteristics. Because of the infrequency of oculomycosis in Europe, no commercial antifungal preparations are available.

Available drugs include the polyene antibiotics (amphotericin B, natamycin and nystatin), the cytostatic 5-fluorocytosines (flucytosine, 5-FC) and the imidazoles (thiabendazole, miconazole, ketoconazole, clotrimazole, econazole, fluconazole and itraconazole).

Amphotericin B is the only truly fungicidal antibiotic, depending on concentration achieved, and is active against a wide range of fungi including *Aspergillus* spp., *Fusarium* spp. and *Candida* spp. It may be given topically as a drop (0.05–0.5%), subconjunctivally and intravitreally. It is toxic by any of these routes, but the use of topical preparations at concentrations of 0.15% or less will minimize toxicity, which relates in part to the presence of deoxycholate in the parenteral preparation. Amphotericin is given parenterally by slow intravenous infusion in the management of endophthalmitis, often on a background of more widespread systemic infection, in addition to intravitreal therapy. Renal (low potassium) and haematological status must be kept under surveillance, and drug levels monitored.

For fungal endophthalmitis, amphotericin (5 µg) or miconazole (10 µg) is usually required intravitreally, together with a vitrectomy. Amphotericin B can be administered intravenously combined with oral flucytosine (100–200 mg kg^{-1} per day) for severe *Candida* infection, or ketoconazole (200–400 mg per day) for other fungal infections. Careful monitoring is required. *Candida* endophthalmitis can be effectively treated with oral fluconazole combined with intravitreal amphotericin B, but vitrectomy and fluconazole alone have also been reported to be successful.

5-FC is only active against *Candida* spp. It is well absorbed by the oral route and achieves high blood and tissue levels. It has been used effectively in the treatment of *Candida* endophthalmitis, in combination with systemic or intravitreal amphotericin B to prevent the otherwise rapid emergence of resistant strains.

19.6 FURTHER READING

Collinge, J. and Palmer, M.S. (1997) *Prion Diseases.* Oxford University Press, Oxford.

Endophthalmitis Vitrectomy Study Group (1995) Results of the Endophthalmitis Vitrectomy Study. *Arch. Ophthalmol.,* **113**, 1479–1496.

Ficker, L.A. and Seal, D.V. (1997) Diseases of the eye. In *The Staphylococci in Human Disease.* Churchill Livingstone, New York, 441–454.

O'Grady, F., Lambert, H., Finch, R.G. and Greenwood, D. (1997) *Antibiotic and Chemotherapy: anti-infective agents and their use in therapy.* Churchill-Livingstone, London.

Pepose, J.S., Holland, G.N. and Wilhelmus, K.R. (1996) *Ocular Infection and Immunity.* Mosby, St. Louis.

Seal, D.V., Bron, A. and Hay, J. (1998) *Ocular Infection – Investigation and Treatment.* Martin Dunitz, London.

20

Infections of the mouth

M.A.O. LEWIS

20.1 GENERAL BACKGROUND

The microbial nature of the adult oral flora is extremely complex and involves a mixture of bacteria, mycoplasma, fungi and protozoa. Furthermore, in certain circumstances viruses may also be present. Bacteria predominate within the flora, and it is estimated that there are usually in excess of 200 different groups of bacteria present. In addition, molecular biology is continuing to reveal that the mouth contains more, as yet, unculturable microorganisms.

The **oral cavity** is lined by stratified squamous cell epithelium, which is modified in particular areas according to function, such as the keratinization that is present on the dorsum of the tongue and hard palate. In addition to mucosal differences, the oral cavity contains a number of specific ecological niches related to the teeth and dentures or prostheses, if worn. Factors that influence the nature of the microbial flora at specific sites within the mouth include local anatomy, saliva, crevicular fluid and specific microbial properties, particularly adhesion. The complex nature of the healthy commensal microflora and variety of tissues within the mouth provides potential for a wide range of microbial infection. Whilst in health, these microorganisms produce no clinical signs of mucosal infection, situations arise when these 'non-pathogenic' commensals can cause opportunistic infection. In addition, the mouth can be affected by recognized pathogenic microorganisms.

20.2 STOMATITIS

Generalised infection of the oral cavity (stomatitis) may occur from a variety of causes and take different forms.

20.2.1 Recurrent aphthous stomatitis

This form of oral ulceration occurs in three forms, minor, major and herpetiform (Figure 20.1). At present, there is no evidence that the aetiology of any form of this condition involves any particular microorganism. However, a form of topical tetracycline therapy was developed due to a proposal that recurrent oral ulceration in some individuals represents an immune reaction to the presence of certain strains of *Streptococcus sanguis*. Many sufferers of recurrent aphthous stomatitis find that reduction of secondary infection of the ulcers by use of an antiseptic mouthwash can assist healing.

Three alternative treatment regimens, all of them satisfactory, are as follows:

- Tetracycline capsule 250 mg broken into 5 ml of water and used as a mouthwash for 3 minutes four times daily for 4 weeks.
- Chlorhexidine gluconate 0.2% mouthwash, 10 ml rinse for 1 minute twice daily when ulcers are present coupled with chlorhexidine gluconate 0.2% spray, up to 12 sprays twice daily.

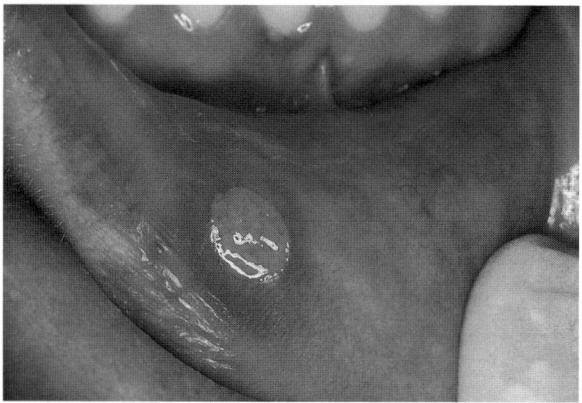

Figure 20.1 *Minor recurrent aphthous stomatitis.*

- Benzydamine hydrochloride 0.15% mouthwash, 15 ml every 1.5–3 hours, as required when ulcers present, but not for longer than 7 consecutive days. This can be used with benzydamine hydrochloride 0.15% spray, 4–8 puffs every 1.5–3 hours, as required.

20.2.2 Herpes simplex virus (HSV)

Primary infection with HSV-1 usually occurs during the first few years of life, and is characterized by the development of widespread oral discomfort (herpetic gingivostomatitis) and mild pyrexia. The symptoms at this time are often mistakenly regarded as an episode of teething in childhood. However, in 5–10% of cases symptoms may be severe and include the presence of blood-crusted lips, gingival swelling, multiple oral ulcers, lymphadenopathy and raised temperature. Regardless of the severity of the primary infection, the symptoms resolve within 10 days. A diagnosis of HSV infection can be confirmed by isolation of the virus during the early symptomatic stage. Large numbers of HSV are present not only on the ulcerated mucosa but also within the saliva; therefore, it is not essential that the swab be taken from the ulcer – which can be difficult in a fractious young patient – as it is easier (and equally effective) to take a swab of saliva from the floor of the patient's mouth. The swab should be placed in viral transport medium containing a mixture of antibiotics, usually penicillin and streptomycin combined with the antifungal amphotericin, to eliminate any bacteria or fungi that are inevitably present in a sample from the mouth. The transport medium should also contain serum and a buffer to maintain virus viability. The presence of HSV is determined in the laboratory by detection of a cytopathic effect in tissue culture (Figure 20.2). The isolation of virus takes up to 10 days to provide a result, by which time the patient is often asymptomatic. Alternatively, diagnosis may be confirmed retrospectively by the detection of a four-fold rise in antibody titre between acute and convalescent sera. Both these techniques have limited clinical benefit in acute diagnosis due to the prolonged time involved in obtaining a result. However, the presence of HSV within a smear from lesional tissue can be demonstrated within 30 minutes by use of commercially available monoclonal antibody kits and immunofluoresence. Fortunately, the signs and symptoms of primary herpetic gingivitis are often sufficiently characteristic that a diagnosis can be made on clinical grounds alone.

Ensuring adequate hydration is a primary factor in patient care, especially if oral ulceration is widespread and fluid intake limited. In addition, a decision must be made on the need to provide the patient with antiviral therapy. Aciclovir is a nucleoside analogue drug that has activity against members of the herpes group of viruses, in particular HSV types 1 and 2. Viral enzymes, within HSV-infected cells, phosphorylate aciclovir to monophosphate and the agent becomes cell bound. Subsequent further phosphorylation to aciclovir triphosphate produces an analogue to deoxyguanosine triphosphate that inhibits viral DNA synthesis and prevents further viral replication. Since aciclovir acts by blocking viral replication, a decision to provide the drug should be made at an early stage, preferably within 48 hours of the onset of acute symptoms. Antiviral therapy started later than this time is unlikely to produce any significant clinical benefit, and therefore is not justified unless the patient is otherwise medically compromised. At present, the agent of choice is aciclovir, – preferably as a suspension, since the tablet form is difficult to swallow in the presence of widespread oral ulceration. Aciclovir (200 mg) should be given five times daily for 5 days; children aged under 2 years should receive a half-dose, while those over 2 years should receive an adult dose. In future, valaciclovir and famciclovir may also be considered for use in primary herpetic gingivostomatitis.

Despite the use of antiviral agents, HSV is not eliminated from the body and the virus remains within the tissues in a latent form. It is traditionally taught that the

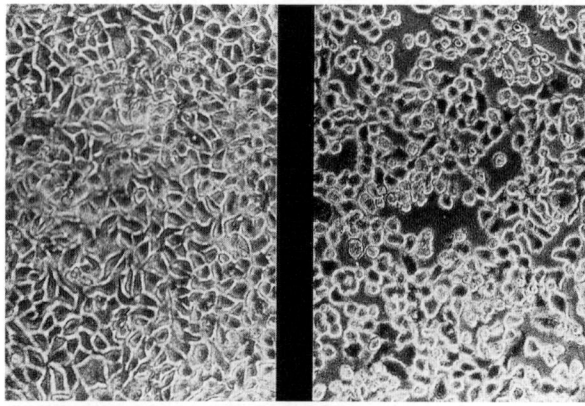

Figure 20.2 *Monolayer of cells in culture prior to (left) and 5 days following (right) inoculation with a swab containing herpes simplex virus.*

virus resides in sensory nerves, but whilst this is likely to be true there is increasing evidence that HSV may also persist locally in the perioral and gingival tissues. Latent HSV may then produce recurrent herpes labialis (see Chapter 18) or intra-oral ulceration, particularly of the hard palate.

20.2.3   Herpes zoster

Primary infection with varicella-zoster virus (VZV) causes chickenpox, whereas subsequent reactivation of latent VZV produces herpes zoster (shingles). The characteristic cutaneous lesions of chickenpox may occasionally be accompanied by the development of small (2- to 4-mm-diameter) oral ulcers in the palate and faucial region. Reactivation of latent VZV in sensory nerve ganglia produces severe pain that is followed within a few days by vesiculobullous cutaneous or mucosal lesions. The trigeminal nerve is affected in about 15% of cases of herpes zoster, and involvement is characteristically limited to one division of the nerve. Although diagnosis can be made on the basis of clinical presentation alone, confirmation of the herpes zoster can be made by isolation of VZV in cell culture. A swab, taken directly from a lesion on the skin or area of ulceration within the mouth, should be sent to the laboratory in viral transport medium. Alternatively, immunofluorescence tests can be applied to a smear of a recent vesicular lesion either on the skin or intra-orally. Antiviral treatment should be instituted as early as possible, preferably within the first 48 hours of symptoms, and should constitute either famciclovir 250 mg every 8 hours (or 750 mg once daily) for 10 days, or valaciclovir 1 g every 8 hours for 10 days.

Post-herpetic neuralgia may be a delayed problem in these patients, and this is why it is recommended that antiviral therapy should be provided for at least 10 days to reduce the risk of this extremely painful condition.

20.2.4   Hand, foot and mouth

Hand, foot and mouth disease is usually caused by Coxsackie virus A16, but may also be due to infection with types A4, A5, A9 and A10. As the name of the condition implies, the distribution of lesions is characteristic, involving macular and vesicular eruptions on the hands, feet and mucosa of the pharynx, soft palate, buccal sulcus or tongue. The cutaneous lesions of hand, foot and mouth disease are transient, lasting only 1–3 days, and may be asymptomatic. The diagnosis of hand, foot and mouth disease is usually made on the basis of the characteristic clinical signs. Viral culture for Coxsackie infections is not widely available, and therefore if confirmatory diagnosis is required this has to be based on demonstration of an increase in convalescent antibody levels. Antimicrobial treatment is rarely required.

20.2.5   Herpangina

Herpangina is due to infection by either Coxsackie virus A2, A4, A5, A6 or A8. This condition occurs predominantly in children, and presents as sudden onset of fever and sore throat with subsequent development of papular, vesicular lesions on the oral mucosa and pharyngeal mucosa. Severity of symptoms is variable, but clinical resolution usually occurs within 7–10 days, even in the absence of treatment. The diagnosis of herpangina is usually made on the basis of the characteristic clinical signs and symptoms. Viral culture for Coxsackie infections is not widely available, and therefore if required confirmatory diagnosis is based on demonstration of an increase in convalescent antibody levels. Treatment consists of bed rest and the use of an antiseptic mouthwash, such as 0.2% chlorhexidine gluconate. Patients should be encouraged to maintain adequate fluid intake.

20.2.6   Candidal (monilial) infection

Approximately 40% of the population harbour *Candida* intra-orally as part of their commensal oral microflora. It is generally accepted that a salivary level of up to 100 colony forming units per millilitre (cfu ml^{-1}) can be accepted as consistent with healthy commensal carriage. Levels of *Candida* above 10^2 cfu ml^{-1} are considered to be indicative of infection, even in the absence of any clinical signs and symptoms. *Candida* species encountered in the oral cavity include *C. albicans, C. glabrata, C. tropicalis, C. dubliniensis, C. pseudotropicalis, C. guillerimondii* and *C. krusei. Saccharomyces* spp. are also occasionally isolated. Although traditionally *C. albicans* is the most commonly reported species, there is an increasing trend for the isolation of non-albicans species.

The presence of *Candida* on the orofacial tissues may be demonstrated simply and rapidly by the use of a smear stained using the Gram method. Such a smear can also differentiate between yeast and hyphal forms (Figure 20.3). Although it was previously believed that

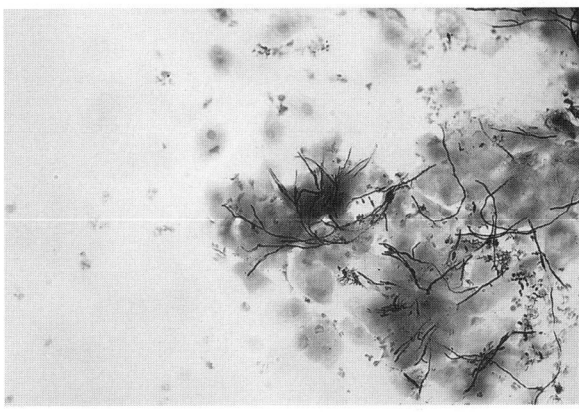

Figure 20.3 *Smear of angular cheilitis stained by Gram's method, demonstrating candidal hyphae and blastospores.*

the presence of hyphae was an indication of pathogenicity, the significance of this finding is now uncertain. *Candida* can also be isolated by the use of a microbiological swab taken from lesional tissue and sent for routine mycological culture.

Due to the peculiar environment of the mouth, a number of specialized methods have been developed to recover *Candida* from the oral cavity. Such investigations include the oral rinse technique and the imprint culture method; each method has its own advantages and disadvantages, and the choice of sampling is often governed by the type of lesion present.

The oral rinse technique involves a patient holding 10 ml of sterile phosphate-buffered saline (0.01 M, pH 7.2) in the mouth for 1 minute. The solution is then concentrated (10-fold) by centrifugation, and 50 μl inoculated on an agar medium by a spiral plating system. After 24–48 hours' incubation at 37°C, the resulting colonies are enumerated to determine the cfu ml^{-1} within the original rinse. Quantification of *Candida* is advantageous since it differentiates between carrier and infected states. This method is not site-specific, and provides an overall assessment of the mouth.

The imprint culture technique utilizes a sterile foam-pad of known size (typically 2.5 cm^2), soaked immediately before use in Sabouraud's broth. The pad is placed firmly on the surface of the lesion for 30 seconds, and then transferred immediately face down onto Sabourand's agar. After 24–48 hours incubation at 37°C, the resulting growth is enumerated to determine the number of colony forming units (Figure 20.4). An advantage of the imprint culture over the oral rinse is that it can be specifically targeted at lesional tissue or a particular oral site.

The most frequently used primary isolation medium for *Candida* is Sabouraud's dextrose agar (SDA), which suppresses the growth of many oral bacteria because of its low pH. *Candida* species appear as cream, convex colonies on SDA, but differentiation between *C. albicans* and non-albicans species is rarely possible.

The germ-tube test is the standard laboratory method for confirming the identity of *C. albicans*. This involves the induction of hyphal outgrowths (germ-tubes) from yeast in serum after 2–4 hours incubation at 37°C (Figure 20.5). Approximately 95% of strains of *C. albicans* produce germ-tubes, although this property is also shared by *C. stellatoidea* and rare isolates of *C. tropicalis*. Chlamydospore production is primarily associated with *C. albicans*, but is also found with *C. stellatoidea* and rare isolates of *C. tropicalis*. Chlamydospores are thick-walled, dormant growth forms that can be induced *in vitro* through culture of *C. albicans* on cornmeal agar supplemented with Tween-80. The inoculated area is overlaid with a coverslip, and the agar incubated at room temperature for 72 hours.

Although *C. albicans* accounts for approximately 90% of clinical isolates from the oral cavity, it has been estimated that one or more non-albicans strains is also present in 10% of samples taken from the oral tissues. There is an increasing amount of evidence that non-albicans species may have specific pathogenicity in certain forms of oral candidosis. Therefore, it is recommended that all specimens from oral lesions should be inoculated not only onto SDA but also onto a differential medium which will increase the likelihood of detection of non-albicans strains.

Pagano–Levin agar distinguishes between *Candida* species based on reduction of triphenyltetrazolium chloride. On this agar, *C. albicans* appears as pale coloured-colonies, while colonies of other *Candida* species exhibit varying degrees of pink coloration. In addition, a number of other commercially available systems are now available that can differentiate between *C. albicans*, *C. tropicalis* and *C. krusei* based on colony colour and appearance.

For a definitive identification of individual strains of *Candida*, the physiological properties need to be examined in conjunction with morphological criteria. Carbohydrate assimilation profiles for *Candida* species can be obtained by examining zones of candidal growth around sugar-impregnated discs or wells, in seeded basal agars. In contrast, fermentation tests are generally performed in liquid media where acid or gas production is detected. These tests are time-consuming and laborious to perform, although the introduction of commercially available systems has greatly reduced analysis time and the ease of *Candida* identification in routine clinical laboratories. Commercial identification systems can be

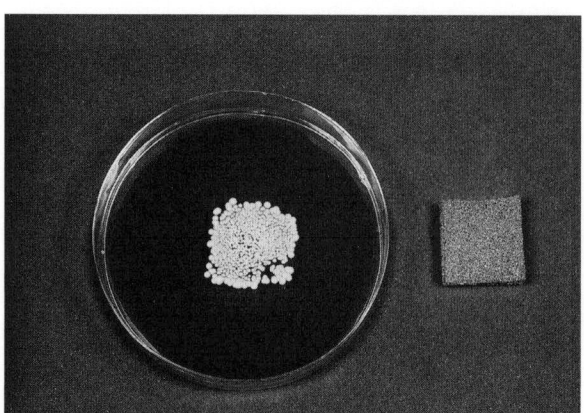

Figure 20.4 *Heavy* Candida *growth on Sabourand's agar which had been inoculated with an imprint method.*

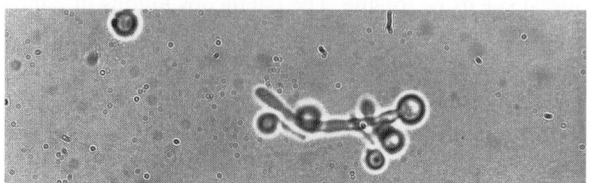

Figure 20.5 *Germ-tube formation by a strain of* Candida albicans.

based on enzyme activity or growth, with the latter typically requiring incubation for 72 hours.

The approaches to *Candida* identification described above are based upon the analysis of phenotypic criteria which may be subject to variable expression. A more stable approach would be one based on genetic variability, as assessed by analysis of electrophoretic karyotypes and restriction fragment length polymorphism (RFLP) using gel electrophoresis or DNA-DNA hybridization. Techniques based on polymerase chain reaction (PCR) amplification of 18s ribosomal DNA (rDNA) that enable discrimination of *C. albicans*, *C. dubliniensis*, *C. glabrata*, *C. tropicalis* and *C. krusei* have been developed, and are likely to play a role in diagnosis in the future. Furthermore, molecular-based methods are now available that permit identification of *Candida* species in formalin-fixed archive tissue sections.

A basic principle in the treatment of oral candidosis is the elimination of any underlying known predisposing factor, such as by improving denture hygiene, by establishing glycaemic control in a diabetic, or by minimizing the effects of steroid inhaler therapy. Occasions do arise however where the use of **antifungal agents** are required. These are of use in the treatment of oral candidosis, and comprise three groups, namely: **polyenes** (nystatin and amphotericin); **imidazoles** (miconazole and ketaconazole); and **triazoles** (fluconazole and itraconazole).

Neither nystatin nor amphotericin is absorbed from the gut and their use is therefore limited to topical preparations, such as lozenges, cream or suspension. Unfortunately, patient compliance with these agents is low due to their unpleasant taste, which may in part explain the poor clinical effectiveness of topical drugs in management of oral candidosis.

Miconazole can be used in topical format, while ketoconazole is given orally, although its use is associated with a number of significant side effects.

Fluconazole and itraconazole, both of which are given orally, have become available, and have dramatically improved the treatment of oral candidosis. Fluconazole achieves good drug levels within the saliva, whilst itraconazole achieves good levels in the tissues.

The proliferation of *Candida* within the oral cavity can produce a number of superficial infections of the oral mucosa, including acute pseudomembranous candidosis (thrush), acute erythematous candidosis (antibiotic sore mouth) chronic hyperplastic candidosis (candidal leukoplakia) and chronic erythematous candidosis (denture stomatitis).

ACUTE PSEUDOMEMBRANOUS CANDIDOSIS

Also known as 'thrush', this is characterized by soft creamy-yellow patches that may affect large areas of the oral mucosa. This plaque is adherent but can occasionally be wiped off to reveal an underlying erythematous mucosa. Diagnosis of pseudomembranous candidosis can be made

in a smear stained by Gram's method to demonstrate large numbers of fungal hyphae or blastospores. A swab or an oral rinse should also be taken and sent for culture. Topical polyene therapy is generally ineffective, and hence an oral antifungal should be prescribed, such as fluconazole 50 mg once daily or itraconazole 100 mg once daily.

ACUTE ERYTHEMATOUS CANDIDOSIS

The oral mucosa in acute erythematous (atrophic) candidosis appears red. Any site of the oral mucosa may be affected, but involvement of the palate and the dorsal surface of the tongue is frequently seen in patients on steroid inhaler therapy. Unlike other forms of oral candidosis, acute erythematous candidosis is often painful. Diagnosis can be confirmed by use of swab or an oral rinse that should be sent for culture. Topical polyene therapy is generally ineffective and patients should be given a systemic agent such as fluconazole 50 mg once daily, or itraconazole 100 mg once daily.

Patients using steroid inhaler therapy should be advised to rinse their mouth with water after inhaler therapy in order to minimize persistence of the drug in the oral cavity, particularly if they are also taking an antibiotic.

CHRONIC HYPERPLASTIC CANDIDOSIS

This condition is characterized by the appearance of speckled white patches. Although this form of candidosis can occur at any intra-oral site, it characteristically presents bilaterally in the commissure region of the buccal mucosa. This form of oral candidosis is associated with severe epithelial dysplasia and malignant transformation. An imprint culture of the affected area should be taken and sent for culture. In addition, a mucosal biopsy of an area of affected mucosa that has not previously been swabbed should be performed. Swabbing of the mucosa prior to biopsy will remove superficial layers containing *Candida*, which may hinder diagnosis. Histological examination should reveal the presence of candidal hyphae within a hyperplastic epithelium (Figure 20.6).

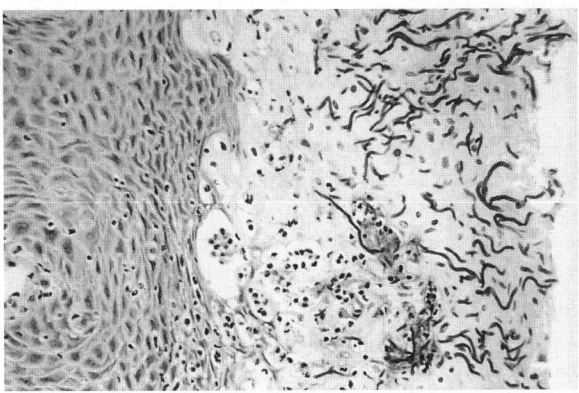

Figure 20.6 Candida *hyphae penetrating the epithelial characteristic for diagnosis of chronic hyperplastic candidosis.*

In the past, the regular use of topical polyene agents was advised over a period of 3 months, but more recently the use of systemic antifungal agents (fluconazole 50 mg once daily for 7–14 days or itraconazole 100 mg once daily for 15 days) has been found to produce both clinical and histological resolution in 2–3 weeks (Figure 20.7). Smoking will encourage recolonization and patients should be advised to stop any tobacco habit.

CHRONIC ERYTHEMATOUS (ATROPHIC) CANDIDOSIS

This is the most frequently occurring form of oral candidosis, and is present in 25–66% of patients who wear dentures. Continuous coverage of the palatal mucosa is a recognized predisposing factor to chronic erythematous candidosis, and clearly the habit of wearing dentures both day and night should be discouraged. In addition, the disease is not infrequent beneath the mucosal coverage area of upper orthodontic appliances. Diagnosis can be made from clinical appearance, and can be confirmed by swabs or imprints taken from areas of affected mucosa and the fitting surface of dentures. Patients should be advised to place their dentures in a dilute solution (1:10) of hypochlorite at night for 2–3 weeks to eliminate any candidal infestation of dentures. Patients who have metal components on their dentures should use 0.2% chlorhexidine gluconate, since hypochlorite will cause corrosion. The use of systemic antifungal

agents is not justified for this form of intra-oral candidosis. However, topical agents applied to the denture may assist elimination of infection, including nystatin ointment 100 000 units g^{-1} applied to the fitting surface of the denture two to four times daily, or miconazole oral 24 mg ml^{-1} gel applied to the fitting surface of the denture two to four times daily.

20.2.7 Angular cheilitis

Angular cheilitis is a common condition which presents as inflammation at either one or both corners of the mouth, and is usually associated with the presence of intra-oral candidosis. *Candida* species can be isolated from approximately two-thirds of patients with angular cheilitis, either alone or in combination with staphylococci or streptococci. Colonization of the angles of the mouth with *Candida* is probably a result of direct spread of the organisms from the oral flora, whilst colonization with *Staphylococcus* spp. is due to spread from commensal carriage in the anterior nares. Diagnosis can be confirmed by smears taken from the angle. In addition, swabs should be taken from each angle of the mouth, each anterior nares, the palate and (if worn) fitting-surface of upper dentures. An oral rinse should be sent for culture if dentures are not worn.

Management of angular cheilitis is based on eradication of chronic reservoir of candidal infection. Systemic antifungals are useful (e.g. fluconazole 50 mg once daily), but the patient should also be instructed in hygiene of dentures, if worn. If staphylococci alone are isolated from both the angles and anterior nares, then a topical antimicrobial may be used (e.g. mupirocin 2% ointment applied up to three times daily up to 10 days, or fusidic acid 2% cream applied two or three times daily). Two tubes of medication should be issued to the patient, since one should be used for the angles and the other for the anterior nares. Miconazole nitrate 2% cream applied twice daily is effective against both candida and staphylococci and is therefore indicated if a mixed infection is detected.

A number of rare forms of systemic mycosis can produce orofacial lesions; such conditions include paracoccidioidomycosis, histoplasmosis, and mucormycosis.

20.2.8 Acute necrotizing ulcerative gingivitis

Acute necrotizing ulcerative gingivitis (ANUG) is associated with the development of fusospirochaetal complex, involving *Fusobacterium nucleatum* and *Treponema* spp., at the gingival margin. Diagnosis is often made on the characteristic clinical symptoms that comprise the combination of painful sloughing ulceration involving the papillae between the teeth and a distinct offensive oral

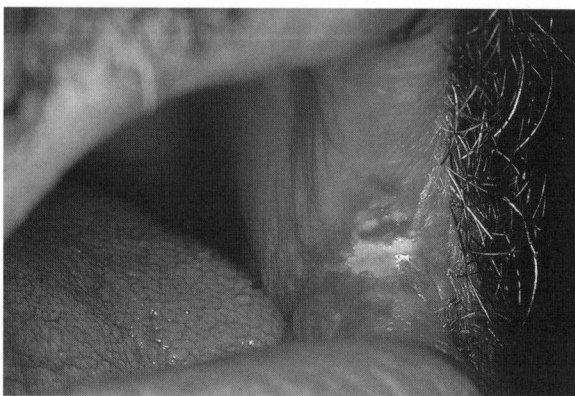

Figure 20.7 *This patient was referred by his general practitioner with a complaint of painful erosive lesions affecting both commisure regions of the mouth. Medical history was unremarkable apart from a smoking habit of 40 cigarettes a day. The patient had been provided with topical antifungal to apply to the affected areas, but these had failed to produce any improvement. A mucosal biopsy revealed chronic hyperplastic candidosis with mild epithelial dysplasia. An imprint culture yielded a heavy growth of* Candida albicans. *A 14-day course of fluconazole 50 mg capsule once daily was prescribed. At review there had been almost complete resolution of the lesions.*

odour. Microbiological confirmation of the condition can be obtained simply by examination of a Gram-stained smear from the lesion for the presence of fuso-bacteria, spirochaetes and leucocytes (Figure 20.8). Management is by local cleaning, preferably with an ultrasonic scaling instrument. A 3-day course of metronidazole (200 mg every 8 hours) is the antimicrobial therapy of choice.

20.2.9 Cancrum oris (noma)

This is a severe form of acute necrotizing ulcerative gingivitis and is occasionally seen in children in developing countries. The child is characteristically less than 10 years of age, malnourished and has a history of recent viral infection such as measles. The initial lesion of ulcerative gingivitis spreads into the cheek, face and neck causing extensive tissue loss. Treatment is with combinations of antibiotics, such as benzylpenicillin with metronidazole, but each combination should include agents active against both Gram-negative and Gram-positive organisms.

20.3 BURNS AND ULCERS

20.3.1 Mucosal burn and traumatic oral ulceration

An injury to the mucosal lining of the mouth becomes colonized by members of the oral microflora, which delays healing. Such secondary infection can be reduced by the use of an antiseptic mouthwash containing 0.2% chlorhexidine gluconate or 0.15% benzydamine hydrochloride. Alternatively, a mouthwash prepared by adding a teaspoon of salt to a cup of warm water is equally effective.

20.3.2 Pyostomatitis vegetans

This condition is associated with the presence of active inflammatory bowel disease, in particular ulcerative colitis but also Crohn's disease. The oral mucosa is diffusely inflamed, with fissured ulcers separating papillary projections. Histological examination reveals suprabasal separation of the epithelium with the formation of eosinophilic abscesses. The severity of pyostomatitis vegetans often mirrors the bowel disease activity. Interestingly, the provision of metronidazole can relieve oral symptoms. Healing occurs when the underlying inflammatory bowel disorder is brought under control.

20.3.3 Tuberculosis

Spread of *Mycobacterium tuberculosis* from the lung can produce characteristically painless (but not invariably) punched out ulcers in the mouth, in particular on the dorsum of the tongue (Figure 20.9). The diagnosis of oral tuberculosis can be made by either histological examination or microbiological culture of biopsy material. Treatment of tuberculosis requires specialized knowledge, particularly where disease involves resistant organisms or non-respiratory organs e.g. kidney. In the UK, management involves two phases – an initial phase involving at least three drugs, and a continuation phase using two drugs. Variations of this approach are used in other countries. Antimicrobial drugs used include isoniazid, rifampicin, pyrazinamide and ethambutol. Treatment failure is often due either to incorrect prescribing by the physician or inadequate compliance by the patient.

20.3.4 Gonorrhoea

Although gonorrhoea, caused by *Neisseria gonorrhoeae*, is essentially a sexually transmitted disease affecting the

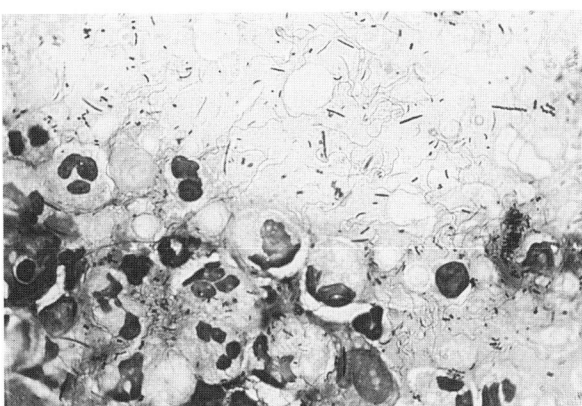

Figure 20.8 *Smear from acute ulcerative gingivitis, stained by Gram's method and showing fusobacteria, spirochaetes and acute inflammatory cells.*

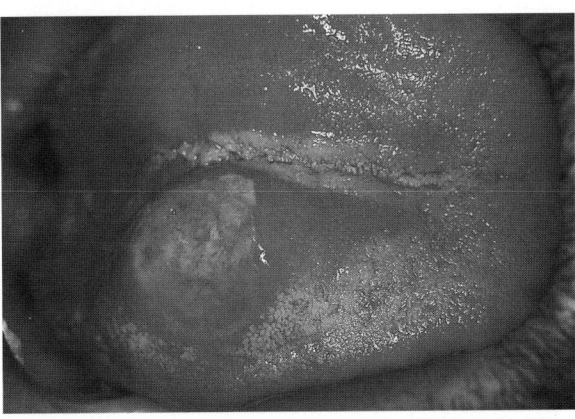

Figure 20.9 *Tuberculous ulcer on the dorsum of the tongue.*

genital mucosa, it may also produce oral lesions, (including tonsillitis and gingivitis) as a result of orogenital contact.

Diagnosis is made by examination of a smear of a lesion, which will show Gram-negative pairs of cocci within neutrophils. Culture on lysed blood or chocolate agar will yield typical translucent colonies of *N. gonorrhoeae*. Treatment should involve provision of intramuscular penicillin or high-dose oral amoxicillin.

20.3.5 Syphilis

Although syphilis usually develops on the genitalia, it can also initially present as an indurated painless area of ulceration on the lips or oral mucosa. The highly infectious primary lesion (chancre) is caused by infection with *Treponema pallidum*, and should be examined with extreme caution. Secondary syphilis appears clinically approximately 6 weeks after the primary infection, and in addition to generalized symptoms may produce oral lesions described as 'snail track ulcers'. Finally, untreated syphilis may become latent and produce tertiary lesions many years after initial infection, including deep ulceration (gumma) in the palate and leukoplakia affecting the dorsal surface of the tongue.

Diagnosis is supported by use of dark-field microscopy to detect numerous spirochaetes, in size and form typical of *T. pallidum*, in a smear taken from either primary or secondary lesions. However, serological investigations (10 ml clotted sample) are the most reliable way of diagnosing syphilis from the late stage of primary infection onwards because *T. pallidum* cannot be cultured routinely *in vitro*. The Venereal Diseases Reference Laboratory (VDRL), *T. pallidum* haemagglutination (TPHA) and fluorescent treponema antibody absorbed (FTA abs) tests should be undertaken.

The most effective treatment of any stage of syphilis is intramuscular procaine penicillin. Patients should be followed up for at least 2 years, and serological examination repeated over this period of time.

20.4 INFECTION-ASSOCIATED TUMOURS OF THE CHEEK AND THE FLOOR OF THE MOUTH

Structures consistent with candidal hyphae are often seen as an incidental finding in mucosal biopsies of squamous cell carcinoma. The true role of *Candida* in the onset of malignant transformation is unknown, and the presence of these organisms may simply represent secondary opportunistic invasion within an altered epithelium rather than a primary factor in malignant change. Interestingly, there is a high incidence of carcinoma in hyperplastic candidosis occurring in the buccal mucosa.

20.5 TONGUE INFECTIONS

20.5.1 Median rhomboid glossitis

The aetiology of this localized lesion is not fully understood, although it is now generally accepted that candidal infection is likely to be involved. *Candida* species can usually be isolated from the surface of the lesion by a swab. It should be remembered that the dorsum of the tongue is a frequent site for commensal carriage of *Candida*, and therefore quantification is helpful to confirm significant levels. The use of an imprint culture (p. 208) can help differentiate between the presence of commensal levels and those representing infection. In addition to being present on the surface, structures consistent with candidal hyphae are seen deep within the epithelium in biopsies of lesional material. Further support for the involvement of *Candida* has been observed in recent years due to the resolution of lesions following the provision of systemic antifungal therapy (fluconazole 50 mg once daily for 14 days or itraconazole 100 mg once daily for 15 days). Topical antifungal agents are ineffective.

20.5.2 Fissured tongue

The dorsum of the tongue may be deeply fissured in some individuals, and although this purely represents a variation of normal structure rather than pathological change, it can occasionally be symptomatic. The fissures may become infected by members of the commensal oral microflora. Topical hygiene using 0.2% chlorhexidine gluconate, applied using cotton bud tips, will lead to improvement of any discomfort.

20.5.3 Hairy leukoplakia

Hairy leukoplakia was first described in the mouths of homosexuals with AIDS in California, and has subsequently become recognized as a specific oral manifestation of HIV infection or immunosuppression. Characteristically, hairy leukoplakia presents as a corrugated white lesion on the lateral border of the tongue, although it has also been described on the dorsum of the tongue and the buccal mucosa. Epstein–Barr virus (EBV) has been demonstrated in lesional tissue by *in-situ* hybridization and DNA probes. Although the exact role of EBV in hairy leukoplakia is still uncertain, temporary clinical resolution of the condition can occur following provision of high doses of aciclovir. Imprint cultures of hairy leukoplakia often yield *Candida* species, but it is likely that this represents opportunistic secondary invasion. It has been observed that the clinical appearance of hairy leukoplakia may improve when the patient is provided with antiviral agents with activity against the herpes group of viruses.

20.6   HYPERKERATOSIS AND LEUKOPLAKIA

Leukoplakia is a clinical term used to describe 'a white patch affecting the oral mucosa that cannot be classified clinically or pathologically as any other disease'. Leukoplakia is extremely common, and infection with *Candida* may play a role in some lesions. A biopsy of leukoplakia may show evidence of dysplasia, and this is often associated with the presence of *Candida* invading the tissues. In the past, treatment with prolonged topical amphotericin or nystatin over a period of 3 months was recommended; however, this approach rarely produced any benefit and such treatment has now been replaced with systemic therapy using the same agents. The systemic delivery of antifungal agents produces a dramatic improvement both clinically and histologically, but should be assisted by the advice of a microbiologist to decide dosage and length of treatment.

20.7   BENIGN NEOPLASMS ASSOCIATED WITH HPV INFECTION

More than 60 distinct types of human papillomavirus (HPV) have been identified. Conditions occurring within the mouth that have been suggested to be related to HPV infection include focal epithelial hyperplasia (Heck's disease), squamous papilloma, condyloma acuminata, verruca vulgaris and leukoplakia. It must be emphasized, however, that involvement of HPV in these lesions is not yet proven and further investigations are being undertaken to establish the role of these viruses in oral disease. The demonstration of HPV requires DNA hybridization, since culture of the virus is not possible, and serology is of little help.

20.8   DENTAL AND PERIODONTAL INFECTIONS

20.8.1   Pericoronitis

The eruption of a tooth into the oral cavity produces a breach of the overlying mucosa. For a period of time a space known as the operculum is created between the crown of the tooth and the overlying flap of tissue (Figure 20.10). Infection of this space with resultant swelling of local tissue is referred to as pericoronitis.

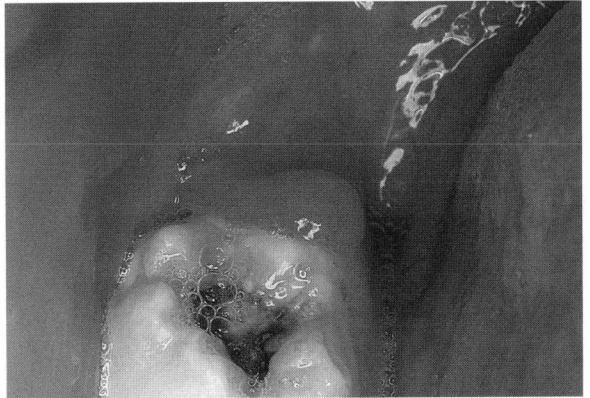

Figure 20.10 *This 21-year-old female presented with a painful swelling of gingivae distal to the lower right third molar. A clinical diagnosis of pericoronitis was made, and the patient was prescribed a 5-day course of metronidazole tablets 200 mg, three times daily. Microbiological sampling of pericoronitis is difficult due to the risk of contamination of the sample from surrounding tissues and saliva. Culture of a dental paper point placed between the crown of the tooth and the inflamed gingivae yielded a mixed growth of* Eubacterium *spp.,* Fusobacterium nucleatum *and anaerobic Gram-positive cocci. At review after 48 hours there had been considerable improvement in the symptoms. It is sometimes helpful to extract the opposing upper third molar if it is non-functional.*

Although pericoronitis could (in theory) affect any tooth, it is almost exclusively limited to the eruption of lower third molars. Accurate microbiological sampling of this condition is difficult due to contamination from the salivary flora. Despite this problem detailed studies have revealed that the microbiology of pericoronitis comprises a mixture of viridans group streptococci, *Prevotella* spp., *Porphyromonas* spp., *Actinomyces* spp. and *Eubacterium* spp.

Treatment includes local measures of antiseptic irrigation (e.g. with chlorhexidine solutions) under the flap, and if symptoms are severe the provision of an antimicrobial agent such as amoxicillin is suggested, although some workers recommend the use of metronidazole due to the predominance of strict anaerobes in this infection. In severe infection, either phenoxymethylpenicillin (penicillin V) (500 mg every 6 hours, increased to 750 mg every 6 hours), amoxicillin (250 mg every 8 hours, increased to 500 mg every 8 hours) or metronidazole (200 mg every 8 hours, increased to 400 mg every 8 hours) are recommended.

20.8.2   Caries

Dental caries is one of the most common diseases of man. Caries is the loss of tooth substance due to demineralization of the surface enamel and subsequently

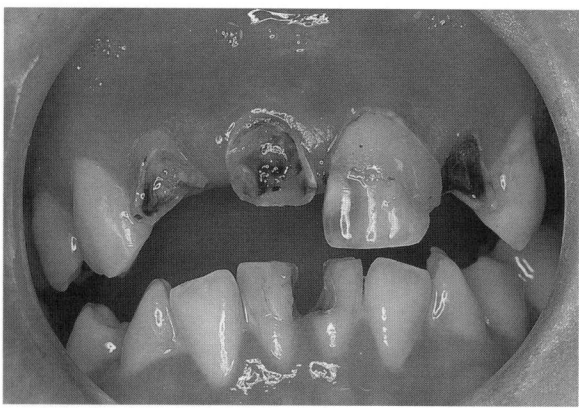

Figure 20.11 *Gross dental caries.*

proteolytic destruction of the underlying tissues (Figure 20.11). It is a chronic process which requires the presence of microorganisms with substrate, usually refined carbohydrate from the diet, acting on the tooth over long periods of time. The microbiology of caries remains uncertain, but *Streptococcus mutans*, *Lactobacillus* spp. and *Actinomyces* spp. are likely to be involved. *Strep. mutans* (which consists of a group of seven species: *Strep. mutans*, *Strep. sobrinus*, *Strep. cricetus*, *Strep. ferus*, *Strep. rattus*, *Strep. macacae* and *Strep. downe*) is one of the primary implicated bacteria. Evidence for the involvement of *Strep. mutans* in caries includes a high prevalence with carious lesions, ability to adhere to tooth surfaces, production of caries in animal experiments and production of acid of low pH. In addition, immunization against *Strep. mutans* in primates has also shown a reduced rates of caries. Lactobacilli are also likely to be involved in the carious process since they are encountered in high numbers within carious lesions, and they are also able to produce lactic acid in low pH conditions. Finally, *Actinomyces* spp., especially *A. viscosus*, is associated with caries occurring on the root surfaces of teeth.

Diagnosis of dental caries is made by clinical and radiographic examination of the teeth. In epidemiological studies, saliva samples can be examined quantitatively on Mitis Salivarius Bacitracin agar for levels of *Strep. mutans* and Rogosa SL agar for levels of *Lactobacillus* spp. A high caries rate correlates with the presence of a *Strep. mutans* count of greater than 10^6 cfu ml^{-1} or a *Lactobacillus* spp. count of 10^5 cfu ml^{-1}.

Treatment of caries is preferably by provision of restorative dental treatment. Untreated or recurrent caries will continue to cause tooth destruction and eventually lead to changes within the pulp. Following inflammation of the pulp (pulpitis), death (necrosis) of the vascular pulp occurs with the result that infection spreads into the apical tissues. Unless there is significant co-incidental soft-tissue (gingival) infection, antibiotics are not indicated for treatment of caries (see below).

20.8.3 Periodontal disease

Few adults manage to go through life without developing a degree of periodontal disease. There are a number of forms of periodontal disease, including: acute necrotizing ulcerative gingivitis, chronic gingivitis, localized juvenile periodontitis, rapidly progressive periodontitis and chronic adult periodontitis. The aetiology of these various conditions is not fully understood, but it involves a relationship between host tissues, defence mechanisms and microorganisms resident within subgingival plaque. Evidence that bacteria are involved in the tissue changes is provided by epidemiological data that correlates plaque levels and severity of disease as well as improvement following removal of plaque and the benefit of application of antimicrobials such as 0.2% chlorhexidine gluconate. The microbiological study of plaque and periodontal disease is extremely complex. Methods used include: (i) dark-field microscopy to estimate different morphological types, in particular spirochaetes; (ii) screening of specific bacteria believed to be 'pathogens'; and (iii) more recently molecular biological based markers, including DNA probes, ELISA and fluorescent antibodies.

In health, the gingival crevice contains a resident microbial flora containing low numbers of spirochaetes and motile rods which, with the onset of different forms of periodontal disease, are accompanied by an increase in the proportion of strict anaerobes, Gram-negative bacteria and motile organisms.

20.8.4 Chronic gingivitis

The gingivae become erythematous, swollen and bleed on tooth brushing (Figure 20.12). Microbiological investigations have implicated the presence of a number of bacterial species, in particular *Prevotella* spp., *Capnocytophaga* spp. and *Fusobacterium nucleatum*.

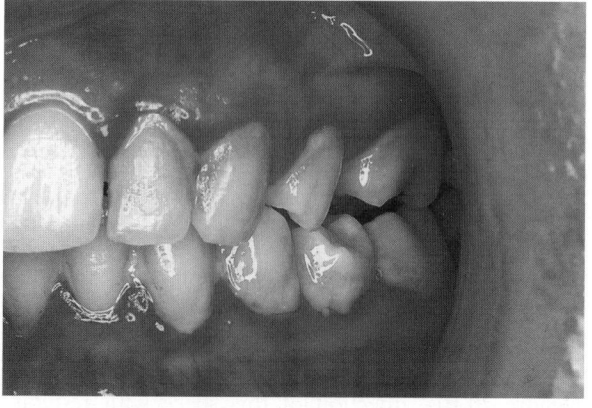

Figure 20.12 *Chronic gingivitis.*

20.8.5 Adult periodontitis

The progression of periodontal disease involves sporadic episodes of tissue destruction with migration of the gingival attachment towards the apex of the tooth. In addition to the bacterial species implicated in gingivitis, other species implicated in the disease process include *Actinobacillus actinomycemcomitans*, spirochaetes, *Porphyromonas* species and *Eikenella corrodens*. Correct attention to oral hygiene combined with efficient plaque removal and a correct (low-carbohydrate) diet are the mainstay of treatment, but metronidazole 200 mg three times daily can assist in achieving rapid control.

20.8.6 Localized juvenile periodontitis: rapidly progressive periodontitis

Localized juvenile periodontitis and rapidly progressive periodontitis are related forms of periodontal disease that affect less than 1% of individuals. A relatively rapid destruction of tissue occurs around the incisors and first permanent molars in the teenage years. Specific bacteria implicated in these conditions include *Actinobacillus actinomycemcomitans*, *Capnocytophaga* spp. and *Porphyromonas gingivalis*. Treatment is based on dietary correction, local hygiene therapy including fluoride-containing preparations combined with systemic tetracycline therapy.

20.8.7 Dentoalveolar abscess

Dentoalveolar abscess (periapical abscess) is by far the most common acute suppurative dental infection, and is associated with the apex of the root of the tooth. The tooth is necrotic with a non-vital pulp, usually as a result of dental caries but occasionally due to trauma, particularly when an anterior tooth is involved. For reasons that are not fully understood, a chronic inflammatory condition (granuloma) at the apex of the root may be present asymptomatically for many months or years before undergoing acute suppurative change. The presence of a longstanding preceding chronic lesion at the apex of the tooth is evident from a radiograph of an abscessed tooth which shows a periapical radiolucency within the alveolar bone (Figure 20.13). Such bone loss will have only occurred over a period of many weeks or months, and this confirms the chronic nature of the condition. Bacteria may gain access to the periapical area via three routes: (i) direct spread from the pulp; (ii) via the vessels of the periodontal ligament; or (iii) via the general circulation (Figure 20.14). Once suppuration occurs, the infection spreads through the tissues by the path of least resistance to present either intra-orally or extra-orally (Figure 20.15). The clinical appearance will involve a swelling either intra-orally or extra-orally.

Microbiological studies carried out between 1974 and 1984 reported that the flora of dentoalveolar abscess comprised either one or two species of viridans streptococci, *Neisseria* spp. and *Staphylococcus* spp. However, it is now generally accepted that these studies were flawed due to contamination of the specimen. Swabs were used which would have inevitably become contaminated with salivary microorganisms. Other problems with the studies included delay in processing, use of inadequate media, lack of anaerobic incubation and culture time limited to 24–48 hours.

It is now appreciated that microbiological investigation of dentoalveolar abscess must involve sampling by aspiration using an 18- or 20-gauge needle. Samples should be transferred to the laboratory promptly for immediate processing within 3 hours onto blood agar. Plates must be incubated either in an anaerobic chamber or anaerobic jar. Duplicate plates should be incubated

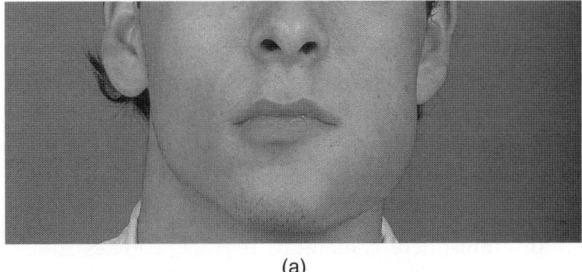

(a)

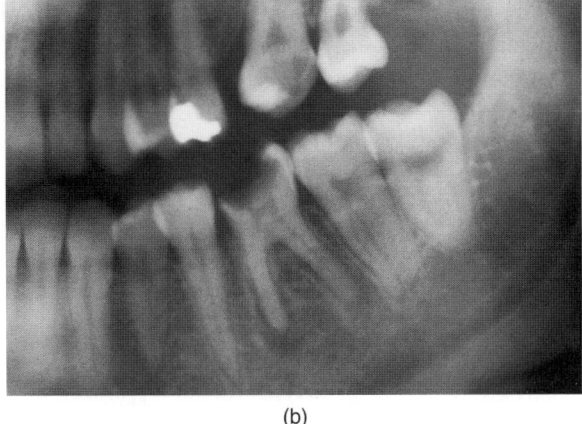

(b)

Figure 20.13 *This adult male presented with swelling of an acute dentoalveolar abscess affecting the left cheek (a). Radiographic examination of the teeth revealed radiolucent areas on the roots of the lower left first molar tooth (b). This case illustrates the fact that an acute abscess may be preceded by a prolonged asymptomatic period of chronic inflammation resulting in bone loss (seen as the radiolucency) prior to the onset of acute symptoms of pain and swelling. An aspirate of pus was obtained prior to incision of the swelling via an intra-oral approach. Pain relief is almost instant once drainage is achieved. The aspirate of pus yielded a mixed growth of Streptococci of the milleri group, Prevotella intermedia and anaerobic Gram-positive cocci. The P. intermedia was resistant to penicillin (MIC > 2 μg ml⁻¹) but sensitive to co-amoxiclav (MIC = 0.016 μg ml⁻¹).*

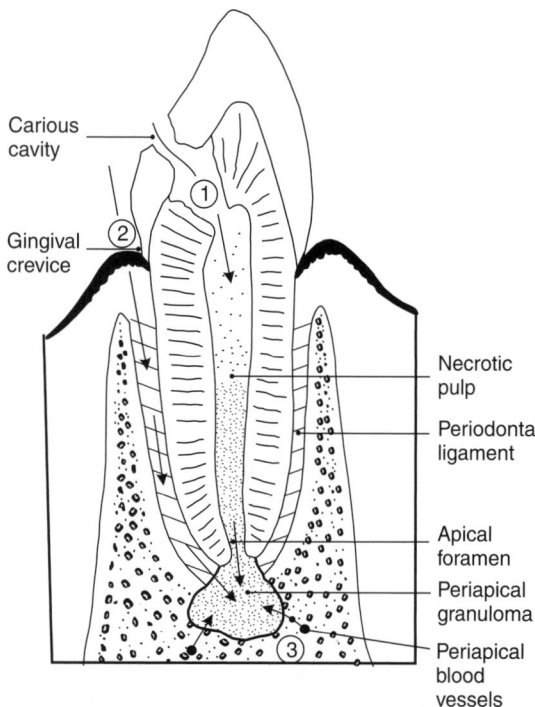

Figure 20.14 *Pathways of bacterial invasion of the periapical tissues. 1, Apical foramen; 2, Periodontal ligament; 3, blood vessels.*

in an atmosphere containing 10% CO_2. Plates should be examined after 48 hours, then daily for a total of 10 days, since many bacteria in these infections are slow growing. Recent studies, involving collection of pus by aspiration and the use of such appropriate methods, have shown that the flora is a mixed one, comprising between four and eight bacterial species. The culturable flora usually include one or more of the following: *Streptococcus milleri* group, *Veillonella* spp., *Actinomyces*

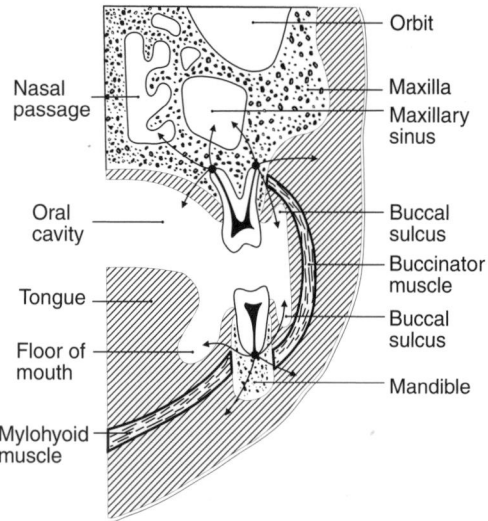

Figure 20.15 *Pathways by which pus may track from acute dentoalveolar abscess.*

spp., *Haemophilus* spp., *Eikenella corrodens*, anaerobic Gram-positive cocci, *Eubacterium* spp., *Prevotella intermedia*, *Prevotella oralis*, *Prevotella melaninogenica* and *Fusobacterium* spp. Quantitative microbiological studies of dentoalveolar abscess have revealed a viable microflora 10^6–10^8 cfu ml^{-1}. In addition, quantification has demonstrated not only a qualitative predominance of strict anaerobes but also that strict anaerobes occupy a larger percentage of the flora than facultative anaerobes. In recent years, molecular techniques, based on PCR amplification of 16s rDNA have been developed that enable the identification of specific bacterial species within the pus from a dentoalveolar abscess. Application of this methodology will, in the future, greatly assist the investigation and treatment of acute dental infections.

Interestingly, all the bacterial species encountered in acute dentoalveolar abscess are also regarded as members of the commensal oral microflora. There is uncertainty why these apparent non-pathogenic strains produce acute suppuration. Suggested mechanisms include the occurrence of specific bacterial combinations or the possession of capsular material. Capsule, demonstrated by use of India ink negative staining, is frequently detected in strains isolated from abscess, but it is absent in strains isolated from healthy oral sites. In addition, capsulate isolates are more pathogenic in experimental abscess models. The capsule does not limit phagocytosis, but may prevent intracellular killing by host polymorphs.

The basic principle in the management of orofacial infection is elimination of the source of causative microorganisms. In the case of dentoalveolar infection this involves establishment of surgical drainage of pus and extirpation of the dental pulp or extraction of the affected tooth. The bacterial species isolated from dentoalveolar abscess are traditionally regarded as being sensitive to the penicillins, and therefore members of this group of antibiotics are used routinely as antimicrobials of first choice. In cases where patients are known to have a hypersensitivity to penicillins then erthyromycin is often used as an alternative drug. In recent years, a growing awareness of the importance of strict anaerobes in dental infection has resulted in the use of metronidazole. The various alternatives for antibiotic treatment (each of which is given for a minimum of 5 days) are as follows:

- Phenoxymethylpenicillin (Penicillin V) 500 mg every 6 hours, increased to 750 mg every 6 hours in severe infection.
- Amoxicillin 250 mg every 8 hours, increased to 500 mg every 8 hours in severe infection.
- Erythromycin 250–500 mg every 6 hours or 0.5–1 g every 12 hours.
- Metronidazole 200 mg every 8 hours.

In recent years an increasing incidence of penicillin-resistant β-lactamase-producing strains in suppurative infection has been noted. Although at present the use of penicillin has rarely been associated with clinical failure, the prescribing of alternative drugs may be necessary in the future. Co-amoxiclav may be used in cases that fail to respond to initial therapy.

The importance of dental and periodontal infection for the promotion of temporary episodes of bacteraemia has been recognized for many years, as it is a prime cause of infective endocarditis (SABE). The organisms adhere to, and destroy, both abnormal valves as well as prostheses. This danger is exacerbated by dental treatment. For this reason, prophylactic treatment using amoxycillin 3.0 g should be given to all at-risk cases before dental treatment is under taken, which can be combined with probenecid.

20.9 INFECTIONS OF MAXILLARY SINUSES

20.9.1 Maxillary sinusitis

Maxillary sinusitis is usually caused by infection spreading from the nasopharynx into the sinus. Sinusitis is often recurrent, and characteristically develops after the common cold. Symptoms are often confused with toothache from the maxillary premolars and molars. The bacteriology usually involves *H. influenzae*, *Strep. pneumoniae* or *Strep. pyogenes*. Treatment should involve the provision of standard dosages of amoxycillin, ampicillin or erythromycin for 2 weeks. Doxycycline is also occasionally used for sinusitis, but this is expensive and should be used only for special indications.

Sinusitis may become chronic, resulting in pathological changes in the tissues and discharge of pus. The microbiology of chronic sinusitis is similar to the acute form, although it may also involve *Staph. aureus*, enterobacteria or *Prevotella* spp. Treatment should be dictated by susceptibility tests on specimens. Rarely, infection in the sinus may be caused by direct spread from a dentoalveolar abscess (see Figure 20.21). In these circumstances, the microbiology of the infection will reflect the abscess and should be managed accordingly.

A communication between the mouth and the sinus may be created during the extraction of premolar or molar teeth. This situation is referred to as an oro-antral fistula and if it occurs the use of antibiotic therapy, such as amoxycillin or erythromycin, is suggested to prevent delay in healing due to infection.

20.10 FURTHER READING

Bagg, J., MacFarlane, T.W., Poxton, I.R., Miller, C.H. and Smith, A.J. (1999) *Essentials of Microbiology for Dental Students*. Oxford University Press, Oxford.

Lamey, P.J. and Lewis M.A.O. (1997) *A Clinical Guide to Oral Medicine*, 2nd edition. British Dental Association, London.

Marsh, P. and Martin, M. (1999) *Oral Microbiology*, 4th edition. Wright, London.

Samaranayake L.P. (1996) *Essential Microbiology for Dentistry*. Churchill Livingstone, London.

Scully, C. and Samaranayake, L.P. (1992) *Clinical Virology in Oral Medicine and Dentistry*. Cambridge University Press, Cambridge.

Infections of the pharynx, neck, larynx and trachea

M.A.O. LEWIS AND G. SHONE

21.1 PHARYNGEAL INFECTIONS

21.1.1 Acute tonsillitis

Acute tonsillitis is a relatively common condition in children and young adults that may be due either to a viral or to a bacterial infection. Viruses implicated in tonsillitis include adenoviruses, herpes simplex virus and Epstein–Barr virus. The bacteria most frequently recovered from tonsillitis include *Streptococcus pyogenes* Lancefield group A, C and G. The tonsils become swollen with pus exuding from within the tonsillar crypts (Figure 21.1). A throat swab is useful. The most effective antibiotic treatment for severe tonsillitis is intramuscular benzylpenicillin. In less severe cases, phenoxymethylpenicillin (penicillin V) (500 mg every 6 hours) or erythromycin (250–500 mg every 6 hours or 0.5–1 g every 12 hours) may be given. Treatment should be given for at least 10 days.

On occasion, acute tonsillitis due to infection with β-haemolytic streptococci may be followed by acute glomerulonephritis or acute rheumatic fever due to the formation of anti-streptococcal antibodies.

21.1.2 Peritonsillar abscess (quinsy)

Occasionally, tonsillitis progresses into an acute abscess, termed quinsy, in the space between the tonsil and the pharyngeal musculature. The clinical presentation in such circumstances is dramatic, with the patient complaining of severe pain and limitation of opening of the mouth. The abscess must be drained as a matter of urgency and an aspirate sample sent for culture. Characteristically, a mixed growth of bacteria, frequently involving β-haemolytic streptococci associated with a variety of strict anaerobes, is obtained. Parenteral antibiotic treatment is required in the form of either benzylpenicillin or a broad-spectrum agent, such as cefuroxime or co-amoxiclav.

Acute tonsillitis or quinsy can progress to a parapharyngeal abscess, which has serious implications due to involvement of the great vessels in the neck and the possibilities of mediastinitis and airway obstruction.

21.1.3 Retropharyngeal abscess

The retropharyngeal space can become infected due to suppuration in a retropharyngeal lymph node as a result of spread of infection from the nose, pharynx or teeth. It may, alternatively, be due to a foreign body that penetrates the pharyngeal wall. The patient presents with severe sore throat and dysphagia, with drooling of saliva, malaise and pyrexia. The airway may become compromised due to secondary oedema. The microbiology is variable, and is influenced by the source of original infection. Urgent surgical drainage is required

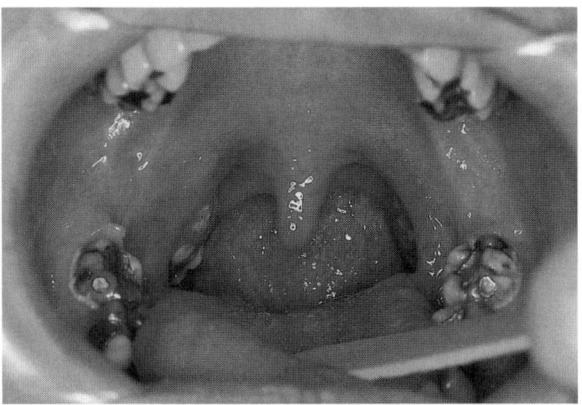

Figure 21.1 *Swollen tonsils with purulent discharge from crypts.*

and a sample of pus (preferably an aspirate) must be sent for culture and sensitivity. Immediate parenteral antibiotic therapy, involving either co-amoxiclav or a combination of amoxycillin and metronidazole, should be provided empirically; these antimicrobial agents can subsequently be modified once the microbiological findings and sensitivities of the organisms become available.

A chronic abscess may develop at this site as a result of spread of infection from a tuberculous infection of the cervical spine. This should be treated by repeated aspiration combined with anti-tuberculous drugs; and surgical drainage should be avoided, except as a last resource.

21.1.4 Adenoid infection

Infection of the lymphoid tissue at the nasopharyngeal interface known as the adenoids occurs frequently in children with upper respiratory tract infection, and is universal in cases of acute tonsillitis. The microbiology of adenoid infection is similar to that of tonsillitis, and treatment is the same (see section 21.1.1). Repeated infection may lead to hypertrophy, with secondary obstructive symptoms in the nose and possibly secondary effects on middle-ear function, due to obstruction or ascending infection of the Eustachian tube. (Surgical removal of the adenoids may be indicated in children with persistent middle-ear problems or severe nasal obstructive symptoms, particularly if this results in obstructive sleep apnoea.) The adenoid tissue regresses naturally after the age of about 7 years.

21.1.5 Pharyngitis

Pharyngitis may be either acute or chronic and occurs in specific and non-specific forms.

ACUTE NON-SPECIFIC PHARYNGITIS

Non-specific pharyngitis usually results in a sore throat, with little in the way of systemic symptoms. The infection may be either bacterial or viral and often it is not possible to distinguish between the two on clinical grounds. The patient is usually improving by the time that the results of culture swabs are available, in which case treatment is symptomatic only. The use of antibiotic therapy is reserved for prolonged infections, in which case 10 days of penicillin V (500 mg every 6 hours) may shorten the duration of the illness.

ACUTE SPECIFIC PHARYNGITIS

This may include several important diseases.

Infectious mononucleosis

Infectious mononucleosis (glandular fever) is caused by the Epstein–Barr virus, and causes a sore throat in association with fever, malaise, cervical lymphadenopathy and hepatosplenomegaly. Diagnosis is made from the typical appearance of the slough on the surface of the tonsil, and is confirmed by the blood film (mononucleosis), Paul Bunnell and/or monospot tests. Severe infection may result in swelling large enough to obstruct the airway, and these patients require systemic hydrocortisone and sometimes temporary intubation.

Diphtheria

This is now rare in countries with an immunization programme, but is still common in parts of Africa and Asia. Early pharyngeal infection is initially associated with malaise and fever and pearly white lesions on the mucosa. Severe symptoms may follow, with the formation of a characteristic grey membranous slough, with a generalized illness due to exotoxaemia, which may cause myocarditis or paralysis of cranial nerves. The pharyngeal involvement may progress to the larynx, with resulting airway impairment that may be life-threatening. The causative microorganism, *Corynebacterium diphtheria*, is sensitive to penicillin and therefore benzylpenicillin should be given intramuscularly 600 mg 6-hourly, in conjunction with antitoxin 10 000–100 000 units depending on the severity of the illness and the age of the patient. Antibiotic treatment should be continued until symptoms resolve.

Vincent's angina

This condition is caused by the development of a microbial fuso-spirochaetal complex, that produces an ulcerative tonsillar infection. Vincent's angina occurs in the presence of poor sanitary conditions and malnutrition. It is often unilateral, but may spread to the mouth to produce acute necrotizing ulcerative gingivitis (trench mouth). Treatment is with penicillin or metronidazole.

Other causes

Acute specific pharyngitis may also be due to herpetic or gonococcal infection. In addition, pharyngitis may develop in association with scarlet fever, measles, chickenpox and a range of other fevers. These causes each have specific treatments, as outlined in other chapters.

CHRONIC NON-SPECIFIC PHARYNGITIS

Chronic sore throat can be due to a wide variety of infective and non-infective agents, often acting in combination. Such non-specific pharyngitis may accompany chronic rhinosinusitis, dental infection, mouth-breathing, vocal abuse (singers mainly), atmospheric pollution, smoking, excessive alcohol ingestion, chronic pulmonary infection and gastro-oesophageal reflux. Treatment is to the primary cause, though this is often difficult to identify.

CHRONIC SPECIFIC PHARYNGITIS

As with acute specific pharyngitis, this condition incorporates several diseases.

Syphilis
The pharynx may be involved in primary, secondary, tertiary or congenital syphilis.

Tuberculosis
Acute miliary tuberculosis can produce an eruption or ulceration in the pharynx that is often painful and haemmorrhagic. Advanced pulmonary tuberculosis may be associated with very painful shallow pharyngeal ulcers. Treatment is for the tuberculous infection as a whole.

Fungal infection
Candidosis is the most frequent fungal disease within the pharynx. However, related organisms, such as blastomycosis, can also cause chronic pharyngitis. Topical antifungal agents are of limited benefit, and the therapy of choice would be systemic administration of either fluconazole or itraconazole.

Scleroma
This condition is caused by infection with *Klebsiella scleromatis*, and spreads from the nose to involve the pharynx. It is endemic in eastern Europe, north Africa, and central America. Although *Klebsiella* spp. have traditionally been regarded as being sensitive to the penicillins, more recently a number of strains have been found to be resistant to this group of antimicrobials due to β-lactamase production. Therefore, the antimicrobial of choice for this infection is co-amoxiclav.

Leprosy
As with scleroma, pharyngeal involvement is secondary to nasal infection. In Western countries, treatment must involve advice from the Panel of Leprosy Opinion (POLO). The World Health Organization has recommended the use of specific combinations of dapsone, rifampicin and clofazimine.

21.2 NECK INFECTIONS

21.2.1 Actinomycosis

Actinomycosis may occur at a number of sites, but the submandibular and neck regions are the most common (Figure 21.2). *Actinomyces israelii* is the characteristic causative microorganism, although *Actinomyces naeslundii* has been isolated in some cases. Diagnosis is achieved by examining pus from the lesion for the presence of 'sulphur granules'. Staining of the pus by Gram's method will reveal characteristic Gram-positive filaments. Culture requires prolonged anaerobic incubation up to 7 days at 37°C, and produces typical 'molar tooth' colonies on blood agar. Treatment should involve the provision of benzylpenicillin in standard doses over a period of 6–8 weeks initially, and continued until all signs of persisting infection have completely resolved. The advice of a microbiologist should be obtained.

21.2.2 Ludwig's angina

Ludwig's angina is defined as a spreading infection involving the sublingual and submandibular spaces. The

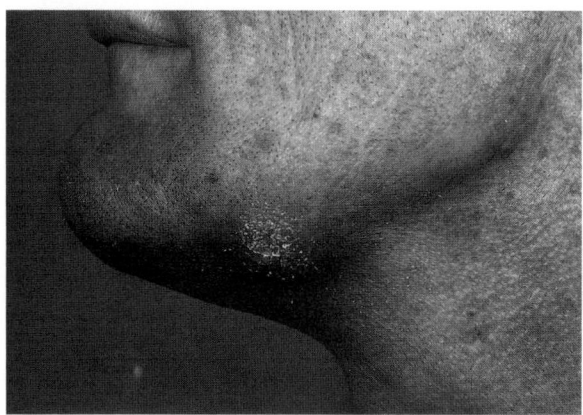

Figure 21.2 *This patient presented 1 month following extraction of a lower molar tooth with a complaint of swelling and discharge on the border of the mandible. Closer examination of the lesion revealed multiple sinus openings suggestive of actinomycosis. It was not possible to obtain an aspirate from the swelling, and therefore a swab was sent for culture. The laboratory was informed of a clinical diagnosis of actinomycosis.* Actinomyces israelii *was cultured after prolonged incubation. Isolation of* A. israelii *should be drawn to the clinician's attention since an extended course of antibiotic therapy over 6 weeks is required. It is generally accepted that actinomyces gains entry to the tissues from the saliva via the extraction socket.*

condition is almost always related to spread of bacteria from an acute dentoalveolar abscess or following post-extraction infection. Occasionally, the source of infection may be a suppurative submandibular sialadenitis, an infected fracture of the mandible or soft tissue lacerations involving the floor of the mouth. Further spread of infection into the pharyngeal spaces can produce a life-threatening situation requiring immediate surgical management. It is usually possible to obtain an aspirate of pus prior to incision and drainage. Culture invariably yields a mixture of strict anaerobes, such as *Prevotella intermedia*, *Prevotella nigrescens*, *Fusobacterium nucleatum* and anaerobic Gram-positive cocci. Empirical intravenous antibiotic therapy consisting of co-amoxiclav or a combination of amoxicillin and metronidazole in high doses should be started immediately, and changed appropriately according to the clinical response and the microbiological data obtained by culture and sensitivity tests.

21.2.3   Necrotizing fasciitis

The neck is a uncommon site for necrotizing fasciitis, but it has been described as a result of dentoalveolar infection. The microbiology of such cases usually involves members of the *Streptococcus milleri* group and strict anaerobes (in particular, the *Prevotella* species). The use of intravenous antibiotics, as advised by a microbiologist, is essential. In addition, administration of hyperbaric oxygen has been shown to be helpful.

21.2.4   Staphylococcal cervical lymphadenitis

Painful swollen submandibular lymph nodes are usually related to streptococcal tonsillitis or dental abscess.

Chronic lymphadenitis can be related to many non-infectious conditions as well as infection due to Epstein-Barr virus, *M. tuberculosis* and general systemic infection.

Children may develop painful localized swelling of facial or submandibular lymph nodes as a result of staphylococcal infection in the adjacent tissues. The most common source of bacterial infection is *Staphylococcus aureus* within the nose. Swabs should be taken of the anterior nares and an antibiotic such as flucloxacillin (250 mg every 6 hours) prescribed for between 3 and 5 days.

21.2.5   Tuberculous lymphadenitis

Evidence of previous tuberculosis may be seen as a coincidental finding on radiographs of the head and neck (Figure 21.3). Chronic tuberculous infection of lymph nodes of the neck producing an abscess or a sinus may require surgical intervention to remove the affected nodes; the operation should be covered by anti-tuberculous drugs.

21.2.6   Infected branchial cyst

Branchial cysts within the neck can become acutely infected and produce symptoms of pain and swelling (Fig. 21.4). An aspirate of the cyst fluid should be taken for culture and sensitivity. If pus is obtained it is likely to contain staphylococci, although the microbiological request should also indicate the possibility of infection involving mycobacteria. Empirical antibiotic therapy should consist of flucloxacillin (250 mg every 6 hours) for 5 days. When the infection has subsided, surgical removal of the cyst should be arranged.

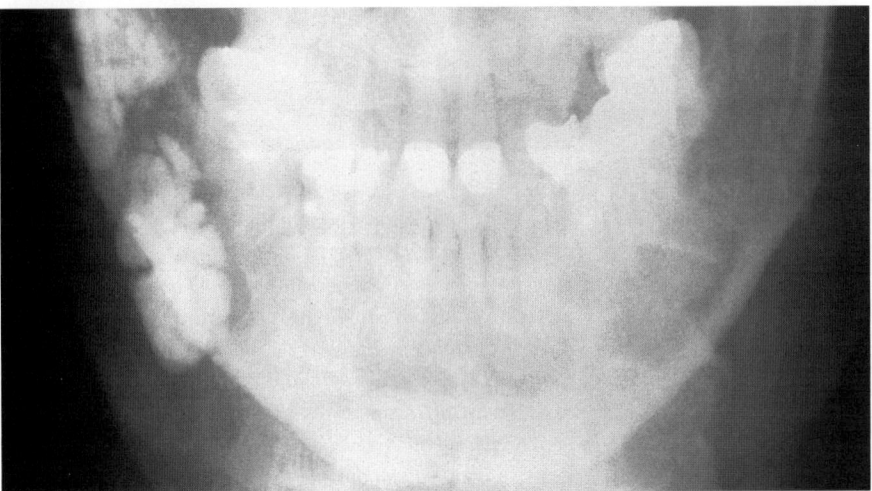

Figure 21.3 *Radio-opacity in the right submandibular region. Such a lesion is often found as an incidental finding on radiographs of this region, and this patient was asymptomatic. However, medical history included tuberculosis some 30 years previously. Calcification of the regional lymph nodes may occur and produce the appearance seen here. Clinical investigation should be undertaken to exclude pathology of the submandibular salivary gland, in particular the presence of sialoliths (stones). No treatment is required in this patient.*

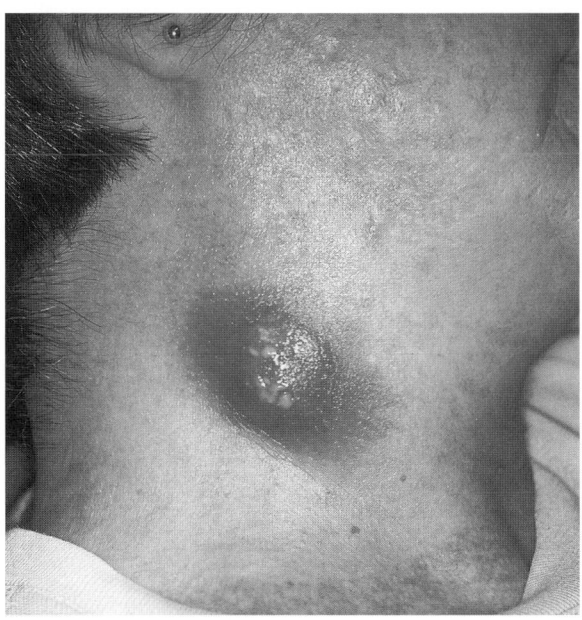

Figure 21.4 *Infected branchial cyst. (Illustration courtesy of Mr. C. Bell, Bristol Dental Hospital.)*

21.3 LARYNGEAL AND TRACHEAL INFECTIONS

21.3.1 Acute epiglottitis

Acute epiglottitis in children leads to a dramatic presentation, with a severe illness of a few hours duration that progresses rapidly to airway obstruction and death if untreated. The child has a sore throat and total dysphagia leading to drooling and a characteristic leaning-forward posture. There is pyrexia and severe malaise due to the accompanying septicaemia. The infection is caused by *H. influenzae* capsular type b. Acute epiglottitis has become rare in countries that have an effective immunization programme against this organism. The clinical picture is highly recognizable, and confirmation of the diagnosis through throat swabs and blood cultures must be carried out *after* the airway has been secured, as fatal asphyxiation can occur at any moment. Immediate empirical treatment should be started with a broad-spectrum antibiotic and changed as indicated by microbiological results from culture and sensitivities. For **children**, first-line antimicrobial treatment should involve either amoxycillin or chloram-

phenicol given systemically on an in-patient basis. **Adult epiglottitis** usually has a less dramatic onset over a slightly longer time course, and a variety of bacterial organisms have been implicated. Initial antibiotic therapy should consist of either amoxycillin or co-amoxyclav.

21.3.2 Acute laryngotracheobronchitis

Infection with respiratory tract viruses, notably the parainfluenzal group, are the most frequent cause of this infection. As with acute epiglottitis, children present with stridor and respiratory obstruction, though usually less acute.

Secondary bacterial infection with *Staph. aureus* may result in a serious worsening of the child's condition. Initial treatment with flucloxacillin is recommended.

21.3.3 Bronchitis

Acute bronchitis is usually a minor viral infection in an otherwise healthy individual. However, acute bronchitis due to secondary bacterial infection of the respiratory mucosa also develops in patients with a history of chronic bronchitis, bronchiectasis or asthma. The microbiology in these circumstances usually involves *Strep. pneumoniae*, *Branhamella catarrhalis* or *Mycoplasma pneumoniae*. Culture of sputum samples should yield the causative bacteria and enable susceptibility testing. Initial antimicrobial therapy should comprise of amoxycillin, erythromycin or tetracycline. Co-trimoxazole comprising of sulphamethoxazole and trimethoprim may be used, but only if indicated by the results of microbiological culture and sensitivity profiles.

21.4 FURTHER READING

Bagg, J., MacFarlane, T.W., Poxton, I.R., Miller, C.H. and Smith, A.J. (1999) *Essentials of Microbiology for Dental Students*. Oxford University Press, Oxford.

Marsh, P. and Martin, M. (1999) *Oral Microbiology*, 4th edition. Wright, London.

Samaranayake, L.P. (1996) *Essential Microbiology for Dentistry*. Churchill Livingstone, London.

22

Post-operative respiratory infection

A.M. SEFTON

22.1 INTRODUCTION

The respiratory tract is the site of the majority of infections in humans, many of which are managed at home by community practitioners, with the remainder being treated by general physicians or chest physicians. Few patients present to surgeons with respiratory tract infections, but many patients develop respiratory problems postoperatively that may be infective in nature. In the intensive care unit (ICU), respiratory tract infections carry a significant mortality, and this is considered in Section 22.2.

22.2 POSTOPERATIVE RESPIRATORY TRACT INFECTIONS

Hospital-acquired (nosocomial) infection occurs in about 5–10% of in-patients overall. Most of these infections are not life-threatening, but they are still likely to lengthen hospital stay, increase cost and cause distress to the patient. Hospital-acquired infections are spread by three main routes: autogenous spread (self-infection), cross-infection, and via the environment. Patients commonly become colonized by these organisms rather than infected.

Urinary tract, wound and respiratory tract infections are the three most common types of hospital-acquired infection. Lower respiratory tract infections are the third most common, but are the ones with the highest morbidity and mortality. They are especially likely to occur in the elderly, debilitated or immunocompromised patients, smokers and in patients with underlying respiratory tract disease. Having a general anaesthetic or a decreased level of consciousness for any reason are also risk factors. Intensive care patients who require ventilation and/or respiratory suction are at a particular risk of developing severe nosocomial pneumonia. Patients with either large surgical wounds or trauma to the chest or abdomen may be frightened of coughing and this, especially if they suffer chronic respiratory problems, may predispose them to developing lower respiratory tract infections. Occasionally, outbreaks of respiratory tract infections due to influenza A or B or other viruses may occur in hospital wards; respiratory syncytial virus is a problem usually associated with paediatric wards.

In addition to developing hospital-acquired respiratory tract infections, patients may occasionally be admitted to hospital with signs of a respiratory tract infection – either upper or lower. In these circumstances elective surgery should be delayed until the patient is better, but the surgeon may have to proceed with emergency surgery. Such patients are likely to be at particular risk of developing a severe postoperative respiratory infection.

22.3 PATHOPHYSIOLOGY

The majority of nosocomial pneumonia probably arises from aspiration of potential pathogens which have previously colonized the mucosal surfaces of the upper airway. Hospitalized patients, and especially those who have received broad-spectrum antibiotics and are in the intensive care setting, often have Gram-negative bacilli colonizing their upper airways. This is in contrast to the predominantly Gram-positive flora of patients in the community. Under the correct conditions, these organisms can then cause infection.

In fit, healthy young adults the 'mucociliary escalator' prevents organisms in the upper respiratory tract from gaining access to the lower airways. The presence of an endotracheal tube prevents this working effectively, and hence predisposes the patient to development of bacterial lower respiratory tract infection. In addition, mechanical trauma of the respiratory mucosa during intubation may also predispose to bacterial colonization of the lower respiratory tract. Smoking and viral upper respiratory tract infections also prevent the mucociliary escalator from functioning properly. Influenza viruses have a particularly strong inhibitory effect in the mucociliary escalator.

Many people, especially the elderly, have occasional micro-aspirations in their sleep. Anything causing a decreased conscious level or a decreased cough reflex – as occurs in patients recovering from anaesthetic or requiring strong analgesics or with neurological problems – makes aspiration of upper respiratory tract flora more common.

22.4 DIAGNOSIS

Before starting antimicrobial therapy, a sputum or respiratory secretion sample should be obtained from any patient in whom a lower respiratory tract infection is suspected. If the patient is already receiving antibiotics, a sample should still be sought, though in this instance the results need to be interpreted with caution.

Care should be taken when obtaining the samples in order to avoid **oropharyngeal contamination**. The patient should be instructed to cough deeply into a sterile pot in order to obtain sputum from deep in the lungs. Some patients with respiratory tract infections find coughing painful, and therefore try to prevent themselves from expectoration. This is likely to be a problem in post-surgical patients who may find that expectoration makes their wound hurt and are worried about splitting it open if they cough too rigorously. Hence,

a physiotherapist may be required to help obtain an optimum sample and to reassure the patient that he/she will not harm themselves by coughing. If the patient is told to 'spit in a pot', he/she is likely to do just this and produce a sample of saliva.

As soon as the sputum is obtained it should be sent to the microbiology laboratory for microscopy, culture and sensitivity. An accompanying form should provide a brief clinical history, including any present/recent antimicrobial therapy. If the patient is on a ventilator, endotracheal secretions will need to be sent instead of sputum. If, for any reason, a bronchoscopy is performed, then bronchoalveolar lavage samples are extremely helpful. *Mycobacterium tuberculosis* does not grow on standard bacterial culture and will not be seen on the Gram-stain and it will not be looked for unless specifically requested. Although *M. tuberculosis* is an uncommon cause of nosocomial respiratory infections it may occasionally cause disease in a postoperative patient who has been previously exposed to this organism and who is immunocompromised by disease or treatment such as chemotherapy or high-dose steroids.

Once in the laboratory the sputum will be examined for the presence of pus cells, epithelial cells and bacteria. The presence of many epithelial cells suggests a poorly taken sample, and the results of such a specimen must be interpreted with caution. Bacteria associated with white blood cells (WBC) are highly suggestive of infection. Potential pathogens such as *Streptococcus pneumoniae* or *Haemophilus influenzae* may be seen on Gram staining. If a patient is already receiving antibiotics when a sputum is taken, the presence of Gram-negative rods in a film may represent merely colonization of the patient, and not be the causative organism.

A chest X-ray should be performed and blood cultures taken in any such patient suspected of having a bacterial pneumonia. A full blood count should also be taken: elevation of the WBC count, although non-specific, may be suggestive of infection. Sputum, nasopharyngeal or bronchoalveolar washings can be taken and sent to the virology department if a viral aetiology is suspected. If atypical pneumonia is suspected – a rare cause of nosocomial pneumonia, except in the immunocompromised patient – acute and convalescent sera should be taken 2 weeks apart for retrospective diagnosis. Further tests such as the detection of *Legionella* antigens in the urine may be available in some centres.

22.5 AETIOLOGY

If a patient develops a lower respiratory tract infection within 2–3 days of admission to hospital, it is likely to be caused by the organisms colonizing their upper respiratory tract while they were still at home, and which cause pneumonia in the community. *Strep. pneumoniae* is the commonest bacterial cause of community-acquired lobar pneumonia, followed by *H. influenzae* or less commonly, *Moraxella catarrhalis*. All of these organisms can cause infective exacerbations of chronic obstructive pulmunory disease. In aspiration pneumonia, either community- or hospital-acquired, anaerobic bacteria are frequently involved as well.

When a patient has been in hospital for longer than 2–3 days, the incidence of Gram-negative pneumonia due to organisms such as enterobacteria and *Pseudomonas* increases greatly. Some of these Gram-negative pneumonias, especially in patients who have recently received broad-spectrum antibiotics, may be resistant to many antimicrobial agents. Knowledge of local resistance patterns is thus extremely helpful for rational empirical prescribing. The X-ray findings in an ICU patient who developed a post-operative Gram-negative pneumonia are shown in Figure 22.1.

Staphylococcus aureus is a rare cause of community-acquired pneumonia except during influenza outbreaks, and can sometimes cause pneumonia in postoperative patients. In this case many Gram-positive cocci in clusters and closely associated with pus cells should be visible in the Gram film of the sputum. *Staph. aureus* tends to cause a severe pneumonia which has been associated with the development of abscesses in the lungs. However, up to about 40% of the population carry *Staph. aureus* in their nares, and so may contaminate a sputum sample.

The presence of *Staph. aureus* in a sputum sample does not necessarily imply that the patient has *Staph. aureus* pneumonia. Pneumonia in severely immunocompromised patients can be caused by a wide variety of organisms, including Gram-positive cocci, Gram-negative rods, *Pneumocystis carinii* and *Aspergillus* spp., but this subject will not be dealt with further here.

22.6 MANAGEMENT

Prevention of postoperative respiratory tract infections is better than cure. Hence every attempt should be made to minimise the risks of a patient developing a respiratory tract infection following surgery. Smokers should be counselled to try and stop prior to an elective operation and smokers/anyone with chronic respiratory disease are likely to need both pre- and post-operative physiotherapy on their chests.

Ideally elective surgery on patients presenting to hospital with a viral/bacterial upper or lower respiratory tract infection should be postponed until the infection has resolved. If a patient with chronically infected sputum is having elective surgery or a patient with an acute chest infection requires emergency surgery they are likely to require antimicrobial treatment for this starting pre-operatively. Treatment (pending results of sputum microscopy and culture) should be as for a patient recently admitted to hospital (see Table 22.1). The possibility of the operation being performed under either local or spinal anaesthesia rather than a general anaesthetic should also be considered.

Full supportive therapy should be given to all patients with postoperative respiratory tract infections, in addition to appropriate antimicrobial therapy. Antimicrobial therapy will most likely need to be started before the aetiological agent causing the respiratory tract infection has been isolated. However, therapy should be modified according to the microbiological results obtained. Some initial treatment strategies are summarized in Table 22.1. Treatment will usually be for about 7–10 days, except in severe pneumonia and pneumonia in the immunocompromised patient for whom longer treatment may be required.

If a patient has only recently been admitted to hospital, a parenteral cephalosporin such as cefotaxime, ceftriaxone or cefuroxime that has good activity against *Strep. pneumoniae*, *H. influenzae* and *M. catarrhalis* (as well as many Gram-negative rods) is a reasonable choice of therapy. Ceftazidime has poor activity against *Strep. pneumoniae*, and should not be used at this stage. Oral or parenteral co-amoxyclav acid would be an alternative. If *Strep. pneumoniae* was thought to be the likely aetiological agent then oral or parenteral amoxycillin (or intravenous benzylpenicillin) could be given.

For sick 'ICU-type' patients who have already received broad-spectrum antimicrobials, an agent with good

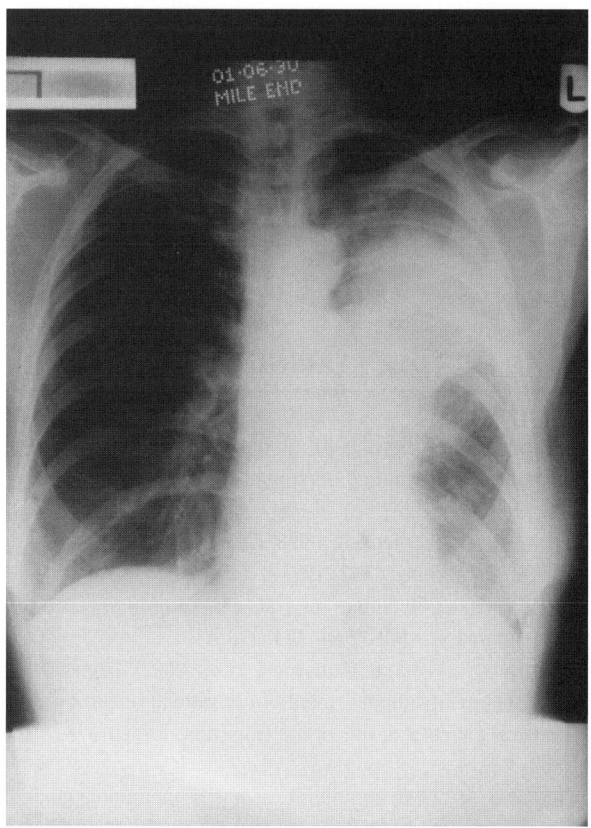

Figure 22.1 *X-ray of a patient with Gram-negative pneumonia*

Table 22.1 *Initial management of respiratory tract infections in postoperative patients*

Patient/infection	Suggested choices
Patient recently admitted to hospital	Cefotaxime/cefuroxime/ceftriaxone (i.v.) or co-amoxyclav (oral/i.v.)
Severe pneumonia in patient who has received antibiotics recently (pending sputum culture)	Piperacillin-tazobactam (i.v.) or Amoxycillin plus ciprofloxacin (oral/i.v.)
Severe pneumonia in a patient with Gram-negative rods seen in sputum/ tracheal secretions	Ceftazidine plus gentamicin (i.v.) or Piperacillin-tazobactam plus gentamicin (i.v.) or Imipenem/meropenem (i.v.)
Aspiration pneumonia	Co-amoxyclav plus gentamicin or Piperacillin-tazobactam plus gentamicin or Amoxycillin plus gentamicin plus metronidazole or cefuroxime plus metronidazole
Staphylococcal pneumonia: (a) thought not to be MRSA (b) MRSA thought to be possible	(a) Flucloxacillin plus gentamicin (b) Vancomycin or teicoplanin
Pneumonia of presumed viral aetiology	Seek specialist advice
Severely immunocompromised patient	Seek specialist advice

anti-Gram negative activity (including activity against *Pseudomonas* spp.) should be given empirically. If the aetiology of the infection is unknown and a sputum/endotracheal tube sample is not obtainable, broad-spectrum cover may be required, e.g. piperacillin-tazobactam (a ureidopenicillin + β-lactamase inhibitor) provides cover against streptococci, staphylococci, most Gram-negative rods including *Pseudomonas* spp. and anaerobes. This would also provide suitable cover if a seriously ill patient was thought to have a significant aspiration pneumonia. However, if the pneumonia is thought to be due to Gram-negative organisms, agents such as ceftazidime, a cephalosporin with anti-pseudomonal activity, together with an aminoglycoside could be used. Ciprofloxacin with an aminoglycoside would be a suitable alternative. Treatment of a presumptive staphylococcal pneumonia arising in hospital would depend on the local incidence of methicillin-resistant *Staph. aureus* (MRSA) in the unit. If it was thought that the pneumonia could be due to MRSA, then treatment with vancomycin or teicoplanin should be started pending susceptibility results. However, in units with an extremely low incidence of MRSA, the regimen should be an anti-staphylococcal penicillin such as flucloxacillin with an aminoglycoside.

Postoperative respiratory tract infections are a common cause of increased in-patient stay, increased morbidity and, occasionally, mortality in surgical patients. Prevention, although better than cure, is not always possible. Perioperative chemoprophylaxis is not recommended in the prevention of respiratory infection. However, early intervention is needed, and every attempt should be made to diagnose and treat these infections promptly in order to minimize risk to the patient.

22.7   FURTHER READING

British Thoracic Society. (2001) Guidelines for the management of community acquired pneumonia in adults. *Thorax*, **56** (suppl 4).

Brown, P.D. and Lerner, S.A. (1998) Community-acquired pneumonia. *Lancet*, **352**, 1295–1302.

Keeley, D. (2002) Guidelines for managing community acquired pneumonia in adults. *BMJ*, **324**, 436–437.

Montravers, P., Veber, B., Auboyer, C. *et al.* (2002) Diagnostic and therapeutic management of nosocomial pneumonia in surgical patients: results of the Eloe study. *Crit Care Med*, **30**, 368–375.

Woodhead, M. (1998) Community acquired pneumonia guidelines – an international comparison: a view from Europe. *Chest*, **113**, suppl. 183S–187S.

23

Infections of the gastrointestinal tract

J.D. WILLIAMS

23.1 BACKGROUND

The key feature of infection in the gastrointestinal system is exposure of the whole system to many different bacteria and other infective agents. These infective agents are either normally resident in different parts of the gastrointestinal tract, or are ingested with food and can attack the mucosa of the tract.

23.1.1 The resident microbial flora

The mouth has a rich flora of bacteria that are continually being swallowed, and these can be found in the oesophagus, stomach and upper small intestine. The organisms found in the oesophagus and stomach are a reflection of the oral flora, so that alteration in the oral flora – for example, after the administration of antibiotics – will lead to similar changes in the flora reaching the stomach.

The commonest species reaching the stomach are viridans streptococci, most of which are non-pathogenic, coagulase-negative staphylococci and anaerobic bacteria such as *Prevotella*, *Bacteroides* and anaerobic streptococci. *Candida albicans* is a minor component of the oral flora, but this increases in ill and elderly patients (particularly following antibiotic therapy) and may reach the stomach in large numbers. Similarly, Gram-negative aerobic bacteria associated with the lower gastrointestinal tract such as enterobacteria and *Pseudomonas* may be present in the oral flora of the ill, the elderly or those receiving antibiotic therapy.

The number of bacteria surviving in the stomach is reduced by the acidity of the gastric secretions, so that in normal persons the number entering the small intestine is low. The protective effect of acidity is of course less effective in achlorhydria. This must be remembered when patients have undergone medical or surgical therapy to reduce acid secretion for the treatment of duodenal ulcer. The microbial flora of the small intestine is also influenced by bacteria in the colon. With obstructive lesions of the lower intestine, retrograde colonization of the small intestine by enterobacteriaceae and anaerobic bacteria occurs.

The colon contains the greatest concentrations of bacteria to be found in the body. The two major classes are enterobacteria (*Escherichia coli*, *Klebsiella* and other related species) and anaerobes (streptococci, *Bacteroides*, *Prevotella*), and these are supplemented by a wide variety of other species such as clostridia, corynebacteria and enterococci. The number of bacteria approach 10^{10} cells per gram of intestinal contents. Once a patient enters hospital, the bacterial flora can change, such changes being greatly influenced by the administration of antibiotics and by the prevalence of Gram-negative bacteria in the hospital environment and in food.

23.1.2 The ingested bacteria

Large numbers of bacteria are ingested daily in food. The majority of these organisms are non-pathogenic and cause no concern. Of pathogenic potential are firstly the food poisoning organisms such as *Salmonella*, *Shigella* and *Campylobacter*; and secondly, for patients in hospital, multi-resistant Gram-negative bacteria such as *Pseudomonas*, *Enterobacter* and related species. The food-poisoning organisms frequently give rise to symptoms, while the multi-resistant hospital bacteria usually give rise to asymptomatic colonization of the gastrointestinal tract.

23.1.3 The impact of resident bacteria on surgery of the gastrointestinal tract

It is inevitable that the normal flora of the gastrointestinal tract will contaminate any operative site that is exposed to its contents. The type of bacteria to which these patients' tissues are exposed will vary with the site of the operation, the condition of the patient, and where the patient has been before the procedure. Under normal conditions the contents will consist mainly of antibiotic-susceptible Gram-negative bacteria and anaerobes. The changes brought about by illness, antibiotic therapy and hospital stay can be profound, and may influence decisions by the surgeons – particularly on choice of chemoprophylaxis.

Operations on the gastrointestinal tract are also open to extraneous organisms such as *Staphylococcus aureus* that can affect all surgical procedures, and contamination of invasive instruments by *Pseudomonas* and related species. These organisms pose fewer problems than those presented by the size and variability of the resident flora in the gastrointestinal tract. Recently, the specific problem of surgical instruments contaminated by HIV has been highlighted.

23.2 CHEMOPROPHYLAXIS

23.2.1 General principles

Most of the useful concepts of chemoprophylaxis are very well established, and the practice is widespread. Many people are, however, worried about antibiotic resistance developing – perhaps as a result of chemoprophylaxis. There is also concern that chemoprophylaxis may be limited or altered due to the high prevalence of resistance. Although we know when, why and how to use chemoprophylaxis, it can be quite difficult to convince surgeons who use antibiotics both therapeutically and chemoprophylactically to adhere to the well-established principles when the fear of antibiotic resistance is so strong. The Scandinavians have been quite successful at maintaining resistance at a low level in their countries, and part of this success is due to the careful use of antibiotics.

23.2.2 The effectiveness of chemoprophylaxis

Chemoprophylaxis is essential for many invasive procedures in surgery. The absence of chemoprophylaxis when it is clearly indicated often results in infection. Because trials of chemoprophylaxis comparing antibiotics with placebo have not been conducted in recent years, it is necessary to go back to data obtained from the early 1970s to illustrate the effectiveness of chemoprophylaxis. Studies at that time showed that elective surgery on the lower gastrointestinal tract without chemoprophylaxis resulted in infection in about one-third of cases, whereas appropriate short-term chemoprophylaxis with the correct agents reduced this rate to about 5%.

A study by Pollock and Evans showed that chemoprophylaxis reduced the postoperative infection rate from 25% to 12% in 'contaminated' surgery. Patients in one group received oral antibiotics, to 'decontaminate' the bowel, while the other group received parenteral cephaloridine during the time of the operation. Primary infection rates show a significant difference. Of the 249 patients who went through contaminated surgery, 25% of those who had bowel preparation had infective complications, but only 8% who received a single dose of cephaloridine became infected.

Their figures for secondary infection rates (which concern infections arising later, and which are probably due to infection acquired in the ward) were almost identical in clean or contaminated surgery with or without chemoprophylaxis. Therefore adequate perioperative chemoprophylaxis protects from infection acquired in the operating theatre, but has no effect on ward-acquired infection. Many other studies have confirmed the usefulness of chemoprophylaxis in perioperative infections, and several different classes of antibiotic have been used with similar outcomes. For colorectal operations (a high-risk group for perioperative infections), chemoprophylaxis should be active against both Gram-positive and Gram-negative bacteria; metronidazole is usually the antibiotic of choice against Gram-negative anaerobes.

23.2.3 Is chemoprophylaxis necessary?

Chemoprophylaxis does contribute to the increasing antibiotic resistance in bacteria. Although it is sometimes difficult to distinguish between therapeutic and chemoprophylactic use, about half of all prescriptions for antibiotics in hospitals are used for chemoprophylaxis. Thus, it is implied that chemoprophylaxis is making significant contributions to antibiotic resistance. A second argument against chemoprophylaxis is that it needs frequent review to take account of resistant bacteria in the hospital environment, and therefore to keep changing the antibiotics. The cost and side effects of chemoprophylaxis are mentioned at times as negative points. However, the validity of all the above arguments are somewhat suspect. In chemoprophylaxis, only a small number of pathogens, staphylococci in the nose or skin is being exposed to the antibiotic. On the other hand, when treating a lesion that has millions of pathogenic bacteria, the antibiotic is exposed to those teeming organisms which encourages the chances for more resistance.

Furthermore, chemoprophylaxis is only given for a very short period of time compared with therapeutic courses. Some patients receive many antibiotics both for treatment and chemoprophylaxis, e.g. in transplant surgery for neutropenia, diabetes, neurosurgery and other forms of clean surgery and, in some instances, it is not necessary. In the intensive care unit, antibiotics are used on catheterized patients to prevent urinary tract infections and on tracheostomy and unconscious patients to prevent respiratory tract infections. Such use rarely prevents infection, however. Surgeons and other medical staff must consider whether such patients should be given broad-spectrum chemoprophylaxis to prevent infections. Many trials have shown that the effects of chemoprophylaxis during the early days are excellent, but after this the problems of the patient are multiplied by resistant organisms. Therefore, ad-hoc speculative use of antibiotics on patients without infections who might possibly become infected must be decreased.

23.2.4 Sources of organisms

Organisms can be contracted from the surgical team and operating procedures, from the hospital environment and ward procedures, from other patients in the hospital, and most importantly from the patient's own microbial flora.

Chemoprophylaxis should not be used against most of these risks. The transmission of infection can be prevented by other methods. Organisms from the surgical team and surgical materials are not a target for chemoprophylaxis. The use of aseptic techniques such as gloves, gowns and masks are the correct alternatives to chemoprophylaxis. Organisms from the hospital environment and ward materials and procedures can be dealt with by disinfection of the operating environment. Patients with dangerous bacteria from other wards should not be mixed with those awaiting an operation. However, because of inadequate control of infection procedures, chemoprophylaxis is sometimes used to cover up defects in hospital hygiene, staff discipline and faults in technique.

Two examples are given to illustrate the misapplication of chemoprophylaxis. A patient may contract septicaemia, usually with *Pseudomonas*, following endoscopy

of the biliary tract. This organism has not originated from the patient's own biliary tract, but from a contaminated endoscope. It is better to disinfect the endoscope to render it free from *Pseudomonas* than to give the patient a course of ceftazidime. For minor surgical procedures, some surgeons use chemoprophylaxis to reduce the incidence of infection rather than pay strict attention to aseptic precautions.

Most organisms infecting surgical wounds come from the patient's own bacterial flora. The main aim of chemoprophylaxis should be to control these organisms – not to eradicate them, but merely to kill those arriving at the operation site. The organisms vary from one patient to another, but many different species of bacteria are present in the bowel, on the skin and in the mouth. Coagulase-negative staphylococci are present in every surgical operation because the organisms are always on the skin. *Staphylococcus aureus* (penicillin-resistant but susceptible to other antibiotics) can be found in the nose, hand and/or skin of 30% of patients. Clostridia, including *Clostridium perfringens* can often be found in the perineal and groin areas, particularly in elderly patients. *E. coli*, *Proteus mirabilis*, enterococci, viridans streptococci, anaerobic streptococci and Gram-negative anaerobes are present in large numbers in the gastrointestinal tract. Provided that the bacteria remain in their own essential ecological niche, they do no harm; only those spilling into sterile tissues require control, and this is best achieved by having a high concentration of antibiotic in the tissue at the time they are incised. This is achieved to best effect by an in-theatre intravenous high dose of the appropriate antibiotic(s) prior to the start of the operation; for a lengthy procedure a further dose can be given after 4 hours (see later).

23.2.5 Hospital organisms, the patient and surgery

Patients in hospital waiting for surgery are exposed to colonisation by hospital bacteria. From the surgical team, nurses and other health care attendants and from other patients they may acquire coagulase-negative staphylococci or *Staph. Aureus* colonising the skin.

From the hospital environment and ward procedures, organisms can colonize patients or cause, for example, infection by multi-resistant *Staph. aureus*, *Klebsiella*, *Enterobacter*, *Serratia*, *Pseudomonas* species and enterococci. Patients who have stayed in hospital for a long period of time, who have had multiple operations, or have had an operation after a long illness, could be exposed to a wide range of multi-resistant species. Chemoprophylaxis is not considered to be an appropriate method of prevention of hospital-acquired colonization or infections, but if it becomes necessary to carry out a subsequent surgical procedure, the chemoprophylactic regimen may have to be modified from that used in patients admitted for surgery directly from home.

23.2.6 Sources of organisms in abdominal surgery

There are three sources of microbiological problems in abdominal surgery. The first source is the patient's endogenous flora, which needs to be considered for almost every patient undergoing such surgery. The main bacteria are the antibiotic-sensitive coliforms such as *E. coli* and *Pr. mirabillis*, antibiotic-sensitive coagulase-negative staphylococci and penicillin-resistant *Staph. aureus*. Anaerobic cocci, *Bacteroides*, respiratory bacteria such as pneumococci and *Haemophilus*, *Candida albicans* and enterococci are also endogenous to the patient.

Secondly, there are the exogenous hospital bacteria that can colonize a patient so heavily as to become an endogenous source. Antibiotic-resistant coagulase-negative staphylococci become colonists of the skin of patients by being transferred from the contaminated hands of nurses and other ward staff. It takes only about 2 days for a patient in hospital to become colonized with coagulase-negative staphylococci. Antibiotic-resistant Gram-negative rods such as *Serratia* and *Pseudomonas*, may take up to 7 days to become colonizers of the respiratory or gastrointestinal tracts. With antibiotic-resistant *Staph. aureus*, the period of a patient's stay in hospital before colonization is variable, and depends on the prevalence of staphylococci in the unit.

Finally, there is the exogenous *Staph. aureus* from the surgical team and from the air expired by other patients. Because of its ubiquity, *Staph. aureus* remains overall the most common organism causing hospital infection.

23.2.7 When and how to employ chemoprophylaxis

Various types of misuse can arise in perioperative chemoprophylaxis. Chemoprophylaxis may be used when not necessary, or omitted when it is necessary, but this is unusual. **Selection of the wrong agent** for chemoprophylaxis is more common. The **timing** of chemoprophylaxis is often wrong and most important of all, the **duration** of chemoprophylaxis may be incorrect and antibiotics given for too long a period of time.

THE CHOICE OF AGENT

In most patients, common simple antibiotics (which are usually cheap) are all that is necessary. Most surgical procedures are elective, and patients are admitted to hospital shortly before surgery. In an emergency situation the operation is carried out shortly after the patient is admitted. Therefore, the organisms causing contamination of the wound are not multi-resistant hospital pathogens but are those present in the community. Although antibiotic resistance is increasing in the community, most organisms are still sensitive to the most commonly used antibiotics. Antibiotic-susceptible coliforms, staphylococci and anaerobic bacteria can be found in the patient's own microbial flora. Anaerobic bacteria are present on oral mucosa, sinuses and periodontal area and in the gastrointestinal tract, with high levels from the jejunum onwards. The female genital tract also harbours high levels of anaerobic bacteria from the cervix outwards, and these can spread to the skin, particularly in the axillae, buttocks, groin and other areas. All of these areas require specific chemoprophylaxis against anaerobes. Penicillins or cephalosporins alone cannot be relied upon when dealing with anaerobic bacteria.

Co-amoxyclav (or ampicillin/sulbactam), gentaicin, metronidazole, and anti-staphylococcal penicillins are the mainstay of chemoprophylaxis, and new antibiotics need not be used. Unfortunately, chemoprophylaxis users often pay great attention to the arrival of new antibiotics and use them for chemoprophylaxis because they believe that the new agents are more effective than the old ones. The indications for use of new broad-spectrum antibiotics are patients having multiple operations and/or spending time in hospital for long periods before operation. For the majority of patients amoxycillin should be used instead of imipenem, cefazolin instead of cefotaxime, and flucloxacillin instead of vancomycin.

TIMING OF CHEMOPROPHYLAXIS

In order to ensure the antibiotic level in the tissue is highest within the desired time frame, the start of chemoprophylaxis is by the parenteral route about 30 minutes before surgery begins. If started too soon, the antibiotic concentration may fall to low levels and resistant bacteria may emerge. If started too late, the wound may be contaminated with bacteria and no antibiotic is present in the tissues to kill them.

DURATION OF PROPHYLAXIS

The main problems with chemoprophylaxis is that the duration of therapy employed is too long. For most operations, only one dose is necessary, though in operations longer than 4 hours, the antibiotic level starts to fall and a second dose may be needed. Current practice that extends antibiotic therapy for several days precipitates all the evils of chemoprophylaxis. The selection of resistant organisms in the hospital environment and replacement of the patient's normal antibiotic-susceptible flora by resistant bacteria are some inevitable consequences of prolonged use of antibiotics. The duration of use must be kept to a minimum, not only because resistant bacteria are being selected, but because side effects occur due to antibiotics being used for too long. The side effects of antimicrobial agents include hypersensitivity, diminished renal function, immunomodulation, and bone marrow suppression, all of which lead to a poor prognosis for the postoperative patient.

The rising prevalence of resistant bacteria in hospitals is due to the acquisition of resistant genes and the subsequent spread of these clones. With one injection of antibiotic there is little or no acquisition of new genes, of mutation of genes to resistance, or of selection of resistant variants. However, even with a single dose of antibiotic, it is inevitable that there is some selection of pre-existing naturally resistant strains, and this occurs with almost all antibiotics. Macrolides affect the mouth flora, β-lactams affect the gut, and aminoglycosides affect bacteria on the skin – allowing selection of resistant strains. The effect of a single dose of chemoprophylaxis has almost no effects for the spread of resistant clones. The production of resistant variants is the normal response of pathogens which are exposed to antibiotics. All organisms do this, and all antimicrobials select resistant variants to a greater or lesser extent. Moreover, the normal flora of humans is very rich in species of which some are naturally resistant to antibiotics. All antimicrobials destroy some of the normal flora, allowing naturally resistant species to overgrow. If an infection does arise after an operation where prolonged use of chemoprophylaxis has occurred, it is likely to be with resistant organisms which have survived chemoprophylaxis. By keeping the chemoprophylaxis to a minimum, the least effect is displayed upon the normal flora.

ANTIBIOTIC COMBINATIONS IN CHEMOPROPHYLAXIS

Because contamination of the operation site is possible by both aerobes and anaerobes, each of the following combinations of antibiotics has been used for chemoprophylaxis of polymicrobial infections of the gastrointestinal tract or the female genital tract. All of them are effective, the range of satisfactory options for gastrointestinal infections being especially wide. However, it is clearly better to use amoxycillin-clavulanate than imipenem for surgical prophylaxis in the vast majority of procedures:

- ampicillin-gentamicin-metronidazole
- ampicillin-metronidazole
- cefuroxime-metronidazole
- piperacillin-metronidazole
- piperacillin-tazobactam
- gentamicin-clindamycin
- amoxicillin-clavulanic acid

- ampicillin-sulbactam
- imipenem-cilastatin.

23.3 INFECTIONS OF THE GASTROINTESTINAL TRACT

23.3.1 The oesophagus

The oesophagus has good resistance to the bacteria that pass continually through it en route to the stomach.

Candida albicans and occasionally non-*albicans Candida* can cause severe oesophagitis in patients with oral candidiasis. These are mainly seen in patients with immunocompromised states, such as AIDS, or in those severely ill patients who have received extensive antibiotic therapy. Treatment with anti-*Candida* drugs such as fluconazole or amphotericin B is usually necessary.

Carcinoma or **penetrating injuries** of the oesophagus may cause leakage of pathogenic bacteria into the mediastinal tissues and give rise to infections. The causative organisms are difficult to determine, but they will be reflected in the oral flora. With normal oral flora for example, in a healthy person with a perforating injury, the organisms are of low pathogenicity, i.e. viridans streptococci, coagulase-negative staphylococci and anaerobes. Antibiotic therapy could be confined in such cases to combined amoxycillin-clavulanic acid or ampicillin-sulbactam. In a hospital patient with malignant disease, the mouth flora can contain multi-resistant Gram-negative bacteria, and antibiotics such as piperacillin-tazobactam would be more appropriate. Underlying the regimen however, is the possibility of candidal infections either from the start or subsequent to antibiotic therapy, and such infection should be considered if there is *Candida* in the mouth and clinical signs of infection persist, in which case systemic anti-candidal preparations should be prescribed.

23.3.2 The stomach

HELICOBACTER PYLORI INFECTION

The most important infection of the stomach is with *Helicobacter pylori*. Much information has been published since the first description of this bacterium and its association with gastritis and peptic ulceration, and conferences are held regularly with the latest findings on epidemiology, pathogenesis, diagnosis and treatment of the condition. Over the course of the past 10 years these diseases have been transformed from one amenable only to surgical intervention to one treated mainly by acid secretory inhibitors and antibiotics. Only a brief outline is given here.

H. pylori is a small, curved Gram-negative bacterium which can resist gastric acid and colonizes the gut mucosa.

It produces ammonia by way of the enzyme urease, which protects the organism against the killing effects of gastric hydrochloric acid (by neutralizing it to NH_4Cl).

Many different practitioners are now involved in management of patients with proven or suspected *H. pylori* infection, including general practitioners, gastroenterologists, general physicians as well as the surgeon. Eradication of the organism appears to be the main objective of most doctors handling these patients, although sometimes the symptoms are not greatly improved and efforts to define more precisely the relation of the organism to symptomology continue. The surgeon still has to deal with the more complicated peptic ulcers and gastric cancer.

Eradication of *H. pylori*

After many trials of antibiotics combined with antacids of various types, there is some consensus over the types of regimen that will eradicate the organism. The general agreement is that 2 weeks' treatment is needed with two antibiotics and one proton-pump inhibitor. Eradication rates of 80–90% are reported, but this still leaves many patients requiring a change of therapy. The appearance of resistance of *Helicobacter* to some antibiotics is a cause of concern, and adjustments in eradication regimens will be needed from time to time.

Surgical intervention in patients with *H. pylori* infection may be necessary in peptic ulcer complicated by stricture or perforation. Surgeons also have patients who were operated on for peptic ulcer disease before *H. pylori* attained prominence. The eradication of *H. pylori* is still necessary in such cases. Persistence of *H. pylori* is very high in patients who had undergone vagotomy only, and fairly high in those who had partial gastrectomy. It is also reported that not all patients with recurrent ulcer still have *H. pylori* infection. Also under debate is whether or not operated patients are in danger of developing gastric cancer because of persistent *H. pylori* colonization. It appears reasonable to try to eradicate these organisms from the stomach, and the following treatment regimens are suggested:

- Omeprazole, 20 mg once daily
- Clarithromycin, 250 mg twice daily
- Tinidazole, 500 mg twice daily for 7 days

As an alternative, tinidazole may be replaced by ampicillin 750 mg three times daily for 10 days, and several other combinations.

INFECTION FOLLOWING GASTRIC SURGERY

Peritonitis

Peritonitis may follow leakage of gastric contents into the peritoneum (i.e. perforation) before or during gastric surgery. The bacteria contaminating the peritoneum will be those present in the normal flora as stated above, together with any additional harmful bacteria that have replaced the oral flora while the patient was in hospital awaiting surgery. With a short wait (i.e. up to 48 hours) before surgery in a patient not receiving antibiotics, the normal flora will be antibiotic-susceptible and contain anaerobes, and co-amoxyclav acid or ampicillin-sulbactam should be effective in these cases. Alternatives for therapy are listed above, together with alternatives for patients at higher risk. Patients who have the normal gastrointestinal flora replaced by hospital bacteria require more broad-spectrum antibiotic prophylaxis.

The risk of *Candida* infection should always be borne in mind in patients who do not respond fully to antibiotic therapy but persist with fever and symptoms. Culture of relevant specimens (blood, fistulae, drainage) may confirm the clinical suspicion of *Candida* and so guide therapy.

Postoperative surgical wound infection

As in all postoperative surgical wound infections, *Staph. aureus* is the commonest primary pathogen. These organisms are introduced into the wound from the skin of the patient, the surgeon, or the surgical team. Improvement in hospital and theatre practice has reduced such infections to relatively low levels. Infected wounds and stitch abscess would most likely be staphylococci in origin, and anti-staphylococci therapy is essential.

Organisms from the stomach which contaminate the wound may also be responsible for postoperative wound infection. Infection with these organisms is more insidious than staphylococcal infection in that they are of less abrupt onset and, if anaerobic, likely to be persistent and chronic. Indeed, they may even arise after the patient has left the hospital. There is controversy over whether chemoprophylaxis is indicated for operations on the stomach and oesophagus, or not. If chemoprophylaxis is to be employed it should be directed against the potential endogenous flora in the stomach or oesophagus, i.e. streptococci and anaerobes. Chemoprophylaxis against staphylococci is not required because the normal aseptic procedures should be sufficient to prevent extraneous transfer of staphylococci to the surgical wound.

STAPHYLOCOCCAL FOOD POISONING

The main symptom of staphylococcal food poisoning is vomiting. Most cases are short-lived and do not come to the doctor's attention; however, staphylococci can give rise to violent, persistent and debilitating vomiting for 24–48 hours, leading to admission to hospital. There, it should be differentiated from other forms of persistent vomiting that lead to dehydration.

The symptoms are caused by ingestion of staphylococcal toxins in food contaminated by staphylococci, in which the organisms have grown and in which poisonous levels of toxins have accumulated. The onset of vomiting and the severity depends on the amount of toxins ingested, and vomiting usually starts within 3–4 hours. Many types of food can be involved; sweet dishes containing cream are common, but meat dishes and pies may also be responsible. Vomiting is preceded by upper abdominal pain, and the vomiting may be forcible. Episodes may continue at 15 to 30-minute intervals until the effects of the toxin wear off. The nature of the vomitus after the first episode is watery, rusty coloured or bile-stained, and quite large amounts of fluid can be lost. Even after 24–48 hours however, the vomitus is not faecal, and normal bowel movements may occur. Although some viable staphylococci may have been ingested, the symptoms are due to the pre-formed toxin, and antibiotic therapy is not considered to contribute to resolution of the symptoms.

If other forms of persistent vomiting have been excluded, oral rehydration with isotonic salt solutions are required; intravenous therapy is seldom needed.

23.3.3 The small intestine

CROHN'S DISEASE

An infective aetiology (*Mycobacterium paratuberculosis*) of Crohn's disease has been proposed on several occasions. The problem is that several other aetiologies have also been suggested (e.g. genetic predisposition or focal ischaemia). The disease poses two problems for the surgeon: first, the aetiology of the disease itself; and second, the infective complications arising from the surgical interventions that may be necessary for treatment.

Aetiology

If the aetiology is due to a bacterium, questions arise over the prevention and antimicrobial treatment of the disease. Johnes bacillus is *Mycobacterium paratuberculosis*, a slow-growing mycobacterium which is responsible for an eponymous wasting disease in cattle and which has some pathological and histological similarities to Crohn's disease. This organism has been found in cows' milk, and is not totally eliminated in the milk by standard pasteurization. Experimental evidence suggests that the organism may be implicated in some cases of Crohn's disease, and eradication of the organism may help to ameliorate the disease. This is still controversial however, and steps have not been taken to prolong the normal pasteurization process for treating milk. Nor has it been possible to agree on a standardized therapy for eradication of the organism.

Treatment of complications

Crohn's disease may be complicated by obstruction (stricture), perforation or abdominal pain related to inflammation. Because Crohn's disease may occur at sites other than the small intestine, the organisms responsible for disease-related infection vary, but in most cases the Gram-negative aerobic flora and anaer-

obes are prominent and are the main target for treatment and perioperative chemoprophylaxis. Although surgery is only undertaken for the most pressing of reasons, repeated surgical intervention for recurrent disease may be needed in some patients, and antibiotic therapy should be tailored to meet the varying needs of such patients – some of whom may have had the normal resident flora widely affected by prior antibiotic therapy. In these cases the microbial aetiology of infection may include *Pseudomonas*, multi-resistant enterobacteria, enterococci and *Candida*. Microbiological cultures are necessary to guide therapy. Peri-anal abscess and fistulae are common in Crohn's disease, in which faecal organisms predominate and for which combination therapy against aerobic and anaerobic bacteria may be indicated.

ABDOMINAL TUBERCULOSIS

Although decreasing in incidence, abdominal tuberculosis still occurs and, unless obstructive lesions arise, is best treated by anti-tuberculous therapy alone. Risk factors for the development of the disease include sex and ethnic origin. In the UK, the young Asian female with abdominal pain is a possible candidate for the disease, and investigations such as the Mantoux test, sedimentation rate and imaging can help to reach the diagnosis without surgical intervention.

WHIPPLES' DISEASE

One of the main symptoms of Whipples' disease is weight loss with chronic diarrhoea and steatorrhoea. These signs are preceded by intermittent joint pain, and patients also have neurological effects such as cranial nerve paralysis. Diagnosis can be made by small intestine biopsy showing enteritis with Periodic acid–Schiff-positive macrophages. The causative agent, *Trophyrema whippelii*, cannot be grown but may be visualized by electron microscopy or detected by polymerase chain reaction analysis.

Treatment is with antibiotics. Several combinations have been used of which demeclocycline combined with either chloramphenicol or ampicillin for 2 months has been most useful.

INFECTIVE DIARRHOEAL DISEASE

Diarrhoea due to food-borne bacteria is common. Most cases (estimated at 80% of occurrences) are not seen by the doctors because the symptoms are relatively mild and self-limiting. About 20% are seen by the general practitioners, and of these a small proportion may reach hospital with abdominal pain as the primary symptom and with diarrhoea less prominent. Such cases may be confused with conditions requiring surgical intervention, such as appendicitis and diverticulitis.

Such differentiation can only be reached on clinical grounds but avoidable interventions are carried out in a small proportion of cases. Nevertheless, the number of cases of food poisoning with *Salmonella* and *Campylobacter* is large, and a significant number present as possible surgical emergencies.

Salmonella and Campylobacter infections

These infections are characterized by watery diarrhoea and abdominal pain, mostly central. Some cases of *Campylobacter* infection may have bloody diarrhoea, but the symptoms are otherwise similar to mild *Salmonella* infection. Both diseases are self-limiting and do not usually require antibiotics. Should patients show evidence of invasive disease, such as high fever or positive blood cultures, a fluoroquinolone such as ciprofloxacin should be given for *Salmonella*, and a macrolide such as erythromycin, for *Campylobacter*.

Typhoid fever

Salmonella typhi and related species such as *S. paratyphi* produce enteric fever, not diarrhoeal disease. After ingestion, the organisms establish themselves in the Peyer's patches of the ileum and spread to other mononuclear cells notably in the liver, spleen and bone marrow. Typhoid fever is a septicaemic condition, and the blood culture is usually positive, the presenting symptoms being fever and abdominal pain. The patient may have a slight looseness of the stool but constipation is equally common. Thus, enteric fever may be present as an acute surgical condition. Diagnostic features include a higher fever than is usual in acute abdomen and a low white blood cell count. Sometimes a sparse rash (rose spots) may be seen. The spleen may be palpable. *S. typhi* is endemic in some parts of the developing world, and most cases in developed countries are contracted abroad; therefore a travel history is essential. The incubation period after ingestion to fever is about 10–21 days.

A definitive diagnosis is made by isolation of *S. typhi* from the blood or bone marrow. The urine may yield *S. typhi*, and a stool specimen (if obtainable) should usually be positive. If typhoid fever is suspected the patient should be transferred to isolation with faeces and blood precautions. Screening of contacts is unnecessary.

Surgical intervention is rarely needed, and then only for severe complications such as haemorrhage from the mucosa or perforation of the intestine.

There are several antibiotics currently in use. Although antibiotic resistance is a recurring problem, the following regimens are widely used: chloramphenicol 2 g daily in four divided doses; ceftriaxone 4 g once daily intravenously for 5 days; and ciprofloxacin or oflaxacin 500 mg twice daily for 7 days. Other alternatives are also available.

After recovery, some patients may become chronic carriers of *S. typhi* with a focus of infection in the gallbladder.

23.3.4 The large intestine

SHIGELLOSIS

Shigellosis is not usually confused with abdominal emergencies because the symptoms all refer to the lowest part of the gastrointestinal tract, i.e. tenesmus, frequent low volume stools with macroscopic blood and mucus prominent.

ESCHERICHIA COLI

Some strains of *E. coli* can cause severe haemorrhagic colitis complicated by haemolytic anaemia and uraemia – (the haemolytic uraemic syndrome, HUS). Such patients require rapid supportive specialist therapy.

ANTIBIOTIC-ASSOCIATED DIARRHOEA/ PSEUDOMEMBRANOUS COLITIS

Antibiotics can cause diarrhoea in several ways. First, they may have a specific pharmacological effect on motility; macrolides such as erythromycin stimulate the motilin receptors in the gut to increase peristaltic action, thus producing abdominal pain and hyperactive bowel movements. Other antibiotics may affect the composition of the bowel flora. In particular, β-lactam drugs can cause a marked reduction in the aerobic bowel flora and allow overgrowth of the other organisms. More severe diarrhoea occurs as a result of overgrowth of *Clostridium difficile*, causing an acute pseudomembranous colitis with bloody diarrhoea and inflammatory infiltration of the mucosa of the large intestine. The pathological effects are due to toxins produced by *Cl. difficile*, which are cytotoxic in action. Some antibiotics such as clindamycin and ampicillin have been associated specifically with this condition, but they are not the only antibiotics which may be responsible. The presence of the toxin-producing organisms is the key precipitating factor.

Cl. difficile is an unusual organism in the bowel flora of adults. Outbreaks of pseudomembranous colitis due to this organism occur in surgical wards of hospitals. Stopping transmission of the organism between patients in the ward is necessary to bring an outbreak to an end. Because the organism is spore-forming and may survive in the environment, the isolation of patients and scrupulous attention to hygiene is essential, as well as curtailing antibiotic use. The organism is susceptible to metronidazole, (400 mg three times daily for 10 days), and this is the first line of antibiotic therapy. Failure to respond to metronidazole may require the administration of oral vancomycin (125 mg four times daily for 10 days), the use of oral vancomycin should be avoided if possible because vancomycin-resistant enterococci are of current concern in hospital-acquired infection and care must be taken not to select out these organisms.

Some patients with pseudomembranous colitis may suffer severe damage to the colon and require extensive surgery.

PARASITIC INFECTIONS

Amoebic dysentery

Bacillary dysentery has been referred to above. Similar symptoms of tenesmus and bloody diarrhoea may occur with amoebae, in particular *Entamoeba histolytica*. Such cases are contracted from faeces-contaminated water supplies, and the onset of illness due to amoebae may occur several weeks after acquiring the organism. If the history suggests that the patient has acquired amoebic dysentery, the diagnosis is best made by examining a very fresh stool under the microscope. The free-living amoebae are very easy to see as they move quite quickly across the microscope field. The encysted forms are more difficult to identify as they are non-motile and can be confused with other non-pathological amoebae found in the gut. In many cases, specific antibodies against amoebae are present in the blood and should be sought in specialist laboratories. Treatment of chronic amoebiasis or acute amoebic dysentery are the same, and are based on metronidazole (750 mg three times daily for 10 days). As alternatives, the use of either tinidazole (2 g daily for 2–3 days) or paramomycin (25 mg kg^{-1} in three doses for 7 days) is recommended.

Amoebic liver abscess

Liver abscess due to *E. histolytica* can follow a stay in an endemic area, and may not have been preceded by a significant episode of diarrhoea. The onset is fairly acute with fever and perhaps liver tenderness. The abscess may rupture and cause peritonitis. Imaging of the liver is the most useful investigation, and serological tests may be confirmative of amoebiasis. Medical treatment is effective and surgical intervention rarely required. Antibiotic treatment is with metronidazole (750 mg three times daily for 10 days) followed by dilanoxide furoate (500 mg three times daily for 10 days). Alternative treatment is with tinidazole (2 g daily for 2–3 days).

Giardiasis

Diarrhoea and other non-specific gastrointestinal symptoms may be due to *Giardia lamblia*. Usually acquired from faulty water supplies (more commonly in Eastern Europe), the organism is a flagellate and also readily recognized in the motile form. The encysted forms can be numerous, but on occasion are not excreted from sites of infection high in the small intestines. A jejunal biopsy may be required for diagnosis.

Diarrhoea and abdominal cramps follow, 7–14 days after ingestion of the cysts. If the infection is prolonged, *Giardia* antigen may be detected in faeces by ELISA. Biopsy of the small intestine shows villous atrophy, and the parasite may be found either in the biopsy or in the duodenal aspirate.

Treatment of amoebiasis and giardiasis can be made with a variety of anti-protozoal drugs, of which the most widely used is metronidazole 400 mg three times daily for 5 days, with the alternative of Mepacrine 100 mg three times daily for 7 days.

23.4   WORM INFESTATIONS

Few worms can cause infestation in temperate zones, but because of the chronicity of many infestations many more varieties can be acquired in tropical areas and may be encountered worldwide in patients who travel extensively.

The worms encountered in temperate zones are *Ascaris lumbricoides*, threadworms and tapeworms. Worm eggs are frequently encountered in the stools of patients presenting with unrelated disease and who have lived in tropical countries. The species most commonly seen include *Trichuris trichura*. Infestations with these organisms may produce little obvious disease, but they are probably best eradicated.

Other parasites do produce more debilitating effects, however. *Ankylostoma* can cause severe anaemia when present in large numbers.

The treatment of worm infestations is often very specialized, and reference should be made to texts that provide the necessary information, of which books on Tropical Medicine are the prime source. Many such patients require referral for specialist treatment.

23.5   FURTHER READING

Anand, A., Bashey, B., Mir, T. and Glatt A.E. (1999) Epidemiology, clinical manifestations and outcome of *Clostridium difficile* associated diarrhoea. *American Journal of Gastroenterology*, **89**, 519–523.

Gyssens, I.C. (1999) Preventing post-operative infections: current treatment recommendations. *Drugs*, **57**(2), 175–185.

Jobe, B.A., Gradey, A., Deveney, K.E., Deveney, C.W., and Sheppard, B.C. (1995) *Clostridium difficile* colitis; an increasing hospital-acquired illness. *American Journal of Surgery*, **169**, 480–483.

Mangram A.J., Horan, T.C., Pearson, M.L., *et al.* (1999) Guidelines for prevention of surgical site infection. Centre for Disease Control and Prevention. Hospital Infection Control Advisory Practices Advisory Committee. *American Journal of Infection Control*, **27**, 97–132.

Platell, C. and Hall, J.C. (2001) The prevention of wound infection inpatients undergoing colo-rectal surgery. *Journal of Hospital Infection*, **49**, 233–238.

Samore, M.H. (1999) Epidemiology of nosocomial clostridium difficile diarrhoea. *Journal of Hospital Infection*, **43**, S183–190.

Schilling, J., Michalopoulos, A., and Gerulanos, S. (1997) Antibiotic prophylaxis in gastroduodenal surgery. *Hepato-Gastroenterology*, **44**, 116–120.

Song, F. and Glenny, A.M. (1998) Antimicrobial prophylaxis in colo-rectal surgery: a systematic review of rendomised controlled trials. *Health Technology Association*, **2**, 1–110.

Wittman, D.H. (1998) Operative and non-operative therapy of intra-abdominal infections. *Infection*, **26**, 335–341.

24

Antibiotic prophylaxis in laparoscopic surgery

M.E.R. WILLIAMSON AND N.S. AMBROSE

24.1 INTRODUCTION

The use of antibiotic prophylaxis in 'open' surgery is now widely established and is indicated for all procedures associated with a high rate of infection, usually when a colonized body cavity is opened, or in situations when postoperative infection, regardless of its incidence, could be severe or even fatal. Although the advent of laparoscopic surgery has brought with it some novel changes to surgical practice, there has been an impetus to mimic the essentials of the equivalent open operation. With the possible exception of wound infections it is therefore likely that most laparoscopic procedures will benefit from the same approach to antibiotic prophylaxis as the equivalent open procedure.

24.2 RATIONALE FOR ANTIBIOTIC PROPHYLAXIS IN LAPAROSCOPIC SURGERY

The aim of antibiotic prophylaxis in all surgical procedures is to reduce the incidence of infective complications by enhancing the body's own defence mechanisms. Transient bacteraemia frequently occurs during surgical procedures, but septicaemic shock is fortunately rare even in the absence of antibiotic prophylaxis. More common are localized infective complications, including intra-abdominal abscesses and wound infections.

During 'clean' laparoscopic operations there is a low risk of infective complications, and antibiotic prophylaxis is not usually warranted. When a prosthetic implant is to be used, prophylactic antibiotics may further reduce the small risk of infection which, if it occurs, may be resolved only by removal of the prosthesis. Patients who already have a prosthetic implant or who have valvular heart disease and are at risk of bacterial endocarditis may also benefit from antibiotic prophylaxis during clean procedures, although the benefits to be gained in these patients are less easy to prove (if they exist at all).

Immunocompromised patients, less equipped to deal with even minor bacterial exposure are also likely to benefit from antibiotic protection in otherwise clean procedures.

All potentially contaminated laparoscopic procedures, whether high or low risk, should receive antibiotic prophylaxis, whilst all 'dirty' procedures should receive preoperative antibiotics continued postoperatively as a therapeutic course.

Bacterial contamination may originate either from exogenous sources such as the surgical team, instruments or environment through a flaw in aseptic technique, or from endogenous sources such as the patient's skin or gastrointestinal tract. For potentially contaminated or dirty laparoscopic procedures the most important source of bacterial contamination is the gastrointestinal tract, and therefore antibiotic prophylaxis is directed at enteric flora during these operations.

24.3 POTENTIAL DIFFERENCES IN INFECTIVE COMPLICATIONS BETWEEN OPEN AND LAPAROSCOPIC SURGERY

A major advantage of laparoscopic surgery is the relatively small size of the skin wounds, although less so for laparoscopy-assisted operations. Laparoscopic techniques are associated with fewer wound infections than open techniques, and when they do occur the wounds are small and therefore present less of a problem. This lower incidence of wound infection can be reduced further by paying careful attention to skin disinfection, particularly at the umbilicus. In all other respects the infective complications would be expected to occur with a similar frequency for both laparoscopic and open procedures, and it would seem prudent to consider the use of the same antibiotic prophylaxis for both.

One potential disadvantage of laparoscopic surgery is the difficulty associated with sterilizing the laparoscope. Their useful life is shortened by autoclaving, and most centres do not have the facilities for gas sterilization. Therefore, in most centres the laparoscopes are disinfected by immersion in glutaraldehyde between cases, but this does not destroy bacterial spores. Although in India there have been a number of cases of tetanus resulting from spore contamination, there is little realistic risk from spore contamination in Western practice. Meticulous physical cleaning should be performed before disinfection, and there appears to be little advantage to increasing glutaraldehyde immersion time beyond 20 minutes. The use of autoclavable autoclaves should avoid the need for disinfection and chemical sterilization.

24.4 SUPPORTIVE EVIDENCE FOR ANTIBIOTIC PROPHYLAXIS IN LAPAROSCOPIC SURGERY

There is now a wealth of experience with the use of antibiotic prophylaxis in open surgery, and this should be the starting point for determining the appropriate use of antibiotics in laparoscopic surgery. Many series of laparoscopic procedures are being reported, extolling the virtues of the new technique; however, in many the role of antibiotic prophylaxis is not stated. It is assumed that for most series antibiotic prophylaxis is used according to the same criteria used in the respective authors' open practice. In the following discussions relating to particular procedures, infection rates for open and laparoscopic techniques are compared, with the relevant conclusions reached.

24.4.1 Biliary tract surgery

Infective complications after routine **cholecystectomy** are rare, but the risk is increased if the biliary tract is opened (for example, during exploration of the common bile duct) or if spillage of bile occurs. Even if spillage does occur there is little risk in the presence of sterile bile; however, **bactibilia** exists in a significant minority of asymptomatic patients and is so likely that it should be assumed present when performing surgery for acute cholecystitis or in the presence of an obstructed biliary system. The existence of bactibilia increases with the age of the patient, and positive bile cultures are present in over 60% of patients aged 70 years or more. The pathogenic organisms most often cultured from bile are the Gram-negative bacteria *E. coli* and *Klebsiella* spp., and Gram-positive enterococci.

OPEN CHOLECYSTECTOMY

Infective complications after open cholecystectomy were observed in 46% of patients with infected bile compared with only 1% in those with sterile bile. In a randomized trial of antibiotic prophylaxis in patients at high risk of bactibilia, based upon the above criteria, preoperative antibiotics reduced infective complications from 24% to 5% after open cholecystectomy. A meta-analysis of 42 studies comparing antibiotic prophylaxis with no antibiotic cover, including more than 4000 patients who had undergone biliary tract surgery, revealed an overall incidence of postoperative infection of 9% for the group with prophylaxis compared with 15% for the group without. This apparent reduction was the same both for patients at 'high risk' and 'low risk' of developing postoperative infection.

It is not practical before surgery to measure whether or not bactibilia exists, and therefore it is reasonable practice that all biliary procedures should be covered with a single preoperative dose of a first-generation cephalosporin.

Infective complications of laparoscopic cholecystectomy are unusual. In a retrospective series of 3603 cases the incidence of wound infections was 0.6%. Chemoprophylaxis with a single dose of '3rd' generation cephalosporin (cefotaxime, ceftriaxone) had been used.

LAPAROSCOPIC CHOLECYSTECTOMY

In a series of 1518 laparoscopic cholecystectomies, reported by the Southern Surgeons Club, USA, there was a 1% incidence of superficial wound infection and only two cases of intra-abdominal abscess requiring drainage. Unfortunately the use, or not, of antibiotic prophylaxis was not stated. In a smaller series of 195 laparoscopic cholecystectomies, in which 95% of patients received antibiotic prophylaxis, there was a 6% incidence of 'wound erythema' resulting in superficial dehiscence in 5%. A similar incidence of wound infection was reported in another series using antibiotic prophylaxis (nine of 164 patients);

however, the same authors subsequently achieved no wound infections in 78 patients using only chlorhexidine skin scrub and no antibiotic prophylaxis.

The incidence of infective complications is likely to be higher in those cases where the gallbladder has ruptured intra-abdominally. Whilst no series report the incidence of this occurrence, one can assume that it is fairly high if the estimates of stone spillage occurring in 15% of laparoscopic cholecystectomy are true. There have been 15 reported cases of intra-abdominal abscess formation as a result of spilled gallstones, and therefore when identified they should be removed. It is more difficult to clear spilled bile, but it should rarely lead to complications – especially if antibiotic prophylaxis has been used.

After reviewing combined series of laparoscopic cholecystectomy, Ponsky (1994) concluded that 'many use antibiotics without evidence of benefit'. In that review he reported an overall incidence of 0.1% for intra-abdominal abscess formation and a 0.4% incidence of wound infection.

Overall, there is little evidence to support the use of antibiotic prophylaxis in routine laparoscopic cholecystectomy, and perhaps more attention should be paid to **skin disinfection**. If the common bile duct is to be explored, antibiotic prophylaxis is justified based upon the evidence from open biliary procedures.

Antibiotic prophylaxis is warranted in high-risk cases such as intra-abdominal rupture of the gall-bladder, or with a history of recurrent attacks of acute cholangitis.

24.4.2 Upper gastrointestinal tract surgery

Significant risk exists only when the stomach and duodenum are opened, with a greater chance existing in the presence of pyloric outlet obstruction or carcinoma. Proton-pump inhibitors and other modulators of gastric acid production raise the pH of the stomach, and this results in significant bacterial contamination.

Antibiotic prophylaxis is not justified if the gastrointestinal tract is not opened, for example during a fundoplication or vagotomy. Even when the upper gastrointestinal tract is entered the risk should in theory be low; however, the presence of the abnormality requiring intervention is likely to increase the potential for bacterial contamination, and antibiotic prophylaxis is therefore warranted. As for open procedures, a single preoperative dose of a third-generation cephalosporin is suggested to cover procedures in which a viscus is opened.

24.4.3 Colorectal surgery

For all colorectal procedures during which the bowel is opened there is a high risk of subsequent infection because of the bacterial load. As early as 1939 the benefit of oral sulphonamide prophylaxis in reducing the incidence of wound infection after colonic surgery was revealed, and the ideal regimen has been sought ever since. The colonic bacteria usually associated with infective complications are *E. coli*, enterococci and mixed anaerobes; hence, antibiotic prophylaxis should be directed at these organisms.

OPEN COLORECTAL SURGERY

Prophylactic antibiotics are highly effective at reducing rates of wound infection after colorectal operations. Many trials, including some prospective randomized trials, reveal a reduction in wound infection rates from up to 40% without antibiotic cover to around 10% with prophylactic antibiotics. It is not clear whether there is any additional benefit in reducing rates of intra-abdominal sepsis or mortality but no trials to date have been large enough to reveal one.

Many of the commonly used combinations, usually metronidazole with a penicillin, cephalosporin or gentamicin, are equally effective and there is no evidence to support more complex or expensive combinations. Furthermore, first generation cephalosporins appear to be as effective as the newer and more expensive cephalosporins. Metronidazole is not as effective when used alone but provides the anaerobic cover in most combination regimens and these combinations appear to be better than most broad-spectrum antibiotics that claim to be effective against both anaerobic and aerobic bacteria. Oral neomycin and erythromycin has been popular in North America but does not appear to be as effective as the intravenous pre-operative regimens, especially if only given on the day before operation.

A single pre-operative dose of antibiotic would appear to be as effective as the more commonly used multi-dose regimens and there is no good evidence to support the widely quoted practice of repeat dosing during long procedures. By restricting the number of doses, the risk of antibiotic resistance could be reduced and substantial cost-savings could be made. There is certainly no benefit in extending prophylaxis beyond 24 hours.

LAPAROSCOPIC COLORECTAL SURGERY

Any laparoscopic procedure that breaches the colonic wall will create a high risk of infective complications and should be covered by antibiotic prophylaxis. Some of the larger series of laparoscopic colorectal procedures reveal that the overall incidence of infective complications is likely to be small if adequate antibiotic prophylaxis is used.

Among 76 laparoscopic bowel resections (25% converted to an open procedure) using oral prophylaxis with neomycin and erythromycin in addition to intravenous prophylaxis with a second-generation cephalosporin, before and for 24 hours after operation, no infective complications were listed. In a series of 110 laparoscopy-assisted bowel procedures, using intravenous cephalosporin and mechanical bowel preparation, the only infective complication was one infected haematoma and one urinary tract infection. Four 'minor' wound infections were reported among 100 patients who received unspecified antibiotic prophylaxis prior to laparoscopic-assisted bowel resection.

Common sense would dictate that antibiotic prophylaxis should be used in laparoscopic colorectal surgery, especially as there is a significant chance of conversion to an open technique, and it is unlikely that significant series will be performed in which they are not used. However, the implications for the patient with infected port sites would appear to be much less than those for infected abdominal incisions and antibiotic prophylaxis to prevent wound infections alone might rationally be questioned in the future.

24.4.4 Appendicectomy

OPEN APPENDICECTOMY

Wound infection rates for uncomplicated appendicectomy can be reduced from between 8 and 27% to less than 1% with antibiotic prophylaxis using a single preoperative dose of a third-generation cephalosporin. Wound infection rates for appendicectomy complicated by necrosis or perforation can be reduced from 80% to between 10 and 25% with appropriate prophylaxis which is continued postoperatively as treatment for up to 5 days. Metronidazole, either alone or in combination with a cephalosporin, has historically been favoured in the UK because of its activity against anaerobes; however, there is no evidence for added efficacy of the combination, and in some studies metronidazole has been shown to be no more effective than placebo when used alone.

LAPAROSCOPIC APPENDICECTOMY

Appendicectomy provides a useful model for evaluating the benefit of antibiotic prophylaxis in contaminated and dirty operations. Overall, laparoscopic appendicectomy is associated with a lower rate of wound infection than the open operation when prophylactic antibiotics are used. This lower incidence may be further reduced with the use of an extraction bag, but this will inevitably increase the cost of the procedure. In one retrospective study comparing 100 laparoscopic appendicectomies with 100 open appendicectomies, using prophylactic antibiotics and the same criteria for their continued use after operation, the wound infection rate was 2% for the laparoscopic procedures compared with 12% for the open procedures. Perhaps more importantly the incidence of intra-abdominal abscesses was only 2% after laparoscopic appendicectomy compared with 6% after open operation.

In a retrospective study comparing 29 laparoscopic appendicectomies with 77 open appendicectomies, sharing the same proportion of inflammation and 'gangrene', either wound infections or intra-abdominal abscesses requiring drainage were found in 10% of the laparoscopic cases compared with 30% after open appendicectomy. The total wound morbidity in terms of those wounds left open or re-opened was 14% for laparoscopic appendicectomy compared with 39% after the open operation.

There is little doubt that antibiotic prophylaxis should continue to be used to cover laparoscopic appendicectomy, and continued as treatment where appropriate because of the relatively high incidence of undiagnosed intra-abdominal septic collections and the significant incidence of wound infection.

24.4.5 Mesh hernia repair

OPEN REPAIR

Open prosthetic mesh repair of inguinal hernias, popularized by Lichtenstein, has now become one of the most frequent methods of repairing groin hernias. Many surgeons choose to use prophylactic antibiotics to cover prosthetic mesh insertion even though hernia repair is essentially a clean procedure, fearing that even a small chance of infection would result in failure of the repair or precipitate mesh removal. A large multi-centre prospective trial comparing the use, or not, of antibiotic prophylaxis in 1834 mesh inguinal hernia repairs revealed an infection rate of 0.6% among the group receiving prophylactic antibiotics and 0.2% in the group without prophylaxis. Furthermore, infective complications were easily managed and did not result in the loss of any meshes, or indeed any recurrent hernias. The routine use of antibiotic prophylaxis in mesh inguinal hernia repair was not recommended. In a further series of 1098 mesh hernia repairs there was a very similar incidence of significant infection of 0.9%; again, in none of these patients was there an associated recurrence or need to remove the mesh.

A study from Scotland reported an incidence of chronic groin sepsis after mesh repair of about 0.1%. All of these cases required removal of the mesh. There was no association of infection with the use or not of chemoprophylaxis peri-operatively.

LAPAROSCOPIC HERNIA REPAIR

If there is little evidence to support a role for antibiotic prophylaxis in open mesh hernia repair, then the arguments for its use in laparoscopic hernia repair must be negligible. In a large multi-centre series in which the use of antibiotic prophylaxis was not stated, there were only two wound infections and one mesh infection (removed at 18 months) among 869 laparoscopic hernia repairs. In a further series no infective complications were reported among 509 transabdominal preperitoneal repairs, although 19 patients developed seromas that required aspiration. No statement was made about the use of prophylactic antibiotics.

24.4.6 Diagnostic laparoscopy

The largest experience with laparoscopy is available from gynaecology series, usually involving 'clean' diagnostic or sterilization procedures. In one large series there were only 19 (0.18%) wound infections among 10 480 open laparoscopies. Hassan – who gave his name to the open laparoscopic technique – reported only two minor wound infections in 630 open laparoscopies. Therefore, there is little evidence to justify using antibiotic prophylaxis for simple diagnostic procedures, and this can probably be extended to all laparoscopic procedures in which contamination does not occur (or is due to a rare unexpected incident).

24.5 PROPHYLAXIS AND IATROGENIC PERFORATION

One potential disadvantage of laparoscopic compared with open procedures is that otherwise clean procedures may be contaminated secondary to iatrogenic viscus perforation. This complication is likely to be under-reported. The largest series of laparoscopy are available from the gynaecological literature, and in two large series the incidences of iatrogenic damage were: in 56 106 Veres needle and trochar insertions, 87 accidental viscus perforations (0.15%) and in 10 480 open laparoscopies, six bowel lacerations (0.06%). Less information is available from surgical series: a single iatrogenic bowel perforation was reported in a series of over 600 patients who underwent transabdominal hernia repair, and a single perforation was reported among 100 patients undergoing laparoscopy-assisted bowel resection, though the significance of such injury will be minimal with respect to antibiotic prophylaxis in an already potentially contaminated procedure.

Whether or not antibiotic prophylaxis can be justified for use in clean laparoscopic operations because of the small risk of iatrogenic bowel perforation is unclear. The likelihood is not, because evidence suggests that prophylactic antibiotics are effective if given within a short time of the exposure occurring; furthermore, they are unlikely to alter the course of an 'occult' perforation that presents after the original procedure.

24.6 THE IDEAL REGIMEN

Selection of the most appropriate agent depends upon a knowledge of the potential infecting organism, resistance patterns and, to some extent, cost. The antibiotic with the narrowest spectrum (but including cover for the potential contaminants) should be used to reduce the morbidity and mortality associated with their use. The antibiotic should achieve adequate levels in the target tissues, and its half-life of activity should cover the at-risk period; otherwise, repeat administration will be required.

Danzinger and Hassan reviewed a large number of randomized controlled trials comparing different regimens of antibiotic prophylaxis in open colorectal procedures. They revealed that most of the frequently used regimens were equally effective: oral neomycin and erythromycin (three doses preoperatively), oral or intravenous metronidazole and intravenous third-generation cephalosporin were all associated with a 5 to 15% wound infection rate. **Intravenous first-generation cephalosporins** were less effective, and resulted in a wound infection rate of between 20% and 30%; hence these should be avoided as prophylaxis for colonic surgery, although they are adequate for most biliary operations. Efficacy in preventing infective complications other than wound infections was not discussed, and neither were the side effects of the different regimens. Therefore, the choice of any one particular regimen over another would be reduced to that of cost. A combination of oral and parenteral antibiotic prophylaxis was not found to be better than either given alone.

Although oral regimens have much to offer in terms of cost and ease of administration, there is a problem in predicting time to operation. This is less important when using antibiotics with a long half-life (e.g. erythromycin); however, it remains unsuited to emergency and urgent procedures, and overall the oral route has never been favoured in the UK. There is a tradition in the UK to combine a third-generation cephalosporin with metronidazole; however, there is little evidence to support any added value for this excess, and the cephalosporin alone is probably adequate.

There is minimal risk from anaerobes in biliary surgery, and a first-generation cephalosporin is adequate.

A single preoperative dose of cephalosporin has been shown to be as effective as multi-dose regimens, and should in theory be associated with fewer side effects. Current recommendations support the efficacy of a single dose, as this also reduces the risks of bacterial resistance and the burden of cost.

Experiments in both animal models and in humans have consistently revealed that, for the best effect, the antibiotic should be in the system before exposure to bacteria occurs. The efficacy of an antibiotic decreases with time if given after inoculation, and it is ineffective as prophylaxis after a few hours. Antibiotics must ideally be given preoperatively to be effective; one study revealed that wound infection was four times higher with postoperative administration and not significantly different to no antibiotic at all! The timing of intravenous administration is ideally a short time (not more than 1–2 hours) before the surgical incision to allow tissue concentrations to peak, but this would be difficult to achieve in most practices. An effective compromise is to delay administration until the induction of anaesthesia and to give the antibiotics intravenously. However, this can sometimes restrict choice and promote thrombosis in the infused vein.

In view of the relatively short half-life of many of the commonly used prophylactic antibiotics, a repeat intravenous dose is recommended if surgery is longer than 3 hours. This is likely in many laparoscopic colorectal procedures, especially at the beginning of a surgeon's learning curve.

Current recommendations for patients at risk of developing bacterial endocarditis are to use amoxycillin or vancomycin, each with gentamicin, to cover gastrointestinal procedures.

24.7 CONCLUSIONS

The benefits of the laparoscopic approach to an increasing number of general surgical procedures are becoming apparent, and randomized trials continue to evaluate and extend the role of laparoscopic surgery for cancer. It is evident that a laparoscopic approach reduces the burden of infective wound complications after 'contaminated' and 'dirty' surgical procedures, and this low incidence can further be reduced by using appropriate antibiotic prophylaxis. This will also maintain a low incidence of other infective complications. There exists an opportunity for laparoscopic surgeons to take the lead once again and to standardize antibiotic prophylaxis. In particular, the opportunity exists to encourage appropriate antibiotic

selection and to reduce the dose regimen to a single preoperative administration.

24.8 FURTHER READING

American Society of Hospital Pharmacists Therapeutic Guidelines on Antimicrobial Prophylaxis in Surgery (1992) *Clin. Pharm.*, **11**, 483–513.

Bernard, H.R. and Cole, W.R. (1964) The prophylaxis of surgical infection; the effect of prophylactic antimicrobial drugs on the incidence of infection following potentially contaminated operations. *Surgery*, **56**, 151–157.

Danzinger, L. and Hassan, E. (1987) Antimicrobial prophylaxis of gastrointestinal surgical procedures and treatment of antimicrobial infections. *Drug Intelligence Clin. Pharm.*, **21**, 406–415.

Karran, S. (1980) *Controversies in Surgical Sepsis*. Praeger, New York.

Meijer, W.S., Schmitz, P.I.M. and Jeeke, J. (1990) Meta-analysis of randomized, controlled trials of antibiotic prophylaxis in biliary tract surgery. *Br. J. Surg.*, **77**, 282–290.

Ponsky, J.L. (1994) The incidence and management of complications of laparoscopic cholecystectomy (Review). *Adv. Surg.*, **27**, 21–41.

Song, F. and Glenny, A.M. (1998) Antimicrobial prophylaxis in colorectal surgery: a systematic review of randomized controlled trials. *Br. J. Surg.*, **85**, 1232–1241.

Wilson, A.P.R. (1995) Antibiotic prophylaxis and infection control measures in minimally invasive surgery. *J. Antimicrob. Chemother.*, **36**, 1–5.

Infections of the liver, spleen, gallbladder and pancreas

J. PHILPOTT-HOWARD

25.1 ROUTES OF SPREAD OF INFECTION

The liver, spleen, gallbladder, biliary tree and pancreas are diverse structures which, although they are closely related anatomically, differ markedly from each other both in the route of infection and in the sequelae of any infective process. The exception is the biliary system, where the pathogenesis and sequelae of bacterial infections are essentially similar throughout the biliary tree and gallbladder.

Organisms may reach these organs by several routes (Figure 25.1). Transient bacteraemia of the portal vein occurs when a few of the very large number of bacteria (10^{10} to 10^{11} organisms per gram of faeces) in the colon and lower small intestine manage to breach the mucosa and submucosal cell-mediated defences, and enter the portal venous system. Ultimately in the normal host they are cleared by the Küppfer cells of the liver. These translocating organisms comprise the more common gut streptococci, enterococci, enterobacteria and anaerobes, although yeasts and other organisms (which are normally present in low numbers) may also translocate from the gut when a patient has acquired an abnormal gut flora, for example after broad-spectrum antibiotic therapy.

In the compromised patient, portocaval bacteraemia may be more frequent when mucosal defences are impaired by mucositis, mucosal ulceration or neutropenia, and normal hepatic clearance may not be sufficient to prevent bacteraemia and subsequent sepsis. In addition, endotoxin and other bacterial constituents may enter the circulation and cause fever, particularly in the neutropenic patient. Patients with an abnormal liver hepatic clearance secondary to acute or chronic liver failure are also more likely to develop bacteraemia and sepsis, even if the integrity of the gut wall is intact. In any patient, focal hepatic abscesses are therefore likely to be derived from the gut flora via the portal vein, as are abscesses caused by amoebae following amoebic dysentery. Other parasites such as *Echinococcus*, which causes hydatid disease, reach the liver parenchyma via the portal venous system. In contrast, a splenic abscess is usually acquired from a systemic bacteraemia, although the original bacteraemia may well be caused by gut pathogens and commensals. The biliary tree and gallbladder become infected when organisms pass directly from the gut through the sphincter of Oddi and ascend the common bile duct. Although in most individuals the duodenal secretions are colonized with only a few Gram-positive bacteria, bacterial overgrowth at this site is common in many debilitating conditions such as diabetes, systemic sclerosis and in patients taking antacids. Ascending infection may then occur, most commonly when there is outflow obstruction secondary to calculi,

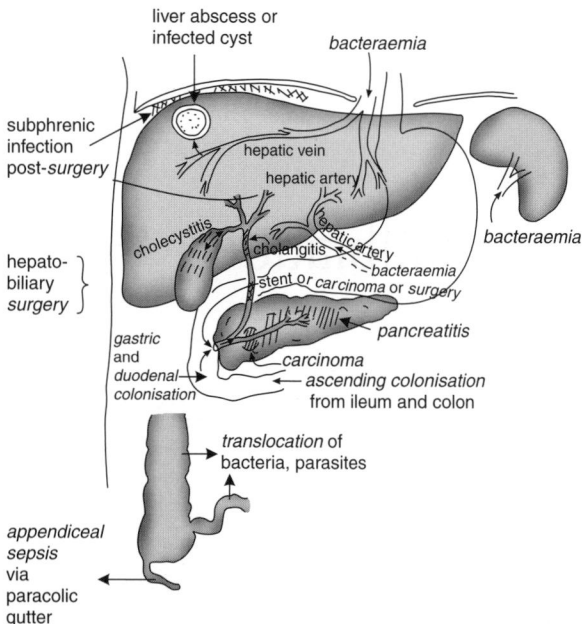

Figure 25.1 *Routes by which organisms reach the liver, gall bladder, pancreas & spleen; & risk factors for infection.*

liver disease or neoplasia, but occasionally in the absence of any local pathology or intervention. Local surgical or endoscopic procedures are also risk factors for the development of infection by this route. Parasites such as nematodes (roundworms) and flukes can ascend the biliary tree and either cause obstruction or a secondary bacterial infection.

Primary bacterial infection of the pancreas seems to be particularly unusual, possibly because of the unfavourable environment of the pancreatic secretions. Acute pancreatitis, especially when caused by pancreatic duct obstruction, is often associated with secondary infection.

Protozoal parasites (other than amoebae), reach the liver or spleen after a primary systemic parasitaemia, for example, *Leishmania*, *Plasmodium* and *Toxoplasma* spp.

Viral infection of the cells of the liver or pancreas are only acquired after viraemia with specific agents that are hepatotropic (hepatitis viruses) or give rise to an incidental pancreatic inflammation as part of a systemic illness (e.g. mumps).

A summary of the laboratory characteristics of bacteria which are associated with infections of the liver, biliary tree, spleen and pancreas is given as an appendix to this chapter.

25.2 INFECTIONS OF THE LIVER

25.2.1 Viral hepatitis

In viral hepatitis, the primary insult is hepatocellular damage following viral replication within the hepato-

cytes. In some cases, particularly hepatitis B, it is the host's immunological response to the virus that causes most of the liver damage. Many viral infections of the liver are subclinical for many years; past infection is a chance finding during routine serological tests, or is found on screening patients presenting with end-stage liver disease.

HEPATITIS A VIRUS (HAV)

This virus has only recently been cultured in cell lines, and has been characterized as a picornavirus (*pico-*, small; *rna*: RNA). It belongs to the heparnavirus genus but unlike other picornaviruses it is hepatotropic. Electron microscopy of faeces from a patient with hepatitis A shows featureless viruses 27 nm in diameter, which are indistinguishable from any other picornavirus. HAV is unrelated to the hepatitis B virus which has a DNA genome, but like hepatitis B virus HAV infects only primate liver cells. Viral gut penetration must occur at some stage since the virus is spread by the faecal–oral route; transfusion-related hepatitis A is extremely rare, as is any other spread through blood contact. HAV causes the disease hepatitis A, which was previously known as 'infectious hepatitis' (as opposed to 'serum hepatitis', hepatitis B). During the acute stage of the infection, virus is present in the faeces. Low concentrations of the virus have also been found in the urine and saliva of infected patients, but the significance of this is unknown.

Infection occurs worldwide, with a slightly higher incidence in autumn and winter. Close contact with faecal–oral spread in a household, and consumption of contaminated food and water in areas of poor quality water supply, account for most cases. There is no true carrier state for HAV. The incubation period after exposure is 2–6 weeks, with an average of 4 weeks. Infectivity occurs during the second half of the incubation period and continues for about a week after the onset of jaundice (or when the liver function tests are most abnormal, if there is no jaundice). Infection is often asymptomatic, particularly in childhood. The patient has a rapid onset of general malaise, nausea, fever and abdominal discomfort followed by jaundice lasting a few days. Many patients with symptoms take 2–6 months to recover fully, and experience convalescent malaise and tiredness. There are no long-term sequelae, and fatality occurs in only 1 in 1000 cases. Rarely, hepatitis A causes acute hepatic failure, but otherwise there are very few serious complications.

HAV infection is **diagnosed** principally by the detection of serum antibody with an ELISA (enzyme-linked immunosorbent assay), or a radioimmunoassay. HAV IgM is found in the acute phase and lasts for about 3 months, whilst HAV IgG without IgM denotes past infection. Immune electron microscopy can reveal the virus in the faeces for about 3–4 weeks around the onset of jaundice, but neither microscopy nor cell culture are used in routine diagnosis.

Passive immunization with normal human immunoglobulin can be given to household contacts of a case, and occasionally to travellers going to areas of poor water hygiene. Active immunization with a high-dose inactivated hepatitis A vaccine is now the preferred method of immunization for persons at risk, especially as titres of anti-hepatitis A antibody in normal human immunoglobulin, which might otherwise be used to confer protection, are declining. A single dose of vaccine provides protection for up to a year, and a booster dose at 12 months gives prolonged antibody levels, probably for up to 10 years.

HEPATITIS B VIRUS (HBV)

Hepatitis B virus is one of the Hepadnavirus family, together with some other hepatitis viruses that affect animals such as the duck and woodchuck. HBV contains circular partially double-stranded DNA, and associated with the DNA is RNA-dependent DNA polymerase ('reverse transcriptase') which is involved in replication. The infective, complete virus particle, the Dane particle, is a sphere 42 nm in diameter. It comprises: (i) an outer lipoprotein envelope of 'hepatitis B surface antigen' (HBsAg); (ii) an inner nucleocapsid core containing DNA and polypeptide core antigen (HBcAg); and e antigen (HBeAg), which is a major subunit of HBcAg. The virus is found exclusively in primates and only infects liver cells. During replication of the virus in liver cells, a large excess of surface antigen is produced in addition to the infective Dane particles. These incomplete viral particles are either spherical, 22 nm in diameter, or tubular, but they have no DNA and so are non-infectious. Dane and HBsAg particles appear in blood, plasma, serum and any blood-stained body fluid, and to a very small extent in vaginal secretions, saliva and tears.

There are four major subtypes of HBsAg, each with a determinant 'a', plus one or more of the determinants d, r, w and y. The common subtypes are adw (commonest in the United Kingdom), adr, ady and ayw. The subtype can be determined using an agar gel diffusion technique and specific antisera. Nucleotide sequence analysis can be used to investigate outbreaks of hepatitis B.

It is estimated that over 200 million people worldwide are carriers of the virus; about 0.05% of all blood donors in the UK are found to be HBV-positive, compared with 1 to 5% or more of injecting drug users in the UK, and about 3–5% of individuals from parts of the world where HBV infection is endemic, such as Africa, the Middle East and Asia. About 10% of chronic carriers will progress to chronic liver disease, and of these a further 10% will develop hepatocellular carcinoma.

Infection occurs after exposure to blood, serum and other body fluids containing infective virus, particularly from a patient whose blood is positive for e antigen or HBV-DNA. The commonest modes of transmission are from mother to neonate, nearly always from blood contamination during birth; sexual contact, especially with blood contamination of mucous membranes, e.g. during anal intercourse; intravenous drug use or transfusion of infected blood and blood products.

After exposure and a very long incubation period (30–90 days), hepatitis B virus infection may have a variety of clinical outcomes. In 80–90% of cases, infection is asymptomatic, especially in infants. Clinical hepatitis may present with jaundice, abdominal discomfort, arthralgia and fevers. Clinical hepatitis usually resolves, but an important outcome of both asymptomatic and symptomatic infection is chronic carriage with a risk later in life of cirrhosis and hepatic carcinoma; the patient is also potentially infective for others.

There is no treatment for the acute infection other than supportive measures; the patient with acute liver failure may require a liver transplant. Chronic carriage has been treated with interferon-alpha and lamivudine with some success.

Analysis of serum by ELISA, haemagglutination or radioimmunoassay during different stages of uncomplicated acute infection shows the hepatitis B 'markers' – HBsAg, HBeAg, anti-HBs, anti-HBe and anti-HBc. HBV-DNA can also be detected in the serum of selected patients, principally those with e antigen, but this test is not performed routinely. The interpretation of patterns of HBV antigens and their corresponding antibodies is shown in Table 25.1.

Patients with the acute infection, and chronic carriers of the virus are infectious and have persistent HBsAg in blood and body fluids. In addition, most patients with acute infection and about 10% of the chronic carriers have large amounts of HBeAg in their serum, and they are much more infectious than patients with HBsAg only. Patients with anti-HBs only are not infectious; they would have had past infection or hepatitis B vaccination. Those with HBsAg are of low infectivity if they are anti-HBe-positive; patients with HBsAg but no e antibody are highly infectious (see Table 25.1). HBV-DNA in the blood is also a marker for infectivity, and a few patients who are normally low-infectivity carriers are found to be HBV-DNA-positive.

The detection of anti-HBc IgM is a useful test when trying to decide if someone who is jaundiced has acute infection with hepatitis B, since a positive HBsAg in a jaundiced patient could reflect coincidental chronic carriage and the patient might have biliary rather than hepatic disease as a cause for the jaundice.

Prevention

The first HBsAg vaccine was derived from the plasma of carriers, but recombinant DNA vaccine produced by yeasts is now used. This consists of purified surface antigen (without core or e antigens or DNA). The vaccine can

Table 25.1 *Antigen and antibody markers in hepatitis B virus (HBV) infection*

Marker	Significance
HBsAg	*Surface antigen*: Produced in great excess in acute HBV infection, and in chronic HBV carriers
HBeAg	*e antigen*: Component of HBcAg; detectable in acute HBV infection for several months and in about 10–20% of chronic carriers. e-antigen-positive individuals are highly infectious
HBcAg	*Core antigen*: Not detectable in blood, present in liver in cells with replicating virus
anti-HBs	Indicates either past infection with HBV or immunization with hepatitis B vaccine
anti-HBe	*Antibody to e antigen*: Appears during recovery phase of acute hepatitis B infection, and replaces HBeAg (i.e. the patient becomes less infectious)
anti-HBc	*Antibody to core antigen*: If anti-HBc IgG is detected, this indicates past infection with HBV. It is not produced after vaccination, so a non-responder to hepatitis B vaccine can be tested to determine whether the individual has had past infection (as, paradoxically, infected patients respond poorly to the vaccine). Anti-HBc IgM can be used to diagnose acute infection, e.g. in an individual who could be a carrier but who also has acute hepatitis
HBV DNA	Serological marker indicating viral replication. Can be positive in some 'low risk' (e-antigen-negative) patients
HBV PCR and sequencing	Used for analysis of HBV genome, e.g. in outbreaks of infection

be given in three doses at 0, 1 and 6 months, or as an accelerated course of four doses at 0, 1, 2 and 12 months. It is offered to healthcare workers who regularly handle blood and body fluids (especially surgical, dental, midwifery and high-risk medical teams; all individuals who perform 'exposure-prone procedures' must have evidence of immunity to hepatitis B); medical laboratory workers; neonates born to HBsAg-positive mothers; and workers in mental handicap institutions. All medical and dental students are immunized, either before starting their training or in the first year of the course. Side effects from the vaccine are rare, but a severe reaction to the first dose means that subsequent doses should not be given. At 1 month after the end of the vaccine course, a serum sample should be sent for anti-HBs assay. If there is a good antibody response, booster doses are given every 5 years. Individuals who do not respond to a course of the vaccine may be given a fourth dose of the vaccine, and if still a non-responder (about 5% of vaccinees) they may benefit from an alternative hepatitis B vaccine which has an extended peptide sequence. Any non-responder may have had past infection with the virus, and the blood should be tested for anti-HBc IgG (which indicates past infection, since vaccinated individuals do not produce anti-HBc). If the anti-core antibody is positive, tests for HBsAg and other markers should be performed since the individual may be a carrier; if so, they are at risk of chronic liver disease and hepatic cancer. The individual should give consent to these tests, but if they perform exposure-prone

procedures on patients these tests must be carried out. In the UK, if permission is not given, the individual is not allowed to perform exposure-prone procedures.

In addition to vaccine, an intramuscular dose of anti-HBs immunoglobulin can sometimes be used to prevent infection after a high-risk exposure to the virus, such as a needle injury contaminated with blood known or suspected to be HBsAg-positive. Anti-HBs immunoglobulin must be given within 48 hours of the exposure (preferably within 24 hours), and this is followed by a full vaccine course starting within 72 hours. Alternatively, a second dose of immunoglobulin can be given a month after the first, for example if the vaccine is contraindicated for some reason. Hepatitis B-positive liver transplant patients are given a large dose of anti-HBs immunoglobulin in order to delay the onset of hepatitis in the new liver.

Occasionally a patient with no obvious risk factors for hepatitis B develops acute infection, and the only risk factor of note is that the individual underwent surgery some months before. Such cases must be investigated fully by the Infection Control Doctor and Consultant in Communicable Disease Control (CCDC) in conjunction with the Consultant Virologist, since the patient may have acquired the infection from a surgeon who is a carrier of hepatitis B virus, or from a contaminated blood or blood product transfusion (although this is very rare in the UK). If the surgeon was the source of the infection, all other patients on whom he or she has performed exposure-prone procedures must be checked to see if they have become infected. This is called a 'look-back' procedure, and it is necessary because the patients exposed to the surgeon's blood during surgery may have had subclinical infection, and they are still at risk of long-term carriage and liver disease; they may also transmit the virus to another individual. The look-back period may extend over several years, depending on the individual circumstances of the case.

In the UK, all healthcare staff who perform 'exposure-prone procedures' must be known to be immune to hepatitis B either through immunization or through natural immunity, provided they are not carriers of the virus. An exposure-prone procedure means any intervention on a patient where an injury to the healthcare worker may result in blood transmission to the patient, i.e. there is a risk of transmitting blood-borne virus infections. Surgeons and others who do not respond to hepatitis B vaccine may be HBsAg-positive, and should be checked for anti-core IgG and hepatitis B antigens. Any infected person may not be allowed to perform exposure-prone procedures, and the employer is obliged to provide re-training in another type of work.

Mutants of hepatitis B

'Escape mutants' of hepatitis B virus are rare strains that have mutated a codon in the region of the pre-S sequence of the genome. They are of concern since current hepatitis vaccines will not protect against infection, although new vaccines under development will include antigenic sequences which will provide protection.

HEPATITIS C

For many years it was recognized that patients developed hepatitis after blood transfusion, and that this infection was not caused by hepatitis A or hepatitis B (hence the name non-A non-B (NANB) hepatitis). Most of these are now known to be due to hepatitis C, a flavivirus with a single-stranded RNA genome.

Once a reliable antibody test for hepatitis C antibody was developed (the first-generation ELISA tests gave a significant number of false-positive results), it was recognized that hepatitis C had some of the characteristics of hepatitis B, particularly its association with chronic hepatitis and subsequent chronic active hepatitis in about 20% of infected individuals; a small percentage of these subsequently develop hepatocellular carcinoma. In the UK and North America the seroprevalence of hepatitis C antibodies ranges from 1 in 250 to 1 in 500 of the population, with a higher proportion of people from Southern Europe and Japan affected (1.5%). Between 30% and 50% of intravenous drug users are seropositive. Now that blood for transfusion is screened for hepatitis C antibody in most countries, infection with hepatitis C occurs mainly through sharing of needles during intravenous drug use, close household contact (although the exact mechanism of transmission is unclear), sexual activity and haemodialysis. Transmission to a surgeon through a needlestick injury has been described; the risk of transmission from an infected 'donor' in these circumstances is thought to be about 3–4%; this is higher than the risk of HIV (0.4%) but lower than from hepatitis B e-antigen-positive blood (20%). Neonatal infection from an infected mother appears to be uncommon. The incubation period is about 6 weeks, but it can be as long as 6 months; during this time, about 25% of patients will be unwell and overall 50% will have abnormal liver function tests. As with hepatitis B, the risk of chronic infection, relapsing infection and hepatic sequelae after exposure to hepatitis C is the same whether the patient has symptoms during the acute attack or not. Rarely, acute hepatic failure may occur during the acute infection; hepatitis C accounts for about one-third of all cases. Alcohol abuse may aggravate liver damage by the virus.

Diagnosis of hepatitis C infection relies on an ELISA screening test for antibody to core and non-structural proteins. Most people infected with hepatitis C virus are antibody-positive by 6 weeks, although a few take 3–4 months to develop antibodies. Viral RNA may also be detected by reverse transcriptase PCR, but this test is used mainly for research and in patients undergoing liver transplantation, or when an individual who is antibody negative is strongly suspected to have had recent infection.

Studies of interferon-alpha plus ribavirin have shown that prolonged treatment can improve hepatic function and reduce viraemia but most patients (including those who have undergone a liver transplant) are at risk of relapse, or re-infection of the new liver in the case of transplants. There is some evidence that of the six genotypes some are associated with worse disease and a poorer response to therapy. Currently there is no licensed specific immunoglobulin or vaccine for the management of exposure to hepatitis C virus, and a healthcare worker who sustains an accidental exposure can only be offered antibody tests to detect infection, at 3 and 6 months. The incidence of hepatitis C in healthcare workers, including surgeons and others who perform exposure-prone procedures, is suprisingly low – and no higher than the general population.

OTHER HEPATITIS VIRUSES

Hepatitis D virus (HDV, delta virus)

Hepatitis D is a defective RNA virus which can only replicate in the presence of hepatitis B virus, i.e. in patients with acute or chronic HBV infection. Hepatitis D virus infection is particularly common in intravenous drug users and others with significant blood exposure, especially in South America, Africa, some Mediterranean countries and the Middle East. Chronic HDV infection is unusual and is seen in less than 5% of cases, when a patient becomes infected with hepatitis B and D viruses simultaneously. The clinical course is similar to that of hepatitis B. However, when hepatitis D infection occurs in a patient who already has established HBV infection, acute HDV infection can lead to severe hepatitis with a mortality rate of 5 to 15%, and a greater risk of cirrhosis. Both HDV antigen and antibody are detectable in the blood, and HDV RNA can also be assayed. All patients with HBV are routinely automatically screened for HDV.

Hepatitis E virus

Hepatitis E is an RNA virus transmitted oro-faecally in a manner similar to hepatitis A. Water-borne outbreaks have been described in India, China and some parts of Central Africa and Central America. Infection results in a hepatitic picture (similar to hepatitis A) which resolves without long-term carriage or other sequelae. Occasionally it may run a fulminant course, particularly in late pregnancy.

Hepatitis G viruses

This recently discovered group of flaviviruses includes the human hepatitis virus 'hepatitis GB virus C' (GBV-C), which is almost certainly identical to an independently identified virus called hepatitis G virus (HGV). The term HGV is now used more commonly. Approximately 0.5% of blood donors and 10% of surgical patients have been reported to be HGV antibody-positive. However, there appears to be no underlying liver disease in seropositive patients, or at least hepatitis is very uncommon with HGV. It may be a co-factor for disease, with other viruses.

Other causes of hepatitis

Yellow fever virus is a primary cause of hepatitis and gives its Latinized name to the group of viruses to which it belongs – the flaviviruses. It causes severe hepatitis, together with gastrointestinal haemorrhage, which is a common feature. The virus is maintained in two ways, amongst monkeys (sylvatic or jungle cycle), and amongst man (urban cycle) in tropical Africa and South America. *Aedes* mosquitoes, particularly *A. aegyptii*, transmit the virus. After mosquito inoculation the virus enters lymph nodes and disseminates after 3–5 days of incubation to the liver, spleen and kidneys where necrotic lesions may occur; histology shows intracellular Councilman bodies. Diagnosis is made with serology (haemagglutinin-inhibition) or by virus isolation in mice. Live attenuated vaccine is available: the 17D strain provides at least 10 years of immunity, and a certificate of immunization is required for entry into a number of tropical countries. Eradication of *Aedes* in urban dwellings has reduced urban yellow fever greatly in South America.

In the immunocompetent individual, other viruses only rarely cause clinical hepatitis with jaundice; these include Epstein–Barr virus (EBV), rubella and cytomegalovirus (CMV). Abnormalities of liver enzymes are not uncommon during infectious mononucleosis infection caused by EBV or CMV, however. Immuno-compromised patients, especially those who have undergone organ transplantation, are at particular risk of CMV hepatitis. They may also have severe infection caused by two other herpesviruses, varicella-zoster virus and herpes simplex virus, as part of disseminated disease.

Granulomatous disease of the liver is effectively a low-grade hepatitis which forms part of a systemic infective process. Classical examples are syphilis, tuberculosis, melioidosis, brucellosis, histoplasmosis and schistosomiasis. These diagnoses should be considered in patients with risk factors for these diseases.

In addition to these specific infections, sepsis anywhere in the abdomen may disturb hepatic function, as may septicaemia and generalized infections such as tuberculosis, the enteric fevers and syphilis. Finally, surgical procedures including transplantation, choledochojejunostomy, Kasai and similar operations radically alter the balance between the microorganism and the liver, usually in favour of the organism so that there is a greater risk of bacteraemia and septicaemia.

25.3 INFECTIONS OF THE GALLBLADDER AND BILE DUCTS

25.3.1 Cholangitis, cholecystitis and the microbiology of bile

Cholangitis is inflammation (primarily infection) of the hepatic and common bile ducts, but it is often associated with infection of the gallbladder. As with other secretory or excretory systems, infection almost invariably arises secondary to complete or partial obstruction of the bile drainage, since such obstruction may damage the endothelium of the biliary tree, and secondary bacterial infection readily occurs. The causes of obstruction are numerous: cholelithiasis; pancreatitis; biliary or pancreatic tumours; surgery including hepatic transplantation, endoscopic retrograde cholangiopancreatography (ERCP) and manipulations such as biliary stent insertion; and parasites such as *Ascaris* (common roundworm) or flukes. Although healthy individuals have a few Gram-positive bacterial species in the duodenum and jejunum, patients with these diseases or interventions (particularly those who have been hospitalized) are likely to have a heavier and mixed Gram-positive and Gram-negative bacterial flora which may opportunistically invade the damaged biliary tree. As specimens of bile are rarely obtained directly from such patients, data on the most common pathogens are derived principally from records of septicaemias secondary to cholangitis and cholecystitis. However, surgical practices such as T-tube drainage have also provided some information on the likely pathogens. In patients who have not undergone hepatobiliary surgery or have recently received antibiotics, the common pathogens are enterobacteria ('coliforms') such as *Escherichia coli*, *Klebsiella* and *Enterobacter* spp., and anaerobes, particularly *Bacteroides fragilis* and *Clostridium perfringens*. Patients who have undergone complex biliary surgery such as the Kasai procedure or anastamoses secondary to transplant surgery are more likely to have had numerous courses of antibiotics. In these patients cholecystitis is likely to be caused by more resistant Gram-negative bacteria such as *Enterobacter* spp., or less commonly *Pseudomonas aeruginosa*; *Enterococcus faecalis* and *Enterococcus faecium* are also common. Some of these will be multiply-resistant strains if the paediatric or adult surgical unit has such organisms. Yeasts and coagulase-negative staphylococci are frequent isolates from patients with biliary stents, but these rarely cause true infection.

At the present time bile specimens are infrequently sent to the laboratory, even from specialist liver units. If a sample from an ERCP or open biliary surgery is sent, there is no value in bile leucocyte counts or a Gram stain, since any positive findings from these tests correlate poorly with the aetiology of the cholangitis or cholecystitis. An exception would be pus obtained from gallbladder empyema when a Gram stain would be useful; even so it is necessary to give broad-spectrum therapy in such cases. Bile samples should be cultured aerobically and anaerobically, but an enrichment culture is of little value. The organisms isolated the next day require some interpretation, as shown in Table 25.2.

Although in other settings *Clostridium perfringens* is associated with serious sepsis such as gas gangrene, in the biliary tree it does not appear to cause anything other than cholangitis and, when isolated from bile draining from a T-tube, can be disregarded if the patient has neither localizing symptoms nor other evidence of sepsis.

The precise antimicrobial therapy varies according to the clinical background and degree of sepsis:

- **Mild cholangitis in a patient with known liver or biliary disease**: oral antibiotic therapy alone is usually sufficient, e.g. trimethoprim; co-amoxiclav (if antibiotics have been given recently ciprofloxacin may be used). In units caring for children with liver disease, ciprofloxacin (normally contraindicated in children) may be considered if resistant enterobacteria are likely to be a cause, if the benefits of therapy outweigh the remote risk of side effects (joint damage has been noted in infant animals). Note also that co-amoxiclav has been associated with cholestasis.

- **Moderate to severe cholangitis and cholecystitis**: intravenous therapy with cefuroxime and metronidazole is suitable for most patients; if there is clinical evidence of sepsis syndrome progressing to shock, or blood cultures with Gram-negative rods, a combination such as gentamicin with piperacillin-tazobactam, or ceftriaxone and metronidazole should be used. Patients who have received recent antimicrobial therapy or have undergone prolonged hospital admission prior to the development of severe sepsis should receive combinations such as piperacillin-tazobactam with or without gentamicin, or ciprofloxacin with amoxycillin, or ceftazidime and amoxycillin. The medical microbiologist should be consulted for advice about the most suitable regimens according to the local microbial resistance patterns in the hospital or unit, and recent cultures from the individual patient. If infection with multiply-resistant enterobacteria is likely, then a carbapenem such as imipenem/cilastatin or meropenem may be indicated. Once the patient has received 48–72 hours of intravenous therapy and if there has been a rapid clinical improvement, then oral therapy may be substituted. Oral trimethoprim with metronidazole, ciprofloxacin with metronidazole, or oral co-amoxiclav alone are suitable regimens for the uncomplicated case. Clearly, antimicrobial therapy is secondary to other

Table 25.2 *Isolation and interpretation of organisms infecting the bile*

Organism	Interpretation	Possible antibiotic therapy
Coliforms, e.g. *E.coli, Klebsiella*	Primary cause of infection	Cefuroxime, ceftriaxone, gentamicin (if septicaemia)
Bacteroides spp., *Clostridium perfringens* and other anaerobes	Primary cause of infection	Metronidazole
Resistant enterobacteria (e.g. cephalosporin-resistant *Enterobacter* or *Klebsiella*)	Hospital-acquired after complex procedures – could be colonization only, if no clinical evidence of infection	If treatment required – consider ciprofloxacin, gentamicin, piperacillin-tazobactam (check susceptibilities)
Resistant enterococci (e.g. vancomycin-resistant strains)	Hospital-acquired after complex procedures – could be colonization only, if no clinical evidence of infection	If treatment required – consider tetracycline, chloramphenicol, linezolid (check susceptibilities)
Yeasts and coagulase-negative staphylococci	Often colonization only	Not indicated unless blood cultures positive or other evidence of infection

interventions such as drainage of an empyema or removal of an obstruction, where these are indicated.

- **Recurrent cholangitis**: this is most common after complex biliary surgery when the biliary tract and its drainage are permanently abnormal, e.g. in a child with a failed Kasai procedure. If attacks of cholangitis are frequent, then oral prophylaxis may be considered. Cycles of 4-weekly oral co-amoxiclav, trimethoprim, ciprofloxacin and cefuroxime, taken twice daily, are convenient regimens for such patients. If 'breakthrough' cholangitis develops then the possibility of resistant organisms should be considered, although in many cases a sensitive organism is isolated from blood cultures.

Carriage of *Salmonella typhi* (also known as *S. enterica* serovar typhi)

Although enteric fever can be readily controlled by antibiotics, the patient may continue to excrete *S. typhi* for several weeks after clinical recovery. The excretion is intermittent, and small numbers of Salmonellae are present in the faeces. However, the infective dose is low and hygienic measures should be emphasized. Some notable outbreaks have been reported when food handlers became long-term excretors.

Should a patient be found to be excreting for several months the possibility of a nidus of infection in the gall-bladder should be considered. Usually, the gallbladder is abnormal with chronic inflammatory changes, scarring and gallstones. Several eradication regimens have been tried, such as 3 months of ampicillin therapy, but failures still occur. The current antibiotic therapy for chronic carriers is ciprofloxacin 750 mg twice daily for 28 days. Failure of this regimen should lead to consideration of whether cholecystectomy is carried out. Such persons should not work as food handlers and should observe good hand hygiene. The risk of transmission is then reduced to a low level.

25.4 HEPATIC, PANCREATIC AND SPLENIC ABSCESSES

Intrahepatic abscesses may be primary lesions found in isolation with no evidence of other pathology in the abdomen or elsewhere. More commonly, the lesion is secondary to infection in sites such as the biliary tree, a colonic diverticulum or an appendix abscess. These abscesses are usually polymicrobial, and the most common organisms isolated are enterobacteria, *Streptococcus intermedius* (Strep. milleri group), and anaerobes such as *Bacteroides fragilis* and *Prevotella* spp. Parasitic causes of hepatic lesions are by nature secondary to invasion from another site such as the gut in the case of amoebic abscess. Bacteraemia or fungaemia from any site may give rise to splenic and hepatic abscesses, most commonly caused by enterobacteria, *Staphylococcus aureus*, *Salmonella* spp.

(more common in developing countries) and yeast-like fungi such as *Candida albicans*. Deep *Candida* infection is seen in the immunocompromised host, but also in patients who have undergone complicated gastrointestinal surgery together with broad-spectrum antibiotic therapy. Oesophageal perforation and surgery is a particular risk for yeast infection. Hepatic abscesses are important complications of liver transplantation, and are a common indication for re-transplantation, especially if the pathogen is multiply antibiotic-resistant and is therefore unlikely to respond to antibiotic therapy and simple drainage. In these patients, organisms such as resistant *Klebsiella* spp., enterococci, methicillin-resistant *Staphylococcus aureus* and *Candida* are of particular concern. Pancreatic abscesses are almost always secondary to pancreatitis, and the organisms responsible are mainly enterobacteria, streptococci and anaerobes. Splenic abscesses should be considered in septic patients with sickle cell disease and in intravenous drug users, when there is evidence of splenomegaly and a poor response to empirical antimicrobial therapy.

Although ultrasonography and computed tomography (CT) scanning are the cornerstones of diagnosis of intra-abdominal lesions, the microbiological diagnosis of any patient with a hepatic, splenic or pancreatic abscess is essential since the mortality is high and a wide range of pathogens may be responsible. Ultrasound-guided aspiration of the lesion or open surgical drainage should yield a reasonable quantity of pus, and if possible at least 10–20 ml should be sent to the laboratory. This facilitates the culture of more fastidious organisms such as anaerobes and microaerophilic streptococci. In addition, blood cultures are essential and must be sent before antibiotics are started. Most of the pathogens listed above are readily grown with good aerobic and anaerobic microbiological techniques. Slow-growing and rarer organisms such as *Nocardia*, *Actinomyces* and *Yersinia* require longer incubation; *Yersinia* infection is best diagnosed by serology, as are parasitic diseases (unless biopsy material, or a worm, is available). Mycobacterial infection is a very rare cause of a solitary abscess, but may need to be considered if multiple small abscesses (microabscesses) are seen on scanning, particularly in an immunocompromised patient. *Candida* may cause a hepatitis in the recovering neutropenic patient (chronic disseminated candidiasis), and the diagnosis is only made on liver biopsy as blood cultures are usually negative. The chronically severely ill patient who has had gut resection and numerous antibiotics is also at risk of disseminated candidiasis, with abscesses in the liver (Figure 25.2). Patients who have been to regions endemic for *Entamoeba histolytica* should have a stool sent for ova, cysts and parasites (see p. 253); it is unlikely that they will have concurrent or recent dysentery, and so the chances of seeing amoebic trophozoites (as opposed to cysts) in faeces are small. However, trophozoites are sometimes seen in a sample

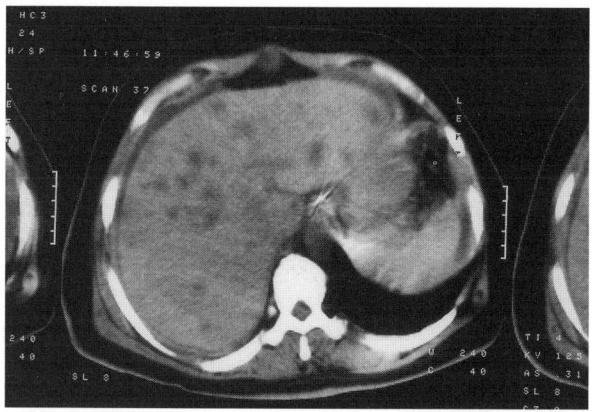

Figure 25.2 *Abdominal CT scan showing multiple hepatic abscesses. Subsequently candida albicans was isolated from abscess pus.*

of the abscess wall – rather than in deep pus – so direct microscopy is worthwhile if this specimen can be obtained. A clotted blood sample for an amoebic fluorescent antibody test (FAT) should also be sent in these patients; this is a very specific test, and if amoebic abscess is likely then a positive test can obviate the need for surgical intervention as antibiotics alone are sufficient in most cases. Reference laboratories can identify amoebic antigens in surgical specimens, and occasionally culture of the amoebae is possible. Patients who have

lived in areas endemic for hydatid disease (see p. 254) should be tested for antibodies to *Echinococcus* spp. before surgical intervention is attempted, otherwise the parasite may be disseminated within the peritoneum. The possibility of secondary bacterial infection of a hydatid cyst may need to be considered in a few cases.

Therapy of abscesses in the liver, spleen or pancreas is obviously dependent on the likely aetiology and the culture and sensitivity results. As empirical therapy, one of the antimicrobial regimens outlined in Table 25.3 should be considered. The duration of intravenous and then oral therapy may need to be continued for several weeks. Expert advice should be sought from a medical microbiologist or infectious disease clinician.

25.5 PARASITIC INFECTIONS ASSOCIATED WITH THE LIVER AND BILIARY TREE

25.5.1 *Entamoeba histolytica*

Entamoeba histolytica is the cause of amoebic dysentery and is also responsible for secondary abscesses at remote sites, particularly the liver and occasionally the lung, bone and brain.

The life cycle is relatively simple: cysts present in contaminated food or water are ingested, after which the amoebae excyst in the small intestine and migrate to the

Table 25.3 *Antimicrobial therapy of hepatic, splenic and pancreatic abscesses*

Clinical setting	Likely pathogen(s)	Empirical or specific therapy
Previously well patient, solitary abscess, no other pathology	Enterobacteria *Strep. intermedius* Anaerobes	Cefuroxime and metronidazole
Previously well patient, visited endemic areas	*Entamoeba histolytica* *Echinococcus granulosus*	Metronidazole followed by diloxanide furoate Albendazole
Patient with other intra-abdominal infection	Enterobacteria *Strep. intermedius* Anaerobes	Cefuroxime, ceftriaxone or cefotaxime plus metronidazole *or* gentamicin, piperacillin-tazobactam (or cefuroxime) and metronidazole
Compromised patient, postoperative	Resistant enterobacteria and enterococci	Ceftriaxone or cefotaxime or ceftazidime or ciprofloxacin plus ampicillin/amoxycillin; *or* Gentamicin and piperacillin-tazobactam
	Candida spp.	Intravenous amphotericin B or fluconazole (N.B. non-*albicans Candida* species may be less susceptible to azole antifungals)

caecum and colon, where they divide by binary fission and infection is established. New cysts are formed and passed in the faeces. Infection at extraintestinal sites does not contribute to the life cycle. There are different subtypes of *E. histolytica* called **zymodenes**, some of which appear to be much more pathogenic than others, but it is likely that the 'non-pathogenic' types are in fact other species of *Entamoeba*. *Entamoeba histolytica* infection of the colon gives rise to abdominal pain, fever and severe diarrhoea with passage of blood and mucus (amoebic dysentery). Flask-shaped ulcers appear in the colonic wall, and a localized pedunculous abscess can develop. Amoebic dysentery may result in systemic invasion, the most common result of which is a single hepatic abscess, but multiple hepatic lesions are sometimes seen. Often, the patient who presents with a hepatic abscess does not recall any diarrhoeal disease. Other abscesses may be found in the lung, brain or bone.

Asymptomatic infection with *E. histolytica* is presumed to occur, since patients may be found to be cyst-passers with no history of amoebiasis. The active amoebae (called **trophozoites** or vegetative forms) are 10 to 30 μm in diameter and can be seen on direct microscopic examination of either liquid faeces, pus from a liver abscess (typically described to have an 'anchovy sauce' appearance) or other abscess; they may also be seen in an abscess wall biopsy. These specimens must be transported rapidly to the laboratory, and the glass microscope slide heated during examination; otherwise the amoebae will form cysts and be more difficult to identify. This is particularly true of the stool specimen (the 'hot stool'), since *E. histolytica* needs to be distinguished from the commensal amoebae. In contrast to the commensals, *E. histolytica* is large, active, and contains ingested red blood cells; the nucleus also has peripheral chromatin on staining. In faeces, cysts may be seen that are 12–15 μm in diameter and contain chromatoid bodies. Although cysts may be seen on direct microscopy of faeces in saline, a formalin-diethyl ether concentration method is usually employed when such parasite cysts are sought. Amoebic cysts are seen in those who are recovering from amoebic dysentery and sometimes in individuals who are completely asymptomatic (cyst passers), as noted above.

Apart from microscopy, *E. histolytica* can be cultured *in vitro* on a 'lawn' of *Escherichia coli*, but this is usually only undertaken in a reference laboratory. Amoebic serology is useful for diagnosis of amoebic abscesses when stool examination is negative and aspiration of pus from a liver abscess or other lesion is difficult; over 95% of patients with an amoebic abscess are antibody-positive after the end of the first 10 days, whereas about 75% of cases of uncomplicated intestinal amoebiasis are antibody-positive. As false-positive serology can occur, a confirmatory test, the cellulose acetate precipitin (CAP) test, is performed on all positive sera. PCR is also available and can be used to identify on-pathogenic anaerobes.

E. histolytica is sensitive to metronidazole given as a 5-day course for treatment of dysentery, extended to 10 days if an abscess is present. Another drug, diloxanide, is used to eradicate the cyst forms in chronic cyst passers or in patients with abscesses. Abscesses do not usually need to be drained surgically. Sewage disposal, food hygiene and the provision of a clean, filtered water supply will prevent the development of endemic amoebiasis within a community.

25.5.2   *Echinococcus*

The most important species, *Echinococcus granulosus*, is the cause of hydatid disease and is found throughout the world in sheep-rearing areas. The adult worm is only a few millimetres long and resides in the gut of dogs and other canines – the definitive hosts. Ova in the faeces may then be ingested by the intermediate hosts, sheep or cattle, or by a human as an accidental host. Within these hosts, the ova release larvae into the gut; these penetrate the gut wall, enter the portal vein and form fluid-filled hydatid cysts in the liver, lungs and other sites. These cysts contain hundreds of scolices, and the life cycle is completed when the dog eats infected viscera of sheep or cattle; when each of the scolices develops into an adult worm. In humans, of course, the life cycle will not be completed and the cysts remain for life.

Hydatid disease, also known as echinococcosis, may involve the liver, lung, bone and central nervous system. Symptoms and signs result from pressure effects at these sites and sometimes from cyst rupture which can rarely cause anaphylaxis; cyst rupture can also result in daughter cysts in the proximal tissues. Hydatid disease may be diagnosed in the laboratory by serological tests such as the hydatid ELISA, or histologically by demonstrating scolices within cyst fluid; however, aspiration of cysts is not a safe procedure. The Casoni skin test is rarely used. The drug that appears to be most active against *E. granulosus* scolices is albendazole, and this can be given as sole therapy. If surgical intervention is planned, albendazole can be given for 3 months preoperatively in order to kill the parasite before the cysts are removed.

Another identified species of *Echinococcus* is *E. multilocularis*, which has a life cycle between that of canines and rodents. When humans are infected, rapidly invasive metastatic cysts develop.

25.5.3   Ascaris ('common roundworm')

This worm is included here as it occasionally ascends the biliary tree from the gut, and causes obstruction. *Ascaris lumbricoides*, which causes ascariasis, is found throughout the world, but particularly in the tropics. The adult worm is about 20–30 cm long, and inhabits the upper and middle small intestine. The female discharges fertilized ova into the faeces, and these may then contaminate either food or water. When the ova are ingested by another individual, larvae hatch out into the small intestine, where they penetrate the bowel wall and migrate through the veins and lymphatics to the lung alveoli. They then ascend to the bronchi, are coughed up and swallowed, thereby returning to the small intestine where they develop into the adult worms. The complete life cycle takes about 3 months.

Ascariasis is diagnosed by finding the ova in faeces; occasionally the worms are vomited or passed in faeces, or found at surgery. The infestation is usually asymptomatic but it can result in malabsorption, intestinal obstruction, biliary colic (due to a worm obstructing the biliary tree) and pneumonitis (due to migrating larvae); rarely, aberrant worms are found in different regions of the body.

The worm is sensitive to mebendazole, but piperazine may also be used, particularly in children aged under 2 years who cannot be treated with mebendazole.

25.6 LIVER FLUKES: *CLONORCHIS, OPISTHORCIS, FASCIOLA*

These three flukes are all animal parasites that occasionally infect humans as an incidental host. Like *Schistosoma* spp., they all have an intermediate stage in water-snails, but the cercariae encyst upon the surface of a second intermediate host, and this second host is then eaten by animals or humans.

25.6.1 *Clonorchis*

Clonorchis sinensis, the oriental liver fluke, is found in China, Japan and other areas of the Far East. The adult worm resides in the biliary tree of fish-eating mammals; the ova enter the faeces and the larvae first infect snails and then encyst on fish scales. If the fish is eaten raw or improperly cooked, both humans and animals may become infected; the cysts (metacercariae) produce larvae in the duodenum, which enter the biliary tree and become adults. Most infected individuals are asymptomatic but cholangitis and (after many years) cholangiocarcinoma can develop.

25.6.2 *Opisthorcis*

This liver fluke of cats and dogs can occasionally infect humans; it is prevalent in the Far East and Eastern Europe; its life cycle is similar to that of *Clonorchis*.

25.6.3 *Fasciola*

Fasciola hepatica affects sheep worldwide, and can infect humans after the ingestion of aquatic plants (the second intermediate host) contaminated with cysts of metacercariae. Biliary colic and hepatomegaly may be features early on in the infection.

25.7 ABNORMAL HEPATIC AND SPLENIC FUNCTION PREDISPOSING TO INFECTION

The role of the normal liver and spleen in the prevention and control of serious infection cannot be underestimated. Abolition of either hepatic or splenic function (or both) places the host at serious risk of overwhelming sepsis. As noted above, hepatocellular damage such as cirrhosis allows the gut bacteria to enter the systemic circulation more readily. However, other, more subtle immunological effects related to liver function are also important, and these are outlined below.

25.7.1 Acute liver failure

In the UK, the main causes of acute liver failure (ALF) are paracetamol overdose, fulminant viral infection (hepatitis B and C) and adverse drug reactions. Patients with ALF are known to have numerous immunological defects that increase their susceptibility to infection, particularly reduced levels of serum complement (mainly C3 and C5 components) and impaired phagocytosis of microorganisms by Küpffer cells. In acute and chronic liver disease, levels of endotoxin in the circulation are raised because the gut-derived endotoxin is not cleared by the liver. Endotoxaemia may have a role in the development of hepatorenal syndrome in ALF since endotoxin (lipopolysaccharide) induces cytokines to be released from macrophages and other cells, and causes haematological disturbances secondary to the activation of complement, kallikrein and coagulation mechanisms. Endotoxaemia also damages the vascular endothelium directly, with subsequent capillary leakage. ALF patients require arterial, central venous pressure and Swanz–Gans line to be inserted, and unfortunately these are all important sources of bacteraemia. Approximately 50% of patients require treatment by haemodialysis, endotracheal intubation and ventilation, all of which increase the risk of bacteraemia and other infections. Cerebral oedema in ALF patients precludes chest physiotherapy, and the subsequent accumulation of secretions may increase the risk of chest infection. Infections are almost inevitable in patients with ALF, and occur in up to 80% of patients who are not given antibiotics on admission. In about one-third, conventional indicators of infection such as pyrexia and an elevated peripheral white blood cell count are absent. The predominant bacterial pathogens are *Staphylococcus aureus*, coagulase-negative staphylococci and *Escherichia coli*. Fungal infection is also common, particularly with *Candida albicans*, often with a concomitant bacterial infection. For these reasons, all patients with ALF should receive antibiotic therapy on diagnosis since this significantly reduces mortality and progression to encephalopathic coma. Patients who proceed to transplantion for ALF have more episodes of infection compared with patients with chronic liver, and the risk of fungal infection is five times greater. These patients should therefore receive intravenous amphotericin B routinely for 21 days after transplantation, whatever the clinical state.

25.7.2 Splenectomy and hyposplenism

Splenic dysfunction or splenectomy is associated with a high level of susceptibility to capsulate bacteria, principally pneumococci, meningococci and haemophili. The precise defect is uncertain, but is probably related to defective major histocompatability complex (MHC) class II-associated presentation of capsular antigens to T cells by macrophages within the spleen.

If a patient is to undergo an elective splenectomy for any reason, they should be immunized at least 2 weeks beforehand (preferably longer) with the following vaccines: pneumococcal 23-valent; *Haemophilus influenzae* type b (Hib), if not given previously; and influenza vaccine. Patients undergoing emergency splenectomy should have the same protocol immediately after the operation, i.e. before leaving hospital. Those who are hyposplenic, mainly patients with sickle cell disease, thalassaemia major, Hodgkin's disease and CLL should receive Hib as part of their childhood schedule (no childhood vaccine is contraindicated in splenic dysfunction). Pneumococcal vaccine is only given after the age of 2 years as it is ineffective below this age (but new conjugate pneumococcal vaccines containing fewer pneumococcal serotypes appear to be suitable for children in this age group). Antibiotic prophylaxis should prevent infection in the first 2 years of life. Meningococcal A + C vaccine must be offered to those travelling to high-risk areas such as the Middle East, Africa and India, or after a close contact with a case of meningococcal infection. All of these patients should also receive oral penicillin V (125 to 500 mg twice daily), the dose depending on age, for *at least* 2 years or until they are 16 years of age, whichever is the longer. However, *lifelong* penicillin prophylaxis is recommended. Erythromycin is an alternative (125 to 500 mg once daily, the dose depending on age). Patients should also be given a supply of amoxycillin to be taken (at home) if there is evidence of a febrile illness, whereupon medical attention should be sought. Penicillin-allergic patients should increase the dose of erythromycin. Such patients must carry a warning card and obtain medical attention if a febrile illness develops.

Re-vaccination with pneumococcal vaccine should be given every 5 to 10 years, and influenza vaccine given annually.

25.8 SURGICAL AND MEDICAL PROCEDURES PROMOTING INFECTION

25.8.1 Biliary tree

As noted earlier, bacterial cholangitis may occur after procedures on the biliary tree such as biliary surgery, ERCP, biliary stent insertion and choledochojejunostomy. Infections may be prevented through good surgical technique and, where indicated, single-dose antibacterial prophylaxis (particularly directed against coliforms and some anaerobes). In the case of ERCP, correct disinfection of the endoscope is essential after each patient, and the instrument and accessories must be stored dry, in compliance with current guidelines. Severe and life-threatening sepsis secondary to endoscope contamination with *Pseudomonas aeruginosa* has been noted when glutaraldehyde disinfection, rinsing and drying have been inadequate. Liver biopsies and transcutaneous aspiration of bile or injection of radiological contrast media are very rarely associated with deep infection, although *Staph. aureus* infection of the skin penetration site may occasionally be seen.

25.8.2 Liver transplantation

The majority of infections in liver transplant patients occur in the first 6–8 weeks after transplant, and are mostly related to the surgical procedure rather than to immunosuppression. These include general infections common to all major surgery, such as wound and urinary tract infection, central and peripheral line sepsis, peritonitis secondary to anastomotic leaks, and lower-respiratory tract infections. In addition there may be cholangitis, and hepatic or perihepatic abscesses. Patients transplanted for ALF are more likely to have these infections and are particularly prone to deep *Candida* infections. In many centres infections in transplant patients are often caused by more resistant pathogens such as MRSA, vancomycin-resistant enterococci and Gram-negative bacteria resistant to most β-lactam antibiotics, such as *Enterobacter*, *Klebsiella* or *Acinetobacter*. Prophylaxis and treatment must therefore be tailored to the microbial flora of the individual transplant unit.

'Late' infections after liver transplant are those infections which arise as a result of the concurrent immunosuppressive therapy: cyclosporin or tacrolimus, and steroids. Acute rejection is also a risk factor for infection. *Pneumocystis* and aspergillosis are in fact quite unusual after transplant, whereas CMV and other herpesvirus infections are common. The requirement for immunizations has been noted earlier, (see p. 246).

Currently, insufficient data are available on infections after pancreatic and small bowel transplant, although it is likely that the infectious problems will be similar to those occurring after liver transplantation.

25.9 INFECTION CAUSING HEPATOSPLENOMEGALY

Numerous infections may give rise to hepatic and/or splenic enlargement, usually with some disturbance of hepatic function evident on blood chemistry. The following are the most important causes:

- **Congenital infections**: these include CMV, rubella, *Listeria*, syphilis and toxoplasma.
- **Children and adults**:
  - *Bacteria*: typhoid and paratyphoid, tuberculosis, *Brucella*, syphilis, relapsing fever, rickettsial infections, tularaemia.
  - *Viruses*: EBV, acute and established HIV.
  - *Fungi*: histoplasmosis.
  - *Parasites*: malaria (splenomegaly), visceral leishmaniasis, African and South American trypanosomiasis, schistosomiasis.

25.10 FURTHER READING

Cook, G. (ed.) (1996) *Manson's Tropical Diseases*, 12th edition. W.B. Saunders, London.

Lee, W.M. and Williams, R. (eds) (1997) *Acute Liver Failure*. Cambridge University Press, Cambridge, UK.

Mandell, G.L., Bennett, J.E. and Dolin, R. (eds) (2000) *Principles and Practice of Infectious Diseases*, 5th edition. Churchill Livingstone, New York.

APPENDIX: SUMMARY OF COMMON ORGANISMS CAUSING BILIARY AND HEPATIC INFECTION

Enterobacteriaceae

These include the lactose fermenters: *Escherichia, Klebsiella, Serratia, Enterobacter* and *Citrobacter* – these genera are sometimes collectively known as 'coliforms'.

Non-lactose fermenters include *Proteus, Providencia, Morganella, Salmonella, Shigella* and *Yersinia*.

These organisms are nearly all large Gram-negative rods, and they may be found in the lower gastrointestinal tract as commensals or pathogens (*Yersinia pestis* is an exception). They are distinguishable from other Gram-negative rods by a number of characteristics: (i) the oxidase test is negative; (ii) they grow aerobically and anaerobically on simple media such as nutrient agar; and (iii) they tolerate bile salts, hence their ability to colonize the gut.

The various genera are differentiated principally by biochemical tests and the detection of surface antigens using serology. They can be broadly divided according to their ability or inability to ferment lactose on MacConkey agar (this agar contains bile salts, lactose and phenol red indicator so that when organisms fermenting lactose produce acid, the indicator colour changes and the colonies appear deep pink or magenta). Examples are *Escherichia* and *Klebsiella*. Colonies of non-lactose fermenters are pale pink or colourless; examples are *Shigella, Salmonella* and *Proteus*.

Further biochemical tests are performed in order to identify the enterobacteria to genus and species level. In addition to the biochemical tests, some enterobacteria can be identified by analysis of their surface antigens. Enterobacteria have a complex antigenic structure; all have O (cell wall) antigens and those that are motile have H (flagellar) antigens. Some strains within a species have a microcapsule – called a K antigen, when it occurs in *Klebsiella* or *E. coli*; and some salmonellae have an equivalent Vi (virulence) antigen. The O antigen is in fact located at the outer end of the molecule **lipopolysaccharide**, otherwise known as endotoxin. This molecule comprises lipid A, which forms part of the outer membrane of all Gram-negative bacteria, and a chain of saccharides terminating in the variable region O-antigen. Endotoxin is released during cell death, and to some extent during replication. It is a very potent cause of fever, sepsis syndrome and shock in the patient infected with a Gram-negative organism.

Some species of enterobacteria are particularly adept at acquiring and transmitting antimicrobial resistance genes borne on plasmids – in particular *Klebsiella* and *Enterobacter* spp. These genera also survive more readily on the hands of staff, and so epidemics of infection may occur unless strict hand hygiene is observed.

Pseudomonas

Members of this genus are motile, strict aerobes, and have a wide temperature range for growth, from below 10°C up to 43°C. Pseudomonads are motile, oxidase-positive and grow easily on nutrient agar; some can even multiply in plain water and mild disinfectants such as cetrimide. This is because they can use the simplest carbon compounds for synthesis of complex organic molecules. On MacConkey agar they are non-lactose fermenters. Pseudomonads are mostly found in wet sites such as rivers, streams, standing water, sink traps, drains and any surfaces wet for long periods of time – including medical equipment.

Pseudomonas aeruginosa is the most important species. It produces a green pigment (pyocyanin) when grown on nutrient agar. Some strains of *Ps. aeruginosa*, particularly those cultured from the sputum of patients with cystic fibrosis, are very mucoid and the colonies almost drip off the agar plate.

Ps. aeruginosa is widely distributed in the environment, especially water, soil and plants, but is rapidly destroyed on drying. It may be carried in small numbers in the colonic or perineal flora (3–5% of individuals, but higher in hospitalized or immunocompromised patients), and it can appear as a commensal in the sputum and in superficial sites of hospitalized patients. Those receiving long-term assisted ventilation who have a tracheostomy can be colonized in their upper respiratory tract, as are patients with severe chronic chest disease such as cystic fibrosis. Food and water may be a source of *Pseudomonas*, and transmission to patients from hospital meals has been documented. In the clinical settings of immunosuppression, intensive care management and chronic chest disease (especially cystic fibrosis), *Ps. aeruginosa* can become invasive and cause opportunist infections with a high mortality, such as pneumonia and septicaemia; these are sometimes accompanied by necrotic skin lesions – echthyma gangrenosum. As a hospital pathogen it may also cause urinary tract infection in catheterized patients; infections of burns and other wounds; and infections of intravenous lines, Hickman lines, shunts and peritoneal dialysis catheters. Rarely, severe eye infections may occur after eye surgery, when *Pseudomonas* contamination of a fluid or instrument should be considered. Patients admitted to hospital from the community may sometimes have a severe infection with *Ps. aeruginosa*, for example 'malignant' otitis externa, an invasive destructive infection seen in diabetics. Individuals with no underlying disease may acquire a *Pseudomonas* dermatitis from contaminated whirlpools and other warm water-jet baths; swimmers may get superficial otitis externa; and eye infections from contaminated eye drops or contact lens fluids are seen rarely.

Outbreaks of *Pseudomonas* infections have been reported and are frequently traced to contaminated fluids; equipment such as ventilator tubing, flexible endoscopes and humidifiers are also a potential source of infection, especially if inadequately disinfected or if left wet for long periods of time.

For diagnosis, *Ps. aeruginosa* is easy to culture from clinical samples, but if grown from a site with a normal flora, e.g. the upper respiratory tract, it should not be regarded as causing infection unless appropriate signs and symptoms of infection are present.

Ps. aeruginosa has a complex cell wall and a slime layer; consequently it is resistant to most of the usual antibiotics. Important anti-pseudomonals are the aminoglycosides, the extended-spectrum penicillins (e.g. piperacillin-tazobactam, azlocillin, ticarcillin), cephalosporins (e.g. ceftazidime), monobactams (e.g. aztreonam) and carbapenems (imipenem or meropenem). Quinolones such as ciprofloxacin are also active, and since they can be given orally are of value in continuation therapy in serious infections.

Clostridium perfringens

C. perfringens is carried as part of the normal bowel flora of both humans and animals. Infants frequently have large numbers of clostridia. The spores are also found in soil and dust.

C. perfringens causes food poisoning and gas gangrene (secondary either to trauma or to amputative surgery); and it is occasionally found in intra-abdominal abscesses or severe wound and pelvic infections, usually mixed with other bowel organisms. Cultures of bile taken at operation for gallbladder disease occasionally grow *C. perfringens*, but this is very unlikely to lead to necrotic infection.

Of the non-type A *C. perfringens*, type C has been identified as the cause of enteritis necroticans (pig-bel). Types B, D and E cause economically important diarrhoeal disease in sheep and cattle.

Bacteroides spp. and Fusobacterium spp.

Bacteroides is involved in a wide range of infections, usually secondary to disease, trauma or surgery of the colon or other sites with an anaerobic flora. Specimens from intra-abdominal infections such as abscesses and faecal peritonitis frequently grow *Bacteroides* spp. together with Gram-positive anaerobes and enterobacteria. In addition, *Bacteroides* is involved in some postoperative wound infections, lung abscess, empyema and necrotizing pneumonia, otitis media, sinusitis, cerebral abscess, intra-oral abscess, osteomyelitis, paronychia, anaerobic vaginosis and pelvic inflammatory disease. It almost never causes urinary tract infection, and only a few cases of *Bacteroides* endocarditis have been reported.

Of the several species, *B. fragilis* is the most pathogenic; it possesses superoxide dismutase to enhance oxygen-tolerance, and has a capsule which promotes abscess formation. In addition it is resistant to penicillin, whereas all other species are sensitive. Some species have been placed in a separate genus, *Prevotella*.

Fusobacterium has a characteristic spindle-shaped appearance on Gram stain, and has a habitat and infective role similar to that of *Bacteroides*. In addition, fusobacteria together with the spirochaete *Borrelia vincentii* cause the infection Vincent's angina (acute necrotizing ulcerative gingivitis, and pharyngeal ulceration). The species *F. necrophorum* is responsible for necrobacillosis, a rare illness affecting young adults who present with a sore throat, septicaemia and disseminated abscesses. It is sensitive to penicillin. *Bacteroides* and *Fusobacterium* are sensitive to a number of antibiotics; with very rare exceptions they are highly sensitive to metronidazole and the related compound tinidazole. Penicillins are active (but not against *B. fragilis*), as are erythromycin, clindamycin and chloramphenicol; many cephalosporins, however, have poor activity (cefoxitin is an exception), and all anaerobes are resistant to the aminoglycosides.

Streptococcus intermedius (formerly part of the *Strep. milleri* group)

Streptococcus intermedius, like enterococci, is often non-haemolytic but possesses Lancefield antigens like those in beta-haemolytic streptococci. Some strains have the Lancefield group F antigen and are identified by other characteristics, such as the caramel odour of agar cultures, the fermentation of sugars and certain enzyme reactions. *Strep. intermedius* is part of the normal gastrointestinal tract flora; it is sometimes associated with abscess formation, in both previously healthy and immunocompromised patients; it may be the sole pathogen, but is more commonly found in mixed culture from abdominal, liver, lung and cerebral abscesses. It is very sensitive to all types of penicillins, and erythromycin. *Strep. anginosis* and *Strep. constellatis* are also members of this group.

Infections in urological surgery

J.D. WILLIAMS AND K.G. NABER

26.1 INTRODUCTION AND CLASSIFICATION

Infection in the normal urinary tract may occur by bacteria spreading up the urethra into the normal bladder, or it may complicate a urinary tract that is already anatomically or physiologically abnormal. Infection may occur throughout life from birth to old age, and any underlying physical disease in the patient may influence the progression of the infection and the response to therapy. It is clear that infections vary widely in their significance for the patient, choice of therapy and outcome. Therefore some form of classification of urinary tract infections is necessary for diagnosis, therapy and follow-up.

It is usual to classify the infections into whether or not they occur in a normal or abnormal urinary tract, although it may not be known at presentation if the urinary tract is abnormal (Table 26.1). Other subdivisions are related to age, and the following age groups have particular points in relation to causation and management: (i) the neonate (especially male); (ii) the young child (especially female); (iii) young women; (iv) pregnant women; (v) patients with diabetes; and (vi) elderly persons of both sexes (especially males).

Because there is such a high prevalence of urinary tract infection in the normal urinary tract of females, the commonest division is into infections of young women (either pregnant or not pregnant) which are labelled as non-complicated; and all other types of urinary tract infection which are called **complicated**. Infections of the urethra, prostate and testicle fall into a special category. Hospital-acquired infections also require special consideration, and may occur in patients with either normal or abnormal urinary tracts.

Most surgical contact is with patients who have abnormal urinary tracts, but at initial consultation it is not known if the urinary tract is abnormal or not and only a minority of patients presenting with urinary tract infection have abnormalities. Surgeons also see urinary tract infection in their hospitalized patients who are in the wards for various forms of surgical intervention other than urological.

Table 26.1 *Classification of urinary tract infections*

1. Non-complicated urinary tract infection
    (i) Young women
    (ii) Young pregnant women

2. Complicated urinary tract infection
    (i) Neonates
    (ii) Small children
    (iii) Adults with anatomically abnormal urinary tract
    (iv) Patients with underlying diseases such as diabetes
    (v) The elderly
    (vi) Patients with prostate obstructions
    (vii) The catheterized patient

3. Special considerations
    (i) Sexually transmitted diseases
    (ii) Prostatitis
    (iii) Epididymo-orchitis

26.2 NON-COMPLICATED URINARY TRACT INFECTIONS

Between 20 and 30% of adult women experience episodes of increased frequency of micturition and dysuria one or more times each year. About half of these episodes are associated with large numbers of bacteria and pus cells in the urine. In some of these patients, risk factors such as vaginal colonization with enterobacteria may be found, while in others there is a relationship to sexual intercourse. Women with recurrent infection may have enhanced adherence of *Escherichia coli* to mucosal epithelial cells, but others may have *E. coli* with enhanced virulence in their faecal flora. Some may have congenital or acquired abnormalities of the urinary tract. Patients with frequent recurrences require investigation in order to exclude any underlying reason for the recurrences and indeed, in the great majority of those with frequent infections, no underlying cause is found. Persistent infections with the same organism which relapse soon after treatment is an indication for early investigation compared with those with infrequent recurrences due to new strains entering the lower urinary tract from the perineal flora. Current evidence suggests that women presenting to the general practitioner with urinary tract infection should be treated first, and that no urine cultures are performed at this stage. Only those with persistent symptoms or frequent recurrences are given the benefit of urine cultures. This is 'cost-effective' because treatment is less expensive than urine culture, and is quicker to initiate.

26.3 BACTERIOLOGICAL DIAGNOSIS OF URINARY TRACT INFECTIONS

Urinary tract infection is defined quantitatively. If bacteria are established in the urine and are growing well, the numbers usually exceed well over 10^6 ml^{-1}; and a level of 10^5 cells ml^{-1} is frequently taken as the cut-off point for infection. This should not be regarded as absolute, however. In the early stages of infection, numbers may be smaller, perhaps 10^3–10^4 cells ml^{-1}, or frequent voiding may help to keep the bacterial population below 10^5 cells ml^{-1}.

26.3.1 Urine cultures

In the interests of economy, as stated earlier, it is often advised that urine cultures of spontaneous uncomplicated infections in young women are unnecessary. As the cost of cultures may be higher than the cost of treatment, it is more cost-effective to treat first and culture afterwards only if symptoms persist. One argument against this policy is that 50% of persons with symptoms suggestive of urinary tract infection have few, if any, bacteria in the urine, and hence half of the patients receive antibiotics unnecessarily. The doctor may also be uncertain as to whether or not the patient had a urinary tract infection or some other condition that might give rise to frequency and dysuria, e.g. early pregnancy or urethritis. One further problem arises in the absence of a urine culture. Antibiotic resistance is increasing among the enterobacteria that are mainly responsible for urinary tract infections. For example, in many places *E. coli* may show a resistance rate of 30% to either trimethoprim or ampicillin, or to both. In such circumstances, other antibiotics, which are perhaps best kept for other purposes, are used instead. Unless good epidemiological data are available, or cultures are made from a consecutive series of urinary infections that has arisen in the local community, it is not possible to establish what the primary therapy should be. There is a suspicion that the rising rate of resistance reported in uropathogens may be distorted because the numerical data are drawn from patients who have already failed a course of treatment; therefore, a preponderance of antibiotic-resistant organisms is isolated.

26.3.2 Interpretation of urine cultures

Infection is accompanied by an excess of pus cells. In patients with asymptomatic bacteriuria, the number of white blood cells may be low, but most symptomatic infections show an excess of white cells in the urine. The finding of many squamous epithelial cells in the urine indicates skin or vaginal contamination, and this may arise from contamination by perineal bacteria. In infected urine, one bacterial species tends to predominate, and the 10^5 ml^{-1} cut-off only applies if a single bacterial species, for example *E. coli*, is present. Patients with chronic catheters *in situ* or other mechanical invasion of the urinary tract may, on occasion, show more than one species at a level of 10^5 ml^{-1} or more, but in other patients, the presence of large numbers of bacteria of different species indicates that the specimens were unsuitable for examination.

26.3.3 Uropathogens

There is little variety of the organisms found in spontaneous infection in patients with a normal urinary tract. *E. coli* accounts for 80–90% of infections, and coagulase-negative staphylococci for up to 10%. Organisms other than these are unusual and are usually contaminants. Some other species do, however, appear. *Proteus mirabilis* is important because its alkalinization of the urine may precipitate crystals, forming a nidus for calculus. Other enterobacteria such as *Klebsiella* are also found in a small percentage of cases. Finding of significant numbers of organisms such as *Pseudomonas* spp. may indicate recent hospitalization, whilst *Enterococcus faecalis* can be seen in elderly men with outflow difficulties.

In patients requiring either hospital care, individual catheterization or urological surgery (especially to the lower urinary tract), infection is common and generally involves a wide variety of organisms. These organisms reflect those found in the ward environment and include various enterobacteria including *Klebsiella*, *Enterobacter*, *Proteus* spp. (other than *mirabilis*), staphylococci and enterococci, pseudomonads and *Acinetobacter* species. Several types of yeasts, mainly *Candida* spp., may also establish themselves in the urine. *E. coli* still accounts for 40–50% of these hospital-acquired infections, although the antibiotic resistance pattern may differ significantly from that seen in community-acquired species.

26.4 COMPLICATED URINARY TRACT INFECTIONS

The major significance of the division between complicated and non-complicated urinary tract infections relates to the prognosis for the renal function of the patient. Non-complicated urinary tract infection is not associated with decline in renal function, even in patients with many recurrences over several years. Complicated infections are those in which such a benign course may not take place and the patient requires careful monitoring. The complication of obstruction plus infection is particularly destructive of kidney function and requires more acute intervention by the surgeon, including more aggressive therapy or chemoprophylaxis.

Some pointers to possible complications are shown in Table 26.2. The categories of patients shown include only those where there is agreement that the risks exist; some lesions in the list are more acute than others. Some categories where the effects of significant renal damage are debatable, (e.g. in the elderly female with anatomically

normal urinary tract and other categories of non-immunocompetent patients) have not been included.

This group of patients can be expected to be very heterogeneous, ranging from severe obstructive acute pyelonephritis with imminent urosepsis up to catheter-associated, postoperative urinary tract infection that might disappear spontaneously as soon as the catheter is removed. The aim of treatment of complicated urinary tract infection is to restore normal urodynamics and renal function as far as possible.

Patients are especially prone to urinary tract infection in the case of an in-dwelling urethral catheter, even if a closed drainage system is used; indeed it is only a matter of time before bacteriuria and urinary tract infection occur. A suprapubic catheter is preferable, but even then this may only postpone the onset of bacteriuria.

The surface of a catheter is uneven and biologically rough, and a biofilm grows on its surface; within this biofilm large amounts of microbial debris bind to cells and to the substratum. Biofilm urinary infection is associated not only with catheters, but also with infected stones, scar tissue and/or necrotic tissue, chronic obstructive uropathies and chronic bacterial prostatitis. Bacteria growing in biofilms differ markedly from planktonic (or floating cells) in the same ecosystem and from cells grown in pure culture for laboratory tests in regard to their vulnerability to treatment. The bactericidal antibiotic dose determined by laboratory tests to be sufficient does not have any effect on bacteria in a biofilm, where the bacteria are also protected from host defence mechanisms and cause intractable chronic persistent urinary tract infection. Underlying disorders of the urinary tract also favour the occurrence of biofilm. The treatment of biofilm infection is prevention by employing scrupulous catheterization procedures (by a 'catheter team' when practical), frequent changes of the catheter, and use of the least irritant catheters available. At present, no effective antibiotic is available, but some fluoroquinolones and macrolides penetrate the biofilm better than others.

Table 26.2 *Possible complications of urinary tract infections*

Group	Pathology	Possible presentation
Neonate male	Urethral valves obstructing urine outflow	Fever, oliguria Swollen abdomen Septicaemia
Young girl	Vesico-ureteric reflux with hydronephrosis	Recurrent infections, low growth rate, anaemia
Pregnant woman	Pelvi-ureteric dilation	Ascending pyelonephritis Fever, loin pain
Diabetes	Chronic nephrosclerosis	Laboratory evidence of diminishing renal function
Elderly male	Prostate hypertrophy	Outflow irregularities
The catheterized patient	Recurrent infections	Fever, anorexia, pyuria

Cross-infection is the major cause for the spread of resistant strains throughout the hospital. Patients with indwelling catheters play an important role as donors as well as recipients of bacteria. *Pseudomonas* spp., coagulase-negative staphylococci and enterococci are not very virulent in the urinary tract, and a substantial proportion disappear without therapy after the catheter is removed or the urodynamics are restored. In one clinic, a spontaneous cure rate was observed of 20% with *Ps. aeruginosa*, 60% with enterococci and 63% with coagulase-negative staphylococci. This suggests that every episode of bacteriuria does not need to be treated with antibiotics, but only if a patient is symptomatic or a urological intervention must to be performed. When urodynamic conditions improve, or the source of biofilm is removed, there is a high chance of spontaneous clearance, although this may take several months.

26.5 TREATMENT OF URINARY TRACT INFECTIONS

Because the symptoms of urinary tract infection may be severe, treatment is often started before the results of culture are known. The choice of presumptive therapy varies and is based on generally available clinical and epidemiological evidence.

26.5.1 Acute urinary tract infections arising in the community

Most of these infections are treated by the general practitioner, though more severe cases may be directed to the emergency departments of hospitals. Patients with evidence of renal involvement such as high fever, denoting possible bacteraemia, and pain and tenderness over one or both kidneys usually find themselves admitted to hospital. The strategy of treatment is shown in Table 26.3. If good epidemiological evidence is available on susceptibility this should play a part in the selection of an antibiotic. A prevalence of resistance of up to 20% to a simple oral antibiotic may be acceptable when treating a mild urinary tract infection, but this is clearly not acceptable for patients with pyelonephritis and high fever.

Many studies have shown that short-term therapy (single dose or treatment up to 3 days) is sufficient. The advantages of such a regimen are good compliance, lower cost, a lower rate of adverse events and a reduced influence on the periurethral, vaginal and rectal flora. Several studies have shown that persistent bacteriuria after 2–3 days' treatment indicate the presence of complicating factors within the urinary tract. In most studies the failure rates are low, and short-term treatment could also be used as a diagnostic tool, in that patients failing short-term therapy with two separate courses of different antibiotics would be considered for further urological investigation.

Evidence-based guidelines for antimicrobial therapy of uncomplicated acute bacterial cystitis and pyelonephritis in women have been devised by a committee of the Infectious Diseases Society of America (IDSA) and the following conclusions were drawn:

- Most antimicrobials given for 3 days are as effective as longer durations. Longer treatment usually showed higher rate of adverse events.
- A 3-day regimen with trimethoprim-sulphamethoxazole (TMP/SMZ) can be considered the standard therapy. Trimethoprim alone was equivalent to TMP/SMZ in eradication and adverse effects. Trimethoprim alone or TMP/SMZ can be recommended as first-line drugs for empirical therapy in communities with rates of uropathogen resistance

Table 26.3 *Strategy for antibiotic therapy for urinary tract infections in the community*

Type of Infection	Management
Mild symptoms, no fever, indefinite diagnosis	Urine culture results should be awaited before treatment.
Moderate symptoms haematuria, no evidence of pyelonephritis	Urine should be taken for culture but treatment started. If urine culture negative (and results received within 3 days) antibiotics should be stopped.
	Choice of antibiotics as for infection in patients with non-specific symptoms and proven culture.
	Patients should be reviewed at 3 days. Patients with persistent symptoms may need an antibiotic from the second choice list.
Severe symptoms with signs of pyelonephritis	Urine and blood cultures should be taken before parenteral antibiotics are given. Parenteral antibiotics can be replaced by oral therapy after 3–5 days but duration of therapy should be for at least 14 days.

to trimethoprim of less than 10%. There is a close correlation between susceptibility and eradication of *E. coli*.

- The fluoroquinolones are probably similarly effective as TMP/SMZ when given as a 3-day regimen. Fluoroquinolones are more expensive than TMP and TMP/SMZ and not recommended as first-line drugs, except in communities with resistance rates to trimethoprim of more than 10%.
- *β*-Lactams as a group are less effective than the foregoing drugs. When oral cephalosporins or aminopenicillins are combined with a *β*-lactamase inhibitor, no large study for comparison with a 3-day trimethoprim or TMP/SMZ is available.
- Nitrofurantoin requires further study and cannot yet be considered a suitable drug for short-term therapy.
- Cystitis in older women and episodes caused by *Staphylococcus saprophyticus* may respond better to longer durations of therapy, for example, 7 days.

CHOICE OF AGENTS

Fluoroquinolones which are excreted in the urine such as ciprofloxacin, ofloxacin and norfloxacin have been extensively used for treatment of all types of urinary tract infection. In uncomplicated cystitis, trimethoprim with or without sulphamethoxazole is an acceptable option. In pyelonephritis, cefuroxime (or an equivalent cephalosporin) or co-amoxiclav are alternatives. In complicated infections, susceptibility of the uropathogen provides a guide to choice of agent which may need to include broader-spectrum cephalosporins, such as cefotaxime, aminoglycosides or even carbapenems and antifungal drugs.

About one-third of the patients with uncomplicated cystitis will become symptom-free within 1 day, and an additional 50% within 2 days. Patients with recurring infections, (i.e. more than twice within 6 months) should be offered antibacterial prophylaxis such as a daily low dose of, for example, either nitrofurantoin (50 mg), trimethoprim (50 mg), or co-trimoxazole (40 mg/200 mg); for pregnant or lactating women, cephalexin 250 mg; for patients with urinary tract infections related to sexual intercourse, a single post-coital dose may be sufficient. In cases of 'break-through' infection, a low dose (125 mg) of ciprofloxacin, for example, is recommended. Some patients with infrequent recurrent urinary tract infection may prefer self-medication when clinical symptoms occur. In post-menopausal women, a hormonal periurethral and intravaginal oestrogen cream may reduce the frequency of recurrences.

The duration of therapy for mild or moderately acute symptomatic infection which is clinically confined to the lower urinary tract is 3 days. For patients with evidence of renal involvement, treatment should be continued for a period of 7–14 days.

26.5.2 Treatment of urinary tract infections arising in hospital

The variety of organisms isolated from infections of the urinary tract in hospital is so wide, and the susceptibility of the organism so varied, that identification of the infecting organism and susceptibility testing are essential to allow correct selection of antibiotic therapy. Such infections are often symptom-free, and may be associated with catheterization and prolonged bladder drainage. Treatment in the absence of symptoms is not necessary, especially when the chances of reinfection are high. Unusually there is no requirement for empirical antibiotic therapy on the suspicion of infection because there is usually time to assess the clinical and bacteriological evidence before deciding therapy.

CHOICE OF AGENTS

If it is considered necessary to treat these infections (provided that the organism is not resistant), the choice of antibiotic for each organism is as follows:

- *Pseudomonas*: Ciprofloxacin is the only oral therapy available. If the organism is resistant, then ceftazidime, cefoperazone/sulbactam, piperacillin/tazobactam, are parenteral alternatives. Carbapenems are the ultimate antibiotics available for cases unresponsive to the former.
- **Multi-resistant enterobacteriaceae**: Ciprofloxacin is often the only oral agent available. Oral cephalosporins such as cefuroxime axetil, cefixime or ceftibuten also may be active, as too may co-amoxiclav. The parenteral choice is as for *Pseudomonas*.
- **Enterococci**: These organisms, especially *Enterococcus faecalis*, are usually fully sensitive to amoxycillin. In some hospitals, multi-resistant enterococci are found in very vulnerable patients including those on renal units. Because they may be resistant to vancomycin as well as other agents, finding a suitable antibiotic may be difficult. Fortunately, such infections often do not require therapy. New antibiotics such as oxazolidinones, and streptogramin combinations are now available should such a need arise.
- *Candida* species: Asymptomatic candiduria in immunocompetent patients is usually found in patients with indwelling catheters, and does not need specific therapy. Symptomatic urinary infections due to *Candida* should be treated because the kidneys may become infected and infection become widespread. The availability of oral azoles such as fluconazole certainly makes treatment easier to manage than with intravenous amphotericin. With the increase in the number of patients with poor immune functions, eradication of *Candida* from the urine should be considered even in the absence of symptoms.

26.6 ACUTE UNCOMPLICATED PYELONEPHRITIS

Effective antibacterial treatment must be initiated as soon as possible in pyelonephritis diagnosed clinically by fever, flank pain, pyuria, and bacteriuria with or without lower-urinary tract symptoms in order to prevent renal parenchymal damage and renal scarring. Anatomical or functional abnormalities must be excluded by ultrasonography. Antibiotics active against *E. coli* when administered by the parenteral route (e.g. cephalosporins, aminoglycosides, fluoroquinolones or aminopenicillins/ β-lactamase inhibitors) are suitable for this purpose. Parenteral therapy should be switched as soon as possible to an oral regimen; a 7- to 14-day course is sufficient. C-reactive protein (CRP) may be used as guidance for the duration of therapy. If pyelonephritis is diffuse, a prompt response can be expected. If focal or abscess-forming pyelonephritis is demonstrated by computed tomography scanning or MAG 3 scintigraphy, then treatment duration of between 4 and 8 weeks may be necessary.

26.7 URETHRITIS

Primary urethritis must be differentiated from secondary urethritis, which occurs in patients with in-dwelling catheters or urethral strictures and is caused by uropathogens or by staphylococci. For primary specific urethritis, infectious causes and also chemical or mechanical damage have to be included. Gonorrhoeal or chlamydial urethritis must to be differentiated from non-specific urethritis. Trichomoniasis in the male develops with relatively few symptoms but is well recognized as a cause. *Ureaplasma urealyticum* sometimes causes urethritis. *Mycoplasma hominis* is probably not a cause of urethritis.

Gonorrhoea responds well to ampicillin, procaine penicillin or cefuroxime, whilst doxycycline and azithromycin are considered to be equally effective in the therapy of chlamydial infections. Doxycycline therapy is required for 7 days, while therapy with a single dose of 1g azithromycin can be performed under supervision. Erythromycin is less effective and causes side effects. If therapy fails, infections by *Trichomonas vaginalis* and/or *Mycoplasma* must be taken into consideration, despite doubts about the virulence of the latter organism.

26.8 PROSTATITIS

There is a clear lack of knowledge concerning the epidemiology, pathophysiology, diagnosis and treatment of prostatitis, though the National Institute of Diabetes and Digestive and Kidney Diseases has proposed the following classification system:

- Category I   Acute bacterial prostatitis
- Category II   Chronic bacterial prostatitis
- Category III Chronic pelvic pain syndrome
  - III A   Inflammatory
  - III B   Non-inflammatory
- Category IV   Asymptomatic inflammatory prostatitis.

Despite reports that less than 10% of prostatitis cases are bacterial, a much higher proportion of men diagnosed with prostatitis receive antimicrobials. Antibiotic therapy is recommended for acute bacterial prostatitis and chronic bacterial prostatitis, but is debatable in patients with inflammatory chronic pelvic pain syndrome.

The **chronic prostatitis syndrome** is difficult to manage, and 35–50% of men are affected at some time. Chronic bacterial prostatitis is a clinical entity defined by two basic features: (i) recurrent urinary tract infection; and (ii) persistence of mainly Gram-negative rods in the prostatic secretion. Sequential bacteriological localization cultures are of critical importance. Usually, four cultures are performed; (i) first voided urine; (ii) midstream urine; (iii) expressed prostatic secretion; and (iv) urine after prostatic massage. The different kinds of lower urinary tract infection and prostatitis are separated according to distinguishing patterns of white blood cells. Chronic bacterial prostatitis is diagnosed if pathogenic bacteria are recovered in significant numbers from purulent prostatic fluid in the absence of concomitant urinary tract infection and any signs of acute bacterial prostatitis.

The frequency of chronic bacterial prostatitis in all patients with complaints suggestive of prostatitis is only about 5–10%. It is, therefore, an important but uncommon disease, and is mainly caused by *E. coli* and to a lesser degree by other enterobacteriaceae and *Pseudomonas* species. The causative roles of Gram-positive cocci, *Ureaplasma urealyticum* and *Chlamydia trachomatis* are still undecided.

26.8.1 Therapy of prostatitis

Few antibiotics are able to penetrate well into prostatic secretions, mainly because of the degree of their ionization in plasma. A weak base such as trimethoprim with a pK_a of 7.4 can be expected to be concentrated about 4- to 5-fold in acid prostatic secretion. However, the pH of prostatic fluid in patients with chronic prostatitis is neutral or alkaline, and hence no concentration of trimethoprim can be expected, which probably explains why trimethoprim-sulphamethoxazole provides only a 50% cure rate.

The fluoroquinolones may be better alternatives as they are zwitterions with one pK_a in the acid milieu and one in the alkaline. The isoelectric point of ciprofloxacin is at pH 7.4, which corresponds to the pH of plasma. At this pH, about 90% of ciprofloxacin is not ionized and thus can penetrate through biological barriers. The concentrations of ciprofloxacin in prostatic tissue obtained from patients undergoing TUR of the prostate also exceeded the corresponding plasma concentration confirming good penetration. The duration of treatment should be for a minimum of 2–4 weeks. In chronic prostatitis, relapse is the main problem and the follow-up period must be at least 6 months.

26.9   EPIDIDYMITIS AND ORCHITIS

Inflammation of the epididymis causes pain and swelling which is almost always unilateral and relatively acute in onset. In many cases, the testicle is involved in the inflammatory process which is consequently known as 'epididymo-orchitis'. Correspondingly inflammatory processes of the testicle, especially viral-induced orchitis, often involve the epididymis.

Inflammatory processes of the testicle (orchitis) and epididymis (epididymitis) are classified into acute and chronic processes. In the case of testicular involvement, chronic inflammation may result in testicular atrophy and destruction of spermatogenesis. Complications of epididymo-orchitis include abscess formation, testicular infarction, testicular atrophy, development of chronic epididymal induration and infertility.

Epididymitis caused by sexually transmitted organisms occurs mainly in sexually active males under the age of 35 years. Overall, the majority of cases (especially in older men) are due to common urinary pathogens, frequently the same organisms that cause bacteriuria. Bladder outlet obstruction and urogenital malformations are risk factors for this type of infection. Epididymitis due to uropathogens or sexually transmitted organisms follows the spread of infection from the urethra or bladder. In non-specific granulomatous orchitis, autoimmune phenomena are assumed to trigger chronic inflammation. Orchitis of childhood and mumps-orchitis are of haematogenous origin. Other systemic infections such as tuberculosis, syphilis, brucellosis and cryptococcal diseases may also affect the epididymis.

It is imperative to make the differential diagnosis between epididymitis and spermatic cord torsion immediately using all information, including the age of the patient, history of urethritis, clinical evaluation and Doppler scanning of testicular blood flow. In children and adolescents, torsion must be assumed unless it is proved otherwise (by surgical exposure if no other means is sufficiently positive).

In younger sexually active men, *Chlamydia trachomatis* is common; in elderly men with prostatic or other micturition disturbances, uropathogens are the usual aetiological agents, and antimicrobials for empirical treatment should be selected accordingly. Microbiological results obtained after puncture of the epididymis and from a urethral swab as well as the urine have shown very good correlation; hence, a urethral swab and midstream urine should be obtained for microbiological investigation, before any antimicrobial therapy is given.

Fluoroquinolones active against *C. trachomatis* (e.g. levofloxacin) should be the first-choice drugs because of their broad antibacterial spectra and their favourable penetration into the urogenital tract tissues. If *C. trachomatis* has been confirmed as the aetiological agent, the treatment should be continued with doxycycline 200 mg per day for at least 2 weeks, with macrolides as alternative agents.

Supportive therapy includes bed-rest, support for the testes and anti-inflammatory agents. Since epididymitis in young men can lead to permanent occlusion of the epididymal canal and thus to infertility, antibiotic therapy should be supported with methylprednisolone starting at 40 mg per day and reducing the dose every second day by half. Any underlying causes of micturition disturbances and abscess-forming epididymitis or orchitis, e.g. benign enlargement of the prostate, must be treated surgically.

26.10   PERIOPERATIVE CHEMOPROPHYLAXIS

The aim of perioperative prophylaxis is to limit infection related to intervention. However, it can never compensate for poor operative technique. The need for prophylaxis depends on the type of intervention and the individual risk for each individual patient. Risk factors such as chronic debility, diabetes mellitus, immunosuppression, poor surgical condition, reoperation and special risk factors, e.g. artificial cardiac valves, must be considered. In the absence of risk factors and if the patient has sterile urine, prophylaxis is not mandatory in urological procedures.

The desired effect of reducing the bacterial load must be balanced against the negative consequences, e.g. drug-induced hypersensitivity and possible selection of resistant strains. Parenteral (preferably intravenous) administration of the antibiotic is recommended to reach sufficient tissue concentrations, particularly in an emergency, although modern antibiotics (e.g. fluoroquinolones) have sufficient bioavailability for oral preparations to be equally effective. Local antibiotic irrigation is not recommended since the effect is not sustained.

Some suggestions for chemoprophylaxis related to the type of surgery being undertaken are given in Table 26.4.

Table 26.4 *Recommendations for perioperative antibacterial prophylaxis in urological interventions*

Procedure	Common pathogen(s)	Antibiotic(s) of choice	Alternative antibiotic(s)	Comments
I. Open operations				
a. Urinary tract with use of bowel segments	enterobacteriaceae enterococci anaerobes staphylococci	aminopenicillin + β-lac inhibitor cefuroxime + metronidazole flucloxacillin	In high-risk patients: ceftriaxone; aminopenicillin + β-lac inhibitor	In all patients
b. Urinary tract without bowel segment use	enterobacteriaceae enterococci staphylococci	fluoroquinolone* cefuroxime aminopenicillin + β-lac inhibitor	In high-risk patients: ceftriaxone; aminopenicillin + β-lac inhibitor	In patients with increased risk of infection
c. Implant/ prosthesis penis sphincter Reconstructive genital operation	staphylococci	cefazolin		In all patients; in secondary operations and in patients with increased risk of infection (e.g. immunosuppressed)
d. Other interventions outside the urinary tract	staphylococci	cefazolin		In patients with increased risk of infection
II. Endoscopic: instrument operations				
Urethra, prostate, bladder, ureter, kidney including percutaneous litholapaxy laparoscopic procedures and ESWL	enterobacteriaceae staphylococci enterococci	fluoroquinolone* aminopenicillin + β-lac inhibitor cefuroxime fosfomycin trometamol	co-trimoxazole aminoglycoside	In patients with increased risk of infection
III. Diagnostic interventions				
a. Transrectal biopsy of the prostate (with thick needle)	enterobacteriaceae enterococci anaerobes streptococci	fluoroquinolone* aminopenicillin + β-lac inhibitor, cefuroxime + metronidazole	aminoglycoside co-trimoxazole	In all patients
b. perineal biopsy of the prostate, urethrocystoscopy pyeloscopy laparoscopic procedures	enterobacteriaceae staphylococci enterococci	fluoroquinolone* aminopenicillin + β-lac inhibitor cefuroxime	co-trimoxazole	In patients with increased risk of infection

*Fluoroquinolone with sufficient renal excretion.
ESWL: Extracorporeal Shock Wave Lithotripsy.

26.10.1 Urological operations outside the urinary tract

Perioperative antibiotic prophylaxis is not generally recommended except in reconstructive operations on the genital area or with implant surgery. It can be achieved with flucloxacillin or cephazolin, since staphylococcal infection predominates.

26.10.2 Urological operations inside the urinary tract

Perioperative prophylaxis is recommended in cases with increased risk of infection. For patients undergoing transurethral resection of the prostate, additional risk factors include the size of prostate (>45 g), operative time (>90 minutes) and acute urinary retention.

Appropriate antibiotic regimens are fluoroquinolones, cephalosporins or aminopenicillins plus β-lactamase inhibitors. Studies of prophylaxis comparing fluoroquinolones and co-trimoxazole are not available; alternatives include aminoglycosides. For laparoscopic operations (e.g. nephrectomy, radial prostatectomy) definitive infection studies are missing, but on current evidence it is reasonable to manage them in the same manner as open clean surgical procedures.

26.10.3   Diagnostic interventions

Perioperative antibacterial prophylaxis (e.g. with an oral fluoroquinolone, an aminoglycoside, a cephalosporin + metronidazole; or aminopenicillin + β-lactamase inhibitor) is recommended to cover a transrectal prostate biopsy with a thick needle. In other diagnostic procedures of the urinary tract, (e.g. cystoscopy) prophylaxis is suggested only in high-risk patients. Oral or parenteral fluoroquinolone or co-trimoxazole are appropriate treatments.

26.11   POSTOPERATIVE URINARY DRAINAGE

When continuous urinary drainage by in-dwelling catheter, stent or nephrostomy is left in place after operation, then prolongation of perioperative antibacterial prophylaxis is contraindicated. If a symptomatic or febrile infection episode occurs, the patient must be treated empirically until culture results are available. Asymptomatic bacteriuria has to be treated only prior to any urinary tract intervention or when the drainage tube is removed.

26.12   FURTHER READING

Blumberg, E.A. and Abrutyn, E. (1997) Methods for reduction of urinary tract infection. *Curr. Opin. Urol.*, **7**, 47–51.

Kapoor, D.A., Klinberg, I.W., Malek, G.H. *et al.* (1998) Single dose oral ciprofloxacin versus placebo for chemoprophylaxis during transrectal biopsy. *Urology*, **52**, 552–558.

Shearman, C.P., Silverman, S.H., Johnson, M. *et al.* (1988) Single dose oral antibiotic care. *Br. J. Urol.*, **62**, 424–438.

Warren, J.W., Abrutyn, E., Hebel, R. *et al.* (1999) Guidelines for antimicrobial treatment of acute bacterial cystitis and acute pyelonephritis in women. *Clin. Infect. Dis.*, **29**, 745–758.

27

Infections in obstetrics

A.P.R. WILSON

27.1 INTRODUCTION

The incidence of Caesarean section is rising in most countries. Public awareness of listeriosis, toxoplasmosis and *Streptococcus* group B infection has resulted in more patients requesting information and screening for possible congenital infection. Diagnosis and treatment of infection are therefore an increasingly important part of obstetric practice. Antibiotic prophylaxis of wound infection following Caesarean section remains an area of controversy despite a large number of controlled trials, not regarding its efficacy but whether it is cost-effective in all populations.

27.2 CHORIOAMNIONITIS

Infection of the uterine contents occurs in up to one-quarter of premature deliveries and in 1% of term deliveries, and is often asymptomatic initially. Prolonged rupture of membranes or repeated vaginal examinations result in an ascending infection of the amniotic fluid. Infection is more common in the young primagravida or following bacterial vaginosis, and can also arise from amniocentesis, fetal blood sampling or by the

haematogenous route (e.g. *Listeria* spp.). Infections are polymicrobial and pathogens include anaerobes, *Streptococcus* group B, mycoplasmas and *Escherichia coli*. Enterobacteriaceae and enterococci suggest a gastrointestinal source.

The mother develops fever, tachycardia and abdominal tenderness and the fetus a raised but variable heart rate. Labour can be disrupted, and oxytocin or Caesarean section are commonly needed. If given as soon as the diagnosis is made, ampicillin and gentamicin are effective against *Streptococcus* group B and *E. coli*, but cure depends on delivery of the baby. Vaginal delivery is preferred unless there are other reasons for Caesarean section to be performed, in which case a regimen active against anaerobes, e.g. clindamycin plus gentamicin, should be used.

27.3 WOUND INFECTION AND ENDOMETRITIS

The increasing proportion of pregnancies ending in Caesarean section ensure that endometritis and wound infections continue to be a significant cause of prolonged hospital stay, increased cost of care and use of antibiotics.

Fever following Caesarean section is common, but estimates vary widely with the definitions used and the risk factors of the population. Rates of surgical wound infection and urinary tract infection after Caesarean section also vary widely between studies. Entry of vaginal flora into the lower uterine segment before or during operation produce the majority of infections. Antibiotic prophylaxis probably reduces the incidence of infection by 50% in emergency section (although controversy exists, see below) but up to 30% of patients can still develop endometritis.

Postpartum endometritis follows vaginal delivery in up to 4% of women compared with 10–50% following Caesarean delivery. The rate is related to maternal age, poverty, prolonged labour or rupture of membranes and repeated vaginal examination. In Caesarean section, failure of prophylaxis is often associated with clinically inapparent infection at the time of delivery, and is related to the number of vaginal examinations, gestational age under 37 weeks and the type of prophylaxis. Primagravida deliveries are more likely to develop infections than multigravida, and emergency sections have been associated with higher rates of endometritis than elective operations. Women having emergency procedures are more likely to be in labour with rupture of membranes and to have the minimum of preoperative preparation. Superficial wound infection is more common in elective than emergency sections. The first Caesarean section is more likely to be associated with endometritis or bacteraemia, but a second section is more likely to develop surgical wound infection (Figure 27.1). Vaginal examinations promote entry of vaginal bacteria into the uterus whether or not antibiotic prophylaxis is used.

Endometritis is caused by a wide variety of bacteria including *Streptococcus* group B, *Gardnerella vaginalis*, enterococci and streptococci, *E. coli* and anaerobes (*Prevotella* spp., *Bacteroides* spp., peptostreptococci). Although mycoplasmas and ureaplasmas may be isolated, their significance is not large as recovery follows antibiotics not active against them. *Chlamydia trachomatis* is associated with delayed endometritis. Caesarean section wounds, as with other clean wounds, are usually infected with *Staphylococcus aureus*, coagulase-negative staphylococci and streptococci, frequently derived from the patient's own skin flora.

Maternal fever 1–2 days after delivery, lower abdominal pain and tenderness with a raised white blood cell count are suggestive of endometritis, and this can be confirmed on bimanual examination. Blood culture is essential and is positive in up to 20% of cases. Cultures via the vagina will be contaminated with commensal flora but may be helpful if treatment fails. Detection of chlamydial antigen should be requested in cases with a delayed onset. Clindamycin and gentamicin is indicated for treatment of severe or post-Caesarean endometritis, while co-amoxiclav or cefuroxime plus metronidazole can be used in moderate infections. Initial administration is by the i.v. route, but once fever has resolved antibiotics can be given orally. Erythromycin or doxycycline for 10 days are effective in chlamydial disease. Enterococci cause failure of treatment if present in heavy growth, but ampicillin, gentamicin and metronidazole can be used to eradicate the infection. Pelvic or wound abscess or venous thrombosis cause persistent fever.

Caesarean wound infection has been reported in between 5% and 85% of patients depending on the population and definitions used. Most studies require the presence of pus to define infection, but serous exudate, erythema or wound separation may be found in any combination or extent of wound involvement. The majority of infections will resolve with daily dressings and an appropriate antibiotic (e.g. flucloxacillin) if surrounding cellulitis is present. Rapidly spreading cellulitis in toxaemic patients suggests infection with *Streptococcus* group A and requires immediate high-dose benzylpenicillin and debridement.

Ovarian vein thrombophlebitis is a rare complication of vaginal or Caesarean delivery, but is usually associated with endometritis following Caesarean section. Patients develop fever and lower abdominal pain 2–4 days after delivery which fail to respond to antibiotics. Tachycardia, ileus and rigors are common. In half the patients, the thrombosed vessel can be felt on examination extending laterally from the right uterine cornua. A computed tomography scan or ultrasound can aid diagnosis. Broad-spectrum antibiotics are given with heparin for 10 days.

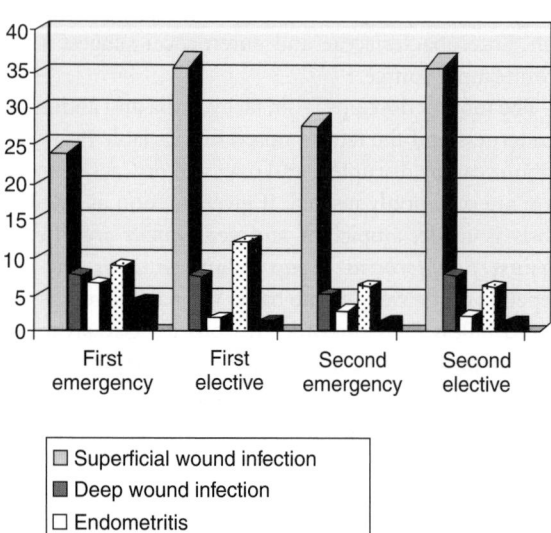

Figure 27.1 *Infections following first and second Caesarean section. Primary sections: emergency* n = 696, *elective* n = 96, *secondary sections: emergency* n = 140, *elective* n = 405. *(From Henderson and Love, 1995.)*

27.4 EPISIOTOMY INFECTION

Episiotomy infection is rare, but can occur in 1–2% of third-degree extensions. Simple infection affects the skin and superficial tissues and is characterized by erythema and swelling of the local tissues. Infection is polymicrobial and includes Enterobacteriaceae, staphylococci and anaerobes, so that treatment requires broad-spectrum antibiotics (e.g. cefuroxime plus metronidazole or clindamycin plus gentamicin). If there is no response after 2 days, the wound should be opened and debrided to confirm that no communication with the rectum exists.

Necrotizing fasciitis is a serious complication in which infection spreads along deep fascial planes, often with few local external signs. There is severe local pain, fever and toxaemia, commonly in a diabetic patient. At surgery, there is marked tissue necrosis in the superficial fascia. Parenteral antibiotics (benzylpenicillin, clindamycin and gentamicin) are combined with urgent radical debridement.

Necrosis of the deep muscles can develop from an infection caused by *Clostridium perfringens*. Extension to the muscles around the hip joint can be caused by deep pudendal injection. Benzylpenicillin in high doses and debridement are required. Hyperbaric oxygen, if available, may be of some benefit.

27.5 PUERPERAL SEPSIS

Puerperal sepsis develops after delivery or abortion when *Streptococcus* group A colonizing the patient's vagina or introduced on the hands of staff infect the endometrium, lymph and blood. Endometritis and bacteraemia ensue with pelvic cellulitis, thrombophlebitis and pelvic abscess. Before the introduction of strict aseptic techniques, puerperal sepsis was a major cause of death following delivery. If it does occur, source isolation and prompt treatment with high-dose benzylpenicillin is essential. An outbreak (two or more cases) requires notification of public health doctors, strict source isolation, screening cultures (nose and throat) of medical and nursing staff, treatment of any carriers, keeping them off work until demonstrated free of the organism, and screening of neonates. The organisms need to be typed to confirm a single source.

27.6 SEPTIC ABORTION

Abortion associated with fever, endometritis and parametritis is rare in countries where induced abortion is legal, but it remains common in areas where abortion is not permitted or too expensive for the majority of the population. Mortality from induced abortion in Europe is less than 1 per 100 000 compared with half of the 500 000 obstetric deaths per year globally due to induced abortion, mostly in the Third World. Infection is the usual cause of death related to illegal abortion, and is most likely in the young unmarried woman with incomplete evacuation of uterine contents. **Perforation** is more likely in more advanced pregnancy. If untreated, the patient develops bacteraemia, pelvic sepsis and thrombophlebitis, septic shock, disseminated intravascular coagulation, and renal failure, with a fatal outcome.

CASE HISTORY

A 40-year-old woman developed fever and mastitis 6 days after a difficult forceps delivery. *Streptococcus* group A was isolated from blood culture. She was source isolated and treated with benzylpenicillin. Cultures of breast milk and cervix were negative. She rapidly improved and was discharged 3 days later, taking oral flucloxacillin and amoxycillin. The baby was not affected.

A 25-year-old-woman had a Caesarean section 2 days after the first woman, attended by the same obstetric registrar. She became febrile 3 days after delivery and a cervical swab produced a growth of *Streptococcus* group A. She was source isolated and treated with benzylpenicillin followed by oral amoxycillin. Her baby was well, but *Streptococcus* group A was found in an umbilical swab and the baby was treated with penicillin V.

A third woman, on a different ward from the other two, had Caesarean section performed at 33 weeks' gestation for pre-eclampsia by the same registrar the day after the second woman. The mother remained well and left hospital a week later. Three days after delivery a throat swab from the baby in the special care baby unit produced *Streptococcus* group A. The baby was source isolated and treated with penicillin.

The registrar had had a sore throat and was sent home for 48 hours, but a throat swab was negative; nevertheless, he was treated with erythromycin. Screening of the nose and throat of the midwives and the medical staff was performed, but no carriers were found. Inspection of the theatre revealed dust on shelves and blood on the floor of the anaesthetic room, but environmental swabs were negative. A departmental meeting was held to encourage better cleaning and hygiene. The isolates of *Streptococcus* group A were all similar (T3, opacity factor negative, M64) but no other cases occurred.

Effective and easily available contraception, legal abortion and correct medical management are highly effective in preventing septic abortion. The most vulnerable for unwanted pregnancies are adolescents who may be persuaded into sexual relationships ignorant or unable to use adequate contraception. Although induced abortion early in pregnancy is safe, adolescents are often reluctant to obtain parental permission for the procedure and continue the pregnancy. In the first trimester, vacuum currettage can be performed as an outpatient, and prophylactic antibiotics should be used in high-risk cases.

When septic abortion does occur, early treatment is essential and the diagnosis must be considered if a woman presents with vaginal bleeding, lower abdominal pain and fever. A pregnancy test will still be positive in a woman who does not reveal she has had an induced abortion. If feasible, the person who performed the procedure should be contacted to find any bacteriological cultures, the procedure performed and investigations of tissue removed. Perforation is most likely if a rigid object has been used to procure abortion. Abdominal tenderness and guarding and whether they are limited in distribution or generalized should be noted, together with any injury to the vagina or cervix. Pus or products of conception in the os, enlargement of the uterus or an adnexal mass make the diagnosis more likely. Fever, tachycardia, hypotension and respiratory distress suggest systemic infection. Free gas in the abdomen can be seen on abdominal X-ray. Incomplete abortion or retention of blood may present as fever, mild abdominal pain and vaginal bleeding. Vacuum currettage is effective in preventing septic abortion in these cases.

Septic abortion is usually caused by organisms from the normal vaginal flora plus, in many cases, sexually transmitted pathogens (*Neisseria gonorrhoeae* and *Chlamydia trachomatis*). *Clostridium perfringens* or *Clostridium tetani* can be associated with illegal abortion. Cultures should be made of blood, urine and cervix. A full blood count and X-ray of the chest, abdomen and pelvis should be taken. Endometrial biopsy is most likely to reveal the true pathogens. Patients with established infection should always be admitted for parenteral treatment in case complications develop such as adult respiratory distress syndrome (ARDS).

As infection is usually polymicrobial, antibiotic treatment is broad spectrum and should include anaerobic activity, for example, clindamycin (2.4 g per day) plus gentamicin. Some would combine this with high-dose penicillin or ampicillin. The uterus must be evacuated as soon as possible, whatever the condition of the patient. Vacuum currettage can be performed under local anaesthesia. In later pregnancy, oxytocin or prostaglandin $F_{2\alpha}$ can be used (not prostaglandin E_2 because of its effect on raising the temperature). Laparotomy is needed if other measures fail or if there is uterine perforation. Closed suction irrigation should be performed and the abdomen closed with interrupted internal stays, but the subcuta-

neous layer and skin should be left open and packed. *Clostridium perfringens* is treated with high-dose benzyl-penicillin, currettage and intensive monitoring. If this fails, or there is air in the uterine wall, then hysterectomy should be performed.

Infection of the endometrium by *Chlamydia trachomatis* may result in spontaneous abortion, but contradictory reports have appeared concerning the relationship between fetal loss or prematurity and the presence of chlamydial infection. One large treatment study compared 1110 untreated women, 1323 women treated with erythromycin and 9111 uninfected women. There was a significant reduction in the rate of premature rupture of membranes in infected women who were treated compared with those who were not.

27.7 URINARY TRACT INFECTION

From the seventh week of pregnancy, dilatation of the ureters and renal pelvis predispose to urinary infection. Bladder tone decreases, and this allows a larger urinary volume. Asymptomatic bacteriuria occurs in 5% of pregnant women, being more common with a past history of infection, diabetes, greater age, or parity, the infection being most frequent at the first antenatal visit. Pyelonephritis develops in one-third of those with bacteriuria in early pregnancy, and three-quarters of cases could be eliminated by treating bacteriuria. Premature labour and low birth weight are associated with pyelonephritis and bacteriuria, but studies differ as to whether elimination of bacteriuria reduces prematurity. Screening is justified because of the severe consequences of pyelonephritis.

Significant bacteriuria should be treated to avoid the risk of pyelonephritis. Amoxycillin, co-amoxiclav or an oral cephalosporin are usually effective unless there is an abnormality of the urinary tract. Nitrofurantoin only reaches therapeutic concentrations in urine and, although it crosses the placenta, amniotic concentrations are very low. It has been used safely in pregnancy including some infants with glucose-6-phosphate dehydrogenase (G6PD) deficiency. Tetracyclines and quinolones should be avoided.

A 3-day course is advisable to reduce exposure to antibiotic in pregnancy. Repeat urine cultures must be taken 1–2 weeks after treatment, and then at regular intervals during the remainder of the pregnancy. Recurrent urinary infection can be prevented using a single daily dose of nitrofurantoin (50 mg) or an oral cephalosporin.

27.8 *STREPTOCOCCUS* GROUP B

Streptococcus agalactiae is a Gram-positive diplococcus which produces a zone of β-haemolysis on blood agar and is a common cause of infection in postpartum women and neonates. The organisms are present in the genital tract of up to one-third of pregnant women, and can cause asymptomatic bacteriuria. Transmission to the fetus may occur by ascending infection into the uterus or during birth in 30–70% of cases. Heavily colonized women are more likely to transmit infection, and their neonates are more likely to develop invasive infection. Prolonged rupture of membranes (>18 h), multiple births, rupture of membranes before 37 weeks of pregnancy, amnionitis, maternal fever, age under 20 years and black race predispose to invasive infection of the offspring.

Neonatal infection (i.e. in first five days) occurs in up to 4 per 1000 live births, usually term infants. A further 1 per 1000 live births develop late-onset infection up to 3 months of age. Meningitis is associated with infections by type III organisms. Maternal infection causes one-fifth of cases of fever after delivery. Infants born before 37 weeks' gestation have a considerably increased risk of symptomatic infection, and premature rupture of membranes may be caused by ascending infection with the organism. Reduced concentrations of anticapsular antibody in the blood of premature infants may result in an increased susceptibility. Complement activation is required in the opsonization and phagocytosis of *Streptococcus* group B, and the low concentrations of complement proteins in infants may explain the greater incidence of disease in the very young. Residues in the capsule of types Ia and III inhibit complement activation and absence of the capsule is associated with loss of virulence.

In early neonatal infection, bacteraemia, pneumonia or meningitis are the common presentations and are usually associated with maternal obstetric complications. Late-onset neonatal infection is usually bacteraemia with meningitis caused by type III strains, and maternal complications are rare. *Streptococcus* group B accounts for one-fifth of cases of maternal bacteraemia but recovery after antibiotic treatment is usual. Endometritis presents within 48 hours of delivery as fever and uterine tenderness with normal lochia and is also associated with Caesarean section, often with wound infection. Pelvic abscess or septic shock are rare. Bacteriuria with cystitis or pyelonephritis can also occur.

Diagnosis is made by isolation of the organism from blood, cerebrospinal fluid (CSF) or the site of soft tissue infection. Antigen detection methods are available for patients already receiving antibiotics but are principally used in neonates. Detection of colonization during labour can be made by a Gram stain of vaginal or cervical swabs, but this is sensitive rather than specific.

Benzylpenicillin (6 g per day for 10 days) is recommended for the treatment of adult bacteraemia, pyelonephritis or soft tissue infection reserving vancomycin or teicoplanin for individuals allergic to β-lactam antibiotics. Urinary infection other than pyelonephritis responds to oral ampicillin. Neonates are treated with ampicillin plus an aminoglycoside.

Oral antibiotic treatment during pregnancy usually fails to eradicate carriage of the organism by the time of delivery. Parenteral ampicillin administered during labour prevents maternal bacteraemia and transmission of infection to the neonate, but administration of penicillin to the neonate does not prevent the onset of infection. A significant reduction in early-onset streptococcal infection of neonates compared with placebo has been reported in colonized women with prolonged rupture of membranes or early labour who were given parenteral ampicillin (1–2 g 4-hourly) until delivery. However, one-quarter of early-onset infections still occur in mothers without symptoms or prolonged rupture of membranes. Late-onset infection is unaffected.

Rapid antigen detection methods have been used at parturition to identify carriers, who are then given benzylpenicillin until delivery. Unfortunately, one-quarter of patients may not have results by the time of delivery, and some infants born to antigen-negative mothers develop *Streptococcus* group B infection. The sensitivity of these methods may be only 50% compared with culture. Vaccination with capsular polysaccharide antigens could provide protective antibodies in susceptible women, but the immunogenicity of the antigens is poor and more effective preparations are awaited.

27.9 LISTERIOSIS

Listeria monocytogenes is a Gram-positive aerobic bacillus identifiable by being motile at room temperature, catalase-positive and hydrolysing aesculin. It is found in asymptomatic carriers, a wide variety of animals, food and sewage. Outbreaks have been associated with the consumption of vegetables, dairy products (notably soft cheeses) or meat. *Listeria* can cross the placenta during bacteraemia, infecting the amniotic fluid and the fetus. Listeriosis is rare (<1 in 100 000 per year), but one-third of cases occur in pregnant women and result in abortion or premature delivery. Infection in the third trimester presents as fever and rigors (sometimes with back pain), but a negative urine culture. Confirmation is only possible by blood culture, so infection is often not diagnosed. Infection of the fetus can cause granulomatosis infantiseptica, in which the fetus develops abscesses in all organs. Amnionitis and fetal circulatory failure may develop. Cultures of fetal and maternal blood, amnion, lochia and the infant's throat or skin lesions will confirm the diagnosis. A lumbar puncture will show meningitis. Mortality for the fetus is high and immediate treatment with ampicillin and gentamicin is indicated. Listeria can also cause a meningitis starting after 3 days of age.

27.10 TUBERCULOSIS

Pregnancy should not be a reason to delay treatment of tuberculosis. Isoniazid, ethambutol and rifampicin are used, but streptomycin must be avoided because of the risk of fetal ototoxicity. Pyrazinamide has not been properly assessed in pregnancy and should be avoided. Isoniazid should be withdrawn if hepatotoxicity develops.

27.11 MALARIA

Despite any potential risk, intravenous quinine to treat malaria must be given as it is life saving and preserves the pregnancy. Fansidar should not be used and quinine needs to be given at least 48 hours beyond the loss of parasitaemia. **Abortion** is a potential risk and babies may have a low birth weight. Congenital infection is well recognized.

27.12 SYPHILIS

Infection of the fetus by untreated maternal syphilis is rare until after the fourth month of pregnancy. Abortion, stillbirth, neonatal death or latent infection can occur. Congenital syphilis can be recognized by early rhinitis, a maculopapular rash with loss of skin on the palms and soles, osteochondritis giving a saddle nose and bowed tibia, splenomegaly, anaemia and jaundice. Serological testing of mothers is required to identify cases at risk.

Treatment of syphilis in pregnancy requires penicillin in the same regimens as used in non-pregnant patients, e.g. procaine penicillin 4 g i.m. daily for 10 days plus probenecid. Doxycycline, tetracycline and chloramphenicol cannot be used. Patients allergic to pencillin require desensitization (exposure to gradually increasing doses) as erythromycin has not been found to be effective. If adequate treatment is given the risk of infection of the fetus is small, but following delivery monthly follow-up examinations of the child are required until serology becomes negative. A child of an inadequately treated mother should be treated quickly with penicillin.

27.13 GONORRHOEA

Although gonorrhoea is associated with perinatal mortality, premature labour or rupture of membranes and abortion, it may be simply that the disease is more common in women liable to have these complications. Pelvic inflammatory disease becomes less likely in later pregnancy because of the physical barrier presented by the uterus. However, there is some evidence that disseminated infection is more likely in pregnancy, and treatment is often conducted as an inpatient. Neonates can acquire gonorrhoea before, during or after delivery, and most commonly it results in ophthalmia neonatorum. A purulent conjunctivitis develops within a week of delivery, the organisms being visible on a Gram-stained smear of the

discharge. Septicaemia can occur in some infants. Screening of women before delivery is therefore essential.

Treatment is usually a single dose of ceftriaxone 250 mg i.m. or an oral dose of amoxycillin 2–3 g plus probenecid 1 g p.o. or cefuroxime 1.5 g i.m. plus probenecid 1 g p.o. Doxycycline and the quinolones are contraindicated, and azithromycin has not been adequately assessed in pregnancy.

27.14 GIARDIASIS

Metronidazole is usually the treatment of choice for giardiasis, but it is recommended that short high-dose regimens be avoided. A dose of 250 mg every 8 hours for 5 days could be used. The drug should, if possible, be avoided in the first trimester. Alternatively, paromomycin, an aminoglycoside, can be given orally (25 mg kg^{-1} per day in three doses) for 5–10 days without significant systemic absorption.

27.15 TOXOPLASMOSIS

Toxoplasma gondii is an intracellular protozoan which commonly infects both patients and animals, but only a minority experience the symptomatic disease, toxoplasmosis. The definitive host is the cat, which excretes the oocysts for 1–3 weeks. Mature oocysts remain viable in the environment for up to 18 months; this allows infection of secondary hosts, including man. The invasive form, the tachyzoite, infects the host cells and multiplies intracellularly. The tissue cysts containing bradyzoites often develop in muscle, myocardium and brain, and if undercooked meat (particularly lamb or pork) is eaten they can infect man. Vegetables contaminated with oocysts are another source. Cooking, irradiation or freezing followed by thawing kill tissue cysts.

Transplacental transmission of infection occurs when a pregnant women develops acute infection or occasionally following acute infection in the 2 months before conception. A woman travelling from an area of high prevalence of the disease is at risk. Only one-fifth of adult infections develop symptoms, although painless lymphadenopathy lasting several months is common. Fever, night sweats, sore throat, rash or myalgia can occur. Up to one-quarter of women infected during the first trimester transmit infection to the fetus, resulting in abortion, stillbirth or granulomatosis infantiseptica. In the second trimester, transplacental infection occurs in 30–50% of cases, up to 80% of whom will have no symptoms, while in the third trimester 60–65% of cases are affected with 90–100% asymptomatic. The infant may have mental retardation, microcephaly, chorioretinitis, blindness, anaemia, jaundice, rash or intracranial calcification. Children without signs at birth commonly develop chorioretinitis during childhood.

Diagnosis of acute infection in pregnancy depends on the identification of IgG and IgM. A latex agglutination test is widely used as a screening test for serum to be examined by more detailed methods. The Dye test is the most sensitive and specific test, but is restricted to reference laboratories. Indirect fluorescent antibody tests detect IgG antibody which reaches a peak at 6–8 weeks after infection and falls over 1–2 years. An ELISA method is also widely used, but some kits do not perform well. IgM antibody appears within a week of infection, peaks and then disappears within a few months. IgM can be detected by an immunofluorescent method, ELISA or by the IgM immunosorbent assay (ISAGA) which is sensitive and specific. The IgG avidity test can provide an estimate of the duration of infection as avidity is time-dependent. If IgG and IgM are absent, the infection is excluded but the patient is at risk. IgG without IgM suggests chronic disease with little risk of congenital infection. The presence of IgM suggests infection within 12 months, but the time of infection can be estimated by a changing titre or the avidity test. In the case of acute infection, ultrasound to show ventricular enlargement, sampling of umbilical blood for antibody testing or of amniotic fluid for polymerase chain reaction studies are helpful in identifying women needing treatment. Congenital toxoplasmosis is then greatly reduced. Fetal blood injected into mice can also be used to isolate toxoplasma.

Treatment does not cure toxoplasmosis in pregnancy but can reduce the risk to the fetus. Urgent treatment is needed if acute infection is established. Spiramycin (3 g per day) is the usual choice to prevent transmission to the fetus, but it does not cross the placenta well. If fetal infection is demonstrated, the mother is treated with sulphadiazine (4 g per day), pyrimethamine (25 mg per day) and folinic acid (5–15 mg per day), pyrimethamine and folinic acid being omitted during the first 16 weeks of pregnancy. Prevention of infection in seronegative women is achieved by ensuring that meat is heated to at least 66°C, eggs are cooked, hands are washed after handling raw meat or vegetables, and milk is not drunk unpasteurized. Gloves must be worn when removing cat litter. Screening depends on the prevalence of the disease and financial constraints. Tests of all patients at 10–12 weeks' gestation will identify seronegative women who require repeat testing at 20 weeks and again at term.

27.16 VIRAL INFECTIONS

27.16.1 Transmission of Hepatitis viruses

The majority (>70%) of neonates born to mothers carrying hepatitis B surface antigen or e antigen develop hepatitis B and usually become chronic carriers. Cirrhosis and hepatic carcinoma are complications in later life in one-quarter of cases. Hepatitis B vaccine or hepatitis B immunoglobulin prevent infection in the majority of infants, and given together reduce the risk of chronic carriage to 10%, even in children born to HBeAg carriers. Vaccine and immunoglobulin are given within 12 hours of delivery with further doses of vaccine at 1 and 6 months. All pregnant women should be screened for hepatitis B at antenatal booking with a second specimen later if the risk of exposure is high. All positive specimens should be confirmed with a second test. Patients presenting for care late in pregnancy, particularly those with a history of drug abuse, have a greater risk of hepatitis B carriage. Hepatitis C can be transmitted from mother to infant in late pregnancy or at delivery at a rate of between 3% and 10%.

Hepatitis E virus is acquired by the faecal oral route predominantly in India, Africa and China, and symptoms resemble hepatitis A. Fulminant hepatitis and disseminated intravascular coagulation are more common in pregnant women than in other patients, with a mortality rate of those with the complication of 25%; however, the reasons are unclear. There is no proven effective antiviral treatment.

Transmission of human immunodeficiency virus from mother to child during pregnancy is second only to intercourse as a means of spread of the disease, with risk estimates of 14 to 30%. Mothers with primary infection or late disease are most likely to infect their offspring. Infection during delivery or by breast feeding are also common. AIDS is diagnosed in 43% of infected children within 1 year. HIV can be demonstrated in fetal tissue as early as 8 weeks' gestation, and early infection allows detection of the virus in the child at birth by molecular methods or culture. Children in whom the virus is not detected at birth may have become infected during late pregnancy or delivery. Most studies suggest that the risk of infection during vaginal and Caesarean delivery is similar, but at least one meta-analysis has suggested perinatal risk to be lower during Caesarean section (14% versus 20%). Breast-fed children have higher rates of HIV than bottle-fed children, and the virus can be demonstrated in breast milk. The risk of transmission by breast feeding is up to 30%.

In areas of high prevalence, routine counselling and screening of HIV should be considered. Treatment of HIV-positive pregnant women with zidovudine from the second trimester up to delivery significantly reduces the risk of perinatal transmission (from 28% to 8%) and is combined with treatment of the infant from 8–12 hours after birth for 6 weeks. The risk of infection was similar for treatment starting at 14–26 weeks of pregnancy as for treatment starting after 26 weeks. Avoidance of intravenous injections in drug abusers is an important preventive measure. Breast feeding should be avoided in areas where safe alternatives to breast milk are available, but in developing countries the benefits of breast feeding outweigh the risks.

Cytomegalovirus (CMV) infection of the cervix becomes more common during pregnancy reaching a prevalence of 11–28% in the third trimester in various studies. Babies born to women not secreting the virus are ten-fold less likely to become infected with CMV than those secreting in the third trimester. If the mother continues to secrete the virus during and after delivery, 57% of babies become infected.

Intrauterine infection with CMV occurs in up to 2% of births and can be diagnosed when viruria in the baby is proven within the first week after birth. Primary infection of the mother during pregnancy is demonstrated by the appearance of CMV antibody or the presence of CMV IgM. Congenital infection occurred in 11 of 21 primary infections in pregnant women, representing 0.3% of all pregnancies in the series, and in three cases, the baby had symptoms. Twenty (0.5%) pregnancies of mothers with past infections also resulted in congenital infections, but all were asymptomatic – presumably because of maternal antibodies.

Infection of the newborn with **herpes simplex virus** occurs in up to 1 in 2000 births, and results from spread of genital HSV-2 infection into the uterus or by passage through the infected birth canal. Fetal scalp monitoring and recent acute maternal infection increase the risks. Primary maternal infection may be asymptomatic but can cause abortion, early labour, rash, growth retardation, microcephaly or chorioretinitis. Skin vesicles, jaundice, hepatosplenomegaly or fits at birth suggest congenital infection, but neonatal infection presents days or weeks later with vesicles, conjunctivitis, fits, cranial nerve palsies and inflammatory cells and a raised protein in the CSF. Mortality in disseminated disease in infants is high. If clinically apparent cervical infection is present before rupture of the membranes, Caesarean section is probably advisable; however, it is of no advantage if rupture has occurred. Vaginal delivery is preferable if there are no visible lesions, but the child will require careful observation.

Influenza during pregnancy has been associated with higher mortality during pandemics. Vaccine is recommended for pregnant women with chronic diseases and/or ill health but not in healthy pregnant women.

Measles during pregnancy is rare but can be severe and has been associated with spontaneous abortion and premature delivery. Half the patients develop pneumonitis. Babies born to mothers with measles should be given immune globulin.

Arenaviruses (e.g. Lassa fever) will infect the fetus and cause abortion. Hydrocephalus and chorioretinitis of the fetus follow infection with lymphocytic choriomeningitis virus. Human polyomaviruses (JC or BK virus) can be detected in the urine of 3% of pregnant women in the third trimester, mainly as the result of reactivation of previous infection. However, evidence for transmission of infection to the fetus is inconclusive.

27.17   USE OF ANTIBIOTICS IN PREGNANCY

Antibiotics given to the mother during pregnancy and lactation are passed, in varying proportions, to the fetus or infant. For most antibiotics, their potential to produce teratogenic effects in humans is not known, but penicillins, cephalosporins and erythromycin have been widely used without adverse effect. Metronidazole and ticarcillin should usually be avoided because of the teratogenic effects in rats. However, metronidazole has often been used to treat trichomoniasis in pregnancy. Trimethoprim (also in co-trimoxazole) is a folate antagonist and there is a theoretical risk of teratogenicity in the first trimester.

Tetracyclines should not be not used in pregnancy because they damage the developing teeth of the fetus and can cause acute fatty necrosis of the liver. Adverse effects are particularly frequent if high or intravenous doses are given to pregnant women with renal impairment (except doxycycline). Aminoglycosides cross the placenta and should be avoided but fetal toxicity has been reported only for the prolonged use of streptomycin in tuberculosis. Neonatal haemolysis and methaemoglobinaemia have been reported following the use of co-trimoxazole in the third trimester. Ciprofloxacin is not recommended for use in pregnancy because of the potential effect on fetal joints, even though no adverse effects could be demonstrated in animal models.

Renal clearance of antibiotics is more rapid in pregnant than non-pregnant women, and plasma volume is increased. Higher dosages – particularly of penicillins – may be needed to maintain therapeutic serum concentrations.

Low concentrations of most antibiotics will be found in breast milk while the mother is treated, depending on the size and solubility of the antibiotic. Breast-feeding infants with G6PD deficiency may be affected by sulphonamides or nalidixic acid given to the mother. Sulphonamides given to the mother can predispose to kernicterus in premature babies who are breast feeding. Chloramphenicol may reach sufficient concentrations in milk to risk idiosyncratic agranulocytosis but not to cause 'grey baby' syndrome. Ciprofloxacin is excreted in breast milk, and its use is contraindicated because of the potential risk of arthropathy in the child. Clindamycin in milk has been reported to cause bloody diarrhoea in an infant; tetracycline in breast milk chelates with calcium and is unlikely to be absorbed.

27.17.1   Antibiotic prophylaxis

Avoidance of wound infection depends on the use of sterile technique, the skill of the operator, a low bacterial inoculum and volume of suture material, and good haemostasis. Antibiotic prophylaxis is not a substitute for good aseptic practice, but extensive literature shows that it reduces the incidence of infection. Research has focused on the duration, timing and choice of antibiotic and type of operation in which it is beneficial. Caesarean sections are frequently covered by perioperative antibiotics, but this depends on the opinion of the consultant obstetrician or the microbiologist.

The antibiotic chosen should be effective against pathogens recovered from the local endogenous flora and from wound infections that have occurred in the recent past. Animal models show the greatest benefit from antibiotics when they are administered a short time before the operation starts. This coincides with general surgical experience. In practice, this is usually at induction of anaesthesia so that peak concentrations coincide with cutting of the skin or mucous membranes. For **Caesarean section**, it is common practice to administer antibiotic after clamping the cord, presumably to avoid exposure of the baby to antibiotic, and this has been shown to be as effective as administering the antibiotic at the start of the procedure.

Clinical trials of antibiotic prophylaxis have demonstrated a few general rules. Effectiveness of different doses is rarely compared, but usually one at the upper limit of therapeutic range is appropriate. There is no benefit of prolonging antibiotics beyond 12 hours, although longer courses remain common in some units. The intravenous route is preferable because high tissue concentrations are achieved at the time of surgery. Intramuscular administration is painful, can cause sterile abscess and does not allow for the operation being delayed. If the operation is prolonged, additional doses should be given at one to two times the half-life; this usually means every 3–4 hours. The antibiotic should be one with few adverse effects and one not routinely used for serious infections.

Compliance with antibiotic prophylactic regimens can be improved by simple measures, for example, a check box on medical records to be completed by the anaesthetist or pre-printed orders. An automatic stop on prescriptions should be made at 24 hours pending review. Procedures should be developed locally with the participation of the surgeons, and a periodic survey undertaken to check compliance. Rates of compliance can then be reported back to the surgeons.

CAESAREAN SECTION

The relationship between amniotic infection and postoperative Caesarean wound infection depends on the type of bacteria, their number and the duration of infection. The wide variety of organisms in the female genital tract means that infections of the surgical wound, placenta, amnion or endometrium are polymicrobial and hence difficult to predict from preoperative cultures. The risk of infection is related to both host factors (e.g. immune defence) and bacterial factors (e.g. the production of a capsule, fimbriae, and collagenases). Antibiotic prophylaxis reduces the bacterial inoculum and the capacity for growth, makes tissues less susceptible to invasion, and improves intracellular killing of bacteria by phagocytes.

There are almost as many definitions of infection as there are trials of antibiotic prophylaxis, resulting in a very wide range of rates of infection (5 to 85%) after Caesarean section. Despite the recruitment of 10 000 patients in reported trials, controversy remains concerning the cost-effectiveness of prophylaxis in Caesarean section. Many trials find emergency surgery and low socioeconomic status to be important risk factors, but are divided on the importance of long duration of rupture of membranes or labour. In a review of 1800 Caesarean deliveries, 766 had prophylaxis of whom 240 (31%) developed fever and uterine tenderness. Prolonged rupture is associated with high bacterial inoculum and an infection rate of 20% in some trials. In a review of trials of all patient groups, 23 placebo-controlled trials suggested a benefit from prophylaxis, but seven placebo-controlled trials suggested no benefit to prophylaxis. Patients with few risk factors also seem to benefit from antibiotic prophylaxis in terms of a significantly reduced incidence of wound infections and febrile morbidity when trials are reviewed together. However, some individual trials find no difference in wound infection when antibiotics are used in these patients. On balance, prophylaxis appears justified but the case is not overwhelming.

Comparison between antibiotic regimens usually shows no significant differences in terms of choice or duration, a single dose being as effective as five doses. In one major trial of 1438 patients, the rate of wound infection following prophylaxis with cefazolin $(3 \times 1$ g$)$$(32/142, 23\%)$ was significantly inferior to 1 cefotetan $\times 1$ g $(9/148, 6\%)$, 1 piperacillin $\times 4$ g $(13/155, 8\%)$, 1 cefazolin $\times 2$ g $(17/161, 11\%)$, or 1 ampicillin $\times 2$ g $(19/148, 13\%)$. Local irrigation using cefamandole (2 g), cefoxitin (2 g), ampicillin (2 g), cefazolin (1 g), cefotaxime (2 g) appears as effective as one to two intravenous doses in controlled trials.

Current US recommendations in high-risk populations are for cefazolin or ampicillin, after clamping and cutting the umbilical cord. This precaution is probably unnecessary (although customary), and it might improve the chances of culturing an infecting organism. Prophylaxis is optional in low-risk patients and if it is an elective procedure with membranes intact, prophylaxis is probably not necessary. However, most trials report significant benefit of prophylaxis in high-risk patients. Although *Staph. aureus* is the most common pathogen in the wound and anaerobes or Gram-negative the most common organisms in endometritis, agents are effective which have no anti-staphylococcal activity (e.g. metronidazole) or no anti-anaerobic activity (e.g. cefazolin).

In the USA, prophylaxis has been found to be cost-effective for all patients because most of those infected are isolated and treated with parenteral antibiotics. Many US trials have a high proportion of emergency sections. In the UK, the cost of management of suspected infection is up to 100 times lower, and prophylaxis may not be cost-effective. Although febrile morbidity is reduced significantly, benefits in terms of serious infections are often found only in emergency cases, and limiting prophylaxis to these cases – especially those with rupture of the membranes – reduces the risk of emergence of bacterial resistance. **Wound infections** are reduced in low-risk patients but many are minor and can be treated as outpatients, so universal prophylaxis may not be cost-effective. Ampicillin, piperacillin, cefotaxime, co-amoxiclav are all effective. Metronidazole alone should be avoided.

PREMATURE RUPTURE OF MEMBRANES

Universal screening for group B streptococci followed by prophylaxis only reduced the rate of infection from 1.5 to 1 per 1000 in one trial. Of 3721 patients, 18% carried the organism, but compliance was only 80% and five failures were due to non-compliance.

ABORTION

Some studies find that the use of antibiotics (e.g. metronidazole or doxycycline) reduce febrile morbidity and infection, but others find no difference compared with placebo. The presence of untreated chlamydial or gonococcal infection trebles the rate of post-abortal infection, so appropriate treatment of sexually transmitted diseases is important. Doxycycline decreases the rate of postoperative chlamydia infections compared with controls, but does not reduce gonorrhoea.

27.18 CONCLUSIONS

Many infections during pregnancy are preventable and can be detected and treated during the antenatal visits.

All healthcare workers conducting antenatal clinics must be aware of the importance of early treatment of, for example, urinary tract infection, before damage to the fetus or complications during delivery result.

27.19 FURTHER READING

Boyer, K.M. and Gotoff, S.P. (1986) Prevention of early onset neonatal group B streptococcal disease with selective intrapartum chemoprophylaxis. *N. Engl. J. Med.*, **314**, 1665–1669.

Chang, P.L. and Newton, E.R. (1992) Predictors of antibiotic failure in post-cesarean endometritis. *Obstet. Gynecol.*, **80**, 117–122.

Faro, S., Martens, M.G., Hammill, H.A., Riddle, G. and Tortolero, G. (1990) Antibiotic prophylaxis: is there a difference? *Am. J. Obstet. Gynecol.*, **162**, 900–909.

Gibbs, R.S., McDuffie, R.S., McNabb, F., Fryer, G.E., Miyoshi, T. and Merenstein, G. (1994) Neonatal group B streptococcal sepsis during 2 years of a universal screening program. *Obstet. Gynecol.*, **84**, 496–500.

Hemsell, D.L. (1991) Prophylactic antibiotics in gynecologic and obstetric surgery. *Rev. Infect. Dis.*, **13** (Suppl. 10), S821–S841.

Henderson, E. and Love, E.J. (1995) Incidence of hospital-acquired infections associated with caesarean section. *J. Hosp. Infect.*, **29**, 245–255.

Ryan, G.M., Abdella, T.N., McNeeley, S.G., Baselski, V.S. and Drummond, D.E. (1990) *Chlamydia trachomatis* infection in pregnancy and the effect of treatment on outcome. *Am. J. Obstet. Gynecol.*, **162**, 34–39.

Smaill, F. (1992) Antibiotic prophylaxis and caesarean section. *Br. J. Obstet. Gynaecol.*, **99**, 789–790.

Stagno, S., Pass, R.F., Dworsky, M.E., Henderson, RE, Moore, E.G., Walton, P.D. and Alford, C.A. (1982) Congenital cytomegalovirus infection: the relative importance of primary and recurrent maternal infection. *N. Engl. J. Med.*, **306**, 945–949.

Stubblefield, P.G. and Grimes, D.A. (1994) Septic abortion. *N. Engl. J. Med.*, **331**, 310–314.

Sexually transmitted and other infections in gynaecology

A.G. LAWRENCE, R. MARWOOD AND E. HOUANG

28.1 BACTERIOLOGICAL DIAGNOSIS

In the investigation of patients with suspected gynaeco-logical infections, specimens of urine, sputum and blood, together with those specimens from appropriate opera-tive sites, should always be obtained for culture before the commencement of therapy. It is important to obtain endo-cervical specimens (and uterine specimens if possi-ble) in all cases of suspected pelvic sepsis. The informa-tion obtained for bacteriological investigation depends upon the quality and appropriateness of the samples sent to the laboratory. Anaerobic organisms are common pathogens in gynaecological patients. Pus in a container rather than on a swab is preferable. The optimal condi-tion for the isolation of these and other fastidious organ-isms requires an appropriate transport system. Transport media such as Stuart's and Amies' contain reducing agents such as sodium thioglycollate and are convenient to use. Nevertheless, the chance of isolating gonococci or anaerobes is reduced when there is a delay of more than 24 hours. Outside normal working hours, agar plates may be inoculated in the theatre or by the bedside and incu-bated in an anaerobic jar using the Gas Pak system if proper laboratory facilities are not available. Similarly, a carbon dioxide Generation Pak or a lidded candle jar offer the correct atmospheric conditions for the isolation of *Neisseria gonorrhoeae*. These simple systems should be considered seriously in centres where transport to the laboratory may incur delay.

Blood culture is invaluable for the diagnosis of infection when the primary site is not accessible to the clinician. Indeed, its value in suspected pelvic infection is underesti-mated. The isolation of microaerophilic or anaerobic organisms from blood culture may suggest the presence of pelvic abscesses. It is important to use culture media which support the wide range of bacteria likely to be encountered in pelvic infection – including the genital mycoplasmas, *N. gonorrhoeae* and anaerobes. Whenever possible, at least two separate sets should be collected before the start of antibiotic therapy. Examination of high vaginal swabs (HVS) is a common test performed in gynaecological practice. This is helpful in early postoperative infections, but is of limited value in the management of upper genital tract infections, including transmitted infections. The high vaginal swab should always be taken under the vision of a Cuscoe's speculum, so as to avoid contamination by organisms of the lower third which may be different from those in the upper third of the vagina and thus give mis-leading results.

The vaginal microflora of healthy, asymptomatic women consists of a variety of anaerobic and aerobic bac-teria, dominated by microaerophilic and anaerobic species of the genus *Lactobacillus*. Although this microbial flora appears to benefit the host by reducing the probability of colonization by exogenous microorganisms, it may play a role in the pathogenesis of various gynaecological infections. The source of bacteria recovered postoperatively from a wound infection is usually endogenous from the flora of the vagina, cervix, skin, respiratory or gastrointestinal tracts. Organisms responsible for hospital-acquired infections such as *Klebsiella* spp., *Enterobacter* spp. or *Pseudomonas* spp., are usually transmitted by the hands of staff from infected patients or inanimate reservoirs. An understanding of the vaginal flora in health and disease and knowledge of locally prevalent organisms and their patterns of susceptibility are necessary to interpret culture results and to choose the appropriate antibiotic(s). Many agents have similar spectra of antimicrobial activity, and more than one regimen of therapy or prophylaxis may be suitable in a given situation.

Indigenous microflora appear to be a major host defence mechanism against invading pathogens. Some of these may become pathogenic under certain circumstances. In menarchal women, there are about 10^8–10^9 anaerobes ml^{-1} of vaginal secretions – ten times more abundant than aerobes. The most frequent isolates in numbers exceeding 10^5 ml^{-1} are facultative and obligate anaerobic lactobacilli, peptostreptococci and peptococi. Anaerobic Gram-negative rods may be recovered from almost 50% of women of reproductive age, the most common species including *Prevotella bivia* and *Prevotella disiens*. Clinically important species such as *Bacteroides fragilis*, members of enterobacteriaceae (e.g. *Escherichia coli*) and *Staphylococcus aureus* may be recovered from 10% of healthy women, but these are usually in low concentrations ($<10^6$ ml^{-1}). Other commonly found anaerobes include *Eubacterium* spp. and *Fusobacterium* spp. *Gardnerella vaginalis*, when sought, may be present in a significant proportion of asymptomatic women, though usually in small numbers. Less common (but by no means unusual) groups of organisms recovered from asymptomatic women include microaerophilic streptococci, such as members of the *Streptococcus milleri* group.

In specimens of pus obtained from the operating theatre and blood cultures of patients admitted with a variety of severe infections of the genital tract, anaerobic bacteria were cultured (using extensive techniques) from all patients, and aerobes from 70%. The most common aerobic and facultative bacteria were *E. coli*, followed by streptococci and *Staphylococcus epidermidis*. *B. fragilis* was the most common anaerobe.

28.1.1 Interpretation of HVS reports

The balanced dynamic ecosystem of the vaginal microbial flora alters frequently in response to known and unknown physiological pressures, the prevalence and population levels of each species varying with frequency and time of sampling during the menstrual cycle. Genital tract surgery, antimicrobial treatment (including that with local disinfectants and antibiotics), immunosuppression, and the presence of invasive cancer are known to alter the normal vaginal microflora. In everyday practice, it is neither cost-effective nor clinically necessary to identify each species isolated from specimens taken from sites where there is a normal commensal flora, such as the vagina. Many laboratories use the term '**normal vaginal flora**' to denote such findings. The clinical significance of the same bacterial species may be interpreted differently in different situations. Enterobacteria may be found in the vagina in significant numbers following antibiotic therapy or the use of antiseptics, but are usually of no clinical significance and are rarely responsible for vaginal discharge. However, in patients with postoperative pelvic infections or after radiation therapy, the isolation of Gram-negative rods is likely to be important and should be taken into account in choosing antimicrobial agents. Adequate clinical information should therefore always be provided to ensure that the laboratory processes HVS and reports its findings appropriately.

28.2 POSTOPERATIVE INFECTIONS

28.2.1 General causes of postoperative pyrexia

General causes of postoperative pyrexia are similar to postoperative pyrexia after procedures at other sites, and hence they will not be elaborated on here. The most common postoperative infection in gynaecology is **urinary tract infection**, associated with catheterization or instrumentation of the bladder. In recent years, the rate of symptomatic urinary tract infection after hysterectomies has been declining to 1–5%, as a result of the routine use of prophylactic antibiotics and diminished use of in-dwelling catheters. *E. coli* is the most common organism found, but other more resistant Gram-negative rods may be involved. Results of antimicrobial susceptibility tests should be used to guide the choice of correct antibiotic(s). It should be remembered that in gynaecological practice, infections commonly occur in women with an intact immune system and are not caused by highly resistant organisms. The exceptions are patients who have undergone surgery for genital malignancy (see Risk factors) and are at a higher risk of infectious morbidity, often caused by multiply resistant Gram-negative organisms. Thus, agents used to treat patients after radical surgery must cover the more resistant aerobic Gram-negative rods (e.g. gentamicin, or a third-generation cephalosporin).

28.2.2 Risk factors

Risk factors that have been consistently identified to increase the general postoperative morbidity following hysterectomies include age, underlying medical conditions, obesity (the depth of subcutaneous tissue), and the approach and duration of the procedure. Wound healing, infection and thromboembolic events are specific problems in the very elderly (>70 years of age). Patients undergoing hysterectomy for cancer have an overall postoperative morbidity rate twice that of patients with benign diseases.

28.2.3 Operative site infection

Operative site infections includes pelvic cellulitis, vaginal cuff abscess, pelvic abscess, wound infection and infected haematoma. In the treatment of vulval cancer, wound breakdown and infection, including sepsis, occurs in approximately 40% of patients after radical vulvectomy. Wound breakdown is primarily due to infection of, and tension on, the wounds. Patients with pelvic infections may complain of pelvic or perineal pain, or of a sensation of needing to defaecate, in addition to the general symptoms of fever and tachycardia. Vaginal examination may reveal an area of pelvic tenderness or a tender mass, and there is usually purulent discharge. It may be difficult to distinguish patients with pelvic cellulitis and low-grade fever from those with unexplained fever and normal postoperative induration of the vaginal cuff. Pelvic ultrasound may be used to identify haematoma or abscesses, but the latter are a relatively uncommon complication. The abscess may discharge through the vagina or rectum, and occasionally may result in a massive postoperative haemorrhage. The examination of HVS may be helpful but is unlikely to reveal the complete picture. Blood culture should be performed and will sometimes help to identify one of the organisms responsible. Antibiotic therapy is usually started after bacteriological samples have been obtained but before the results are available. The choice of agent(s) will be determined by the severity of the infection and the sensitivity of the most likely organisms in that hospital. Appropriate regimens include amoxycillin and clavulanic acid, cefuroxime plus metronidazole, ampicillin, gentamicin plus metronidazole. If *Staph. aureus* is suspected, then cloxacillin should be used.

While antibiotics and conservative therapy will settle most cases of postoperative pelvic sepsis, drainage through an incision in the vagina or the rectum may sometimes be necessary. Patients who fail to respond to standard therapy or who develop signs of peritonitis will require a laparotomy in order to rule out previously unsuspected damage to the bowel or urinary tract. The subdiaphragmatic spaces and the entire intestinal tract should be examined to exclude multiloculated abscesses. Severe postoperative pelvic infections may be followed by adhesions involving the bowel, resulting in intermittent subacute obstruction. Many patients also experience chronic pelvic pain and suffer from impaired fertility if there has been tubo-ovarian damage.

28.2.4 Infection following legal or criminal abortion

Infection following legal or criminal abortion may be serious. Abdominal pain, a purulent discharge, – sometimes with vaginal bleeding and systemic signs of infection – are the usual presentation. An enlarged, tender uterus and tender adnexal masses are common findings. The cervix may be open and there may be evidence of trauma to it and/or the vagina, and the patient may be serious ill if septicaemia is well established. These patients require evacuation of the uterus and repair of laceration after rapid correction of hypovolaemia and institution of antimicrobial therapy – which must be broad-spectrum to cover the likely polymicrobal aetiology. A combination of ampicillin, an aminoglycoside (or a third-generation cephalosporin) and metronidazole may be given. If the patient presents with shock or peripheral circulatory failure, one should be mindful of *Clostridium perfringens* infection and treat with high doses of penicillin in place of ampicillin. Hysterectomy is necessary if there is evidence of perforation of the uterus or evidence of gas gangrene.

28.2.5 Necrotizing fasciitis (NF)

Necrotizing fasciitis is a rare but serious condition which presents like a subcutaneous infection. In gynaecology, it is seen most commonly in the vulval, perineal or gluteal skin, or in the skin of the thigh. The subcutaneous infection spreads widely under apparently normal-looking skin; signs of toxicity worsen and are out of proportion to the apparent extent of the superficial lesion. Diagnosis of NF is difficult and is often delayed. The mortality rate for cases of NF in the perineal and pelvic areas is higher than in other sites. Although diabetes mellitus is an important predisposing factor, the condition may present itself after a straightforward surgical procedure in a previously healthy woman. It is now recognized that these infections are polymicrobial and that bacterial synergism is a key factor in the pathogenesis.

The key to a successful outcome is early diagnosis, together with radical excision of affected skin and tissues – 'cut until it bleeds'. Treatment with antibiotics alone or with antibiotics plus incision and drainage is associated with 100% mortality. A diverting colostomy should be fashioned if the involvement of perineal tissues and anal sphincter is extensive. Nutritional support of these patients may improve survival. Aggressive re-exploration is indicated any time there is not rapid clinical improvement or continuous wound healing.

28.2.6 Infections following conization and insertion of intrauterine contraceptive devices

In the management of patients with an abnormal Papanicolaou test, the traditional surgical technique of cold knife conization is being replaced by laser conization, and more recently by the loop electrosurgical excisional procedure (LEEP). This latter treatment modality has been suggested as suitable in the primary care setting. Data on postoperative infectious complications of these procedures are limited. Postoperative bleeding, commonly regarded as a result of infection, occurs mainly between 6 and 14 days after surgery and is seen in about 5% of patients, irrespective of the method used of conization.

The risk of developing **pelvic inflammatory disease** (PID) is increased in women using an intrauterine contraceptive device (IUCD). There is some evidence suggesting that the risk of developing an IUCD-related pelvic inflammatory disease may be reduced if the device thread is inserted into the uterine cavity. The long-term use of copper or levonorgestrel IUCDs has been shown to be associated with low and declining annual incidences of side effects, including pelvic infection. Extended use of the same IUCD for ≥7 years minimizes the risk of pelvic infection, as higher risks are associated with IUCD insertion, and decreasing rates of PID with long-term use.

28.2.7 Failure to respond to antibiotic therapy

In gynaecology, failure to respond to antibiotic therapy is often associated with the presence of a substantial collection of pus which needs to be located and surgically drained. Infected pelvic thrombophlebitis, an uncommon diagnosis, may be responsible for persistent fever, in spite of adequate antimicrobial treatment and the absence of a collection; dull lower abdominal pain may also be present. Pelvic examination reveals tenderness along the lateral pelvic wall, and there is no localizing sign. A therapeutic test of heparin (24 000 units daily) should bring about a response within 48 hours; this should be followed by oral anticoagulation for a further 3–4 weeks. Other possible causes of a failure of treatment include incorrect clinical or microbiological diagnoses. *Mycoplasma hominis*, an uncommon cause of postoperative infection, may be responsible for high fever and tachycardia after a hysterectomy. *M. hominis* may be isolated from blood cultures and/or in heavy growth from HVS. The patient will respond to a course of tetracycline, initially given parenterally if indicated. Another cause of treatment failure may be incorrect choice or dosage of antibiotics. An antibiotic such as nitrofurantoin is not suitable for systemic infection as increased drug elimination as a result of improved renal function may lead to inadequate plasma concentrations of the drug. When the condition of a patient deteriorates after a satisfactory initial response to antimicrobial therapy, superinfection by a resistant organism should be excluded. Opportunistic infection caused by microbes such as resistant aerobic Gram-negative rods, fungi or protozoa may occur in patients treated with corticosteroids, immunosuppressants, amino acid or lipid infusions, or a parental iron preparation.

28.3 ANTIBIOTIC PROPHYLAXIS IN GYNAECOLOGY

Abdominal procedures involving only clean wounds, such as infertility-related or reconstructive surgery, do not benefit from antibiotic prophylaxis. Nevertheless, some surgeons argue that reconstructive Fallopian tube surgery on previously infected tissues warrants prophylaxis. Prophylactic antibiotic therapy is usually valuable in operations involving clean contaminated wounds, such as hysterectomies, where microbial contamination from the vagina invariably takes place. The mechanism by which chemoprophylaxis functions is unclear, although it is generally believed that the antibiotic present during the operation reduces the contaminating organisms and also renders tissue fluid less suitable as a culture medium. Upon entering the peritoneal cavity during an abdominal hysterectomy, contamination by skin organisms occurs in most patients; the bacterial count of the fluid in the Pouch of Douglas may contain $10–10^4$ colony-forming units (cfu) ml^{-1} of skin organisms. After opening the vault, bacterial contamination by vaginal organisms increases markedly, may be $>10^5$ cfu ml^{-1}. The magnitude of the contamination has been shown to correlate with the likelihood of postoperative infectious morbidity, and is likely to be determined by many factors, including the technical difficulty of the procedure, the surgeon's skill and the duration of the operation. In comparative studies, it is often difficult to demonstrate a significant difference between regimens used because of low infection rates in both chemoprophylactic groups. Single-dose prophylaxis given at the induction of anaesthesia is as effective as multiple-dose regimens. If the surgical procedure is prolonged, a further dose may be given at the end of the operation if the half-life of the agent used is short. The newer cephalosporins with a longer half-life (e.g., cefotetan and ceftriaxone) have been reported to cause increased colonization of the vagina or bowel by resistant organisms such as *Streptococcus faecalis*, *Enterobacter* and yeasts. It is not certain whether postoperative infection following use of these prophylactic agents would be caused by resistant organisms.

28.3.1 Vaginal hysterectomy

Chemoprophylaxis has been shown consistently to reduce pelvic infections and febrile morbidity and also to be cost-effective in prospective, double-blind and placebo-controlled studies. A significant reduction of postoperative urinary tract infection is more difficult to achieve. It is generally agreed that chemoprophylaxis should be used in vaginal hysterectomy.

28.3.2 Abdominal hysterectomy

The benefit of chemoprophylaxis in abdominal hysterectomy has been less uniformly demonstrated. A significant reduction in wound and pelvic infections has been observed in those studies in which the infection rate in the placebo-treated group was relatively high (>15%). Whether the vaginal vault is left open or closed does not seemingly affect postoperative morbidity. Experience of laparoscopic hysterectomy techniques in the UK is still limited, and no comment can be made.

28.3.3 Therapeutic abortion

Although a recent meta-analysis revealed a substantial protective effect from antibiotics in all subgroups of women undergoing therapeutic abortion – even women in low-risk groups – some problems remain unresolved. The optimal antibiotic and dosing regimens are unclear, although tetracyclines and nitro-imidazoles are the most common agents used. There is a lack of uniform definitions and diagnostic criteria of pelvic infections as well as difficulties in completing postoperative follow-up. An alternative approach to universal prophylaxis is to screen for established infection in at-risk women. Risk factors include a previous history of pelvic inflammatory diseases, an age of less than 20 years, two or more sexual partners within a year, nulligravidity and sexually transmitted diseases. Ideally, the local risk profile of genital infections in the catchment population should first be determined locally. Nowadays, using rapid diagnostic techniques in the laboratory, it is possible to carry out preoperative screening for gonorrhoea, chlamydial infections or bacterial vaginosis and to provide appropriate therapy before the termination procedure. In the UK, chlamydial positivity rates of 5–9% have been reported in women seeking a termination of pregnancy at different centres. Screening permits not only active follow-up of infected women but also contact tracing to help prevent reinfection and to identify further cases.

28.3.4 Hysterosalpingography

In 90% of all hysterosalpingography procedures, bacteria from the lower genital tract are injected with a dye into the previously sterile peritoneal cavity. Although the frequency of subsequent acute pelvic infections is low (<3%), the consequences are particularly serious for the population of women undergoing this procedure. It is therefore recommended that dye should not be injected if bilateral hydrosalpinges are clearly seen, as tuboplasty is not indicated. If a unilateral hydrosalpinx is seen and dye is injected to elucidate the state of the other tube, antibotic prophylaxis should be given as soon as possible. The best choice of agents is not certain. The single-dose perioperative regimens, together with a course of doxy-cycline, may suffice.

28.3.5 Patients at risk of infective endocarditis

Patients who are at risk of developing endocarditis may not be identified prior to the procedure. The Endocarditis Working party of the British Society for Antimicrobial Chemotherapy does not recommend routine antibiotic prophylaxis for minor procedures such as cervical dilation and curettage of the uterus or the insertion or removal of IUCDs, except for patients with prosthetic valves or patients who have had a previous attack of endocarditis. Others hold more conservative views because of appreciable morbidity and mortality from endocarditis. Patients with cardiac abnormalities should receive chemoprophylaxis for all surgical, alimentary and genitourinary procedures. IUCDs are contraindicated in women with a history of PID or infective endocarditis. The device is also not advisable in women who have had previous cardiac surgery, have prosthetic heart valves or are drug abusers. In any prophylactic regimen to prevent endocarditis in genitourinary surgery, an agent active against *Strep. faecalis* must be included.

28.4 SEXUALLY TRANSMITTED INFECTIONS

Among the sexually transmitted infections, only those that are likely to be encountered in surgical practice will be discussed here. These include genital ulcers and sexually transmitted diseases that are commonly seen in gynaecological patients. The therapeutic regimens suggested largely follow those recommended by the Centers for Disease Control and Prevention (CDC), Atlanta, USA in 1993: Recommendations for the Prevention and Management of *Chlamydia trachomatis* Infections, and 1993 Sexually Transmitted Diseases Treatment Guidelines. Quinolones are contraindicated in adolescents ≤17 years of age, and also in pregnant and lactating women.

28.4.1 Genital ulcers

Medical conditions associated with genital lesions, for example Behcet's syndrome or Zonn's vulvitis, will not be described here. Lymphgranuloma venereum – caused by serovars L_1, L_2, or L_3 of C. trachomatis – is rare except in some tropical countries and will not be discussed, since most patients who seek care no longer have the self-limited genital ulcer that usually occurs at the site of inoculation. Most genital ulcers are caused by genital herpes, syphilis or chancroid. Their relative frequencies may vary in different geographic areas and patient populations. Each disease has been associated with an increased risk of HIV infection which should therefore always be considered, especially in those with syphilis or chancroid. More than one sexually transmitted infection (including causers of genital ulcers) may be present in patients with genital ulcers. These patients should always be referred to specialists in genitourinary medicine who have the facilities and special skills, not only for clinical management but also the follow-up and counselling of patients and their sexual partners.

A diagnosis based only on history and physical examination is often inaccurate. All evaluations of persons with genital ulcers should include a serological test for syphilis. Other tests include a darkfield examination or a direct immunofluorescence test for *Treponema pallidum*; a culture or antigen test for herpes simplex virus and a culture for *Haemophilus ducreyi*; and HVS, cervical and urethral swabs to exclude other sexually transmitted infections. HIV testing should be considered, especially for those with syphilis or chancroid.

28.4.2 Chancroid

A presumptive diagnosis of chancroid is often based on the clinical appearance of **genital ulceration**. Confirmation of the diagnosis should always be sought by cultural isolation of *H. ducreyi*, although the technique is not widely available. Ideally, swabs of the ulcer exudate taken prior to saline cleansing of the lesion should be inoculated directly onto special culture plates (for which the laboratory usually requires notice to prepare). Chancroid may be suggested by the presence of unilateral tender inguinal adenopathy and one or more painful genital ulcers if *T. pallidum* and syphilis have already been ruled out: the former by darkfield examination of ulcer exudate, and the latter by serology performed at least 7 days after onset of the ulcer. HSV should also be excluded. The incubation period is usually 7 days but may be longer in women. Vaginal introitus is

a common site of presentation, but lesions on other genital sites have been described. Classically, chancroid ulcers have scalloped and undermined edges and there is a purulent exudate overlying a non-indurated base of granulation tissue which bleeds on manipulation. Other appearances are possible: hypertrophic vegetation (commonly associated with peri-anal lesions); multiple shallow ulcers resembling those of HSV lesions; or less destructive ulcers without the undermined edges. One week after the appearance of the ulcer(s), the inguinal lymph gland (usually unilateral) may become a painful swollen red mass in one-third of patients; suppuration follows later. Ulcer infection concomitant with other sexually transmitted diseases (STDs) is well recognized in chancroid. When *T. pallidum* is present, the lesion becomes less painful but more indurated with time. Coexisting herpes infection is common in Europe.

THERAPY

Therapy of chancroid may involve the following:

- Ciprofloxacin 500 mg orally twice daily for 3 days; or
- Azithromycin 1 g orally in a single dose; or
- Ceftriaxone 250 mg intramuscularly (i.m.) in a single dose; or
- Amoxycillin 500 mg plus clavulanic acid 125 mg orally three times daily for 7 days; or
- Erythromycin base 500 mg orally four times daily for 7 days.

Since 1989, *H. ducreyi* has become less susceptible *in vitro* to trimethoprim-sulfamethozaxole, and there is a corresponding decrease in their clinical efficacy. Successful treatment brings about symptomatic improvement within 3 days, though large ulcers may take up to 4 weeks to heal completely and scarring may result. Needle aspiration through adjacent intact skin is recommended for large (>5 cm) fluctuant bubos to prevent spontaneous rupture, even during successful therapy.

SEXUAL PARTNERS

All the sexual partners from the period of 10 days preceding the onset of the chancroid symptoms should be examined and treated, even if they do not have symptoms.

28.4.3 Syphilis

Only the diagnosis of primary syphilis, as a differential diagnosis of genital ulcers, will be discussed here. The incubation period is generally around 28 days, or 10 to 90 days at the extremes. Although the primary stage appears clinically as a localized cutaneous ulcer (chancre), *T. pallidum* organisms disseminate widely throughout the body. By the time of presentation, chancre is commonly seen as a single, small, painless round or oval ulcer with a regular, clearly defined and bright red edge. The floor is rarely infected secondarily and consists of clean-looking granulation tissue. Most chancres occur on the vulva, the labia and rarely on the cervix, where they are likely to be missed. The regional lymph nodes are involved, usually bilaterally, and become enlarged, firm, discrete, mobile and painless. Darkfield examinations or direct immuno-fluorescence tests of lesion exudate or tissue are the defin-itive methods for diagnosing early syphilis. The results of two types of serological tests (non-treponemal and trepo-nemal) may give a presumptive diagnosis. Commonly used non-treponemal tests include the Venereal Disease Research Laboratory (VDRL) and the rapid plasma rea-gin (RPR) tests. The fluorescent treponemal antibody absorbed test (FTA-ABS), a treponemal test, is the first to become positive, followed by the VDRL and then the *T. pallidum* haemagglutination reaction (TPHA). The results of non-treponemal tests are normally reported quantitatively, and a four-fold rise or fall in titre indicates a change in the disease activity, provided that the sequen-tial tests have been performed using the same testing method by the same laboratory. They become negative within 6 months in 90% of patients after adequate treat-ment. Treponemal tests (e.g. FTA-ABS and TPHA) may continue to give a positive result regardless of disease activity. A small proportion (15–25%) of patients, if treated early, i.e. during the primary stage, may have a non-reactive result 2–3 years later.

For patients presenting with **primary syphilis**, an HIV test should be carried out at the time of presenta-tion and then 3 months later. For the vast majority of HIV-infected patients, serological tests are satisfactory for the diagnosis of syphilis and for the evaluation of treatment response.

TREATMENT OF PRIMARY SYPHILIS

Treatment may include the following:

- Benzathine penicillin G, 2.4×10^6 units intramuscularly in a single dose; or
- Aqueous procaine penicillin G 600 mg intramuscu-larly, daily single dose for 10 days; or
- for penicillin-allergic patients, tetracycline 500 mg orally four times daily for 2 weeks.

Patients should be re-examined clinically and serologically at 1, 3, 6, and 12 months after treatment. Failure of non-treponemal test titres to decline four-fold by 3 months after therapy for primary syphilis may indicate treatment failure. If further follow-up cannot be assured, re-treatment is recommended. The patients should always be managed by specialists in genitourinary medicine.

The Jarisch–Herxheimer reaction may occur in 50% of patients with primary syphilis; this begins 4–12 hours after the first injection of penicillin and lasts for a few hours. It is usually mild and harmless, but patients should

be warned about it and advised to rest for a few hours and to take two aspirin or paracetamol tablets when it occurs. It should not prevent or delay therapy for syphilis.

SEXUAL PARTNERS

Sexual partners from the period of 3 months prior to the onset of symptoms plus the symptoms' duration are identified as at risk for primary syphilis, with a 50% chance of infection. Pre-emptive therapy is therefore generally recommended, even if the partners are seronegative. For sexual contact >90 days before examin-ation, the partners should also be treated presump-tively if serological test results are not available immediately, and the opportunity for follow-up is uncertain. Presumptive therapy is also given to partners of patients who have syphilis of unknown duration and who have high non-treponemal serological test titres ($\geq$1:32) and should therefore be regarded as having early syphilis.

28.4.4 Genital herpes simplex virus (HSV) infections

Genital herpetic lesions are usually quite easy to recog-nize. In primary infection, symptoms develop usually in the 5–7 days after sexual contact (extremes: 4–14 days). There may be systemic upsets such as fever, or malaise with myalgia and headache. Lesions are seen on the mucosal surfaces of the labia minora and clitoral hood, frequently spreading to involve the neighbouring skin. The first clinical lesions present as a group or groups of erythematous, painful papules which develop into characteristic herpetic lesions of greyish-yellow vesicles containing clear fluid within 1–2 days. Mild primary attacks of a few vesicles may easily be over-looked. Viral culture from the cervix is often positive in primary infections, particularly if type 2 is involved. Periurethral or perianal lesions cause a great deal of pain and difficulty in voiding or defaecating. The lesions on the cervix may vary from a few classical vesi-cles to extensive necrotic cervicitis which heals readily. Occasionally, the cervix may be the only site involved in a primary infection.

The presence of oral ulceration, iridocyclitis, erythemanodosum-like skin lesions and other features may help to distinguish Behcet's syndrome from genital herpes. However, these features of the syndrome may be absent particularly in the first episode of the disease, and thus pose diagnostic problems. Vulval aphthosis, which is a rare condition, involves the skin of the labia majora and produces painful, short-lived ulcers and may be associated with drug hypersensitivities such as non-steroidal, anti-inflammatory drugs (NSAIDs). The her-pes viral culture result will be negative. In herpes zoster involving the genital area, there is usually marked local pain with eruption occuring in a band over a distribution of one dermatome.

SPECIMEN COLLECTION

For viral isolation, the lesion should be rubbed with a cotton- or Dacron-tipped swab, in order to obtain infected cells. Vesicular fluid should be collected if available as it may contain up to 10^9 HSV particles mm^{-3}. When obtaining specimens from the cervix, the exocervix and the endocervical canal should also be swabbed. The swab should be sent to the laboratory in a viral transport medium. It can be stored for 48 hours at 4°C or for a longer period at -70°C. Viral isolation remains the 'gold standard' method by which other tests are measured. Rapid diagnostic tests relying on the detection of HSV antigen include direct immunofluorescent test and enzyme-linked immunosorbent assay (ELISA). The sensitivity of these tests vary from 70 to 95% compared with culture.

TREATMENT

Acyclovir neither eradicates latent virus nor affects subsequent risk, frequency, severity or recurrences after administration of the drug is discontinued. Episodes of HSV infection among HIV-infected patients may require more aggressive therapy. Immunocompromised persons may have prolonged episodes with extensive disease. For these persons, one should be mindful of infections caused by acyclovir-resistant strains.

First clinical episode

Acyclovir 200 mg should be given five times daily for 5–10 days or until clinical resolution is attained. The dose should be doubled for the first clinical episode of herpes proctitis.

Recurrent episodes

For most immunocompetent patients with recurrent disease, acyclovir therapy is not recommended for recurrent attacks of HSV infections. To be beneficial, therapy must be administered during the prodrome or within 2 days of the onset of lesions. Daily suppressive therapy should be considered if recurrences are frequent and affect the patient's quality of life.

Suppressive therapy

Among patients with attacks on six or more occasions per year, daily suppressive acyclovir therapy reduces the frequency of recurrences by at least 75%, but it may not totally eliminate symptomatic or asymptomatic viral shedding or the potential for transmission. It is normal practice to discontinue suppressive therapy after 1 year to allow assessment of the patient's rate of recurrent episodes. The patient may commence with 400 mg orally twice daily. The regimen may be adjusted to achieve the lowest dose that provides relief.

SEXUAL PARTNERS

Sexual partners of patients with HSV infection may benefit from evaluation and counselling.

28.4.5 Pelvic inflammatory disease (PID)

This clinical syndrome is attributed to the ascending spread of organisms from the vagina and cervix to the endometrium, Fallopian tube and/or contiguous structures. Of the sexually transmitted organisms, *N. gonorrhoeae* and *C. trachomatis* are implicated in the majority of cases. A wide range of microorganisms that can form part of the vaginal flora, such as anaerobes, *G. vaginalis*, *H. influenzae*, enteric Gram-negative rods, Group B *Streptococcus*, alpha-haemolytic streptococci, *M. hominis* and *U. urealyticum* have been isolated from operative specimens. The precise mechanisms determining the spread of microorganisms from the lower to the upper genital tract are poorly understood. The uterus is particularly vulnerable to ascending infections for a few days after childbirth or miscarriage when the cervix remains relatively open, or after surgical instrumentation. A previous episode of PID predisposes the patient to a second attack. The presence of an intrauterine device appears to increase the risk of developing PID by ten-fold. Bacteriospermia in males and adherence of bacteria to spermatozoa suggest that bacteria can be 'carried' to the Fallopian tubes. Retrograde menstruation may also play a part. Direct spread of an infection from a contiguous structure may occur occasionally (e.g. from an inflamed appendix to the right Fallopian tube). Haematological spread is rare; examples include tuberculosis salpingitis and mumps oophoritis.

Women with past chlamydial or gonococcal infections or both are significantly more likely to have bilateral tubal occlusion. Once the gonococcus ascends to the Fallopian tube, it adheres to non-ciliated mucus-secreting cells. However, cytokine release in response to the toxic components of the gonococcus surface structures – lipo-oligosaccharides and peptidoglycan – results in the major damage occurring in uninfected cilated epithelial cells. In addition, there is an inflammatory response which causes extensive cell death and tissue damage, resulting in scarring and tubal adhesions. In chlamydial tubal infection, the tissue damage may be related to delayed hyperimmune reaction in some immunologically 'primed' women. The chronic exposure to *C. trachomatis* that occurs in asymptomatic women with 'silent' chlamydial tubal infection might be especially conducive to the development of this immune response. Furthermore, there are homologous regions in the chlamydial 57 kDa protein and the human 60 kDa heat shock protein. Once an autoimmune response has become set up to the human protein, host tissue damage may continue, even if *C. trachomatis* is no longer present.

The important grave late sequelae of PID are ectopic pregnancy and infertility. Women in the post-PID state have a seven- to ten-fold increased risk of ectopic pregnancy as compared with women who have never had the disease. One mild attack of laparoscopically verified PID has been shown to be associated with a 10–20% chance of tubal infertility. After three or more attacks, 50–60% of women will become infertile; this demonstrates the importance of the early institution of effective therapy, in order to prevent the ascension of the infection and subsequent damage.

The severity of salpingitis may vary from symptomless or self-limiting, to a serious life-threatening condition. Patients usually complain of lower abdominal pain and deep dyspareunia, often with vaginal discharge and sometimes intermenstrual bleeding. Two-thirds of cases develop the symptoms close to a menstrual period. The pain is usually bilateral, often described as a 'bad period pain' which may be made worse upon activities such as running or walking downstairs. The patient may complain of anorexia, nausea and vomiting. Common findings on examination include a purulent cervical discharge, adnexal tenderness and tenderness when the cervix is moved. Fever, leukocytosis and a raised erythrocyte sedimentation rate (ESR) are usually present, as may be signs and symptoms of peritoneal involvement. Gonococcal-associated PID has a more rapid onset than chlamydial infections. Fitz-Hugh–Curtis syndrome (see p. 291, Chlamydial infections) may be found in 5% of patients with salpingitis, who may present with pain and discomfort in the upper right abdominal quadrant.

Many patients present with mild or non-specific symptoms which may not warrant the invasive diagnostic procedure of a laparoscopy immediately, unless another differential diagnosis such as appendicitis or ectopic pregnancy is also suspected. Although the procedure offers a more accurate clinical and microbiological diagnosis, it is not helpful when inflammation of the Fallopian tubes is not visually present, or when the uterus is mainly involved. The diagnosis of PID is therefore often made on clinical grounds,which have been shown to offer 65–90% of the positive predictive values for salpingitis derived from a laparoscopy. Nevertheless, because of the potentially serious effect on fertility, a low diagnostic threshold has been advocated. It is recommended that empirical treatment of PID should be given when lower abdominal tenderness, adnexal tenderness and cervical motion tenderness are present and in the absence of an established cause other than PID. For patients presenting with severe clinical signs, the specificity of the diagnosis can be improved by the presence of fever, abnormal cervical or vaginal discharge, raised ESR, C-reactive protein (CRP) and a positive cervical culture result for *N. gonorrhoeae* and/or *C. trachomatis*. Elaborate criteria for diagnosing PID include histopathological evidence of infection on endometrial biopsy, tubo-ovarian abscesses found by ultrasound or other radiological tests, and laparoscopic evidence consistent with PID.

INVESTIGATIONS

The commonly used indicators for infection, such as neutrophilia, elevated ESR or serum CRP, cannot discriminate mild tubal infections from lower genital tract infections. The serum or urine levels of beta-human chorionic gonadotrophin should always be measured to exclude ectopic pregnancy. Microbiological specimens to screen for the presence of sexually transmitted diseases should be taken before the commencement of antimicrobial therapy. The results of microscopic examination of Gram-stained cervical and urethral smears can be obtained rapidly for the diagnosis of gonococcal infections. Rapid diagnosis of chlamydial infection is also available nowadays (see p. 291, Chlamydial infections). **Blood cultures** should be obtained from febrile patients. In patients whose serious condition warrants a laparoscopy or laparotomy, microbiological specimens such as tubal swabs, pus from a tubo-ovarian abscess or turbid fluid from the Pouch of Douglas should be sent, even if antibiotic therapy has already been instituted.

TREATMENT

For most patients, bed-rest and antibiotics may suffice. There is a trend in developed countries to hospitalize patients, in order to ensure optimal therapy, at least until a satisfactory response to treatment has been obtained. The extent of compliance to the hospitalization guidelines described by the Center for Disease Control – CDC(1993) – will very much depend upon the availability of local resources. These guidelines are:

- Uncertain diagnosis where surgical emergencies such as appendicitis and ectopic pregnancy cannot be excluded;
- Pelvic abscess is suspected;
- The patient is pregnant;
- The effectiveness of outpatient therapy is uncertain because of unreliable compliance, (e.g. among adolescents) or the patient being unable to follow or tolerate the oral therapy;
- The patient has failed to respond clinically to the outpatient therapy within 48 hours; and
- The patient is unreliable to return for follow-up in 48 hours.

The antibiotics chosen should provide a broad spectrum cover of likely organisms, active against mixed infections caused by *N. gonorrhoeae*, *C. trachomatis*, Gram-negative facultative bacteria, anaerobes and streptococci. In young women who are not users of IUCDs, the disease is often sexually transmitted and therapy must cover *N. gonorrhoeae* and *C. trachomatis*. The actual choice will depend on local factors, such as availability, cost and regional differences in antimicrobial susceptibility.

Patients should show significant clinical improvement within 3–5 days of the commencement of antimicrobial therapy. If not, further diagnostic work-up and/or surgical intervention are indicated. Surgery is necessary when the patient presents with generalized peritonitis, does not respond to antimicrobial therapy within 48 hours, or when the pelvic abscess is pointing into the vagina, rectum or through the abdominal wall.

Rescreening for *C. trachomatis* and *N. gonorrhoeae* is indicated 3 weeks after the completion of therapy if the tests have been positive before therapy. Evaluation and treatment of sexual partners of women with PID is important. Some experts recommend that the partners should be treated empirically for possible *N. gonorrhoeae* and *C. trachomatis* infections.

Outpatient regimens

All patients must be reviewed after 48 hours to ensure the lowest possible incidence of sequelae. There is a wide range of recommended regimens, as follows:

- Amoxycillin 3 g orally plus probenecid 1 g by mouth [in areas of low incidence of penicillinase-producing *N. gomorrhoeae* (PPNG)]; or
- Spectinomycin 2 g i.m. (for penicillinase-producing strains, patients allergic to penicillin or pregnant patients); or
- Ciprofloxacin 500 mg orally; or
- Cefoxitin 2 g i.m. plus probenecid 1 g by mouth; or
- Ceftriaxone 250 mg i.m.

Plus

- Doxycycline 100 mg twice daily for 7 days; or
- Tetracycline 500 mg 6-hourly for 14 days; or
- Erythromycin 500 mg 6-hourly for 14 days (for pregnant patients).

Plus

- Metronidazole 500 mg twice daily for 14 days; or
- Clindamycin 450 mg 6-hourly, orally for 14 days.

When parenteral therapy is warranted, the following regimens are recommended:

- Cefoxitin 2 g i.v. 6 hourly; or
- Cefotetan 2 g 12-hourly; or
- Cefuroxime 1.5 g i.v. 6-hourly or cefotaxime 2 g i.v. 8-hourly to be used together with metronidazole i.v. or rectally 500 mg 8-hourly or 1 g 12-hourly for 14 days.

Plus

- Doxycycline 100 mg i.v. or orally 12-hourly for a total of 14 days.

Alternative regimen

- Clindamycin 900 mg i.v. 8-hourly plus gentamicin i.v. or i.m. (2 mg kg^{-1} body weight for the loading dose and 1.5 mg for the maintenance dose) plus doxycycline as above; or
- Co-amoxyclav (Augmentin) 1.2 g 8-hourly plus doxycycline as above.

28.4.6 *Chlamydia trachomatis* infections

In the UK, the prevalence of chlamydial infection varies from 5 to 9% in women attending antenatal, gynaecology or family-planning clinics. In women attending genito-urinary clinics, the prevalence may be as high as 20%. Demographic factors associated with an increased risk of positive cervical isolation include young age (15–22 years), non-white race, single marital status, and use of oral contraceptives. The prevalence of serum antibodies to *C. trachomatis* increases with age until about 30 years, when it plateaus at approximately 50%. The infection is insidious, and most of the infected women do not complain of symptoms. As a result, there is a large reservoir of the organism sustained by asymptomatic (but infectious) persons in the community, who are at risk of acute illness and possible serious long-term sequelae.

CERVICITIS

The site of initial infection is most often the cervix; the urethra and the rectum may also be infected. Cervical ectopia may influence the acquisition, transmission, or effects of sexually transmitted agents, such as *C. trachomatis*, *N. gonorrhoeae*, herpes simplex virus and cytomegalovirus. Ectopia has also been found to be associated with oral contraception, young age, smoking, and douching. About one-third of patients have local signs of infection: mucopurulent discharge, contact bleeding and oedema of the area of ectopy. Clinical recognition of chlamydial cervicitis depends upon a high index of suspicion and a careful cervical examination, as many women are asymptomatic. Sequential culturing of untreated women has shown that the infection may persist for months without development of symptoms, or it may resolve spontaneously.

URETHRITIS

Chlamydia is an important cause of acute urethral syndrome – dysuria and frequency without bacteriuria in young, sexually active women. There is no haematuria or suprapubic tenderness, and the urethra may be the only positive site for chlamydial isolation. Signs of urethritis, such as urethral discharge, meatal redness or swelling are, however, infrequent. Nevertheless, the majority of female STD clinic patients with urethral chlamydial infection do not have dysuria or frequency.

PELVIC INFLAMMATORY DISEASE

See pp. 288–290.

PERIHEPATITIS (FITZ-HUGH–CURTIS SYNDROME)

Chlamydial perihepatitis is more common than gonococcal perihepatitis. The condition should be suspected in young, sexually active women who develop right-upper-quadrant pain, fever, nausea or vomiting. In most cases, there is evidence of a concurrent attack of PID, which may precede or follow the development of hepatitis; there may also be referred pain in the right shoulder region. Examination may show only tenderness under the right costal margin on inspiration, suggesting a disease of the gallbladder. In severe cases, signs of peritonitis may be present. Areas of patchy inflammation with a little exudate develop on the peritoneum, covering the liver as well as the local parietal peritoneum. Laparoscopy may show typical 'violin string' adhesions. The liver is not directly involved, however. The differential diagnoses include gallbladder disease, pneumonia, pleurisy, liver disease and perforated peptic ulcer.

OTHER CHLAMYDIAL INFECTIONS

Reiter's syndrome (reactive arthritis, conjunctivitis and urethritis) occurs primarily among men. The urethritis component is less obvious in women. Chlamydia is receiving greater emphasis in the differential diagnosis of arthritis in young women. Ocular or ophthalmic infections may result from exposure to infectious genital secretions during oral–genital sexual contact, or by autoinoculation. *C. trachomatis* has not been established as a cause of pharyngitis.

LABORATORY DIAGNOSIS

Because chlamydiae are obligate intracellular organisms that infect the columnar epithelium, it is important to ensure that columnar epithelial cells from the endocervix or the urethra are only obtained after removing all secretions and discharge from the cervical os. Urethral specimens should be obtained at least 2 hours after the patient has voided.

Culture method

Laboratory diagnosis may be achieved by cell culture and/or antigen detection. The cell culture system remains the standard for the quality assurance of non-culture tests and the evaluation of new diagnostic methods. It is recommended for urethral specimens from female and asymptomatic patients, nasopharyngeal specimens from infants, all rectal specimens and vaginal specimens from prepubertal girls. In the transport medium, the specimen should be kept at 4°C if inoculated within 24 hours, or stored at −70°C for later inoculation. Cycloheximide-treated McCoy cells are commonly used to culture *C. trachomatis*, *C. pneumoniae* and *C. psittaci*, which grow and produce intracytoplasmic inclusions. The *C. trachomatis* are recognized using monoclonal fluorescein-labelled antibodies for their outer membrane protein, thus giving the 100% specificity of the cell culture method. Alternative antibodies that bind to chlamydia lipopolysaccharide will stain the *C. psittaci* and *C. pneumoniae* inclusions. However, because of the high cost of monoclonal antibodies, iodine staining of cytoplasmic inclusions is satisfactory and widely used by many laboratories when culturing genital specimens. Culture sensitivity is approximately 70–90% in experienced laboratories, and a result takes 3–7 days. A second passage of the culture is required to achieve optimal sensitivity.

Non-culture methods

Non-culture methods allow rapid diagnosis and high-volume throughput of specimens. Much evaluated methods include MicroTrak DFA(Syva) a direct fluorescent antibody test (DFA) and Chlamydiazyme EIA (Abbott) test, an enzyme immunoassay (EIA). DFAs use antigens of the major outer membrane protein or the lipopolysaccharide (LPS). After the slide has dried and the fixative has been applied, it can be stored at ambient temperature and processed by the destination laboratory within 7 days. Stained elementary bodies are identified by fluorescence microscopy. The total processing time may be 30–40 minutes. Cross-reactions can occur between the anti-LPS antibodies used in commercial kits and *C. pneumoniae*, *C. psittaci* and other bacterial species. DFA is particularly suitable for small volume testing such as in an outpatient setting during the patient's visit.

Enzyme immunoassay (EIA) tests

These methods may be automated and are therefore suitable for high-volume testing, provided that a quality control system can be implemented. Specimens for EIA testing are collected by using specimen collection kits supplied by the manufacturers. Monoclonal or polyclonal antibodies labelled with an enzyme detect chlamydial LPS. Specimens can be stored and transported at ambient temperature, and the total processing time may be 3–4 hours. Non-culture methods may be used for adult urethral and cervical specimens as well as for conjunctival specimens from all ages.

Contamination of cervical specimens with vaginal secretions is responsible for some false-positive tests when using Chlamydiazyme. The polyclonal anti-LPS antibody cross-reacts with the LPS of other bacteria found in the vagina and urinary tract of these patients. Verification should routinely be carried out, particularly if the patient has low risk factors, e.g. monogamous relationship, no history of STD or is a member of low prevalence (<5%) patient populations. A second non-culture method may be employed on the same specimens: for example, some EIA test manufacturers recommend a DFA test on the excess of the specimen to verify a positive EIA result. For Chlamydiazyme, a positive test should be verified with the addition of a monoclonal antibody specific for *Chlamydia* LPS which competitively inhibits *Chlamydia*-specific binding by the enzyme-labelled antibody. Initial positive test results can be verified by a negative result from a repeat test using the blocking antibody. However, culture is the most sensitive and specific method of verification.

There is little place for chlamydial serology in the routine clinical diagnosis of genital infections, because the long-lasting antibodies from previous infection cannot easily be distinguished from the antibodies produced in a current infection.

TREATMENT

For uncomplicated urethral, endocervical or rectal chlamydial infections among adults, the following regimens are satisfactory:

- Doxycycline 100 mg orally twice daily for 7 days; or
- Azithromycin 1 g in a single dose; or
- Erythromycin stearate 500 mg twice daily for 14 days; or
- Ofloxacin 300 mg orally twice daily for 7 days.

Unless symptoms persist or reinfection is suspected, no repeat testing is necessary after doxycycline or azithromycin therapy. Re-testing may be considered 3 weeks after the last dose of erythromycin or ofloxacin therapy.

SEXUAL PARTNERS

All sexual partners of an index patient from the period of 30 days preceding the onset of symptoms should be evaluated and treated for chlamydial infection. If the infected index patient is asymptomatic, the interval should be extended to 60 days. It has also been advocated that the last sexual partner of an infected patient should always be treated, even if the last sexual contact took place before 60 days. Sexual abstinence should be observed until the completion of therapy and the disappearance of symptoms.

28.4.7   Gonococcal infections

Gonococcal infection in men gives rise to early symptoms (with an incubation period of 2–5 days) which cause them to seek early medical advice. In women, the lack of early symptoms makes it difficult to estimate the incubation period. The disease is infectious and there is

a 20% risk of a woman's sexual partner developing urethral infection per episode of vaginal intercourse. Without treatment, women may develop serious complications; hence an important measure for controlling gonorrhoea has been the screening of women at risk.

Fresh clinical isolates of *N. gonorrhoeae* initially form colony types P+ and P++ that have numerous pili extending from the cell surface. Expression of pili is a function of the *pil* gene. After 20–24 hours of growth, P⁻ colonies come to predominate. Pilated gonococci are better able to attach themselves to human mucosal surfaces and are more virulent than non-pilated bacteria in animal and organ culture models and in human inoculation experiments. Pili also contribute to resistance to killing by neutrophils. In the Fallopian tube mucosa model, pili mediate attachment to non-ciliated epithelial cells and damage the nearby cilated cells. Non-pilated gonococci show attachment and damage to mucosal cells at a lower rate. Pilated commensal *Neisseria* neither attach nor cause damage in the experimental model. Pili traverse the outer membrane of the gonococcus and are composed of repeating protein subunits (pilin) which have areas of extreme antigenic variability near the carboxy terminus. In addition, different antigenic compositions may be found in a single strain; these variations in antigenic composition have prevented the production of an effective pilus-based vaccine. The outer membrane of gonococcus contains a variety of proteins. Porin (Por) provides channels through which aqueous solutes can pass through the otherwise hydrophobic outer membrane, and is believed to play an important role in pathogenesis. Por shows stable interstrain antigenic variation and is the basis of the most commonly employed gonococcal serotyping system. Certain Por serovars are associated with resistance to the bactericidal effect of normal (non-immune) human serum and is thus endowed with an enhanced propensity to cause bacteraemia. A gonococcal vaccine based on Por is being sought.

Opacity proteins (Opa) are other outer membrane proteins, the expression of which varies considerably during natural infection. For example, mucosal isolates whose colonies are opaque express Opa, whereas cervical isolates obtained during menstruation and isolates from normally sterile sites, such as the Fallopian tubes, blood and synovial fluid, lack Opa and form transparent colonies. Opa proteins increase adherence between gonococci and also increase their adherence to a variety of eukaryotic cells, including phagocytes. Reduction-modifiable protein (Rmp) is present in all gonococci in close association with Por and LOS and shows little interstrain antigenic variation. Rmp can stimulate blocking antibodies that reduce serum bactericidal activity against *N. gonorrhoeae*, which may potentiate reinfection after sexual exposure to an infected partner. Other outer membrane proteins have been identified as necessary for the acquisition of iron from transferrin and lactoferrin *in vivo*. *N. gonorrhoeae* can grow anaerobically, and this may contribute to secondary invasion by strict anaerobes in the development of pelvic inflammatory disease.

Characterization of *N. gonorrhoeae* strains is by **auxotyping** and **serotyping**. Auxotyping is based on the strains' genetically stable requirements for specific nutrients or cofactors, as defined by their ability to grow on chemically defined media that lack these factors. The common auxotypes include protoptrophic (Proto) or wild-type; proline-requiring (Pro-); and the AHU- types (arginine-, hypoxanthine- and uracil-requiring). The most widely used serotyping system is based on Por; this is antigenically classified into the groups IA and IB, which are in turn divided into serovars. Serovars are determined by the patterns of coagglutination reactions using panels of monoclonal antibodies that react with various epitopes of Por IA or IB. Auxotyping and Por serotyping are often used together for epidemiological studies.

GENITAL INFECTIONS

N. gonorrhoeae has a predilection for columnar epithelium in the urethra, cervix, rectum, accessory ducts and glands and conjunctivae. Skin is rarely involved except in the prepubertal vulva and vagina. Attachment to mucosal epithelium, mediated in part by pili and Opa, is followed within 24–48 hours by penetration of the organisms between and through epithelial cells to the submucosal tissues. This results in a vigorous response by neutrophils, and stained smears usually reveal large number of gonococci within a few neutrophils.

The cervix and urethra are infected in most patients. The organism can be recovered from the cervix in 90% of cases, and from both sites in 75% of cases. Urethritis may give rise to some dysuria or frequency. Cervicitis may be completely asymptomatic, with the cervix appearing normal, although the woman may sometimes complain of excessive discharge. The glands of Bartholin may be involved and the ducts may discharge pus when pressed. Occasionally, an abscess is formed, causing severe pain and a tender, inflammatory swelling in the lower third of the labia. Gonococcal proctitis frequently causes no symptoms.

DISSEMINATED GONORRHOEA

Disseminated gonorrhoea is seen in <1% of patients with gonorrhoea in developed countries, more frequently in women. In about half of affected female patients, symptoms of the disseminated infection occur within 7 days of onset of menses. Complement deficiency is also a risk factor. The onset is acute with fever, muscle pains and arthralgia. An additive, asymmetrical arthritis with tenosynovitis may develop in the knee, small joints of the hands and feet, followed by the wrist, ankle, elbow and shoulder joints. Wrist involvement is

common. Effusion may be present, but the fluid may not be positive when cultured. Less common is the development of acute septic arthritis in single large joints such as knee, wrist or ankle. The joint fluid is purulent and gonococci can usually be isolated. Skin lesions, seen in one-third of patients, may appear in crops, usually on the extremities near the affected joints. They appear as red papules at first and later become pustular with a purplish haemorrhagic (or sometimes ulcerative) centre and usually occur in small numbers. The appearance of lesions in large numbers (>20) is said to correlate with the extension of the infection, for example with cardiac (usually the aortic valve) or meningitis involvement. Gonococci may be isolated from skin lesions. Overall, only about half of patients with disseminated gonococcal infection have positive cultures of blood or synovial fluid, whereas mucosal sites may be positive in 80% of cases.

Strains of *N. gonorrhoeae* classically associated with disseminated disease tend to be specific Por IA serovars and of AHU- auxotype, show a tendency to resist the bactericidal action of non-immune human serum, and have a marked sensitivity to penicillin. However, an increasing proportion of disseminated cases has been caused by other auxotypes or serovars. There may be host factors that may predispose the person to gonococcal bacteraemia. These include complement deficiency, female sex, menstruation, pregnancy and perhaps pharyngeal infection.

PERIHEPATITIS (FITZ-HUGH–CURTIS SYNDROME)

See under Chlamydial Infections, p. 290.

ANTIMICROBIAL SUSCEPTIBILITIES

By the early 1980s, the PPNG, which were first described in 1975–76, accounted for nearly 50% of isolates in some parts of the developing world. Both the 4.4-mDa plasmid that was prevalent in resistant strains from Asia and the Philippines and the 3.2-mDa plasmid that predominated in Europe and Africa had by then become common worldwide. PPNG strains now account for about 10% in the USA and UK, with substantially higher rates in many local areas. Tetracycline-resistant *N. gonorrhoeae* associated with a 24.5 mDa plasmid were first documented in the USA in 1985, the resistance often being associated with penicillin and spectinomycin resistance. The prevalence of gonococci with clinically significant chromosomal resistance to the penicillins and tetracyclines has risen steadily in much of the world. Although the minimum inhibitory concentrations (MICs) of ceftriaxone for many such strains are higher than for fully susceptible gonococci, the routinely recommended ceftriazone regimens achieve a higher level and are effective. Most strains with chromosomally mediated resistance belong to Por IB serovars, although other auxotype/serovar may be involved. Decreased susceptibility or resistance to fluoroquinolones has been reported only sporadically, and treatment failure associated with *in-vitro* resistance has not been described. There are, however, recent occurrences of resistant cases in Denver and Seattle, suggesting that clinically important resistance to the fluoroquinolones may be emerging.

TREATMENT

Uncomplicated gonococcal infection

Many antimicrobials are active against *N. gonorrhoeae*. The choice of agents used should take into consideration of the site of infection, the local pattern of antimicrobial resistance, the possible presence of other sexually transmitted infections, and the side effects and costs of the various treatment regimens. Because coinfection with *C. trachomatis* is common, the regimen for gonococcal infection should include an effective anti-chlamydial therapy (see above).

- Ceftriaxone 125 mg or 250 mg i.m. in a single dose; or
- Ciprofloxacin 500 mg orally in a single dose; or
- Cefixime 400 mg in a single dose.

The results of clinical studies indicate that these regimens can cure >90% of pharyngeal infections. Ceftriaxone also may abort incubating syphilis, whereas ciprofloxacin is not active against *T. pallidum*. Strains with decreased susceptibility to some quinolones are becoming common in Asia. Other quinolones such as ofloxacin 400 mg, enoxacin 400 mg, lomefloxacin 400 mg and norfloxacin 800 mg orally in a single dose appear safe and effective for anal and genital infections. However, experience with pharyngeal infections is limited.

Gonococcal conjunctivitis
- Ceftriaxone 1 g single dose.

Disseminated gonococcal infection

Initial phase:
- Ceftriaxone 1 g i.m. or i.v. every 24 hours; or
- Cefotaxime 1 g i.v. every 8 hours; or
- Spectinomycin 2 g every 12 hours.

Once improvement evident:
- Cefixime 400 mg orally twice daily for 7 days; or
- Ciprofloxacin 500 mg orally twice daily for 7 days.

LABORATORY DIAGNOSIS

It is important to use a Cuscoe's speculum under good lighting when obtaining cervical or vaginal specimens. Disposable proctoscopes are convenient for the examin-

ation of rectal gonococcal or chlamydial infection. A pharyngeal specimen should also be obtained for gonococcal culture if oral sex is practised. The swab should be placed in a transport medium and sent to the laboratory for examination on the same day. The sensitivity and specificity of the Gram-stained smear of endocervical swabs and rectal swabs are similar, about 50% and 95% respectively by trained personnel. **Culture remains the routine and 'gold standard' for the diagnosis of gonorrhoea**. Rapid diagnostic techniques under development include the ligase chain reaction, an *in-vitro* nucleic acid amplification technique that exponentially amplifies targeted DNA sequences. Nucleic acid-based tests (PACE 2C) for simultaneous detection of *C. trachomatis* and *N. gonorrhoeae* in endocervical specimens are also under development. Urine testing for the diagnosis of STDs has the potential to simplify and expand the opportunities for STD screening and surveillance of women.

28.5 VAGINITIS

In population-based studies, one in four young women aged between 19 and 25 years may complain of symptoms from the lower genital tract. The most commonly reported are itching, followed by discharge, and soreness. The three common infections associated with these symptoms are trichomoniasis, bacterial vaginosis and candidiasis. The last two conditions may not be sexually transmitted. Uncommonly, patients with gonococcal or chlamydial cervicitis may complain of these symptoms. It should be appreciated that among an appreciable number of symptomatic women, no infectious agent can be identified. One should be mindful of mechanical or chemical irritation of the lower genital tract as a cause for the signs of vaginitis when no genital pathogen has been isolated.

28.5.1 Bacterial vaginosis

Bacterial vaginosis is the most prevalent cause of vaginal discharge or malodor, resulting from disturbance of the normal vaginal microbial flora – the normal H_2O_2-producing *Lactobacillus* spp. being replaced with high concentrations of anaerobic bacteria, e.g. *Bacteroides* spp., *Mobiluncus* spp., *G. vaginalis* and *Mycoplasma hominis*. The condition may be recurrent, and treatment of sexual partners does not improve the therapeutic response. Bacterial vaginosis has been found to be associated with endometritis, PID or pelvic infection following invasive procedures such as a hysterectomy, placement of IUCD, and therapeutic abortion. It may be reasonable to consider treatment of bacterial vaginosis before these surgical procedures. Some patients, however, may not complain of symptoms despite clinical findings.

Clinical diagnosis is usually made by the presence of at least three of the following:

- A homogeneous, white, non-inflammatory discharge that adheres to the vaginal walls.
- The presence of clue cells on microscopic examination.
- pH of vaginal fluid >4.5.
- A fishy odour of vaginal discharge before or after addition of 10% KOH (Whiff test).

The relative concentration of the bacterial morphotypes characteristic of the altered flora of bacterial vaginosis may also be used for the diagnosis of the condition.

TREATMENT

Treatment of bacterial vaginosis may include the following:

- Metronidazole 500 mg orally twice times daily for 7 days; or
- Clindamycin cream (2%), 5 g intravaginally at bedtime for 7 days; or
- Metronidazole gel (0.75%) 5 g intravaginally, twice daily for 5 days.

28.5.2 Trichomoniasis

Trichomoniasis is caused by the protozoan *T. vaginalis*, the condition being characterized by a diffuse, malodorous, yellow-green discharge with vulvovaginal irritation. On examination, copious purulent discharge is usually seen bathing the cervix which often has 'strawberry' markings. Very occasionally, patients may present with minimal symptoms. Sexual partners should be treated.

TREATMENT

Treatment should be based on Metronidazole 2 g orally in a single dose, or 500 mg twice daily for 7 days.

28.5.3 Vulvovaginal candidiasis

Vulvovaginal candidiasis is usually not sexually acquired. The yeast most frequently responsible for vulvovaginal candidiasis is *Candida albicans*, followed by *Torulopsis glabrata*, *C. tropicalis* and *C. krusei*. An estimated 75% of women will experience at least one attack of vulvovaginal infection during their lifetime. Symptoms include pruritus, vaginal discharge, soreness or burning and sometimes superficial dyspareunia and dysuria. The diagnosis should always be confirmed by laboratory findings, as the symptoms are not specific for yeast infections. It is uncertain whether an asymptomatic carriage of *C. albicans* should always be treated. Topical therapy

relies on imidazole preparations, all of which give similar average mycological cure rates, in the region of 84–90%. There are also more expensive oral preparations, such as fluconazole and itraconazole, which have similar efficacy.

28.6 GENITAL WARTS

Human papillomaviruses (HPV) infect the stratified epithelium of many sites in the body. There are approximately 70 types of papillomaviruses, and there seems a predilection for certain types to infect certain sites of the body. Genital warts are generally benign growths (condyloma acuminatum) that cause minor symptoms, and are most commonly caused by HPV types 6 or 11. The premalignant lesions associated with HPV can arise on the same areas as the warts, although the cervix is where malignant conversion occurs most often. Under the recently introduced Bethesda system, low-grade squamous intraepithelial lesions (low SIL) include previous atypias and Cervical Intraepithelial Neoplasia I (CIN I). High-grade SIL include CIN II and CIN III. The incidence of HPV-negative cancers is 5–10%. HPVs 6 and 11, and newer isolates 42, 43 and 44 are found in low-grade SIL, whereas the oncogenic types, HPVs 16 and 18, and the less frequently found 31, 33, 45, and 56 are found in all grades of SIL and importantly in malignant disease. HPV 16 and 18 are detected in over 80% of malignant disease of the cervix.

In **cervical cancer**, HPV DNA is usually integrated into the host cell genome, whereas in premalignant lesions, the viral DNA is free and unintegrated, and able to produce infectious virus particles. It has been established that integration can take place in a few cells at the premalignant phase of the disease, and it is probable that these cells acquire the potential to invade. Although HPVs 6 and 11 have not been found in malignant diseases of the cervix, they have been isolated from locally invading lesions of the vulva, such as verrucous carcinoma and Buschke–Lowenstein's tumours. The natural history of HPV infection is uncertain. In longitudinal studies, HPV DNA may disappear but reappear again in subsequent testing. Prevalence studies have found that precursor lesions for cervical cancer occur approximately five times more often among women attending STD clinics than among women attending family-planning clinics. A Papanicolaou (pap) smear should be obtained as part of the routine pelvic examination if the patient has not had one performed during the previous 12 months. Patients with abnormal smears should be referred to specialists for further investigation. Pap smear diagnosis of HPV generally does not correlate well with detection of HPV DNA in cervical cells. Cell changes attributed to HPV in the cervix are similar to those of mild dysplasia and often regress spontaneously without treatment. Although tests for the detection of several types of HPV DNA in cervical cell scrapes are now available, the clinical utility of these tests for managing the patient is not clear. Screening for subclinical genital HPV infection using DNA tests is therefore not recommended. It is not known whether patients with subclinical HPV infection are as contagious as patients with exophytic warts.

TREATMENT

No therapy has been shown to eradicate HPV. The currently available therapeutic methods are 22–94% effective in clearing external exophytic lesions; better results are obtained if the lesions are small and the history is less than 1 year. Recurrence rates are high, at least 25% within 3 months, probably resulting from reactivation of the subclinical infection rather than reinfection by a sexual partner. If left untreated, genital warts may either resolve on their own, remain unchanged, or grow.

External genital/perianal warts

- Cryotherapy with liquid nitrogen or cryoprobe.
- Podophyllin 10–25%, not more than 0.5 ml and covering total lesion areas of not more than 10 cm each session. Wash off after 4 hours. Contraindicated during pregnancy.
- Podofilox 0.5% for self-treatment. Four cycles of 3 days of treatment followed by 4 days of no therapy.
- Trichloroacetic acid (TCA) 80–90%. Apply to warts and remove the excess acid by powdering the lesions with talc. Weekly therapy if necessary for up to 6 weeks.
- Electrodesiccation or electrocautery.

Vaginal warts

- Cryotherapy with liquid nitrogen.
- TCA (see above).
- Podophyllin (see above). The treatment area must be dry before removing the speculum to avoid causing damage to the healthy mucosa. Some experts warn against vaginal application of podophyllin.

Cervical warts

Management should be carried out in consultation with an expert in genitourinary medicine.

SEXUAL PARTNERS

The majority of partners are probably already subclinically infected with HPV, even if they do not have visible warts. The use of condoms may reduce transmission to partners likely to be uninfected, such as new partners. However, the period of communicability is unknown. HPV infection may persist throughout a patient's lifetime in a dormant state and become infectious intermittently.

28.7 FURTHER READING

1993 Sexually Transmitted Diseases Treatment Guidelines (1993) *MMWR*, **42**, RR-14.

Critchlow, C.W., Hanssen-Wolner, P., Eschenbach, D.A., Kiviat, N.B., Koutsky, L.A., Stevens, C.E. and Holmes King, K. (1995) Determinants of cervical ectopia and of cervicitis: age, oral contraception, specific cervical infection, smoking, and douching. *Am. J. Obstet. Gynecol.*, **173**, 534–543.

Csonka, G.W. and Oates, J.K. (eds) (1990) *Sexually Transmitted Diseases*. Bailliere Tindall, London.

Farley T.M.M., Rosengerg M.J, Rowe P.J, Chen J.H. and Meirik O. Intrauterine devices and pelvic inflammatory disease: an international perspective. (1992) *Lancet*, **339**, 785–788.

Holmes King, K., Mardh, P.-A., Sparling, P.F. and Wiesner, J.P. (eds) (1990) *Sexually Transmitted Diseases*. McGraw-Hill, New York.

Houang, E.T. and Sutter, W.P. (1992) Principles of antibiotic therapy, prophylaxis and treatment of postoperative infection. In, *Gynaecology*, ed. R.W. Shaw, W.P. Soutter and L.S. Stanton, Churchill Livingstone, London.

Mathevet, P., Dargent, D., Roy, M. and Beau, G. (1994) A randomized prospective study comparing three techniques of conization: cold knife, laser and LEEP. *Gynecol. Oncol.*, **54**, 175–179.

McCance, D.J. (1994) Human papillomaviruses. *Infect. Dis. Clin. North Am.* **8**, 751–768.

Nolan, T.E., King, L.A., Smith, R.P. and Gallup, D.C. (1993) Necrotizing surgical infection and necrotizing fasciitis in obstetric and gynecologic patients. *South. Med. J.*, **86**, 1363–1367.

Recommendations for the Prevention and Management of Chlamydia trachomatis *Infections.* (1993) *MMWR*, **42**, RR-12.

Sawaya, G.F., Grady, D., Kerlikowske, K. and Grimes, D.A. (1996) Antibiotics at the time of induced abortion: the case for universal prophylaxis based on a meta-analysis. *Obstet. Gynecol.*, **87**, 884–890.

Simmons, N.A., Ball, A.P., Cawson, R.A., *et al.* (1992) Antibiotic practice and infective endocarditis. *Lancet*, **339**, 1292–1293.

Sivin, I., Stern, J., McCarthy, T. *et al.* (1994) Health during prolonged use of levonorgestrel 20 μ g / d and the Copper T Cu 380 Ag intrauterine contraceptive devices: a multicenter study. *Fertility and Sterility*, **61**, 70–77.

Westrom, L. (1980) Impact of sexually transmitted diseases on human reproduction: Swedish studies of infertility and ectopic pregnancy. In *Sexually Transmitted Diseases Status Report, NIAID Study Group*. NIH Publications, Washington, DC. **81**-2213, p. 43.

29

Paediatric surgical infections

E.H. PRICE

29.1 INTRODUCTION

This chapter is only concerned with infections presenting to the surgeon that frequently or specifically relate to paediatric age groups. For further information regarding infections that involve both paediatric and adult age groups, please refer to the relevant chapters.

Paediatric surgical infections will be considered under the following headings:

- General factors of significance
- Community-acquired infections
- Hospital-acquired infections
- Problems of ward cross-infection
- Antibiotic therapy
- Prophylaxis.

29.2 GENERAL FACTORS

29.2.1 Influence of age on infections

Neonates – and premature neonates in particular – are more susceptible to infection than older age groups. As well as poor physical barriers to infection a neonate of 32 weeks' gestation has half the immunoglobulin G level of a full term neonate, they have impaired plasma opsonizing activity, and their complement levels reduced. Neonates with suspected sepsis should be investigated by taking blood, urine, wound, cerebrospinal fluid (CSF) when indicated and possible and other relevant cultures including deep ear and umbilical swabs. Results of maternal cultures, especially vaginal swabs, should be reviewed. The child should be treated promptly with intravenous antibiotics while awaiting the laboratory results.

Young infants requiring surgery should be looked after when possible by specialist paediatric surgeons and nurses, the aim being to reduce infection rates.

29.2.2 The spectrum of organisms

In general, children have a wider spectrum of infecting organisms than adults. Before birth the foetus is sterile, and colonizing organisms are initially from the mother's genital and gastrointestinal tract. Subsequently, these organisms come from the hospital or home environment. Some hospital-acquired organisms may be resistant to a number of antibiotics.

Examples of infecting organisms which are seen more commonly in children than in adults include the following: group B haemolytic streptococci, which cause septicaemia and meningitis in neonates; *Haemophilus influenzae*, Pittman type b which may cause septicaemia, meningitis, facial cellulitis and osteomyelitis in children under 5 years of age who have not had Hib vaccine; and rotavirus and respiratory syncytial virus which cause gastroenteritis and bronchiolitis respectively and can result in cross infection on hospital wards.

When dealing with infection problems in childhood, an up-to-date knowledge of local pathogens is essential, and close collaboration with the on-site medical microbiologist is recommended.

29.2.3 Clinical history

There will be little or no history available from young infants, and it is important never to disregard history from the mother, grandmother or any other close relative. If this suggests recent or ongoing infection, it should be taken seriously, even in the presence of non-specific clinical signs. Regular review of an infant is mandatory, as the clinical condition may deteriorate rapidly. Details of travel, exposure to animals, contact with infectious diseases (especially tuberculosis) and an immunization history are essential information.

Non-specific laboratory indicators of infection, such as estimation of C-reactive protein (CRP) may be useful in differential diagnosis of an infection or inflammatory condition. However, neonates may not make CRP as well as do older children and low levels may be clinically significant.

29.3 COMMUNITY-ACQUIRED INFECTIONS

29.3.1 Abdominal infections

PEPTIC ULCER

There is a strong association between *Helicobacter pylori* infection and antral gastritis in children. Epidemiological studies of this organism suggest that the initial infection may occur in childhood. Breast feeding may provide protection from *H. pylori* colonization.

Investigations include a gastric biopsy and eradication may be checked by a urea breath test. Appropriate treatment is with a triple therapy regimen, depending on local choice, but most include two antibiotics and a proton pump inhibitor such as omeprazole. Treatment of asymptomatic *H. pylori* is not indicated.

RECURRENT ABDOMINAL PAIN

H. pylori is not considered to be a factor in the production of recurrent abdominal pain in childhood in the absence of a peptic ulcer or gastritis.

ACUTE APPENDICITIS

Rupture of the appendix is more common in children and the elderly. An intra-abdominal abscess may occur secondary to perforation. In some cases the differential diagnosis between infectious gastroenteritis and retrocaecal appendicitis can cause difficulties, particularly in young children. Presentation of Meckel's diverticulitis may be identical to acute appendicitis, and both require antibiotics. A combination of penicillin, gentamicin and metronidazole is often used in treatment but a variety of other regimens have also been employed. Culture of pus at laparotomy is useful. Late presentation may occur with an appendix mass. This may settle on antibiotics but appendicectomy will be required 6–8 weeks later; the patient should be managed by a paediatric surgeon.

MESENTERIC ADENITIS

Yersinia spp. can cause mesenteric lymphadenitis and severe enterocolitis, though an initial differential diagnosis may also include appendicitis. Patients who are particularly susceptible to severe infection with this organism include those with thalassaemia and others with high tissue iron levels. Use of the chelating agent, desferrioxamine, in thalassaemic patients will procure iron and act as a growth factor for *Yersinia* spp.; hence this treatment should be stopped immediately and suitable antibiotic therapy initiated. Main options for serious infections include ciprofloxacin (see 29.6.3) and the cephalosporins. Although *Yersinia enterocolitica* shows *in-vitro* sensitivity to gentamicin, this should not be the primary choice for treatment because of reported failure of this antibiotic to eradicate systemic infection. The advice of a microbiologist should be sought regarding the sensitivity of specific organisms.

Adenoviruses and other viral infections have also been associated with mesenteric lymphadenitis.

PRIMARY PERITONITIS

Particularly susceptible children include those with splenectomy or with nephrotic syndrome. Usual pathogens are *E. coli*, streptococci or klebsiella spp. Cefotaxime or piperacillin-tazobactamis are usually an adequate treatment.

INTUSSUSCEPTION

Adenoviruses sometomes have been implicated aetiologically in this condition in children, and many patients have an associated respiratory infection. However, antibody titre rises to adenovirus have not been demonstrated consistently.

PSEUDOMEMBRANOUS/ANTIBIOTIC-ASSOCIATED COLITIS

This potentially serious condition is usually associated with overgrowth of toxin-producing *Clostridium difficile* following antibiotic therapy. It has not been described frequently in children other than in the immune suppressed. In infancy, the isolation of *C. difficile* from stools and identification of toxin is not usually considered of clinical significance because both may be found in the normal gut flora. This contrasts with the situation in adults where the toxin is rarely found in normal faecal specimens. However, in the absence of other pathogens, detection of toxin in the stool of infants with severe diarrhoea may be of clinical significance. Use of anticholinergic drugs which influence gut motility may exacerbate the symptoms. If the organism has a pathogenic role, early institution of oral metronidazole will alleviate symptoms. Oral vancomycin is effective but may predispose to development of vancomycin-resistant enterococci (see also 29.5).

DIARRHOEA IN CHILDREN WITH HIRSCHSPRUNG'S DISEASE

Although a causal role cannot be established for *C. difficile*, an association has been found between prolonged intestinal carriage of this organism in children over 12 months of age who have Hirschsprung's disease with continuing diarrhoea. Such an association was not seen in children with Hirschsprung's disease without diarrhoea, or in control children. In one report of a seriously ill infant with Hirschsprung's disease (Figs 29.1 and 29.2), the presence of a very high *C. difficile* toxin titre was difficult to detect because of a prozone phenomenon.

Life-threatening enterocolitis, usually described as necrotizing enterocolitis, can occur rapidly in children with Hirschsprung's disease and is treated with antibiotics, usually penicillin, gentamicin and metronidazole initially. Enterocolitis complicating Hirchsprung's disease is becoming rarer than previously because of early diagnosis and early colostomy construction.

ULCERATIVE COLITIS

Although usually not considered to be associated with a primary infective cause, all paediatric patients should

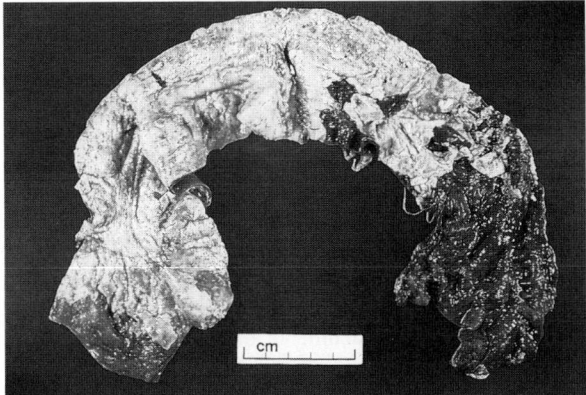

Figure 29.1 *Post-mortem colon specimen from a 4-week-old infant with Hirschsprung's disease and pseudomembranous colitis. An opaque yellow membrane is present with underlying ulcerated red granular mucosa.*

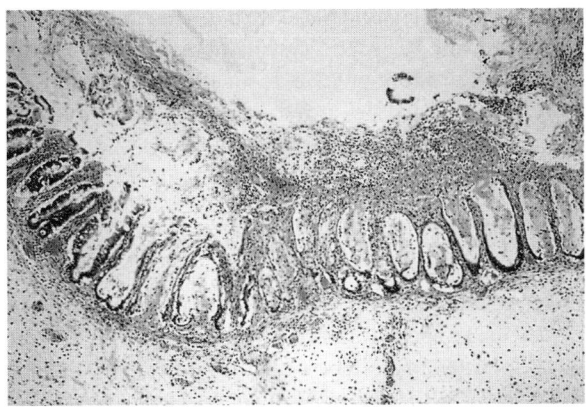

Figure 29.2 *Histology from specimen in Figure 29.1, demonstrating the appearance of pseudomembranous colitis. Fibrinopurulent mucoid substance is erupting from the ulcerated mucosal surface. Polymorphonuclear infiltration and dilated glands are present. Haematoxylin and eosin staining.*

have amoebic serology carried out prior to surgery or starting steroids. This is necessary even in the absence of a history of foreign travel.

PERIANAL ABSCESS

This occurs not uncommonly in infant boys. Antibiotic treatment is rarely required unless infection with *Streptococcus pyogenes* is suspected. Where indicated, surgical incision and drainage is the standard treatment.

PYOGENIC LIVER ABSCESS

This may occur secondary to portal pyaemia associated with intra-abdominal infection, or as a result of spreading infection from the biliary tract. It has been described in infants following the ingestion of sharp foreign bodies such as needles and pins. Haematogenous spread from a focus elsewhere in the body may occur. In many cases no obvious precipitating cause is found. The right lobe of the liver is more frequently affected than the left.

The presenting clinical sign may be a pyrexia of unknown origin (PUO). Chest manifestations are frequent, including cough and right basal pleural effusion. Preferably three sets of blood cultures should be collected, each just as the temperature is beginning to rise. Isolation of anaerobes such as *Bacteroides fragilis*, anaerobic cocci (possibly mixed with *E. coli*) or *Streptococcus milleri* suggests the presence of a collection of pus. Gas-liquid chromatography examination of pus may reveal the presence of anaerobes, and prolonged culture may be necessary.

Amoebic liver abscesses can occasionally be confused with pyogenic liver abscesses and a history of foreign travel is important in such cases. Both conditions may respond initially to metronidazole treatment. Rarely, amoebiases may occur in a child who has not been abroad and serological tests to exclude amoebiasis should be carried out. A hydatid cyst may become secondarily infected and history of travel to an endemic area (which includes parts of Wales as well as areas outside the UK), and contact with dogs, should be sought.

29.3.2 Urinary tract infections

Preferably at least two well-taken midstream (or clean catch) urine specimens are investigations which must not be omitted in any febrile child with no other obvious diagnosis. Up to 40% of positive cultures from 'urine bag' specimens collected from children may be false positive. In neonates, urinary tract infection occurs more often in boys, and jaundice is one possible presentation. Outside this age group, only 1% of boys develop a urine infection, whereas the incidence is three-fold higher in girls. Early diagnosis and treatment are important and most infections with renal involvement occur in the first 12 months of life. Patients with confirmed infection should always be referred for further investigation with regard to the possibility of vesicoureteric reflux (which accompanies infection in children in 8–40% of cases) and surgically correctable congenital abnormalities. Suitable prophylactic antibiotic therapy is recommended, usually long-term, low-dose trimethoprim or nitrofurantoin. Infants and young children are at much greater risk of renal damage secondary to urine infection than adults. If the diagnosis is missed, there is a risk of scarring in the developing kidney. Conversely, incorrect diagnosis of a urinary infection subjects the child to inappropriate and prolonged antibiotic therapy, together with unnecessary radiological investigation, which may sometimes be distressing. General measures for parents which might help to limit recurrences of infection are listed in the Royal College of Physicians guidelines (see further reading).

A travel history should always be sought from a patient with terminal haematuria as **schistosomiasis** is a possibility. Urine specimens, 'terminal' and 'post-exercise', for microscopy after centrifugation and routine culture should be sent to the laboratory. Travel and clinical presentation details should be specified on the request form.

29.3.3 Genital infections

Paediatric surgeons may be asked to carry out genital examinations on young children under anaesthesia. The possibility of child sexual abuse may be under consideration, and suitable specimens for investigation of sexually transmitted diseases should be taken (including specimens from a suspected assailant, if possible). No attempt should be made to take a high vaginal swab from a child: specimens should be taken from the lower vagina only.

Interpretation of the significance of potential pathogens isolated from genital specimens in children is not straightforward, and should be referred to experts in the field. Children from whom *Neisseria gonorrhoea* is isolated should be reviewed with regard to the likelihood of sexual abuse. Presence of this organism indicates the need to look for other sexually-transmitted diseases such as *Chlamydia trachomatis*. However, infection with this organism acquired at birth may persist for months or years. An investigation protocol agreed by all interested parties is necessary. This prevents unnecessary distress for the child by avoiding the need to take repeat specimens. In cases where there is a significant risk of sexual abuse, a written chain of evidence should be available to prove that the specimen taken is the same specimen that has been processed and reported on. Specimens and cultures should be kept until all possibility of legal action is over.

Purulent vaginal discharge more commonly occurs as a result of secondary infection due to the presence of foreign bodies. Less severe vaginal discharge and irritation may follow an extension of threadworm infection from the perianal area to the vagina. Autoinfection as a result of hand transfer of organisms from the mouth to the genital area may also occur with organisms such as *Streptococcus pyogenes* (group A haemolytic streptococcus) and non-typable *Haemophilus influenzae*. Symptoms should be treated with appropriate antibiotics. A study of children presenting to a paediatric casualty department with vulvovaginitis showed that the major causes were poor hygiene and threadworms.

Male neonatal circumcision wounds occasionally become infected, and *Staphylococcus aureus* is the most common infecting organism. *Strep. pyogenes* is sometimes involved and faecal organisms may also be isolated. If oral therapy is appropriate, co-amoxyclav or a combination of amoxycillin and flucloxacillin may be considered.

29.3.4 Skin and soft tissue infections

ABSCESSES

These are usually caused by *Staph. aureus*, sometimes in combination with *Strep. pyogenes*. For children with large abscesses, surgical drainage may be required. A short course of an antibiotic is frequently given and co-amoxyclav or a combination of ampicillin plus flucloxacillin is a suitable oral choice. These may also be given intravenously if necessary. Other intravenous alternatives include cefuroxime or a combination of benzylpenicillin plus flucloxacillin. If an anaerobic infection is also considered possible, metronidazole may be added. Alternatively, intravenous co-amoxyclav or piperacillin/tazobactam are both active against *Staph. aureus* (other than methicillin-resistant *Staph. aureus*, MRSA), *Strep. pyogenes* and anaerobes. If MRSA is present, vancomycin or teicoplanin will be indicated.

OMPHALITIS

Neonatal omphalitis is inflammation of the skin around the umbilicus. It may range from slight redness to a more widespread erythema with purulent discharge. Spreading necrosis of tissues (necrotizing fasciitis) may occur. *Staph. aureus* is commonly grown, but Gram-negative bacteria, streptococci and anaerobes may also be implicated. Severe infection may spread to involve the liver via the umbilical vein.

Broad-spectrum antibiotic combinations are required. These should include staphylococcal and streptococcal cover, often with penicillin and flucloxacillin, anaerobic cover with metronidazole and for Gram-negative organisms, gentamicin and/or a cephalosporin may be given. See also necrotizing fasciitis below.

WOUND INFECTION (CELLULITIS)

A wound infection or spreading cellulitis with lymphangitis and lymphadenitis is usually caused by infection with *Strep. pyogenes*. A sore throat caused by this organism may be the original source. Either auto (self) infection or cross-infection from one child to another may have occurred. Fatalities from *Strep. pyogenes* septicaemia are documented every year in otherwise healthy patients. Antibiotic treatment should include both intravenous penicillin and flucloxacillin. The latter is added to give cover against β-lactamase-producing *Staph. aureus*, which can inactivate penicillin. Cefuroxime is a suitable alternative. Neutropenic patients may develop severe cellulitis due to Gram-negative organisms, including *Ps. aeruginosa*, and at least two appropriate intravenous antibiotics are essential. Anaerobic cover with metronidazole may be added.

PERIORBITAL CELLULITIS

The causative organisms include *Strep. pyogenes*, *Staph. aureus* pneumococci and *H. influenzae* Pittman type b (the latter in a child who has not had Hib vaccine). In patients who have had Hib vaccine, intravenous penicillin or flucloxacillin alone will usually suffice. Intravenous cefuroxime, piperacillin-tazobactam or co-amoxyclav are alternatives. Occasionally, periorbital cellulitis is secondary to orbital cellulitis caused by sinusitis and is a much more serious infection. Mixed infections with aerobic organisms (usually streptococci) and anaerobic organisms should be covered in the antibiotic therapy chosen. Piperacillin-tazobactam and co-amoxyclav have significant anaerobic action themselves, but in orbital cellulitis metronidazole should be added. Sometimes progression of infection results in a subdural empyema or frontal lobe cerebral abscess (see p. 304, Subdural empyema).

NEONATAL OPHTHALMIAL

In neonates, significant swelling around the eye with purulent discharge may occur secondary to neonatal ophthalmia with *N. gonorrhoea*. This condition usually becomes apparent during the first few days of life and should respond to high-dose intravenous cefotaxime which may be changed to intravenous penicillin once susceptibility is confirmed. Hourly saline eyewashes are necessary together with topical antibiotics and the advice of an ophthalmologist is required. Some 50% of infants with *N. gonorrhoea* will also be positive for *Chlamydia trachomatis*. The latter infection may present towards the end of the first week of life, often with marked swelling around the eye, and should be treated with oral erythromycin for 3 weeks. Many specialists also recommend topical tetracycline. For both these infections in neonates, a sensitive approach is required, so that appropriate investigation of both parents can be arranged.

Other infections that may cause eye infections in neonates include *Staph. aureus*, pneumococci and *Haemophilus* species.

INFECTED SKIN LESIONS FOLLOWING CHICKENPOX

Following chickenpox, children are particularly susceptible to secondary infection of their skin lesions with *Staph. aureus* and/or *Strep. pyogenes*. There is probably a temporary impairment of immune function after this viral infection, and secondary bacterial infection may sometimes progress rapidly. Antibiotics discussed for the treatment of abscesses (see p. 300) are usually appropriate, but if the area involved extends with no evidence of early response to treatment, the possibility of anaerobic infection should also be covered and necrotizing fasciitis may occur.

NECROTIZING FASCIITIS

This is an uncommon, rapidly progressive and severe infection involving the subcutaneous soft tissues. In the newborn, it can occur as a complication of omphalitis. Swelling and erythema may develop over several hours or days. Consideration of early surgical excision extending beyond the affected area is required. High-dose antibiotic therapy is urgently required and should cover anaerobes as well as aerobes. For patients in whom antibiotic resistance organisms are unlikely, the combination of high-dose cefuroxime, gentamicin and metronidazole has been recommended; another possible alternative is piperacillin-tazobactam and gentamicin with metronidazole. The advice of a consultant microbiologist should be sought. The presence of antibiotic-resistant organisms such as MRSA should be particularly considered if a patient has been in hospital for some length of time.

Where *Streptococcus pyogenes* is a possible infecting organism, the urgent addition of clindamycin plus intravenous immunoglobulin is indicated especially if initial response to beta-lactams is poor.

BURNS

Infected burns are a common reason for presentation of a young child to a casualty department, and *Staph. aureus* is the usual infecting organism. Occasional cases of staphylococcal toxic shock syndrome have occurred following a mild to moderate infection with a *Staph. aureus* strain producing the relevant toxin (Fig. 29.3). Treatment should be directed towards resuscitation of the patient and general support. Antibiotics are of secondary importance in this condition. *Strep. pyogenes* is another possible infecting organism of burns, and suitable antibiotics have been discussed above.

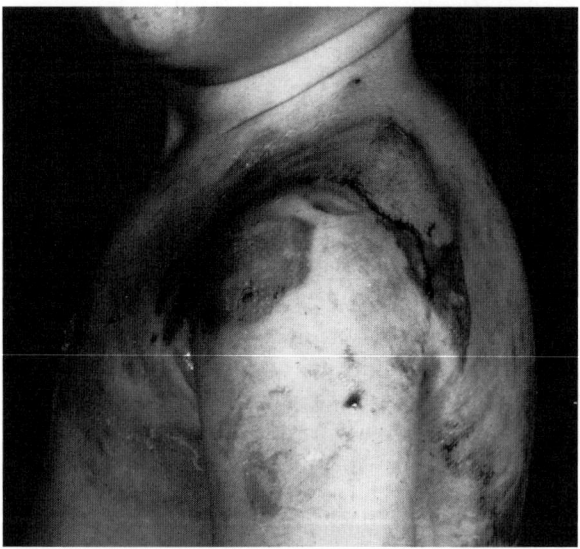

Figure 29.3 *A child with a burn who subsequently developed staphylococcal toxic shock syndrome.*

Both *Strep. pyogenes* and *Pseudomonas aeruginosa* infections can reduce the chances of a skin graft taking successfully and may cause serious septicaemia in burned patients. The use of topical silver compounds may limit the development of pseudomonas infection but gentamicin should not be applied topically to burns as it promotes the emergence of gentamicin-resistant organisms.

BITES

For human bites, a variety of aerobic and anaerobic organisms may cause infection, including streptococci and *Staph. aureus*. Bites from dogs and cats also run the risk of infection with *Pasteurella multicida*, streptococci and *Staph. aureus*. (Also Capnocytophaga from dogs may cause serious illness in immune suppressed patients, especially those who are asplenic.) Co-amoxiclav is appropriate empirical treatment in non-penicillin allergic patients. An assessment should be made of the risk of hepatitis B or human immunodeficiency virus from human bites and of rabies from animal bites in patients bitten in endemic areas. Further specialist advice may be required and tetanus immunisation status should be assessed.

Pyomyositis

In this condition the child presents with a fever and muscle pain and there may be a history of trauma. Visible masses may be present and needle aspiration is sometimes possible. *Staph. aureus* and *Str. pyogenes* are the commonest pathogens; appropriate treatment for these organisms is discussed above.

INFECTION WITH HERPES SIMPLEX (FIG. 29.4)

As children frequently suck their thumbs and fingers, the possibility of herpes simplex infections, secondary to herpetic gingivostomatitis requires consideration. The mouth should be inspected and a swab sent in viral trans-

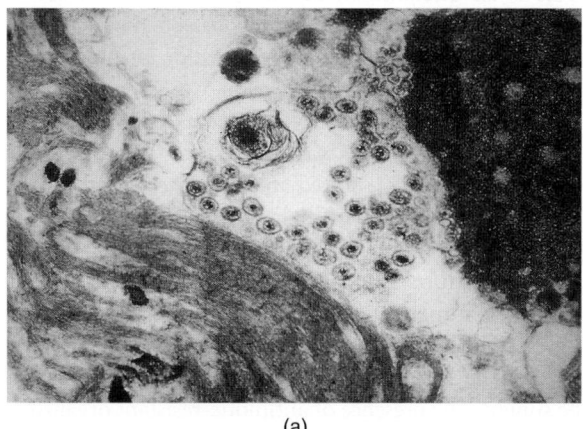

(a)

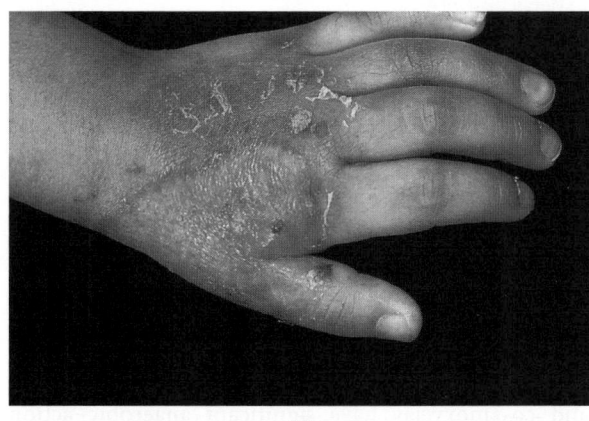

(b)

Figure 29.4 *(a) Electron micrograph of debrided skin from the thumb of a 2-year-old girl with herpes simplex infection. Herpes virus particles are visible. (With kind permission of Dr. A. Phillips, Electron Microscopy Dept., Academic Dept. of Paediatric Gastroenterology, Royal Free Hospital.) (b) Healed thumb of same patient, demonstrating the area involved.*

port medium. Swabs for viral culture should also be taken from the fingers or thumbs involved. Lesions appear as vesicles containing clear fluid. Swabs taken for bacterial culture may not yield growth of any clinical significance. There is sometimes secondary infection with *Staph. aureus* or *Strep. pyogenes*.

29.3.5   Lymphadenitis

As well as acute infections with organisms such as *Staph. aureus*, *Strep. pyogenes*, *Mycobacterium tuberculosis*, *Toxoplasma gondii* cytomegalovirus, *Bartonella henselae* (the cause of cat-scratch fever) or Epstein-Barr virus, lymph nodes may become enlarged as a result of infection with atypical mycobacteria especially *M. avium* complex. This may occur in immune-competent children and often a cervical lymph node is involved without systemic upset. The organisms are usually highly resistant to many of the chemotherapeutic agents used against mycobacteria, and complete surgical excision is the treatment of choice in the absence of impaired immunity. For occasional children where complete excision is difficult effective chemotherapy is also indicated. Careful differentiation must first be made between infections due to atypical mycobacteria and lesions due to *M. tuberculosis*. The child (or parent) should be asked whether he/she has had a BCG immunization and if so, a scar should be detectable. A biopsy specimen should be taken and the histological appearances are the same as those caused by *Myco. tuberculosis*. Specific methods for rapid mycobacterial culture may be useful. Chest X-ray and Mantoux tests should be carried out. An alternative to the Mantoux test is the multiple puncture (Heaf) test. If the latter is employed, an apparatus with either disposable heads or a self-contained single-use device is necessary. Appropriate apparatus for paediatric age group should be used. Specific skin tests against atypical mycobacteria have been used in the past and may help to confirm the diagnosis. However some experts now question their reliability for accurate diagnosis. They should not be used until the Mantoux test has been completed. Management guidelines are available from the British Thoracic Society and advice from a tuberculosis expert should be sought.

29.3.6   Osteomyelitis/infective arthritis

Staph. aureus is the most common causative organism at all ages. Children under 4 years of age who have not had Hib vaccine may be susceptible to infection with *H. influenzae* Pittman type b. The latter organism will not respond to flucloxacillin, which would comprise part of the treatment of choice for *Staph. aureus* infection (usually in combination with intravenous or oral rifampicin or oral fusidic acid). Both *Staph. aureus* and *H. influenzae* Pittman type b are sensitive to intravenous cefuroxime. Clindamycin may be an effective alternative to flucloxacillin in *S. aureus* infections especially in patients hyper-sensitive to beta-lactam antibiotics. Parents should be advised to watch for diarrhoea – a potentially serious side-effect. For infection with non β-lactamase-producing, ampicillin-susceptible *H. influenzae*, amoxycillin may be given orally. Approximately 10% *H. influenzae* Pittman type b produce β-lactamase, and this enzyme breaks down β-lactam antibiotics, such as amoxycillin. For infection with these more resistant organisms, co-amoxyclav is an oral option, but treatment should be discussed with the medical microbiologist. It should be noted that erythromycin does not have good activity against *H. influenzae*, even if the organism shows *in-vitro* sensitivity. Infection with Group B haemolytic streptococci generally occurs in the first 2 months of life, and treatment with a combination of intravenous penicillin and gentamicin is usual. *Strep. pyogenes* and pneumococci may also be causative organisms and intravenous penicillin is indicated. Gonococcal infection is a possibility in older adolescents. Antibiotic-resistant organisms including MRSA require individual discussion with a microbiologist.

In general, treatment is continued for 4–6 weeks for acute osteomyelitis and 3–4 weeks for acute septic arthritis. The initial therapy is given intravenously. There have been reports of successful treatment with shorter courses. Relapse due to poor compliance with oral therapy at home has been described. CRP levels should be monitored during treatment.

Investigations should include blood cultures and culture of pus if available. Anti-streptolysin, anti-staphylolysin titres and serum antigen screens for group B haemolytic streptococcus, *H. influenzae* Pittman type b, and pneumococci may sometimes be useful.

Children with sickle cell disease may develop osteomyelitis, and *Salmonella spp.* are generally the most common cause. Prolonged therapy, usually with ciprofloxacin, is advisable; up to 6 months maybe necessary in severe infection (see 29.6.3). Bone pain also occurs in these patients as a result of infarction and may cause diagnostic difficulty. *Salmonella* osteomyelitis is more common in younger age groups and may involve multiple sites. The extremities are frequently involved in infants, mimicking hand-foot syndrome. In older children, the long bones are more often involved.

29.3.7   Complications of ear, nose and throat (ENT) infections

SORE THROATS AND 'QUINSY'

Sore throats in children are more likely to be caused by *Strep. pyogenes* than in adults, where viruses are the most common cause. (It is not always possible to be certain that *Strep. pyogenes* is the cause of a sore throat in a child because asymptomatic throat carriage of this organism has been described in 10–20% or more patients in this age group.) The possibility of both acute and chronic sequelae of *Strep. pyogenes* infection necessitates appropriate antibiotic treatment. Patients on surgical wards who have *Strep. pyogenes* detected in any swabs should be isolated to prevent spread of infection. Treatment is usually with penicillin or amoxicillin; the latter antibiotic provides higher serum levels. Glandular fever should be excluded before using aminopenicillins because a rash may develop when treatment is started. For patients who are allergic to penicillin, a macrolide such as erythromycin or clarithromycin is a possible alternative, but sensitivity testing is important as resistance of *Strep. pyogenes* to erythromycin has been increasing in recent years.

Untreated streptococcal tonsillitis may become complicated by the development of a peritonsillar abscess or 'quinsy', but this is much less common than in the past. The abscess may require surgical drainage under penicillin or amoxycillin cover. Mixed bacterial flora including anaerobes may be grown; co-amoxiclav will provide cover for staphylococci, streptococci and anaerobes. Alternatively metronidazole may be added to the other beta-lactam antibiotics.

MASTOIDITIS AND SUBDURAL EMPYEMA

Otitis media may occasionally result in mastoiditis, and antibiotic therapy for the latter should cover both aerobic and anaerobic organisms. Co-amoxyclav or piperacillin-tazobactam have good anaerobic activity, but if a cephalosporin such as cefotaxime is chosen, then metronidazole should be added. Extension of infection may result in subdural empyema and/or a temporal lobe cerebral abscess, requiring surgical drainage. A suitable antibiotic combination could include cefotaxime or ceftriaxone with metronidazole. Guidelines on therapy are available and individual patients should be discussed with a microbiologist.

PAROTITIS

This infection may be caused by viruses especially the mumps virus in the non-immunised child. A variety of mouth organisms including anaerobes could be involved in bacterial parotitis, although *Staph. aureus* remains the commonest cause. Gram-negative rods may be involved, especially in neonates and debilitated children. Pus may be expressed from the parotid duct for culture.

EPIGLOTTITIS

This may occur as a result of infection with *H. influenzae* Pittman type b in children who have not had Hib vaccine. Urgent expert intervention to establish an airway is the first requirement. Until then, the child should be kept as

quiet as possible and no upset should be caused by taking blood for culture or other investigations. The mother or close relative should remain near the child.

Other infective conditions where airways may need to be urgently established include laryngeal **diphtheria** and **viral laryngo-tracheobronchitis**. The latter may be caused by parainfluenza viruses. For diphtheria, the presence of a membrane in the throat should be sought together with a history of recent travel (or contact with a recent traveller) to an endemic area. The vaccine history should be checked. In outbreaks of diphtheria in the UK, the first case is often missed as the diagnosis is not considered.

TRACHEITIS

Tracheitis due to *Staph. aureus* occurs occasionally.

INFECTED EMBRYOLOGICAL CYSTS

These include pharyngeal and branchial cleft cysts as well as thyroglossal duct cysts. Secondary bacterial infection, often with oral flora, may occur, and treatment will depend on the infecting organism and its sensitivity. Surgical excision to prevent recurrence should be carried out after the infection has completely resolved.

29.4   HOSPITAL-ACQUIRED INFECTIONS

29.4.1   Prevalence

Prevalence at different ages of the four main hospital-acquired infections (urinary tract, surgical wound, lower respiratory tract and skin infection) is shown in Table 29.1 (with figures for community-acquired infection included for comparison). Increased infection risk in children has been associated with multiple disease processes and multiple operations. Local contamination of wounds is also an important factor. Neonates, in particular birth weight neonates, are at low risk of developing postoperative sepsis.

29.4.2   Hospital-acquired infections

INTRAVENOUS LINE INFECTION

Even short-term intravenous lines may produced thrombophlebitis requiring antibiotics. However, infection in long-term lines, such as Hickman lines, may cause more serious problems. Such lines are frequently used in children who are particularly susceptible to infection because of their underlying illness. Traditionally infected intravenous lines should be removed especially if there is an exit site or tunnel infection. Uncomplicated *Staph. aureus* i.v. line infections should be treated for at least 14 days after line removal and for longer if fever persists or

Table 29.1 *Prevalence of the four main hospital-acquired infections (HAI) by age and sex*

Infection	Age (years) and sex							
	0–≤1		>1–≤14		>14–≤44		>44–≤65	
	M	F	M	F	M	F	M	F
CAI*	10.7	7.8	25.6	28.1	17.5	10.6	13.7	12.1
HAI	8.5	8.4	4.2	5.8	8.2	4.6	9.1	9.9
Urinary tract	0.4	0.3	0.9	1.4	0.8	1.0	1.7	3.1
Surgical wound	0.2	0.2	0.3	0.5	1.0	0.8	1.5	1.5
Lower respiratory tract	2.1	1.5	0.9	1.2	2.2	0.6	2.9	2.0
Skin	1.2	1.7	0.5	0.5	0.8	0.5	0.7	1.2

*Included for comparison.
CAI, community-acquired infection; M, male; F, female.
From Second National Prevalence Survey of Infection in Hospitals: an overview of the results. *J. Hosp. Infect.*, **32**, 175–190 (1996).

there is evidence of complications such as a distant focus of infection or endocarditis. Minimizing the length of the bacteraemic period is particularly important for patients who have in-dwelling foreign material, which may become infected (such as Gore-Tex® patches in the heart). Attempts at antibiotic sterilization without removal of the line may be considered in a limited number of sick patients, without *Staph. aureus*, candida or Pseudomonas infection, for whom changing the line would be very difficult. The risk–benefit ratio of retaining a source of sepsis should be carefully considered. For such patients, it may be possible to prevent bacteraemia for a period of days or weeks, but this may be sufficient to complete a course of chemotherapy or other essential treatment. If there is more than one lumen in a long line, the antibiotics used should be rotated through each lumen, as far as possible. The greatest success is likely to be achieved if the antibiotic has longer and more frequent contact with the infected area in the line. Some studies have shown that antibiotic 'line locks', given in addition to systemic antibiotics, can enhance cure rates. If infection recurs following a course of treatment, further consideration should be given to early removal of the line. This should be undertaken at a peak level of a suitable antibiotic, and it is important to leave as long a period of time as possible with peripheral lines before a new long line is inserted. Arterial lines that become infected are difficult to sterilize, antibiotics cannot be given through them and they should be removed urgently. As well as scrupulous asepsis with regard to intravenous line insertion and daily management, care should be taken that arm splints for neonates and young infants do not carry infection. Cases of infection with a fungus (*Rhizopus* spp.) have been described as a result of using infected throat spatulas for this purpose.

CANDIDA INFECTION

Children receiving antibiotics (especially broad spectrum therapy) for any significant length of time may be given oral and/or topical nystatin to prevent build-up of gastrointestinal and skin *Candida* sp. This build-up could eventually result in infection of intravenous lines and other sites. When a significant growth of *Candida albicans* is detected on surface swabs (and/or in urine specimens) in an unwell patient in spite of nystatin, consideration should be given to whether antifungal therapy such as fluconazole is indicated (as long as the liver function tests are normal). Blood cultures should be taken. Where a urinary catheter is consistently infected with *Candida* sp. it should be removed preferably, or changed and left out as long as possible. Blood cultures should be taken. If candidaemia associated with a long line occurs, the line should be removed urgently and the patient treated for at least 14 days after the last positive blood culture. Amphotericin should be given or fluconazole (if the organism is sensitive to it). In renal failure, a lipid amphotericin preparation is indicated.

PSEUDO-OUTBREAKS OF SEPTICAEMIA

These occur when contaminating organisms are introduced into blood culture bottles as a result of incorrect procedures. Blood culture bottles should always be inoculated before non-sterile tubes or collection bottles. If blood is injected into non-sterile collection bottles for haematological or biochemical investigation (e.g. sequestrine or citrate bottles) before blood cultures are inoculated, contaminating organisms from these non-sterile bottles may be picked up on the tip of the needle or syringe. They are subsequently injected into the blood culture bottles where they grow and falsely indicate a positive blood culture. An alternative way of causing a pseudo-outbreak is by using a blood-filled syringe in a blood gas analyser before inoculating the blood culture bottles. The organisms grown are often unusual varieties of environmental organisms, such as *Pseudomonas* or *Serratia* species.

GRAM-NEGATIVE SEPTICAEMIA IN NEONATES

Neonates, who develop Gram-negative septicaemia as a result of surgery or primary gut pathology, have a higher risk of developing Gram-negative meningitis than older age groups. A CSF specimen for microbiological investigation should be taken where possible. As well as CSF protein, both CSF and blood glucose should be estimated and the ratio compared. In the absence of meningitis, CSF glucose is approximately 60–70% of the blood glucose value, but this figure will decrease in infection since actively metabolizing organisms utilize glucose in the CSF. If presence of infection is indicated, appropriate blood–brain barrier-passing antibiotics (e.g. ceftazidime, cefotaxime or meropenem) should be continued for a minimum of 3 weeks after a repeat negative CSF culture has been obtained. If brain abscess develops, treatment should continue for 4 weeks or more. Specialist advice should be obtained.

NECROTIZING ENTEROCOLITIS

The cause of this serious condition, which leads to significant morbidity and mortality especially in the neonatal and premature age group, is unknown. Bacteria are probably secondary invaders rather than primary instigators of the condition. Oral feeding should be stopped and antibiotic therapy is necessary, usually penicillin, gentamicin and metronidazole in the first instance. It is rare for a child who has not been fed by mouth to acquire this condition. Breast feeding appears to give some protection.

CSF SHUNT INFECTIONS

Hydrocephalus may be congenital or secondary to intraventricular haemorrhage or meningitis in a neonate. The insertion of a CSF shunt (usually a ventriculoperitoneal shunt) should be carried out at a recognized paediatric neurosurgical centre. Infective complications have been described in up to 10% or more of patients in some units. Classically, the organisms involved are skin organisms, particularly coagulase-negative staphylococci including *Staph. epidermidis*, which generally enter the shunt system during operation. The patient's own skin staphylococci are thought to be the usual source. Operations on premature infants and neonates are particularly prone to complications, including infection and blockage. Revision operations following infection have a higher infection risk than the primary operation. Whether or not the experience of the surgeon is an important factor with regard to infection risk is controversial. Where infection with involvement of the ventricular CSF has occurred, the best strategy for eradication is removal of the infected shunt system and insertion of a drain into the ventricles. A course of antibiotics may then be introduced into the ventricles as well as given intravenously. Appropriate doses of intraventricular antibiotics should be provided from the pharmacy department rather than being made up on the ward or the operating theatre. Vancomycin is the usual initial antibiotic used in coagulase-negative staphylococcal infections. Intravenous rifampicin may be added, especially if there is no local access for administration of intraventricular antibiotics.

29.5 CROSS-INFECTION IN PAEDIATRIC SURGICAL WARDS

It has been estimated that 5–8% of children without diarrhoea will develop **gastrointestinal symptoms** 72 hours or more after hospital admission. Rotavirus accounts for about 40% of these, and infection can spread very quickly in the susceptible age group (i.e. children under 2 years of age). Infants with diarrhoea and vomiting should be isolated and barrier nursed. Transmission is most commonly by direct contact and the stability of the virus, together with the large amounts excreted (10^9–10^{10} particles per gram of faeces during the acute phase), makes environmental contamination inevitable. Emphasis should be on scrupulous hygiene, use of gloves, aprons and careful handwashing with alcoholic handwashes for staff. Detergent cleaning and disinfection of surfaces is necessary. A number of other viral agents cause diarrhoea including adeno-, calici-, astro- and small round structured viruses, such as Norwalk agent. Infection with the latter may spread quickly and cause significant symptoms in adults as well as children. Infected staff should be discouraged from returning to work while still symptomatic, as they may be a source of infection.

Outbreaks of **respiratory syncytial virus** and other respiratory virus infections may occur in surgical patients on paediatric wards. The patients should be isolated or cohort nursed, and particular attention paid to handwashing and protection of clothes from respiratory secretions. Young visitors and staff with colds may be a source of infection. The virus survives for up to 20 minutes on skin and up to 6 hours on fomites. Patients with chronic lung disease of prematurity or congenital heart disease are at increased risk, and should be kept away from other child patients with respiratory infections. The potential dangers of proceeding with anaesthesia in a child with respiratory syncytial virus infection are significant, and the risks should be carefully assessed.

29.5.1 Other infectious agents which may cause problems on paediatric surgical wards

These include viral rashes, such as measles and chickenpox. Patients with suspect rashes should be isolated.

Susceptible patients with compromised immunity who have been in contact with suspect cases may require relevant protective immunoglobulin, and this should be given without significant delay. Advice should be sought urgently from the consultant microbiologist or virologist, and national guidelines are available. It should be remembered that immunoglobulin may prolong both the incubation period and also the period of potential infectivity, during which the patient should be isolated if he/she remains in hospital.

29.6 ANTIBIOTIC THERAPY

29.6.1 Antibiotic doses in children

In general, children's doses should not be calculated as though they are 'little adults'; rather, reference to a standard text is necessary. Up to approximately 10–12 years of age (or approximately 30–35 kg body weight), the doses are calculated on a mg per kg basis. For children older than 12 years of age (or slightly younger children who weigh approximately 30–35 kg or more), calculations using a mg per kg basis may result in doses larger than would normally be given to an adult. In such cases, a dose appropriate for a small adult should be used. Neonates, especially prematures, may require different doses from other paediatric age groups because elimination takes longer.

29.6.2 Antibiotic levels

As for adults, levels of aminoglycosides such as gentamicin, amikacin or tobramycin and glycopeptides such as vancomycin, should be assayed. Children with normal renal function should have trough levels checked twice weekly, and those on multiple dosing regimens should have at least one acceptable peak level document during a course of treatment. The once-a-day gentamicin regimens avoid unnecessary assays and clinical results indicate that they are safe, effective and acceptable to patients and staff. Particularly for children, unnecessary blood taking for antibiotic assays should be avoided. If blood is taken from the intravenous line through which the antibiotic has been given and without adequate flushing, the results may be incorrectly high. Renal function and the dose should be checked and a repeat peripheral blood specimen taken before a further dose is given. Children in renal failure require therapeutic dose monitoring dose by dose.

29.6.3 Antibiotics used in paediatrics

Attempts should be made to avoid painful intramuscular injections in children. A temporary iv line may allow the child to receive home therapy when stabilized. Where appropriate there are many suitable and safe oral agents such as macrolides, penicillins and cephalosporins. Some should be avoided, such as tetracyclines, which are deposited in growing bones and teeth, causing staining. They should not be given to children under 8 years, preferably 12 years, or to pregnant or nursing women. In children with cystic fibrosis, required antibiotic doses are high due to rapid drug metabolism. Where indicated, in specific instances, antibiotics not routinely used in children may be recommended by the medical microbiologist. For example, this may include ciprofloxacin for children. (Ciprofloxacin has not yet been licensed for use in children because of its potential for causing arthropathy in young animals.) There are exception, however, such as the treatment of Pseudomonas infection in cystic fibrosis. Ciprofloxacin could be considered in some other serious infections such as invasive salmonellosis, where the potential benefits outweigh the risks.

29.6.4 Compliance

Poor compliance, particularly with oral antibiotic therapy outside hospital, may be one cause of failed treatment or relapse of infection in children. Frequent doses may be difficult to arrange, especially if the child is in school. Where appropriate, antibiotics that can be given once or twice daily are preferable.

29.7 PROPHYLAXIS

29.7.1 Children with cardiac disease

If a child has congenital or acquired heart disease, antibiotic prophylaxis is required for any procedure from which bacteraemia may result. Although classically this applies to dental treatment, other procedures included are surgery or instrumentation of the upper respiratory or genitourinary tracts. Patients undergoing obstetric, gynaecological or gastrointestinal procedures, who have in-dwelling prosthetic material or who have had a previous attack of endocarditis, should also be given prophylactic antibiotics. Minimizing the risk from dental sepsis is of particular importance for children with heart disease, and avoidance of caries promoting sugars important. Medicine should also be checked to avoid this problem.

29.7.2 Post-splenectomy prophylaxis

Asplenic children are at risk of infection with pneumococci and other encapsulated bacteria. Pneumoccal vaccine is recommended and re-immunization may be necessary after 5–10 years. Such children should also receive Hib and meningococcal vaccine. Twice daily penicillin prophylaxis is required. 'Alert' cards and bracelets are also available.

29.8 FURTHER READING

Control and prevention of tuberculosis in the United Kingdom: Recommendations (1998) *Thorax*, **53**, 536–648.

Davies, E.G., Elliman, D., Hart, C.A., Nicoll, A. and Rudd, P.T. (2001) *Manual of Childhood Infections.* Royal College of Paediatrics and Child Health. WB Saunders, London, Edinburgh, New York.

Department of Health (1996) *Immunisation Against Infectious Disease.* HMSO, London.

Hardy, S.P., Bayston, R. and Spitz, L. (1993) Prolonged carriage of *Clostridium difficile* in Hirschsprung's disease. *Arch. Dis. Child.*, **69**, 221–224.

Issacs, D. and Moxon, R. (2000) *Handbook of Neonatal Infections. A Practical Guide.* WB Saunders, London, Edinburgh, New York.

Mackenzie, J.R., Murphy, A.V., Beattie, T.J. *et al.* (1991) Guidelines for the management of acute urinary tract infection in childhood *J. R. Coll. Phys. Lond.*, **25**(3), 263.

Madden, N.P., Levinsky, R., Bayston, R., Harvey, B., Turner, M. and Spitz, L. (1989) Surgery, sepsis and non-specific immune function in neonates. *J. Paediatr. Surg.*, **24**, 562–566.

Management of opportunistic mycobacterial infections: Code of practice (2000) *Thorax*, **55**, 887–901.

Managing bloodstream infections associated with intravascular catheters. *Drug and Therapeutics Bulletin*, Vol.39 No.10, Oct 2001.

Neonatal Formulary (The Northern Neonatal Pharmacopoeia) 3rd edition, 2000. Compiled by the Northern Neonatal Network. BMJ Publishing Group.

Physical signs of sexual abuse in children (1997) 2nd edition. A Report of The Royal College of Physicians.

Pierce, A.M. and Hart, C.A. (1992) Vulvovaginitis: causes and management. *Arch. Dis. Child.*, **67**, 509–512.

Price, E., Wright, V.M., Walker-Smith, J. and Tabaqchali, S. (1988) *Clostridum difficile* and acute enterocolitis. *Arch. Dis. Child.*, **63**, 543–545.

Price, E.H., Borriello, S.P., Ward, H., Brereton, R., Risdon, R.A. and Tabaqchali, S. (1990) *Clostridium difficile and severe enterocolitis in three infants. Clinical and Molecular Aspects of Anaerobes,(ed)* S.P. Borriello. Wrightson Biomedical Publishing Ltd.

Simmons, N.A. (1993) Recommendations for endocarditis prophylaxis. *J. Antimicrob. Chemother.*, **31**, 437–453.

Sinatra, F.R. and Pietzak, M.M. (1996) *Helicobacter pylori* infection in children. *Curr. Opin. Infect. Dis.*, **9**, 187–190.

The management of neurosurgical patients with postoperative bacterial or aseptic meningitis or external ventricular drain associated ventriculitis. Report by the Infection in Neurosurgery Working Part of the BSAC (2000) *Brit. J. Neurosurgery*, **14**, 7–12.

The management of urinary tract infection in children. *Drug and Therapeutics Bulletin*, Vol.35 No.9, September 1997, 65–69.

The rational use of antibiotics in the treatment of brain abscess. Report by the Infection in Neurosurgery Working Party of the BSAC (2000) *Brit. J. Neurosurgery*, **14**, 525–530.

Verrier Jones, K. (1999) Prognosis for vesicoureteric reflux. *Arch. Dis. Child.* **81**, 287–294.

Index

Page references in **bold** indicate tables, page references in *italics* indicate figures.